AF680416

Endocrine Disruption and Human Health

Endocrine Disruption and Human Health

Editor: Calvin Lane

AMERICAN
MEDICAL PUBLISHERS
www.americanmedicalpublishers.com

AMERICAN
MEDICAL PUBLISHERS
www.americanmedicalpublishers.com

Cataloging-in-Publication Data

Endocrine disruption and human health / edited by Calvin Lane.
p. cm.
Includes bibliographical references and index.
ISBN 979-8-88740-093-8
1. Endocrine disrupting chemicals. 2. Endocrine disrupting chemicals--Health aspects.
3. Endocrine glands--Effect of chemicals on. 4. Endocrine toxicology.
5. Endocrine disrupting chemicals--Environmental aspects. I. Lane, Calvin.
RA1270.E53 E53 2023
616.407 1--dc23

© American Medical Publishers, 2023

American Medical Publishers,
41 Flatbush Avenue,
1st Floor, New York,
NY 11217, USA

ISBN 979-8-88740-093-8 (Hardback)

This book contains information obtained from authentic and highly regarded sources. Copyright for all individual chapters remain with the respective authors as indicated. All chapters are published with permission under the Creative Commons Attribution License or equivalent. A wide variety of references are listed. Permission and sources are indicated; for detailed attributions, please refer to the permissions page and list of contributors. Reasonable efforts have been made to publish reliable data and information, but the authors, editors and publisher cannot assume any responsibility for the validity of all materials or the consequences of their use.

Trademark Notice: Registered trademark of products or corporate names are used only for explanation and identification without intent to infringe.

Contents

Preface

The compounds of natural or human-made origin that are capable of interfering with the endocrine system of an organism are called endocrine disrupting compounds (EDCs). These compounds disrupt the normal physiology and homeostatic processes of the organism by mimicking or inhibiting naturally occurring hormones. EDCs are found in low levels in a lot of items due to which all people are exposed to compounds having estrogenic effects in their daily lives. DDT, polychlorinated biphenyls (PCBs), bisphenol A (BPA), polybrominated diphenyl ethers (PBDEs), and a range of phthalates are among the chemicals regularly found in individuals. Endocrine-disrupting substances bind classical nuclear hormone receptors by disrupting other pathways regulating hormone synthesis or action processes of the organism. EDCs severely affect the cellular and whole-body metabolism. They may also act as causative agents in a wide spectrum of metabolic disorders in humans, including obesity, diabetes, dyslipidemia, nonalcoholic fatty liver disease (NAFLD), and cardiovascular dysfunction. This book includes some of the vital pieces of work being conducted across the world, on various topics related to endocrine disruption and its effects on human health. It will prove to be immensely beneficial to students and researchers engaged in this area of study.

This book unites the global concepts and researches in an organized manner for a comprehensive understanding of the subject. It is a ripe text for all researchers, students, scientists or anyone else who is interested in acquiring a better knowledge of this dynamic field.

I extend my sincere thanks to the contributors for such eloquent research chapters. Finally, I thank my family for being a source of support and help.

Editor

1

An Untargeted Metabolomics Approach to Investigate the Metabolic Modulations of HepG2 Cells Exposed to Low Doses of Bisphenol A and 17β-Estradiol

Nicolas J. Cabaton[1†], Nathalie Poupin[1†], Cécile Canlet[1,2], Marie Tremblay-Franco[1,2], Marc Audebert[1], Jean-Pierre Cravedi[1], Anne Riu[1], Fabien Jourdan[1] and Daniel Zalko[1]*

[1] *Toxalim (Research Centre in Food Toxicology), Université de Toulouse, INRA, ENVT, INP-Purpan, UPS, Toulouse, France,*
[2] *Axiom Platform, MetaToul-MetaboHub, National Infrastructure for Metabolomics and Fluxomics, Toulouse, France*

Correspondence:
Nicolas J. Cabaton
nicolas.cabaton@inra.fr

† These authors have contributed equally to this work

The model xeno-estrogen bisphenol A (BPA) has been extensively studied over the past two decades, contributing to major advances in the field of endocrine disrupting chemicals research. Besides its well documented adverse effects on reproduction and development observed in rodents, latest studies strongly suggest that BPA disrupts several endogenous metabolic pathways, with suspected steatogenic and obesogenic effects. BPA's adverse effects on reproduction are attributed to its ability to activate estrogen receptors (ERs), but its effects on metabolism and its mechanism(s) of action at low doses are so far only marginally understood. Metabolomics based approaches are increasingly used in toxicology to investigate the biological changes induced by model toxicants and chemical mixtures, to identify markers of toxicity and biological effects. In this study, we used proton nuclear magnetic resonance (^{1}H-NMR) based untargeted metabolite profiling, followed by multivariate statistics and computational analysis of metabolic networks to examine the metabolic modulation induced in human hepatic cells (HepG2) by an exposure to low and very low doses of BPA (10^{-6}M, 10^{-9}M, and 10^{-12}M), vs. the female reference hormone 17β-estradiol (E2, 10^{-9}M, 10^{-12}M, and 10^{-15}M). Metabolomic analysis combined to metabolic network reconstruction highlighted different mechanisms at lower doses of exposure. At the highest dose, our results evidence that BPA shares with E2 the capability to modulate several major metabolic routes that ensure cellular functions and detoxification processes, although the effects of the model xeno-estrogen and of the natural hormone can still be distinguished.

Keywords: HepG2, metabolomics, BPA, 17β-estradiol, endocrine disruption, metabolic network, multivariate statistics

INTRODUCTION

In the field of endocrine disrupting chemicals (EDCs), bisphenol A (BPA) is among the xeno-estrogens that have been the subject of the most extensive studies over the past two decades. In addition to its adverse effects on reproduction and development observed in rodents, BPA was found to disturb several metabolic pathways, resulting in steatogenic and obesogenic effects (1). Effects of BPA on metabolism and obesity have been assessed in several European reports. Studies carried out in rodents pre- and postnatally exposed to BPA have demonstrated significant changes in metabolic functions, evidenced by effects on lipogenesis, glucose, or insulin regulation, and body weight gain (2). Although these endpoints were not taken so far into account in the final risk characterization of BPA exposure, they have been clearly mentioned in the EFSA opinion on the risks to public health related to the presence of BPA in foodstuffs. The metabolic endpoint was not taken forward for assessing the toxicological reference point, but was taken into account in the evaluation of uncertainty for hazard and risk characterizations (2). EFSA recommended further research on the potential adverse effects of BPA for which there are uncertainties, in particular metabolic endpoints (2). In its opinion on BPA, the European Chemicals Agency (ECHA) considered it prudent to take the metabolic effects into account in hazard and risk assessment and in health impact assessment (3). In 2017, the French agency for food, environmental and occupational health and safety (ANSES) submitted a proposal to ECHA to classify BPA as a substance of very high concern within the framework of the European REACh regulation, based on its endocrine disrupting properties, including metabolic effects, which may cause serious effects to human health (4). This proposal has been adopted by ECHA's member state committee.

Although part of BPA adverse effects are attributed to its ability to activate estrogen receptors (ERs), its mechanism(s) of action at low doses remain(s) incompletely known (5). In particular, the effects of BPA on metabolism have been found to be connected with glycaemia and insulin regulation as well as lipogenesis, but little is known on the impact of BPA on biochemical mechanisms underlying observed changes in metabolic profiles, which likely involve other metabolic pathways as well (6–8).

Metabolomics based approaches are increasingly used in toxicology to investigate the biological changes induced by single toxicants or chemical mixtures, to identify markers of toxicity, and achieve a better understanding of the adverse outcome pathways (AOP) of selected chemicals (9). We previously demonstrated in CD1 mice and Sprague Dawley rats, that the metabolome is modulated in these animals following perinatal exposure to low doses of BPA (10–12). In the context of the implementation of the REACh regulation, and given the need to reduce animal experiments, *in vitro* studies become a priority in toxicity testing. High throughput assays that use cells or cell lines, preferably of human origin, are required to assess relevant disruptions in key toxicity pathways (13, 14). The development of metabolomics, and, in parallel, of bio-informatics modeling based on omics data, opens new possibilities to assess cell response to external stimuli. Combined with appropriate multivariate statistical approaches, metabolomics allows discriminating between sub-populations (of individuals or cells) according to their exposure conditions and evidencing endogenous metabolites which have significantly different levels between these groups, and therefore constitute a metabolic fingerprint of the metabolic modulations induced by the exposure. Several studies reported biomarkers discovery using such approach (15, 16).

In the present study, we used proton nuclear magnetic resonance (^{1}H-NMR) based untargeted metabolite profiling followed by multivariate statistics and computational analysis of metabolic networks to examine the metabolic modulation produced in human hepatic cells (HepG2) by an exposure to low and very low doses of BPA, vs. the female reference hormone 17β-estradiol (E2). The HepG2 cell line is derived from a human hepatoblastoma. This cell line expresses biotransformation capacities for numerous xenobiotics, notably BPA (17). Expression of the estrogen receptor (ER) isoform α was established in different publications (18, 19). Specific biological effects of E2, a ligand of the estrogen receptor, were demonstrated in this cell line as well (18–21). The HepG2 cell line was selected as a cell line model broadly used in toxicology as well as metabolomic studies (16, 22, 23).

The objective of this work was to identify and compare the metabolic consequences of an exposure to low doses of the xeno-estrogen BPA and the reference hormone E2 using proton NMR metabolomics approach combined with *in silico* network reconstruction, to identify the cellular pathways most significantly modulated by these two molecules, and seek for their commonalities and differences.

MATERIALS AND METHODS

Chemicals

Bisphenol A (4,4'-isopropylidenediphenol, BPA), 17β-estradiol (E2) and dimethyl sulfoxide (DMSO) (with chemical purity > 99%) were obtained from Sigma-Aldrich (Saint Quentin Fallavier, France). Penicillin, streptomycin, trypsin, and PBS were also purchased from Sigma-Aldrich. The concentration of the stock solutions was 50 mM in DMSO.

Cell-Line

HepG2 human hepatoblastoma cells (ATCC N° HB-8065) were cultured in monolayer culture in phenol red-free αMEM (Fisher Scientific, France) supplemented with 10% fetal calf serum v/v (PAN biotech), penicillin (100 U mL^{-1}), and streptomycin (100 μg mL^{-1}) (Fisher Scientific), in a humidified atmosphere of 5% CO_2 at 37°C. Continuous cultures were maintained by sub-culturing flasks every 3–5 days.

Cells Treatments and Sample Preparation for ^{1}H NMR Spectroscopy

HepG2 cells, 1×10^6 cells per well, were grown in six well-plates containing 4 mL medium per well. Only one concentration was assessed per plate. Each experiment was repeated at least three times to get a final number of 18 samples per treatment.

After 24 h, cells were washed in PBS and medium was replaced by serum-free and phenol red-free medium. Cells were exposed to 0.25% (v/v) DMSO in the culture medium (controls) and supplemented with BPA (10^{-6}M, 10^{-9}M, or 10^{-12}M) or E2 (10^{-9}M, 10^{-12}M, or 10^{-15}M) or DMSO (0.25%, control). At the end of the 24-h treatment period, cells were washed in ice cold PBS and were recovered by scraping each well twice with 1 mL ice cold water/acetonitrile (90/10, v/v). After each water/acetonitrile addition, cells were agitated with a vortex for 1 min. Samples were then centrifuged at 7000 g for 15 min at 4°C. The supernatant was then evaporated to dryness. The lyophilisates were reconstituted in 600 μL of D_2O containing 0.25 mM TMSP (as a chemical shift reference at 0 ppm). The reconstituted solutions were transferred to NMR tubes.

^{1}H Nuclear Magnetic Resonance (NMR) Analyses

All ^{1}H-NMR spectra were obtained on a Bruker DRX-600-Avance NMR spectrometer operating at 600.13 MHz for ^{1}H resonance frequency using an inverse detection 5 mm ^{1}H-^{13}C-^{15}N cryoprobe attached to a CryoPlatform (the preamplifier cooling unit).

The ^{1}H-NMR spectra were acquired at 300 K using the Carr-Purcell-Meiboom-Gill (CPMG) spin-echo pulse sequence with pre-saturation, with a total spin-echo delay ($2n\tau$) of 320 ms to attenuate broad signals from proteins and lipoproteins. A total of 128 transients were collected into 32 k data points using a spectral width of 12 ppm, a relaxation delay of 2.5 s and an acquisition time of 2.28 s. Prior to Fourier Transformation, an exponential line broadening function of 0.3 Hz was applied to the FID.

To confirm the chemical structure of metabolites of interest, 2D ^{1}H-^{1}H COSY (Correlation Spectroscopy) and 2D ^{1}H-^{13}C-HSQC (Heteronuclear Single Quantum Coherence Spectroscopy) NMR experiments were performed on selected samples.

Data Reduction and Multivariate Statistical Analyses to Create Metabolic Fingerprints

Multidimensional statistical analyses of NMR data were performed using Simca-P12 software (Umetrics, Umeå, Sweden). Principal Component Analysis (PCA) was first used to detect intrinsic clusters and eventual outliers. Then Partial Least Squares—Discriminant Analysis (PLS–DA) was used to study the effect of the treatment on the cell metabolome (BPA or E_2). This supervised method maximizes the separation between treatment groups. The number of components in the PLS models was chosen by cross validation (7-fold). The R^2 parameter represents the explained variance. The predictive performance of the model was evaluated using the Q^2 parameter (predictive capacity), calculated by cross-validation. Typically a robust model is characterized by a $R^2 > 50\%$ and a $Q^2 > 0.4$ (24).

To remove confounding variation (experimental or instrumental) not linked to the studied factor (treatment), OSC filtering was applied to the data, as such variations may overshadow the variability due to the factor under study (25). The treatment was used as a corrective factor. Filtered data were mean-centered and/or Pareto scaled.

In addition, the statistical significance and validity of the PLS-DA models were assessed using a permutation test (200 permutations). This test determines whether the specific classification of individuals in the designated groups is significantly better than any other random classification in two arbitrary groups (26).

VIP (Variable Importance in the Projection) was used to determine the most important NMR variables for the separation observed between experimental groups. VIP is a global measure of the influence of each variable on the PLS components. An arbitrary threshold of VIP > 1.5 was chosen to select the variables. The Kruskal–Wallis test, a non-parametric version of Analysis of Variance, was then used to determine variables that differed significantly between groups (e.g., "discriminant" metabolites), with 0.05 being chosen as the level of significance. The set of discriminant metabolites identified from the comparison of a given treatment condition (for instance BPA 10^{-6}M) vs. control conditions is considered as a "metabolic fingerprint" of the impact of this treatment exposure.

Extraction of Modulated Metabolic Network

Genome Scale Metabolic Networks (GSMN) aim at gathering in a single formalism all metabolic reactions which can occur in an organism (27). Each reaction is described by its substrates and products (metabolites), its stoichiometry, the enzyme(s) catalyzing it and the genes encoding the enzyme. We used the Recon2 human GSMN (28) which contains 7,440 reactions and 5,063 metabolites. In this network, metabolites are assigned to cellular compartments (mitochondria, cytoplasm...). Nevertheless, current global and untargeted metabolomics approaches do not provide information on cellular localization of metabolites. Hence, we created a modified version of Recon2 network by considering any metabolite belonging to several compartments as a single metabolite. The final modified "one-compartment" version of Recon2 that we used in our analyses contains 4,210 reactions and 2,592 metabolites.

We performed metabolic sub-network extraction from the discriminant metabolites identified from the statistical analyses. Metabolic sub-network extraction consists in computationally identifying among the 4,210 reactions, the ones that are more likely to be related to the metabolic fingerprint of each exposure. The algorithm computes the lightest path between each pair of metabolites in the fingerprint. The lightest path is a sequence of reactions and metabolites connecting two metabolites and minimizing a topological criterion in the network (29). For one metabolic fingerprint, the related sub-network is thus the union of all the lightest paths between metabolites in the fingerprint. Metabolic sub-networks were generated from the metabolic fingerprints obtained under exposure to the different doses of BPA (e.g., for instance, "BPA 10^{-6}M metabolic subnetwork" for the higher dose of BPA) and E2 (for instance, the "E2 10^{-9}M metabolic subnetwork").

In order to compare the specificity of the metabolic sub-networks obtained under various exposure conditions, we compared the set of reactions and metabolites belonging to the different sub-networks. In particular, we created a sub-network specific to the effects of a BPA 10^{-6} exposure by subtracting, from the BPA 10^{-6}M metabolic subnetwork, the metabolites and reactions belonging to the E2 10^{-9}M metabolic sub-network. All computational and visualization tasks were performed within MetExplore web server based on the modified Recon2 metabolic network (biosource id 3223) (30, 31).

RESULTS

BPA Effects

A two-component PLS-DA model was constructed based on all BPA-exposed groups data (4 groups: DMSO, BPA 10^{-6}M, BPA 10^{-9}M, and BPA 10^{-12}M). This model explained 62.2% of the variability (R^2) with a predictive ability ($Q^2 = 0.561$) validating the robustness of this model (24). The score plot is presented in **Figure 1**, showing a clear separation between the control (DMSO) group and all BPA exposed cells along axis 1 (X axis, 1st latent variable among 2). The highest BPA dose (10^{-6}M) group was discriminated from the BPA 10^{-9}M and BPA 10^{-12}M groups, respectively, along the 2nd axis (Y axis, 2nd latent variable). However, no significant discrimination between these two lowest BPA exposure groups (10^{-9}M and 10^{-12}M) was evidenced in this 4-group comparison. Twenty metabolites were found to be responsible for the separation between BPA exposed groups and the control group (**Table 1**). This PLS-DA model was validated by the Permutation test, confirming a robust model (32). Main metabolites involved in observed differences were amino acids, with a significant modulation of arginine, isoleucine, leucine, lysine, proline, and valine. Interestingly, specific metabolites such as glycerol, glycerophosphocholine, succinate and serine were significantly discriminant for the BPA 10^{-6}M group only. Reduced glutathione was modulated in the lowest BPA dose group only, as well as AMP.

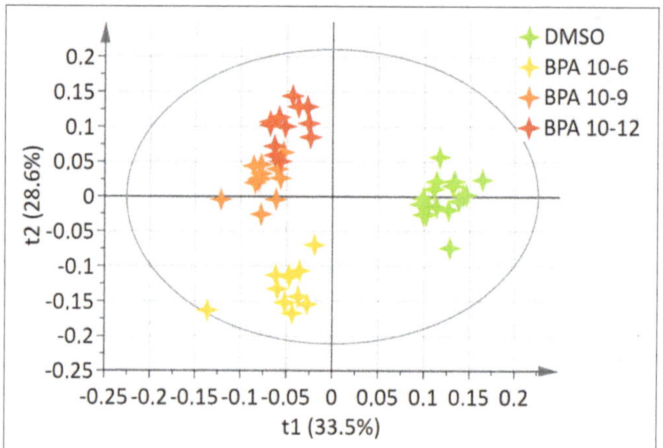

FIGURE 1 | Two-dimensional PLS-DA score plot of HepG2 cell extracts integrated ^{1}H-NMR spectra for BPA exposure. Each star represents an observation projected onto the first (horizontal axis) and the second (vertical axis) PLS-DA latent variables. BPA doses are shown in different colors: DMSO (green; $N = 17$), BPA 10^{-6} (light orange; $N = 12$), BPA 10^{-9} (dark orange; $N = 12$), BPA 10^{-12} (dark red; $N = 12$) (R^2Y= 62.2% and $Q^2 = 0.561$).

17β-Estradiol (E2) Effects

Using an identical approach, a two-component model was constructed for E2-exposed cells, based on the whole set of data. This model explained 81.6% of the variability (R^2) and demonstrated a high predictive ability ($Q^2 = 0.635$). The score plot showed a clear separation between the DMSO and E2 doses groups (E2 10^{-12}M and E2 10^{-15}M) and the E2 10^{-9}M group along axis 1 (**Figure 2**). The "lowest" doses of E2 groups, namely E2 10^{-12}M and E2 10^{-15}M were discriminated from the DMSO group along the 2nd axis. No discrimination between the E2 10^{-12}M and E2 10^{-15}M groups was found in this four-group comparison. The PLS-DA models were validated by the permutation test (32).

Twenty-four metabolites were significantly increased or decreased and were found to be responsible for the separation between groups (**Table 2**). Some amino acids, namely alanine, glycine, lysine, proline, tyrosine, and valine, were identified as discriminant only for the highest dose of E2, whereas other metabolites (including acetate, formate, and isopropanol) were modulated only for the 2 lowest doses. Reduced glutathione was also modulated for the highest tested dose of E2, contrary to BPA. Choline and ethanolamine were significantly modulated at the 3 tested doses.

Comparison of BPA and E_2 Effects

The 7-group comparison generated a 4-component PLS-DA model, explaining 59.5% of the treatment variability and having a Q^2 value of 0.508 (robust model). **Figure 3** displays the projection of the 2 first latent variables (out of 4), demonstrating a marked separation between the effects of "low" estrogenic doses (BPA 10^{-9}M, BPA 10^{-12}M, E2 10^{-12}M, and E2 10^{-15}M) and that of higher doses (BPA 10^{-6}M and E2 10^{-9}M), along axis 1. In addition, a marked discrimination between the effects of the xeno-estrogenic model compound BPA and that of the natural hormone E2 was observed along axis 2. All these groups were clearly separated from the DMSO (control) group. This 7-group comparison model was further validated by the permutation test step. As detailed in **Table 3**, 19 metabolites were found to be discriminant between the 6 exposed groups and the control group (DSMO), respectively. Some of these discriminant metabolites, for instance arginine and glutamine, were found to be similar for all BPA and E2 exposed groups, whatever the dose. Conversely, the modulation of metabolites such as creatinine, citrate and leucine (BPA, all doses) and ethanolamine (E2, all doses) appeared to be molecule specific.

Finally, we proceeded to network analysis based on ^{1}H-NMR data, to further investigate the effects shared by the two molecules.

Network of BPA and E2 Effects

Multivariate analysis revealed that BPA 10^{-6}M and E2 10^{-9}M appear to share some metabolic effects (axis 2) but also have specific effects (axis 1), suggesting both common and molecule-specific mechanisms of action. In order to further distinguish

TABLE 1 | Endogenous metabolite variations induced by BPA exposure (BPA samples compared to DMSO samples) in HepG2 cells.

Metabolites	^{1}H NMR chemical shifts (ppm)	BPA 10^{-6} M	BPA 10^{-9} M	BPA 10^{-12} M
Alanine	1.48 (d,7.2); 3.79(q,7.2)		x	
AMP	4.03(m); 4.38(m); 4.51(m);6.14(d,5.9);8.27(s); 8.61(s)			x
Arginine	1.66(m); 1.74(m); 1.93(m); 3.25(t, 6.9)	x	x	x
Asparagine	2.85(dd, 16.8 and 7.4); 2.95(dd, 16.8 and 4.3); 4.01(dd, 7.4 and 4.3)			x
Citrate	2.66(d,18.1); 2.81(d,18.1)		x	x
Creatine	3.04(s); 3.93(s)	x	x	x
Dimethylglycine	2.93(s)			x
Glutamine	2.14(m); 2.46(m); 3.78(t,6.2)	x	x	x
Reduced glutathione	2.17(m); 2.56(m); 2.96(m); 3.78(m); 4.58(m)			x
Glycerol	3.57(m); 3.66(m); 3.79(m)	x		
Glycerophosphocholine	3.23(s); 3.62(m); 3.68(m);3.89(m); 3.94(m); 4.33(m)	x		
Isoleucine	0.94(t,7.4); 1.01(d,7), 1.27(m); 1.47(m); 1.98(m); 3.68(d,4)	x	x	x
Isopropanol	1.16(d,6.11); 4.01(m)		x	
Lactate	1.33(d,6.9); 4.12(q,6.9)		x	x
Leucine	0.96(t,6.3); 1.71(m); 3.74(m)	x	x	x
Lysine	1.45(m); 1.52(m); 1.73(m); 1.91(m); 3.02(t, 7.5)	x	x	x
Proline	2.01(m); 2.08(m); 2.35(m); 3.35(m); 3.42(m); 4.14(dd, 6.7 and 8.7)	x	x	
Serine	3.84(m); 3.94(dd,12.4 and 5.8); 3.98(dd, 12.4 and 3.7)	x		
Succinate	2.41(s)	x		
Valine	0.995(d,7); 1,045(d,7); 2.28(m);3,62(d,4.4)	x	x	x

Chemical shifts (ppm) are relative to TMSP (^{1}H, δ, 0 ppm). Multiplicity of signals is indicated within brackets: s, singlet; d, doublet; dd, doublet of doublet; t, triplet; q, quadruplet and m, multiplet. Values into brackets are ^{1}H–^{1}H splittings (Hz) in cases where these are clearly resolved. "x" represents significantly modultated concentration compared to DMSO samples.

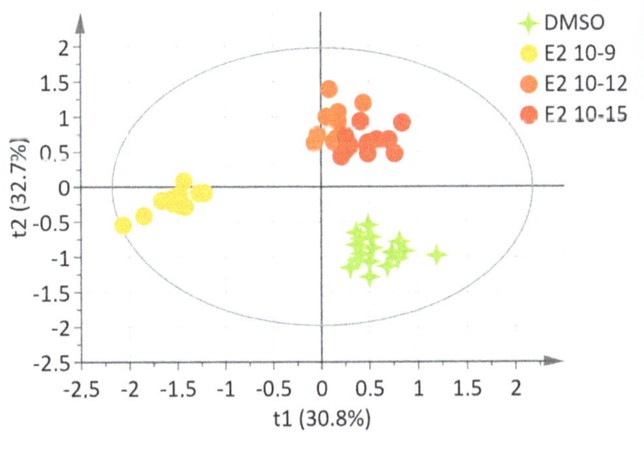

FIGURE 2 | Two-dimensional PLS-DA scores plot of HepG2 cell extracts integrated ^{1}H-NMR spectra for E2 exposure. Each dot or star represents an observation projected onto the first (horizontal axis) and the second (vertical axis) PLS-DA latent variables. E2 doses are shown in different colors: DMSO (green; $N = 17$), E2 10^{-9} M (light orange; $N = 12$), E2 10^{-12} M (dark orange; $N = 12$), E2 10^{-15} M (dark red; $N = 12$) ($R^2Y= 81.6\%$ and $Q^2 = 0.635$).

between shared mechanisms (which likely reflect an estrogenic effect) from the effects specific to BPA 10^{-6}M, we performed a network analysis. Two networks were reconstructed based on metabolic fingerprints obtained in the 7-group analysis (see **Supplemental Figures 1, 2, Supplemental Tables 1, 2,** and the Material and Methods section for sub-network extraction). We extracted the common part for these two subnetworks, resulting in a common BPA-E2 sub-network (**Figure 4**). This sub-network strongly suggests that the common target between BPA and E2, as regards metabolome modulation, relies on the modulation of metabolic pathways involving specific amino acids, namely valine, proline, lysine, and glutamine and, notably, the pathways involving the production/degradation of apolipoprotein C3 (ApoC3) and apolipoprotein C1 (ApoC1). Other key biochemical pathways likely modulated both by BPA and E2 high exposure doses were identified following network reconstruction, including metabolites and reactions involved in the urea cycle (citrulline, arginine, argino-succinate, and ornithine) and in the Krebs cycle (isocitrate, citrate, oxaloacetate, pyruvate).

Finally, with the aim to explore the specific effects of BPA, we subtracted from the BPA network the part shared with E2. In accordance with the metabolomic data that evidenced isoleucine and leucine as specifically discriminant in BPA-exposed groups (but not in E2 exposed groups), these two amino acids were highlighted as major endogenous metabolites modulated by BPA in the BPA-specific subnetwork. Network reconstruction also identified some intermediates in the metabolism of leucine and isoleucine, namely isovaleryl CoA and methylbutanoyl-CoA, that are therefore likely to be specifically modulated by BPA exposure.

DISCUSSION

In this study, we used a proton NMR global metabolomics approach, with no *a priori*, to compare the effects of a

TABLE 2 | Endogenous metabolite variations induced by E2 exposure (E2 samples compared to DMSO samples) in HepG2 cells.

Metabolites	^{1}H NMR chemical shifts (ppm)	E2 10^{-9} M	E2 10^{-12} M	E2 10^{-15} M
Acetate	1.91(s)		x	x
Alanine	1.48 (d,7.2); 3.79(q,7.2)	x		
Asparagine	2.85(dd, 16.8 and 7.4); 2.95(dd, 16.8 and 4.3); 4.01(dd, 7.4 and 4.3)	x	x	
Choline	3.20(s); 3.52(m);4.07(m)	x	x	x
Citrate	2.66(d,18.1); 2.81(d,18.1)	x		
Ethanolamine	3.14(m); 3.82(m)	x	x	x
Formate	8.45(s)		x	x
Glucose	3.25(dd,7.3 and 7.9); 3.42(m); 3.47(m); 3.51(m); 3.54(m); 3.72(m); 3.73(m); 3.77(m); 3.84(m); 3.90(m); 4.65(d,8); 5.24(d,3.8)	x		
Glutamine	2.14(m); 2.46(m); 3.78(t,6.2)	x	x	
Glutamate	2.06(m); 2.13(m); 2.35(m); 3.77(dd,7.5 and 4.9)	x	x	
Reduced glutathione	2.17(m); 2.56(m); 2.96(m); 3.78(m); 4.58(m)	x		
Glycerol	3.57(m); 3.66(m); 3.79(m)		x	
Glycerophosphocholine	3.23(s); 3.62(m); 3.68(m);3.89(m); 3.94(m); 4.33(m)		x	x
Glycine	3.55(s)	x		
Isoleucine	0.94(t,7.4); 1.01(d,7), 1.27(m); 1.47(m); 1.98(m); 3.68(d,4)		x	x
Isopropanol	1.16(d,6.11); 4.01(m)		x	x
Lactate	1.33(d,6.9); 4.12(q,6.9)	x	x	
Lysine	1.45(m); 1.52(m); 1.73(m); 1.91(m); 3.02(t, 7.5)	x		
Phosphocholine	3.22(s); 3.58(m); 4.17(m)	x	x	
Proline	2.01(m); 2.08(m); 2.35(m); 3.35(m); 3.42(m); 4.14(dd, 6.7 and 8.7)	x		
Serine	3.84(m); 3.94(dd,12.4 and 5.8); 3.98(dd, 12.4 and 3.7)		x	
Succinate	2.41(s)		x	
Tyrosine	3.09(dd,14.5 and 7.5); 3.21(dd,14.5 and 5,1); 3.95(dd,7.5 and 5.1); 6.9(d,8.5); 7.20(d,8.5)	x		
Valine	0.995(d,7); 1,045(d,7); 2.28(m);3,62(d,4.4)	x		

Chemical shifts (ppm) are relative to TMSP (^{1}H, δ, 0 ppm). Multiplicity of signals is indicated within brackets: s, singlet; d, doublet; dd, doublet of doublet; t, triplet; q, quadruplet and m, multiplet. Values into brackets are ^{1}H–^{1}H splittings (Hz) in cases where these are clearly resolved. "x" represents significantly modultated concentration compared to DMSO samples.

range of concentrations of E2 and BPA on a broadly used human hepatic cell line (HepG2). Then, we used bioinformatics (Metabolic Network modeling) methods to further investigate the biological pathways modulated by these estrogens: E2 as the reference hormone, and BPA as a model xeno-estrogen with well-documented endocrine disrupting properties, but also strongly suspected metabolic effects. Many EDCs with xeno-estrogenic properties can act as metabolic modulators (1, 33, 34). We previously demonstrated metabolic changes in the liver and brain of mice exposed during *intra-utero* development and lactation, to low doses of BPA (10). However, assessing the effects of EDCs using metabolomics approaches requires substantial resources, especially *in vivo*. The number of chemicals that need to be assessed as regards their potential to induce metabolic changes, and the necessity to comply with the "Three Rs" (3Rs) guiding principles for more ethical use of animals in testing, require developing alternative *in vitro* bioassays, preferably based on human models. The implementation of metabolomics and bioinformatics on the bases of *in vitro* bioassays first needs to be validated with model molecules. It also opens the road for a better understanding of the mechanisms of action of EDCs. These approaches should be as sensitive and relevant as possible to further examine the reliability of biomarkers of effects of EDCs. Experiments carried out to seek for these biomarkers should also link to low, environmentally relevant, exposure levels of EDCs in human body, as mentioned for xeno-estrogens by Wang et al. regarding BPA (35).

The HepG2 cell line, derived from a human hepatoblastoma, was selected to perform this work as it is broadly used in toxicology, including in studies combining *in vitro* cell systems and metabolomics for the identification of the mode of action (MoA) (16, 22). Although this cell line is of limited metabolic capacity compared to human hepatocytes, it has been demonstrated to be efficient in the biotransformation of BPA and the metabolic pathways were found to be similar to those observed in humans (17, 36, 37). Expression of the estrogen receptor (ER) isoform α was established in different publications (18, 38). Likewise, specific biological effects of 17β-Estradiol (E2), a ligand of the estrogen receptors, were demonstrated in this cell line (18–21, 38). These cells were exposed to environmental relevant concentrations of BPA and E2. The selected doses (10^{-6}M, 10^{-9}M, and 10^{-12}M for BPA, and 10^{-9}M, 10^{-12}M, and 10^{-15}M for E2) were in accordance with the bibliography regarding their respective estrogenic potency, as it is estimated that the estrogenic potency of E2 is approximately 1 000 to

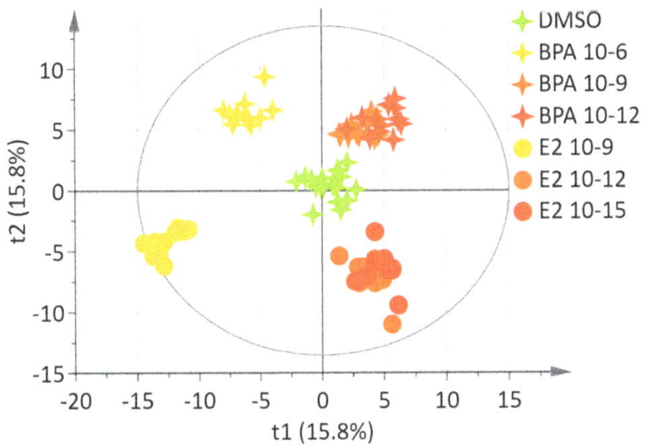

FIGURE 3 | Two-dimensional PLS-DA scores plot (Axis 1 and 2) of HepG2 cell extracts integrated ^{1}H-NMR spectra for BPA and E2 exposure. Each dot or star represents an observation projected onto the first (horizontal axis) and the second (vertical axis) PLS-DA latent variables. Different symbols are used for BPA (4-point star) and E2 (circle) exposure. Doses are shown as follow: DMSO: green (*N* = 17), BPA 10^{-6}M: light orange (*N* = 11), BPA 10^{-9}M: dark orange; (*N* = 12), BPA 10^{-12}M: dark red (*N* = 12), E2 10^{-9}M: light orange (*N* = 11), E2 10^{-12}M: dark orange (*N* = 12), E2 10^{-15}M: dark red (*N* = 12); (R^2Y = 59.5% and Q^2 = 0.508).

10 000 time greater that BPA' s estrogenic potency *in vitro* (39, 40).

Although few papers already reported the effects of low doses of BPA exposure on HepG2 cells, these studies mainly used targeted approaches, providing results on hepatotoxic endpoints, such as serum aspartate aminotransferase (AST) and alanine transferase (ALT) measurements, or inflammatory genes analyzed by RT-qPCR (41, 42). In our study, we applied non targeted ^{1}H-NMR metabolomics approach to HepG2 cells extracts to evidence the impact of BPA on the whole metabolism, in order to gain a more "global picture" and with no *a priori* hypothesis regarding the effect of this endocrine disruptor. The same methodology was applied to estradiol as the reference estrogenic compound, to identify common and specific metabolic pathways modulated by both molecules, with the benefit of bioinformatics and network reconstruction to help identifying metabolites not detected directly during analyses, but yet playing a role in the metabolic pathways modulated by BPA and/or E2.

Several studies have reported that BPA and E2 are acting the same way *in vitro*. For instance, BPA and E2 were both shown to promote HepG2 cell proliferation by inhibition of apoptosis and stimulation of telomerase activity via an estrogen receptor-dependent pathway (43). In our study, metabolomics revealed modulations of the HepG2 metabolome that are molecule specific (discrimination between the BPA exposed groups and the E2 exposed group). Although some metabolic pathways are common to BPA and E2, it is interesting to note that parts of the metabolic fingerprints are different between the 2 molecules at the highest tested concentration (10^{-6}M for BPA and 10^{-9}M for E2, respectively). This specific concentration of BPA was reported to be estrogenic *in vitro* in several models such as MCF-7 cells and ZELH-zfERs cell lines (44, 45). However, our results suggest that BPA is able to induce a metabolic modulatory effect, even at higher and estrogenic doses, which is different from the metabolic modulation at the estrogenic dose of E2 (10^{-9}M). According to Gould et al., BPA interacts with the ERα in a distinct manner from estradiol. BPA is not merely a weak estrogen mimic but exhibits a distinct mechanism of action at the level of ERα. The distinct activity of BPA is most likely due to an induction of a conformation of the activated ERα by BPA that differs from these other known classes of ER ligands. Generally, BPA is considered as a weak estrogenic compound (46). Nevertheless, and despite its relatively low affinity for ERα, an increasing number of studies have demonstrated that BPA can promote estrogen-like activities that are similar (or even stronger) than the ones elicited by 17β-estradiol (47). These low-dose responses result in part from the activation of rapid responses via non-classical ER pathways or by a different BPA recruitment of co-activators or co-repressors (48, 49). For instance, low doses of BPA only induce gene expression related to lipid synthesis and trigger triglyceride accumulation in adult mouse liver (8).

Metabolomics has already been applied to *in vivo* samples from mice and rats. In both cases, we already revealed modulations of energy metabolism (10, 12), which was also observed in other organisms such as Daphnia magna, together with a modulation of part of the same amino acids (such as arginine, glutamine, lysine, valine), and lactate (50). In our case, we also observed changes in many amino acids, as well as in metabolites involved in energy metabolism. The modulation of cholines suggest a modulation in the lipids composition in the cell and in the membrane fluidity at the estrogenic dose (10^{-6}M BPA), which is not the case for the two other BPA doses tested. Interestingly, reduced glutathione was modulated in the lowest BPA dose group only, which may suggest a change in the capacity of detoxification of the cells through this specific biochemical pathway. More importantly, differences in reduced glutathione levels also determine the expressed mode of cell death, being either apoptosis or cell necrosis. Lower levels of reduced glutathione may result in the systematic breakage of the cell which may lead to cell death (51). The metabolic network reconstruction highlighted paths of metabolic reactions specifically modulated by BPA exposure but not by E2 exposure. These paths include leucine and isoleucine, but also intermediary metabolites of the metabolism of these 2 amino acids (isovaleryl-coenzyme A and 2-methylbutanoyl-CoA), suggesting that the metabolism of branched-chain amino acids might be modulated by BPA with possible consequences in the promotion of protein synthesis and turnover, signaling pathways, and the metabolism of glucose (52). Isoleucine, like the other branched-chain amino acids, is associated with insulin resistance: higher levels of isoleucine are observed in the blood of diabetic mice, rats, and humans (53). Also, oxidation of such amino acids may increase fatty acid oxidation and play a role in obesity, which is consistent with the fact that BPA is a candidate "obesogen" (54).

Regarding the specific identification of the commonly modulated parts of the BPA and E2 metabolic networks, it is interesting to note the presence of the urea cycle,

TABLE 3 | Endogenous metabolite variations induced by BPA or E2 exposure (BPA or E2 samples compared to DMSO samples) in HepG2 cells.

Metabolites	^{1}H NMR Chemical shifts δ (ppm)	BPA 10^{-6}M	BPA 10^{-9} M	BPA 10^{-12} M	E2 10^{-9} M	E2 10^{-12} M	E2 10^{-15} M
Arginine	1.66(m); 1.74(m); 1.93(m); 3.25(t, 6.9)	x	x	x	x	x	x
Asparagine	2.85(dd, 16.8 and 7.4); 2.95(dd, 16.8 and 4.3); 4.01(dd, 7.4 and 4.3)				x		
Choline	3.20(s); 3.52(m);4.07(m)				x		
Citrate	2.66(d,18.1); 2.81(d,18.1)	x		x			
Creatine	3.04(s); 3.93(s)	x	x	x			
Ethanolamine	3.14(m); 3.82(m)				x	x	x
Glutamate	2.06(m); 2.13(m); 2.35(m); 3.77(dd,7.5 and 4.9)				x	x	
Glutamine	2.14(m); 2.46(m); 3.78(t,6.2)	x	x	x	x	x	x
Reduced glutathione	2.17(m); 2.56(m); 2.96(m); 3.78(m); 4.58(m)			x	x		
Glycero phosphocholine	3.23(s); 3.62(m); 3.68(m);3.89(m); 3.94(m); 4.33(m)					x	x
glycine	3.55(s)				x		
Isoleucine	0.94(t,7.4); 1.01(d,7), 1.27(m); 1.47(m); 1.98(m); 3.68(d,4)	x	x	x			x
Leucine	0.96(t,6.3); 1.71(m); 3.74(m)	x	x	x			
Lysine	1.45(m); 1.52(m); 1.73(m); 1.91(m); 3.02(t, 7.5)	x	x	x	x	x	
Phosphocholine	3.22(s); 3.58(m); 4.17(m)				x	x	
Proline	2.01(m); 2.08(m); 2.35(m); 3.35(m); 3.42(m); 4.14(dd, 6.7 and 8.7)	x	x		x		
Succinate	2.41(s)				x	x	
Tyrosine	3.09(dd,14.5 and 7.5); 3.21(dd,14.5 and 5,1); 3.95(dd,7.5 and 5.1); 6.9(d,8.5); 7.20(d,8.5)			x	x		
Valine	0.995(d,7); 1,045(d,7); 2.28(m);3,62(d,4.4)	x	x	x	x		

Chemical shifts (ppm) are relative to TMSP (^{1}H, δ, 0 ppm). Multiplicity of signals is indicated within brackets: s, singlet; d, doublet; dd, doublet of doublet t, triplet; q, quadruplet and m, multiplet. Values within brackets are ^{1}H–^{1}H splittings (Hz) in cases where these are clearly resolved. "x" represents significantly modulated concentration compared to DMSO samples.

including metabolites such as citrulline, ornithine and argino-succinate, not evidenced by the metabolomic analyses but highlighted by the metabolic network comparison. This finding is in agreement with published data on a subset of ToxCast chemicals including BPA (55).

Another interesting outcome of the metabolic network analysis is the presence of apolipoprotein C1 (ApoC1) and apolipoprotein C3 (ApoC3) pathways in the shared mechanism between E2 and BPA. These components of high density lipoproteins (HDL) and very low density lipoproteins (VLDL) respectively, are in charge of the uptake, transport and catabolism of lipids. It has already been reported that ApoC3 was affected by BPA exposure, as is the expression of the APOC3 gene, which was found to be decreased in the liver of BPA-exposed C57BL/6 mice (56, 57). It was also reported that BPA modulates novel binding sites for SREBP-1 in genes directly or indirectly involved in cholesterol metabolism, such as APOC3(57). BPA exposure was also reported to be driving the upregulation of SREBP-1 and SREBP-2 *in vivo* (C57/Bl6 mice) and *in vitro* (HepG2 and Caco cells) (56, 58). In intestinal cells, SREBP-2 may be involved in the BPA-induced cholesterol absorption, leading consequently to hypercholesterolaemia (58). Some metabolites (isocitrate, oxaloacetate, and pyruvate) and reactions (citrate synthase, aconitase, and pyruvate carboxylase) involved in energy metabolism, and more specifically in the first steps of the Krebs cycle, were also pointed out as a potential common target for BPA and E2 according to the network analysis. The Krebs cycle was already identified *in vivo* after a perinatal exposure of CD1 mice, as well as for a longitudinal study in Sprague Dawley rats exposed perinatally, all of them to low doses of BPA (10, 12, 35). Although it will be necessary to confirm these *in silico* suggestions by more targeted biochemical assays, these results once again reinforce the fact that BPA and E2 may be considered as metabolic modulator chemicals that are interfering with the energy metabolism.

Network analysis allows identifying reactions that are likely to be modulated by the various exposure conditions. One of the key challenge in metabolic network analysis is the quality of the metabolic network reconstruction used. In fact, since these networks are built based on genomic information they may contain false positive reactions (reactions which

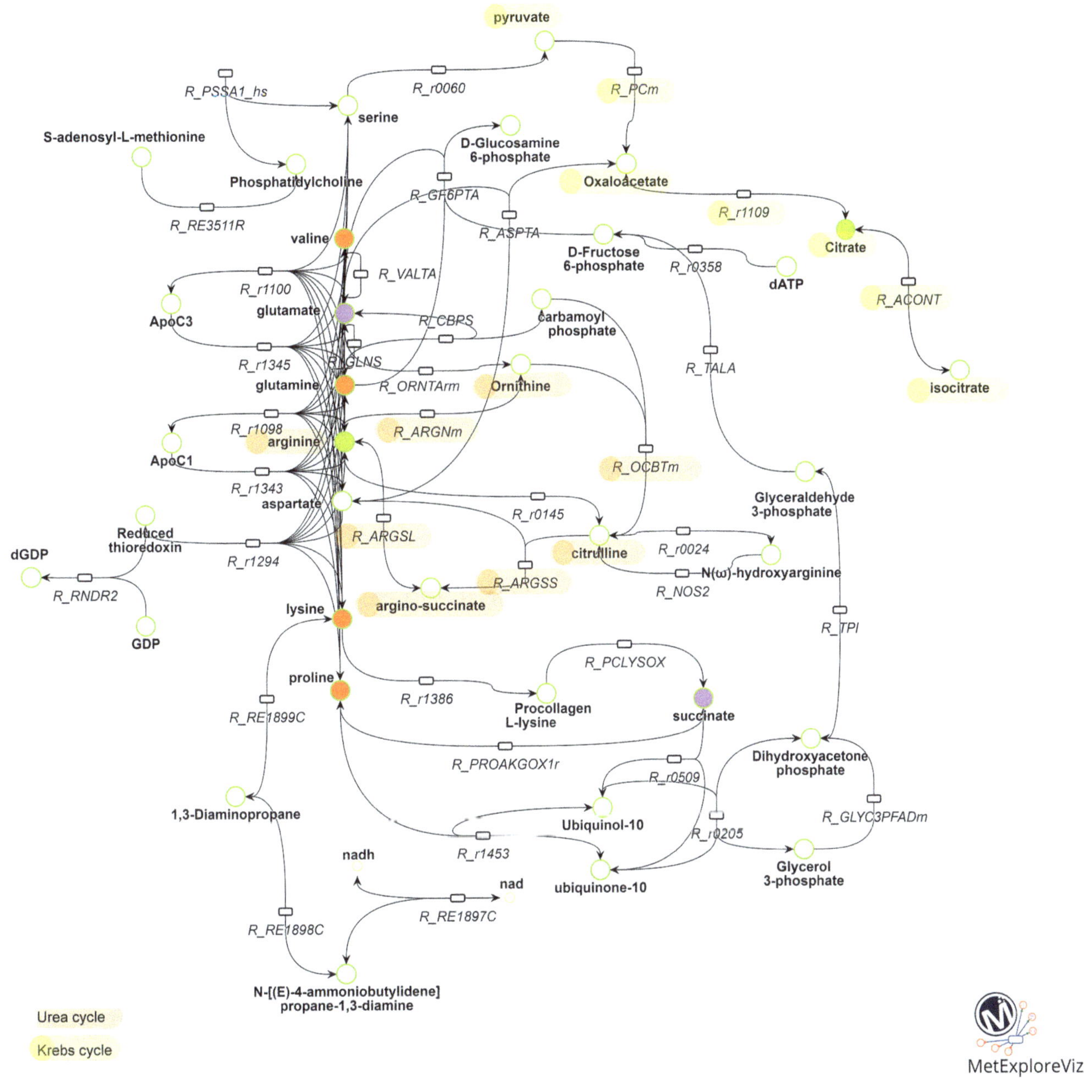

FIGURE 4 | Metabolic pathways commonly modulated by BPA 10^{-6}M and E2 10^{-9}M exposure. Reactions and metabolites belonging to both the BPA 10^{-6}M and E2 10^{-9}M metabolic sub-networks are represented. Reactions are represented by rectangles and metabolites by circles. Metabolites identified as discriminant in the BPA 10^{-6}M (resp. E2 10^{-9}M) group compared to the control group according to the PLS-DA model are colored in green (resp. purple). Metabolites identified as discriminant in the both BPA 10^{-6}M and E2 10^{-9}M groups are colored in orange. Reactions corresponding to biologically non-relevant paths between metabolites were filtered out. For clarity, substrates and products of the reactions, not specifically belonging to the BPA 10^{-6}M and E2 10^{-9}M metabolic sub-networks, are not represented. The whole list of reaction and metabolite names is presented in **Supplemental Table 3**.

should not be included) and false negatives (missing reactions). Recon2 is a highly curated reconstruction for the human metabolic network applied in many studies, but improved versions are regularly released, such as Recon3D, which has been recently introduced but has still not been used in the field of metabolomics (59–62). The other challenge is the algorithm choice to extract sub-networks. As discussed in Frainay and Jourdan (2017), there are several options to extract paths connecting metabolites and their efficiency largely depends on the application: the lightest path option, chosen here, proved to be specifically relevant and efficient to be used in metabolomics (29).

To go further with these findings, it would be interesting to perform non-targeted lipidomics to identify which family of lipids are modulated by BPA and to complete these identifications using targeted lipidomics for specific lipid families. To complete our metabolomics set of data, and to improve the quality of the metabolic networks, mass spectrometry metabolomics could be performed in order to get access to a larger set of discriminant metabolites in complement of the NMR generated list.

In summary, our study highlights that BPA, not only behaves as a xeno-estrogen as regards its potential to impact fertility and reproduction, but also shares with the natural hormone E2, the capability to modulate major metabolic routes that ensure cellular functioning and detoxification processes. We also evidenced that BPA and E2 both exert distinct effects at low and high concentrations in HepG2 cells and may act through different mechanisms. This is consistent with many reports about the non-monotonic dose effects of BPA and with our current understanding of the functioning of natural hormones, which can trigger different responses in the organism, depending on their circulating level (34, 63). Moreover, the results of this study, consistent with our previous *in vivo* results, provide first proofs of evidence that metabolomics combined with network reconstruction can be used *in vitro* (here on the human HepG2 model) as relevant approaches to investigate commonalities and differences in MoA. An even greater added value of metabolic network will come with a metabolite list as complete and specific as possible to identify the most impacted pathways associated with BPA exposure. Connecting these biochemical pathways with MoA will help to identify AOP and to facilitate the hazard characterization of other compounds (61).

AUTHOR CONTRIBUTIONS

NC and NP contributed to synthesize and interpret the data, and writing this manuscript (MS). MA contributed to supervising the cell work to generate the data, and contributed to revising the manuscript. CC was responsible of the NMR analyses and contributed in the writing of this specific section. MT-F was in charge of the statistical analyses and contributed to the writing of this section. J-PC contributed to the writing of this MS, AR contributed in supervising the experiments and revising this MS, FJ contributed in performing the metabolic networks and the writing of the MS. DZ contributed in supervising all this work, including the writing of this MS.

FUNDING

This study was partly supported by the French funding program ANR (CESA 008 01, KISMET).

ACKNOWLEDGMENTS

The authors would like to thank Claire Lapeyre for her excellent work in performing a part of the experiments during her Master training, Adrien Rohan, and Maxime Chazalviel for their contribution to metabolic network visualizations.

REFERENCES

1. Lind L, Monica Lind P, Lejonklou MH, Dunder L, Bergman Å, Guerrero-Bosagna C, et al. Uppsala consensus statement on environmental contaminants and the global obesity epidemic. *Environ Health Perspect.* (2016) 124:A81–3. doi: 10.1289/ehp.1511115
2. ESFA. Scientific Opinion on the risks to public health related to the presence of bisphenol A (BPA) in foodstuffs. *EFSA J.* (2015) 13:3978. doi: 10.2903/j.efsa.2015.3978
3. ECHA. *Committee for Risk Assessment—ECHA—Opinion on an Annex XV Dossier Proposing Restrictions on Bisphenol A.* ECHA/RAC/RES-O-0000001412-86-56/F (2015) Available online at: https://echa.europa.eu/documents/10162/d52d2c6b-2f1c-4ddf-bb44-4e3e42ea1820 (Accessed June 28, 2018).
4. ANSES. *Avis Relatif à L'identification en Tant Que Substance Extrêmement Préoccupante (SHVC) du Bisphénol A Pour Son Caractère de Perturbateur Endocrinien.* (2017). Available online at: https://www.anses.fr/fr/system/files/REACH2016SA01
5. Vandenberg LN, Colborn T, Hayes TB, Heindel JJ, Jacobs Jr. DR, Lee DH, et al. Hormones and endocrine-disrupting chemicals: low-dose effects and nonmonotonic dose responses. *Endocr Rev.* (2012) 33:378–455. doi: 10.1210/er.2011-1050
6. Alonso-Magdalena P, Vieira E, Soriano S, Menes L, Burks D, Quesada I, et al. Bisphenol A exposure during pregnancy disrupts glucose homeostasis in mothers and adult male offspring. *Env Heal Perspect* (2010) 118:1243–50.
7. Soriano S, Alonso-Magdalena P, Garcia-Arevalo M, Novials A, Muhammed SJ, Salehi A, et al. Rapid insulinotropic action of low doses of bisphenol-A on mouse and human islets of langerhans: role of estrogen receptor β. *PLoS ONE* (2012) 7:e31109.
8. Marmugi A, Ducheix S, Lasserre F, Polizzi A, Paris A, Priymenko N, et al. Low doses of bisphenol a induce gene expression related to lipid synthesis and trigger triglyceride accumulation in adult mouse liver. *Hepatology* (2012) 55:395–407. doi: 10.1002/hep.24685
9. Johnson CH, Ivanisevic J, Siuzdak G. Metabolomics: beyond biomarkers and towards mechanisms. *Nat Rev Mol Cell Biol.* (2016) 17:451–9. doi: 10.1038/nrm.2016.25
10. Cabaton NJ, Canlet C, Wadia PR, Tremblay-Franco M, Gautier R, Molina J, et al. Effects of low doses of bisphenol A on the metabolome of perinatally exposed CD-1 mice. *Env Heal Perspect.* (2013) 121:586–93. doi: 10.1289/ehp.1205588
11. Zalko D, Soto AM, Canlet C, Tremblay-Franco M, Jourdan F, Cabaton NJ. Bisphenol a exposure disrupts neurotransmitters through modulation of transaminase activity in the brain of rodents. *Endocrinology* (2016) 157:1736–9. doi: 10.1210/en.2016-1207
12. Tremblay-Franco M, Cabaton NJ, Canlet C, Gautier R, Schaeberle CM, Jourdan F, et al. Dynamic metabolic disruption in rats perinatally exposed to low doses of bisphenol-A. *PLoS ONE* (2015) 10:e0141698. doi: 10.1371/journal.pone.0141698
13. Hartung T, Luechtefeld T, Maertens A, Kleensang A. Integrated testing strategies for safety assessments. *ALTEX* (2013) 30:3–18. doi: 10.14573/altex.2013.1.003
14. Davis M, Boekelheide K, Boverhof DR, Eichenbaum G, Hartung T, Holsapple MP, et al. The new revolution in toxicology: the good, the bad, and the ugly. *Ann N Y Acad Sci.* (2013) 1278:11–24. doi: 10.1111/nyas.12086

15. Brown MV, Compton SA, Milburn MV, Lawton KA, Cheatham B. Metabolomic signatures in lipid-loaded HepaRGs reveal pathways involved in steatotic progression. *Obesity* (2013) 21:E561–70. doi: 10.1002/oby.20440
16. García- Cañaveras JC, Castell J V, Donato MT, Lahoz A. A metabolomics cell-based approach for anticipating and investigating drug-induced liver injury. *Sci Rep.* (2016) 6:27239. doi: 10.1038/srep27239
17. Audebert M, Dolo L, Perdu E, Cravedi J, Zalko D. Use of the γH2AX assay for assessing the genotoxicity of bisphenol A and bisphenol F in human cell lines. *Arch Toxicol.* (2011) 85:1463–73. doi: 10.1007/s00204-011-0721-2
18. Acconcia F, Totta P, Ogawa S, Cardillo I, Inoue S, Leone S, et al. Survival versus apoptotic 17beta-estradiol effect: role of ER alpha and ER beta activated non-genomic signaling. *J Cell Physiol.* (2005) 203:193–201. doi: 10.1002/jcp. 20219
19. Marino M, Acconcia F, Bresciani F, Weisz A, Trentalance A. Distinct nongenomic signal transduction pathways controlled by 17beta-estradiol regulate DNA synthesis and cyclin D(1) gene transcription in HepG2 cells. *Mol Biol Cell* (2002) 13:3720–9. doi: 10.1091/mbc.E02-03-0153
20. Higashi E, Fukami T, Itoh M, Kyo S, Inoue M, Yokoi T, et al. Human CYP2A6 is induced by estrogen via estrogen receptor. *Drug Metab Dispos.* (2007) 35:1935–41. doi: 10.1124/dmd.107.016568
21. Marino M, Distefano E, Caporali S, Ceracchi G, Pallottini V, Trentalance A. beta-estradiol stimulation of DNA synthesis requires different PKC isoforms in HepG2 and MCF7 cells. *J Cell Physiol.* (2001) 188:170–7. doi: 10.1002/jcp.1105
22. Ramirez T, Strigun A, Verlohner A, Huener HA, Peter E, Herold M, et al. Prediction of liver toxicity and mode of action using metabolomics in vitro in HepG2 cells. *Arch Toxicol.* (2018) 92:893–906. doi: 10.1007/s00204-017-2079-6
23. Gerets HHJ, Tilmant K, Gerin B, Chanteux H, Depelchin BO, Dhalluin S, et al. Characterization of primary human hepatocytes, HepG2 cells, and HepaRG cells at the mRNA level and CYP activity in response to inducers and their predictivity for the detection of human hepatotoxins. *Cell Biol Toxicol.* (2012) 28:69–87. doi: 10.1007/s10565-011-9208-4
24. McCombie G, Browning LM, Titman CM, Song M, Shockcor J, Jebb SA, et al. Omega-3 oil intake during weight loss in obese women results in remodelling of plasma triglyceride and fatty acids. *Metabolomics* (2009) 5:363–74. doi: 10.1007/s11306-009-0161-7
25. Wold S, Antti H, Lindgren F, Ohman J. Orthogonal signal correction of near-infrared spectra. *Chemom Intell Lab.* (1998) 44:175–185.
26. Westerhuis J, Hoefsloot H, Smit S, Vis D, Smilde A, van Velzen E, et al. Assessment of PLSDA cross validation. *Metabolomics* (2008) 4:81–9. doi: 10.1007/s11306-007-0099-6
27. Thiele I, Palsson BØ. A protocol for generating a high-quality genome-scale metabolic reconstruction. *Nat Protoc.* (2010) 5:93–121. doi: 10.1038/nprot.2009.203
28. Thiele I, Swainston N, Fleming RMT, Hoppe A, Sahoo S, Aurich MK, et al. A community-driven global reconstruction of human metabolism. *Nat Biotechnol.* (2013) 31:419–25. doi: 10.1038/nbt.2488
29. Frainay C, Jourdan F. Computational methods to identify metabolic sub-networks based on metabolomic profiles. *Brief Bioinform.* (2017) 18:43–56. doi: 10.1093/bib/bbv115
30. Cottret L, Frainay C, Chazalviel M, Cabanettes F, Gloaguen Y, Camenen E, et al. MetExplore: collaborative edition and exploration of metabolic networks. *Nucleic Acids Res.* (2018) 46:W495–502. doi: 10.1093/nar/gky301
31. Chazalviel M, Frainay C, Poupin N, Vinson F, Merlet B, Gloaguen Y, et al. MetExploreViz: Web component for interactive metabolic network visualization. *Bioinformatics* (2018) 34:312–3. doi: 10.1093/bioinformatics/btx588
32. Lapins M, Eklund M, Spjuth O, Prusis P, Wikberg JE. Proteochemometric modeling of HIV protease susceptibility. *BMC Bioinform.* (2008) 9:181. doi: 10.1186/1471-2105-9-181
33. Lejonklou MH, Dunder L, Bladin E, Pettersson V, Rönn M, Lind L, et al. Effects of low-dose developmental bisphenol a exposure on metabolic parameters and gene expression in male and female fischer 344 rat offspring. *Environ Health Perspect.* (2017) 125:067018. doi: 10.1289/EHP505
34. Heindel JJ, Blumberg B, Cave M, Machtinger R, Mantovani A, Mendez MA, et al. Metabolism disrupting chemicals and metabolic disorders. *Reprod Toxicol.* (2017) 68:3–33. doi: 10.1016/j.reprotox.2016.10.001
35. Wang M, Rang O, Liu F, Xia W, Li Y, Zhang Y, et al. A systematic review of metabolomics biomarkers for Bisphenol A exposure. *Metabolomics* (2018) 14:45. doi: 10.1007/s11306-018-1342-z
36. Wilkening S, Bader A. Influence of culture time on the expression of drug-metabolizing enzymes in primary human hepatocytes and hepatoma cell line HepG2. *J Biochem Mol Toxicol.* (2003) 17:207–13. doi: 10.1002/jbt.10085
37. Völkel W, Colnot T, Csanady GA, Filser JG, Dekant W. Metabolism and kinetics of bisphenol A in humans at low doses following oral administration. *Chem Res Toxicol.* (2002) 15:1281–7. doi: 10.1021/tx025548t
38. Marino M, Distefano E, Trentalance A, Smith CL. Estradiol-induced IP(3) mediates the estrogen receptor activity expressed in human cells. *Mol Cell Endocrinol.* (2001) 182:19–26. doi: 10.1016/S0303-7207(01)00556-1
39. Kim HS, Han SY, Yoo SD, Lee BM, Park KL. Potential estrogenic effects of bisphenol-A estimated by *in vitro* and *in vivo* combination assays. *J Toxicol Sci.* (2001) 26:111–8. doi: 10.2131/jts.26.111
40. Lee HK, Kim TS, Kim CY, Kang IH, Kim MG, Jung KK, et al. Evaluation of *in vitro* screening system for estrogenicity: comparison of stably transfected human estrogen receptor-α transcriptional activation (OECD TG455) assay and estrogen receptor (ER) binding assay. *J Toxicol Sci.* (2012) 37:431–7. doi: 10.2131/jts.37.431
41. Moon MK, Kim MJ, Jung IK, Koo Y Do, Ann HY, Lee KJ, et al. Bisphenol A impairs mitochondrial function in the liver at doses below the no observed adverse effect level. *J Korean Med Sci.* (2012) 27:644. doi: 10.3346/jkms.2012.27.6.644
42. Fang C, Ning B, Waqar AB, Niimi M, Li S, Satoh K, et al. Bisphenol A exposure induces metabolic disorders and enhances atherosclerosis in hyperlipidemic rabbits. *J Appl Toxicol.* (2015) 35:1058–70. doi: 10.1002/jat.3103
43. Xu BL, Zhao QZ, Gao XY, Hou GJ. Effect of estradiol and bisphenol A on human hepatoblastoma cell viability and telomerase activity. *Brazilian J Med Biol Res.* (2015) 48:1004–9. doi: 10.1590/1414-431X20154400
44. Stroheker T, Chagnon MC, Pinnert MF, Berges R, Canivenc-Lavier MC. Estrogenic effects of food wrap packaging xenoestrogens and flavonoids in female Wistar rats: a comparative study. *Reprod Toxicol.* (2003) 17:421–32. doi: 10.1016/S0890-6238(03)00044-3
45. Le Fol V, Aït-Aïssa S, Sonavane M, Porcher J-M, Balaguer P, Cravedi J-P, et al. *In vitro* and *in vivo* estrogenic activity of BPA, BPF and BPS in zebrafish-specific assays. *Ecotoxicol Environ Saf.* (2017) 142:150–6. doi: 10.1016/J.ECOENV.2017.04.009
46. Gould JC, Leonard LS, Maness SC, Wagner BL, Conner K, Zacharewski T, et al. Bisphenol A interacts with the estrogen receptor alpha in a distinct manner from estradiol. *Mol Cell Endocrinol.* (1998) 142:203–14.
47. Alonso-Magdalena P, Rivera FJ, Guerrero-Bosagna C. Bisphenol-A and metabolic diseases: epigenetic, developmental and transgenerational basis. *Environ Epigenetics* (2016) 2:dvw022. doi: 10.1093/eep/dvw022
48. Alonso-Magdalena P, Ropero AB, Soriano S, Garcia-Arevalo M, Ripoll C, Fuentes E, et al. Bisphenol-A acts as a potent estrogen via non-classical estrogen triggered pathways. *Mol Cel Endocrinol.* (2012) 355:201–7. doi: 10.1016/j.mce.2011.12.012
49. Welshons W V, Nagel SC, vom Saal FS. Large effects from small exposures. III. Endocrine mechanisms mediating effects of bisphenol A at levels of human exposure. *Endocrinology* (2006) 147:s56–69. doi: 10.1210/en.2005-1159
50. Nagato EG, Simpson AJ, Simpson MJ. Metabolomics reveals energetic impairments in Daphnia magna exposed to diazinon, malathion and bisphenol-A. *Aquat Toxicol.* (2016) 170:175–86. doi: 10.1016/j.aquatox.2015.11.023
51. Hall AG. The role of glutathione in the regulation of apoptosis. *Eur J Clin Invest.* (1999) 29:238–45. doi: 10.1046/j.1365-2362.1999.00447.x
52. Monirujjaman M, Ferdouse A. Metabolic and physiological roles of branched-chain amino acids. *Adv Mol Biol.* (2014) 2014:1–6. doi: 10.1155/2014/364976
53. Lynch CJ, Adams SH. Branched-chain amino acids in metabolic signalling and insulin resistance. *Nat Rev Endocrinol.* (2014) 10:723–36. doi: 10.1038/nrendo.2014.171
54. Heindel JJ, vom Saal FS, Blumberg B, Bovolin P, Calamandrei G, Ceresini G, et al. Parma consensus statement on metabolic disruptors. *Environ Health* (2015) 14:54. doi: 10.1186/s12940-015-0042-7
55. Kleinstreuer NC, Smith AM, West PR, Conard KR, Fontaine BR, Weir-Hauptman AM, et al. Identifying developmental toxicity pathways for a subset of ToxCast chemicals using human embryonic stem cells and metabolomics.

Toxicol Appl Pharmacol. (2011) 257:111–21. doi: 10.1016/j.taap.2011.08.025

56. Lin Y, Ding D, Huang Q, Liu Q, Lu H, Lu Y, et al. Downregulation of miR-192 causes hepatic steatosis and lipid accumulation by inducing SREBF1: novel mechanism for bisphenol A-triggered non-alcoholic fatty liver disease. *Biochim Biophys Acta* (2017) 1862:869–82. doi: 10.1016/j.bbalip.2017.05.001
57. Motallebipour M, Enroth S, Punga T, Ameur A, Koch C, Dunham I, et al. Novel genes in cell cycle control and lipid metabolism with dynamically regulated binding sites for sterol regulatory element-binding protein 1 and RNA polymerase II in HepG2 cells detected by chromatin immunoprecipitation with microarray detection. *FEBS J.* (2009) 276:1878–90. doi: 10.1111/j.1742-4658.2009.06914.x
58. Feng D, Zou J, Zhang S, Li X, Li P, Lu M. Bisphenol A promotes cholesterol absorption in Caco-2 cells by up-regulation of NPC1L1 expression. *Lipids Health Dis.* (2017) 16:1–7. doi: 10.1186/s12944-016-0395-0
59. Gonçalves E, Sciacovelli M, Costa ASH, Tran MGB, Johnson TI, Machado D, et al. Post-translational regulation of metabolism in fumarate hydratase deficient cancer cells. *Metab Eng.* (2018) 45:149–57. doi: 10.1016/j.ymben.2017.11.011
60. Aurich MK, Paglia G, Rolfsson Ó, Hrafnsdóttir S, Magnúsdóttir M, Stefaniak MM, et al. Prediction of intracellular metabolic states from extracellular metabolomic data. *Metabolomics* (2015) 11:603–19. doi: 10.1007/s11306-014-0721-3
61. Ramirez AK, Lynes MD, Shamsi F, Xue R, Tseng Y-H, Kahn CR, et al. Integrating extracellular flux measurements and genome-scale modeling reveals differences between brown and white adipocytes. *Cell Rep.* (2017) 21:3040–8. doi: 10.1016/j.celrep.2017.11.065
62. Brunk E, Sahoo S, Zielinski DC, Altunkaya A, Dräger A, Mih N, et al. Recon3D enables a three-dimensional view of gene variation in human metabolism. *Nat Biotechnol.* (2018) 36:272–81. doi: 10.1038/nbt.4072
63. Vandenberg LN, Ehrlich S, Belcher SM, Ben-Jonathan N, Dolinoy DC, Hugo ER, et al. Low dose effects of bisphenol A. *Endocr Disruptors* (2015) 1:e26490. doi: 10.4161/endo.26490

2

Timing of Exposure and Bisphenol-A: Implications for Diabetes Development

*Eva Tudurí, Laura Marroqui, Reinaldo S. Dos Santos, Iván Quesada, Esther Fuentes and Paloma Alonso-Magdalena**

Centro de Investigación Biomédica en Red de Diabetes y Enfermedades Metabólicas Asociadas and Instituto de Biología Molecular y Celular, Universidad Miguel Hernández de Elche, Alicante, Spain

Correspondence:
Paloma Alonso-Magdalena
palonso@umh.es

Bisphenol-A (BPA) is one of the most widespread endocrine disrupting chemicals (EDCs). It is used as the base compound in the production of polycarbonate and other plastics present in many consumer products. It is also used as a building block in epoxy can coating and the thermal paper of cash register receipts. Humans are consistently exposed to BPA and, in consequence, this compound has been detected in the majority of individuals examined. Over the last decade, an enlarging body of evidence has provided a strong support for the role of BPA in the etiology of diabetes and other metabolic disorders. Timing of exposure to EDCs results crucial since it has important implications on the resulting adverse effects. It is now well established that the developing organisms are particularly sensitive to environmental influences. Exposure to EDCs during early life may result in permanent adverse consequences, which increases the risk of developing chronic diseases like diabetes in adult life. In addition to that, developmental abnormalities can be transmitted from one generation to the next, thus affecting future generations. More recently, it has been proposed that gestational environment may also program long-term susceptibility to metabolic disorders in the mother. In the present review, we will comment and discuss the contributing role of BPA in the etiology of diabetes. We will address the metabolic consequences of BPA exposure at different stages of life and comment on the final phenotype observed in different whole-animal models of study.

Keywords: Bisphenol-A, diabetes, pancreatic β-cell, timing of exposure, metabolic programming

Diabetes mellitus is among the most prevalent metabolic disorders and the current number of cases is approaching epidemic proportions. According to the latest Global Burden Disease report (2015), the prevalence of diabetes has risen from 333 million people in 2005 to approximately 435 million in 2015 (1). The predictions suggest that it will be the seventh leading cause of death in 2030 (2). As proposed by the American Diabetes Association (ADA), the classification of this pathology includes type 1 (T1DM), type 2 (T2DM) and gestational diabetes mellitus (GDM), as well as other forms of diabetes (3). Despite differences on the underlying causing factors, all of them lead to hyperglycemia, which results from defects on insulin secretion, insulin resistance or a combination of both (4).

More than 90% of patients with diabetes have T2DM (5). The etiology of T2DM is multifactorial with a clear genetic background but also with an important environmental compound (6). Poor nutrition, lack of exercise and overweight are commonly seen as contributing factors to cause T2DM but other environmental factors like endocrine disrupting chemicals (EDCs) are also key. EDCs are defined as any chemical or mixture of chemicals able to disrupt any aspect of endocrine function (7). They constitute a heterogeneous range of compounds widely used in consumer products including food packaging, personal care products, pesticides or building materials, among others. General population is exposed to EDCs through different routes, mainly the oral, dermal or inhalation ones (8). From a mechanistic point of view, it is well described that they can interfere with hormonal signaling pathways principally by binding to hormone receptors and/or altering hormone production, metabolism and transport (8, 9). Over the last decade, burgeoning scientific evidence have disclosed that a subset of EDCs are able to modify sensitive metabolic processes leading to altered energy homeostasis and/or glucose and lipid metabolism (10–12). One of the best documented example is the case of bisphenol-A (BPA), firstly synthetized by Dianin in 1891 and reported to show estrogenic properties in 1930s (13). BPA is a monomer that is used as the base compound in the manufacture of polycarbonate and other plastics, and it is also employed as a building block in epoxy can coating and the thermal paper of cash register receipts. It became one of the most pervasive chemical in modern life from the moment it was introduced in the plastic industry in the 50s. Today, it constitutes one of the highest volume chemical produced widespread, with over 6 billion pounds manufactured every year. BPA has been found to migrate from polycarbonate containers and leach into food or water because of overheat, the presence of acidic or basic conditions and/or a repetitive use. Thermal paper has also been shown to constitute an important source of exposure to this EDC (14). The ubiquitous nature of BPA makes human exposure to occur on a virtually constant basis. In consequence, it has been detected in the majority of individuals examined (15, 16).

As regards the regulatory aspects, back in the 80s the Environmental Protection Agency (EPA) established the lowest adverse effect level (LOAEL) for BPA at 50 mg/kg/day and, based on that, the safety level was set on 50 μg/kg/day (17). Although many studies have shown deleterious effects of BPA at doses below the calculated safe dose (8, 18), the reference value of 50 μg/kg/day is still in force. For the European Food Safety Authority the tolerable daily intake has been recently established in 4 μg/kg/day (19). Remarkably, both the reference dose and the tolerable daily intake are higher than the 95th percentile BPA intake level for adults (1.5 μg/kg/day) estimated by the World Health Organization (WHO). This estimation has been done based on published exposure estimation in several countries and regions, as well as taking into account the information available regarding information on food consumption patterns, and BPA presence in foods relevant to the population groups (20).

OVERVIEW OF THE MOLECULAR MECHANISMS LINKING BPA EXPOSURE AND DIABETES

Current molecular and cellular evidence support that BPA may augment diabetes risk by affecting pancreatic β-cell function and/or insulin action in different metabolically active tissues (8, 10, 21). Before commenting on that, we will briefly described some general aspects of BPA mode of action.

BPA is mainly considered a xenoestrogen due to its capacity to promote estrogen-like activities. Structurally, BPA has two phenolic and two (4, 40)-OH substituents that confer the ability to join into the ER-binding structure. Thus, BPA can bind to both estrogen receptor α (ERα) and β (ERβ) although with 1,000 to 2,000-fold less affinity than the natural hormone 17-β-estradiol (E2) (22, 23). Based on that, BPA was considered a weak estrogen for many years. Nevertheless, today we know that, when acting through non-classical ER pathways, BPA can elicit responses with the same potency than E2. Non-classical ER pathways mainly include nuclear mechanisms of estrogen responses elicited by recruiting different transcriptional co-activators or co-repressors, as well as extranuclear-initiated signaling pathways which regulate different cellular pathways such as, gene transcription as well as ion channel and kinase activity. We here summarize some of the principal mechanisms behind BPA action triggered via non-classical estrogen pathways. For more information readers are referred to the following reviews (24–28).

Scientific evidence support that BPA-dependent estrogenic activity flows, at least in part, through rapid, non-genomic alterations of Ca^{2+} handling. Both BPA and E2, in the pico and nanomolar range, have shown to rapidly increase $[Ca^{2+}]$ in GH3/B6 pituitary tumor cells resulting in prolactin secretion (29). In a similar manner, BPA, at exactly the same doses than E2 (100 pM-1nM), potentiated Ca^{2+} signaling and insulin release in pancreatic β-cells (30, 31), while in pancreatic α-cells BPA mimicked E2 action by inhibiting low-glucose induced $[Ca^{2+}]$ oscillations (32). Importantly, *in vivo* studies also reported rapid insulin release in response to low doses of BPA (33). Rapid effects of BPA have also been observed in cardio myocytes. Low dose concentrations of BPA and E2 induced arrhythmic actions in isolated ventricular myocytes from female rats by altering Ca^{2+} handling (34); an effect that depends on the balance between ERα and ERβ (35). These BPA actions on cardio myocytes were characterized by non-monotonic dose responses (36).

Another major mechanism of BPA-induced extranuclear signaling pathways involves the activation of ERK/MAPK kinases. A wide range of BPA concentrations have been shown to rapidly increase the phosphorylation state of ERK1/2 in developing cerebellar neurons (37). In pancreatic islets of Langerhans BPA increased insulin content with the same potency than E2 acting through ERα. This was not an acute but a long-term effect which required the activation of ERK (38).

Furthermore, BPA showed binding affinities for GPR30, a relatively novel 7-transmembrane estrogen receptor (39). Several data support BPA action within nanomolar range via GPR30 in several systems. For example, BPA led to testicular seminoma cell proliferation through GPR30 (40). In pancreatic cells, BPA promoted insulin secretion dysfunction which was connected with inhibition of Pdx-1 and decreased expression of miR-338 (41).

Overall, it has been proposed that these plethora of mechanisms could account for the low dose effects of BPA that have been defined as "any biological change occurring in the range of typical human exposures or at doses lower than tested in traditional toxicological assessments" (42). Hundreds of studies have been published over the years providing strong evidence for low dose BPA effects having the potential to pose health hazards. These low dose effects have been observed for a variety of endpoints including metabolic parameters but also prostate weight, spermatogenesis, brain and mammary gland development as well as hormone levels, among others (18, 43). In addition, it is important to highlight that BPA, like hormones, do not obey the Paracelsus principle of "the dose makes the poison." On the contrary, a typical feature of BPA actions includes non-monotonic dose response curves (NMDRCs) often manifested as U- or inverted U-shaped curves. The mechanisms behind these NMDRCs are typically related to cytotoxicity, receptor selectivity, receptor down regulation or competition with endogenous hormones (44). In addition to its estrogenic activity, BPA may act as an antagonist of androgenic (at doses in the range of 100 nM-10 μM) (45) and thyroid (1–100 μM) (46) activity, and may also activate the human estrogen-related receptor (26 nM) (47), pregnane receptor (2 μM) (48) and the glucocorticoid receptor (1 μM) (49).

A large number of cellular studies have demonstrated that BPA targets pancreatic β-cells. Environmental relevant doses of BPA have been shown to modulate K_{ATP} channel activity, which is key in the stimulus-secretion coupling process that culminates with insulin secretion. In both mouse and human islets, BPA provoked a rapid closure of the K_{ATP} channel and subsequently, increased insulin release. This effect was mediated by the extranuclear activation of the estrogen receptor beta (ERβ) (30, 50). Additionally, BPA may enhance glucose-induced insulin biosynthesis and content via binding to extranuclear ERα (38). In several models of β-cell lines, BPA has also been reported to affect insulin release. In the nanomolar range, it enhances basal (51, 52) and glucose-stimulated insulin secretion (GSIS), leading to ER stress. Conversely, at higher doses in the micromolar range, it displays the opposite effect (53). Furthermore, BPA treatment has been shown to increase reactive oxygen species production and DNA damage (54) as well as to augment apoptosis (53).

BPA may also alter glucose regulation by disrupting insulin action in different peripheral metabolic tissues. In the murine adipose cell line 3T3-L1 and in human adipocytes, BPA impaired insulin-stimulated receptor phosphorylation and signaling, which led to decreased insulin sensitivity and glucose disposal (55, 56). BPA treatment also provoked an up-regulation of inflammatory signaling pathways (56) and induced adipogenesis (57–59).

BPA has also been reported to exert direct effects on hepatocyte physiology. In different hepatic cell lines, BPA has been shown to induce lipid accumulation, favoring the development of hepatic steatosis (58, 60).

RELEVANCE OF EXPOSURE TIMING: THE CONCEPT OF METABOLIC PROGRAMMING

David Barker and colleagues suggested for the first time that early-life nutrition is associated with a number of offspring health outcomes including coronary heart disease, hypertension and T2DM (61–63). These first observations established the bases of the fetal origins of adult disease hypothesis, which states that events occurring during early development may increase the risk of specific diseases later in life. This concept was later expanded to other aspects of developmental plasticity such as early postnatal period and intergenerational influences, and set the framework of the Developmental Origins of Health and Disease (DOHaD) theory (64).

Overall, this paradigm relies on the fact that there exist specific developmental periods whereby an organism is more sensitive to environmental insults. While those insults were initially referred to nutritional imbalance, today it is well demonstrated that the exposure to some environmental chemicals during development may also lead to increased incidence to non-communicable diseases like T2DM (65). The understanding of the molecular mechanisms behind this phenomenon is far to be complete. Nevertheless, it has been proposed that environmental agents acting during specific windows of sensitivity may promote changes in gene expression, cell metabolism, hormone regulation or cellular plasticity, among others. Such functional changes might permanently modify the organism's physiologic and metabolic homeostatic set points, programming the individual to later risk for metabolic diseases (11).

So far, epigenetics processes have been proposed to be the major driving mechanism in the altered programming during development. These epigenetic changes entail chemical modifications of DNA which are heritable and reversible but with no changes in the underlying DNA sequence. Rather, epigenetic marks are capable to alter DNA accessibility and chromatin structure and, therefore, regulate gene expression patterns. They comprise DNA methylation, histone modification, states of chromatin condensation or non-coding RNA-associated gene silencing (66–69). As it will be described later, early life exposure to BPA has been shown to induce epigenetic alterations associated with diabetogenic outcomes.

METABOLIC CONSEQUENCES OF DEVELOPMENTAL EXPOSURE TO BPA

A review of the currently available literature reveals increasing number of animal studies exploring BPA effects on metabolic developmental programming. Although most of the studies differ in the route and timing of BPA exposure (gestation or gestation and lactation), dose, and animal strain used, they generally strengthen the evidence of the diabetogenic action of BPA. Here we review studies reported in the literature addressing the contributing role of BPA in the etiology of diabetes. Detailed information on dosage, age, gender and timing of exposure can be found in **Supplemental Table 1**.

Initial observations came in 2010 when it was shown that the treatment of pregnant dams on days 9–16 of gestation with two different doses of BPA (10 or 100 µg/kg/day) resulted in impaired glucose homeostasis in male adult offspring. Of note, the metabolic phenotype observed was different depending on the BPA dose administered. Thus, animals intrauterine exposed to the lowest dose showed marked insulin resistance, hyperinsulinemia, altered glucose tolerance and increased triglyceride levels. Pancreatic β-cell function was also found to be affected as reflected by enhanced GSIS, both *in vivo* and *in vitro*, probably as a compensatory mechanism for the insulin resistance developed. On the contrary, animals exposed to the highest dose showed mild glucose intolerance with no changes on insulin sensitivity (70).

Later on, a wider BPA dose range study came out with doses tested from 10-fold below EPA reference dose (50 µg/kg/day) to 10-fold above the no-observed-adverse-effect level (NOAEL, 5,000 µg/kg/day). Offspring's metabolic changes following oral exposure of pregnant dams to BPA (5, 50, 500, 5,000, and 50,000 µg/kg/day, days 9–18 of gestation) were evaluated in CD1 mice. The authors found a non-monotonic dose response for body weight changes and increased adipocyte number and volume in the offspring. In addition, offspring from all BPA groups, except for the highest dose one, developed glucose intolerance. Intrauterine BPA-exposed animals to 5 µg/kg/day displayed higher plasma insulin levels, and those treated with the doses of 5 and 5,000 µg/kg/day showed insulin resistance (71).

A similar study by Liu and collaborators focused on a range of timing of exposure instead of on a range of doses. Preimplantation (days 1–6 of pregnancy), fetal (P6-PND0), neonatal (PND0-PND21) or fetal and neonatal (P6-PND21) periods were explored with the same dose of BPA (100 µg/kg/day by subcutaneous injection). The authors reported changes on body weight that were dependent on the animal gender and the exposure timing to BPA. Regarding glucose metabolism, female mice exposed to BPA during fetal and preimplantation periods manifested glucose intolerance at the age of 3 and 6 months. In the case of male offspring, glucose intolerance was observed in fetal, neonatal, and fetal and neonatal exposed-groups at 3 months of age and persisted at 6 and 8 months of age in the first group. Insulin sensitivity was also altered. Reduced insulinogenic index was observed in the 3 month-old female fetally BPA-exposed as well as in males receiving BPA in the fetal, neonatal and fetal and neonatal periods. Together with changes in the insulinogenic index, these animals showed attenuated response to insulin that only persisted in the male fetally exposed-group up to 8 months of age. A transient impairment of pancreatic β-cell function was observed in *in vitro* assays, which was thought to be a functional issue rather than morphological abnormalities, since pancreatic β-cell mass remained invariable or even increased. Isolated islets released less insulin in response to glucose in the fetal female as well as in the fetal, neonatal, and fetal and neonatal male exposed groups. Nevertheless, no changes on insulin secretion were observed when animals reached 8 months of age (72). Of note, in a similar experimental animal model, BPA promoted impaired insulin signaling and glucose transport expression in the prefrontal cortex at 8 months of age (73). Furthermore, glucose intolerance in adult BPA offspring has also been connected with alterations in the structure of hypothalamic energy balance circuitry (74, 75).

In another study, pregnant rats were exposed to 1 and 10 µg/mL BPA (drinking water) from gestation day 6 through lactation, and then male offspring was studied at postnatal days 50 (PND50) and 100 (PND100). Increased body weight was manifested on PND7 and persisted at PND100 together with hyperglycemia, insulin resistance, decreased adiponectin levels and increased oxidative stress (76).

Not only murine but also large-animal model-based studies have found postnatal metabolic outcomes related to fetal exposure to BPA at a level relevant to human exposure. In line with this, Veiga-Lopez and collaborators explored pregnancy as a critical period for BPA exposure by treating female sheep with 50, 500, or 5,000 µg/kg/day (subcutaneous injection) from days 30–90 of gestation. Increased fasting blood glucose in the lowest BPA dose group and a marked tendency to decreased insulin sensitivity in all BPA groups were found in the female offspring at 6 weeks of age. In the postpubertal period (13 months of age), insulin resistance was observed in the 500 µg/kg/day BPA-exposed group. Moreover, enhanced mean adipocyte area and diameter in the visceral adipose tissue, as well as increased inflammation in the subcutaneous adipose tissue depot were reported (77).

It should be mentioned that some reports did not find developmental BPA effects on glucose regulation. This is the case of Ryan and collaborators' article, in which perinatal pregnant CD-1 mice were exposed to BPA (1 ppb via the diet) from embryonic day 0 until weaning. The authors observed that BPA mice were heavier and longer at the moment of weaning but the body weight returned to normal levels in adulthood compared to controls. They did not find any effects on glucose tolerance neither at 8 nor 15 weeks of age. No other metabolic parameters such as insulin sensitivity or GSIS were analyzed. It is remarkable that the authors did not explore more advanced ages in which metabolic abnormalities were revealed in other animal studies (78). In a similar manner, no impairment on glucose tolerance was observed in male 20 week-old offspring after BPA perinatal exposure, although dose-dependent increases of body weight were reported with no changes on global hepatic DNA methylation (79, 80).

Intrauterine exposure to low BPA doses has been shown to affect not only pancreatic β-cell function in the adult offspring but also pancreas development. Increased pancreatic β-cell mass has been found in BPA-exposed animals at the moment of birth, which was also observed at the moment of weaning and PND30. This early life alteration was mainly related to overexpression of cell cycle genes, culminating with a rise in β-cell division as well as decreased apoptosis. All together, these abnormalities led to marked hyperinsulinemia. It is noteworthy to mention that this excessive insulin signaling has been proposed to be crucial for the metabolic phenotype observed in BPA animals later in life (81). Furthermore, BPA has been shown to have an impact on pancreas morphology with a greater number of islet-cell clusters at embryonic day 18.5 (82).

In order to reveal and/or exacerbate any underlying metabolic disorder that accounts for BPA action, the so-called high fat diets (HFD) have been used in several laboratory studies. This approach has helped to shed some light into the metabolic derangements following prenatal BPA exposure. In one study, pregnant rats were exposed to BPA at doses of 50, 250, or 1,250 μg/kg/day by oral gavage through gestation and lactation, and later, offspring was fed with either standard diet (STD) or HFD from the moment of weaning. While some detrimental effects were observed at 26 weeks of age on the BPA animals fed with STD, those effects were accelerated and exacerbated by HFD and became apparent at the age of 15 weeks. Increments in body weight, insulin plasma levels, GSIS and pancreatic β-cell mass were observed in the BPA lowest dose fed with STD group. The same group of animals challenged with HFD exhibited glucose intolerance, hyperglycemia, dyslipidemia and hyperleptinemia. Remarkably, no adverse effects were observed at the highest doses (83). In a different report, pregnant dams were subcutaneously treated with BPA (10 μg/kg/day) from day 9 to 16 of gestation and then 1-month-old male offspring were maintained during 13 or 24 weeks on STD or HFD. In BPA-treated mice, body weight at birth was decreased followed by catch-up growth with similar weight than HFD mice at 22 weeks of age. At the 17th week, BPA animals showed fasting hyperglycemia, increased NEFA and insulin levels, and a tendency to be glucose intolerant, which was severely impaired at the 28th week in STD. In addition, intrauterine exposure to BPA led to changes in the expression of genes involved in glucose and lipid metabolism in liver and adipose tissue as well as in pancreatic β-cell function that were similar to those observed with HFD treatment (84). Similar metabolic outcomes have also been observed in sheep, including insulin resistance, increased adipocyte size and deposition, and inflammation in BPA-exposed and postnatal overfeeding groups (77). Furthermore, metabolomic analysis revealed changes in metabolic profiling related to prenatal BPA exposure, such as variations in glucose, pyruvate, some amino acids and neurotransmitters, which were evident soon after birth (85, 86).

As stated before, epigenetics has been outlined as one of the major links between genes, environment, and developmental outcomes. Several articles have shown that gestational exposure to environmentally relevant BPA doses are able to promote epigenetic changes in the progeny that correlate to adverse multigenerational health effects. Thus, at the age of 3 weeks, male offspring perinatally exposed to BPA (50 μg/kg/day) exhibited overexpression of the methyltransferase 3B mRNA. This phenomenon was related to decreased hepatic global DNA methylation and resulted in reduced hepatic glucokinase gene expression. No changes in insulin sensitivity were found at this age. However, at 21 weeks of age, impaired glucose tolerance and insulin resistance showed up, suggesting that the global methylation changes contributed to the metabolic disarrangement observed in adulthood (87). Epigenetic changes have been connected not only with F1 generation but with subsequent generational effects. In line with this, decreased insulin sensitivity and glucose intolerance were found in F2 generation. These effects were proposed to be transmitted through the male germ line and to be associated with changes in glucokinase DNA methylation (88). Later on, more evidence came out confirming multigenerational phenotypic inheritance upon perinatal BPA exposure. Pregnant mice were treated with two different doses of BPA (10 μg/kg/d and 10 mg/kg/day) and the effects on the offspring were studied. Overall, increased body weight, glucose intolerance and reduced GSIS were observed in both F1 and F2 male offspring. Importantly, it was demonstrated for the first time that maternal glucose homeostasis was affected in F0 but not in F1 pregnant mice, suggesting that the alterations observed were not caused by an abnormal maternal metabolic milieu but were rather related to epigenetic changes. In particular, the authors reported fetal increased expression of the imprinted Igf2 gene and enhanced DNA methylation at the Igf2 differentially methylated region 1 both in F1 and F2 embryos (89). In the same year, another report confirmed the presence of glucose intolerance and pancreatic β-cell dysfunction in male BPA F2 generation; abnormalities that were associated with the dysregulation of Igf2/H19 in the islets of Langerhans (90). More recently, relying on the same epigenetic bases, metabolic effects found in F1 and F2 generation have been extended to impaired mitochondrial function and insulin secretion, reduced β-cell mass and islet inflammation (91).

These above-mentioned multigenerational effects differ from the transgenerational ones. While the former has been defined as "an exposure that directly influences multiple generations", the latter implies transmission across generations but with no direct exposure or involvement, and are manifested from F3 generation. Up to date, much of the work has focused on outcomes in the BPA-exposed F1 generation or the intergenerational F2, but little is known about the transgenerational (F3 and beyond) outcomes, with just some evidence of embryonic exposure to BPA and obesogenic effects in F3 (92, 93).

Contrary to the case of T2DM, the experimental data supporting the contributing role of BPA in the developmental programming of T1DM is still very scarce. One study published in 2014 addressed this issue by using non-obese diabetic (NOD) mice, an animal model of T1DM. The study described how transmaternal orally-exposed female offspring (10 mg/L drinking water) showed aggravated severity of insulitis together with increased apoptosis and decreased number of resident macrophages at 11 weeks of age. This determined increased prevalence of diabetes later at 20 weeks of age (94).

Regarding the possible interactions with the immune system, perinatal exposure to BPA (50 μg/kg/day) has also been shown to promote systemic immune imbalances in male adult mice offspring. Remarkably, these alterations occurred in parallel to microbial disturbances and impaired glucose tolerance. The authors proposed that these disturbances precede the development of obese phenotype as the animals get old (95).

METABOLIC CONSEQUENCES OF ADULT EXPOSURE TO BPA

Multiple studies conducted in adult animal models have observed alterations in glucose and lipid metabolism following BPA treatment. Firstly, one of the most described outcomes is the insulinotropic action of BPA, i.e. its ability to stimulate insulin release from pancreatic β-cells. A single injection of BPA at a low dose of 10 μg/kg of body weight potentiated plasma insulin levels in mice within just 30 min (33). Likewise, BPA treatments with different durations and a wide range of doses, from 5 μg/kg/day to 20 mg/kg/day, also increased plasma insulin levels (33, 41, 96–99). Accordingly, further studies in islets from BPA-treated mice showed an increase in several parameters including GSIS (96), enhanced insulin content (33, 41), improved β-cell area and mass (41), and augmented islet Pdx1 transcript and protein levels, and NeuroD mRNA levels (41). It is important to note that hyperinsulinemia may eventually lead to insulin resistance and, therefore, may contribute to obesity and T2DM development (33, 100). In contrast, other reports described decreased plasma insulin levels after exposing mice to 100 μg/kg/day BPA for 20 days (101) or 28 days (102), or even unchanged plasma insulin levels after 8 months of BPA administration (5–5,000 μg/kg/day) (103). These discrepancies in the observed outcomes might be due to the use of different mouse strains and/or variations in the administration protocol. Secondly, BPA-treated adult mice displayed impaired glucose tolerance after 4 days receiving BPA at 100 μg/kg/day (33) and after 2 months of BPA treatment with 500 μg/kg/day (41) and 5,000 μg/kg/day (103). One study reported no changes in the glucose excursions in response to a glucose load after 8 days of treatment with BPA 100 μg/kg/day (96). Furthermore, some reports also described insulin resistance following BPA exposure (33, 41, 96). Overall, these effects on glucose homeostasis suggested that, besides the endocrine pancreas, other tissues involved in the regulation of glucose metabolism also displayed alterations. In fact, the insulin signaling pathway was altered in skeletal muscle and liver from BPA-treated mice, which showed diminished insulin-stimulated phosphorylation of the insulin receptor β subunit and Akt phosphorylation (96, 97, 104). Such failure in hepatic insulin signaling seems to be responsible for the impaired hepatic glucose oxidation and glycogen content found in rats treated with high doses of BPA (20 and 200 mg/kg/day) for 30 days (97). Furthermore, hepatic glucokinase activity was acutely (2 h) suppressed in response to an oral BPA bolus of 50 μg/kg (105). Additional analysis with liver samples showed that long-term exposure to BPA (20–200 mg/kg/day) potentiated the mRNA and protein levels of GLUT2 (97), as well as important factors involved in lipogenesis and biosynthesis of cholesterol when employing doses in the range of 5–5,000 μg/kg/day BPA (99, 103). Accordingly, augmented plasma triglycerides and cholesterol have been detected following BPA administration (0.5 and 2 mg/kg/day) during 4 weeks (103, 106), and hypercholesteronemia remained after 8 months of BPA exposure (5–5,000 μg/kg/day) (103). Finally, experimental studies employing T1DM animal models reported increased diabetes incidence following BPA treatment (107–109). In NOD mice, 1 mg/L BPA in drinking water accelerated spontaneous diabetes development, insulitis and islet apoptosis, and decreased numbers of tissue resident macrophages prior to insulitis (107, 108). Similarly to what has been previously described in other studies regarding the BPA non-monotonic dose response, the authors reported that the highest BPA dose (100 mg/L) did produce less severe insulitis than the lowest one (1 mg/L) (107). In parallel, in streptozotocin (STZ)-treated mice, drinking water containing BPA at 1 and 10 mg/L promoted diabetes incidence and affected T-cell immunity (109). Oral gavage administration of BPA 5 mg/kg for 5 days also increased the insulin positive area and transcript expression of estrogen receptors in pancreas, and the hepatic expression of inflammation-related genes in STZ-induced diabetic mice (98).

A NEW PERSPECTIVE FOR THE CONCEPT OF METABOLIC PROGRAMMING

Over the years steroid hormone research has set the framework for addressing how EDCs may cause endocrine actions. Many biological principles that operate for natural hormones are also central for the mode of action of EDCs. This applies for the activational and organizational concepts. As originally described, organizational effects refer to permanent changes occurring during critical periods of development. They are precisely time-dependent, and affect morphogenesis and differentiation processes of organ systems. It is important to note that some of the organizational effects are not manifested up to later in life, which is in line with the concept of developmental programming. For example, intrauterine exposure to estrogenic compounds is well known to promote abnormalities in the reproductive tract as well as functional changes at puberty and throughout adulthood. This is well exemplified by the case of diethylstilbestrol (DES). Animal studies have shown that perinatal exposure to DES promote a wide range of gene expression changes that have been associated with the increased incidence of neoplasm and vaginal clear cell carcinoma observed in the DES-daughters (110–112). Although initial studies were focused on the reproductive tract, metabolic disturbances may also encompass organizational effects. By contrast, activational effects typically occur in adulthood, are transient in nature, and commonly persist as long as the stimulus is present. An example of this is the effect of abnormal estrogenic activity on adult female fertility (113).

Under this paradigm, we would expect that pregnancy exposure to BPA affect maternal metabolism in a temporary manner whenever the metabolic disruptor were present but this was not the case. We will describe how BPA exposure during pregnancy promotes long-lasting effects in the mothers that were visible months after delivery.

BPA exposed dams (10 or 100 μg/kg/day) from day 9 to 16 of gestation developed glucose intolerance that was more evident in the lowest exposed dose group (70). Moreover, they showed increased insulin resistance, which underlied defects on the insulin signaling cascade. In particular, decreased Akt phosphorylation in response to insulin was found both in liver and skeletal muscle of BPA mums (70, 114). Interestingly, gestational glucose intolerance related to BPA exposure was found to be associated with abnormalities in the tryptophan catabolism. Diet supplementation with vitamin B6 rescued the disrupted metabolic phenotype in the dams (115). It is important to highlight that any degree of glucose intolerance first recognized during pregnancy is diagnosed as GDM. Thus, we can conclude that exposure to low doses of BPA during pregnancy may compromise maternal metabolic status similarly to GDM.

It has also been reported that metabolic disturbances were resolved after parturition but appeared again months later. At 3 months postpartum no differences on glucose tolerance or insulin sensitivity were found between BPA and control dams. However, at 4 months postpartum early symptoms of altered glucose homeostasis showed up. The metabolic status of BPA mice got worse over time and 7 months postpartum animals exhibited enhanced glucose intolerance, severe insulin resistance together with decreased pancreatic β-cell function and mass (114). These findings demonstrate for the first time that a brief exposure to an EDC during pregnancy could have long-term effects on the mother's metabolism and defined a new window of susceptibility for increased incidence of diabetes.

In view of this data, we should keep in mind that metabolic programming induced by EDC exposure could be extended to other critical periods of life as it is the case of pregnancy for the mother. Hence, we should be cautious when considering the importance of the disruption of normal signaling pathways for metabolic memory beyond early development.

CONCLUSIONS

BPA is one of the most pervasive and ubiquitous EDCs. Laboratory animal and human epidemiological studies have revealed the importance of BPA as a contributing factor in the etiology of T2DM. We know that timing of exposure is critical for determining the consequences of exposure to BPA. Developmental period has been outlined as an extremely sensitive window of vulnerability since early-life exposure to this EDC can program the risk for metabolic disorders in adult life. An additional aspect of concern is that the incidence of metabolic abnormalities may increase not only in the exposed individuals but also in the subsequent generations. Some of these multigenerational and transgenerational effects may have an epigenetic origin.

Evidence described here also underscore the importance of examining pregnancy, an often understudied critical exposure window for long-term metabolic effects in the mother. Gestational exposure to BPA has been linked to metabolic programming of maternal T2DM, yet more research is needed to understand the molecular mechanisms underlying this phenomenon.

AUTHOR CONTRIBUTIONS

ET and PA-M wrote the manuscript. RDS, LM, IQ, and EF contributed to the discussion and reviewed and edited the manuscript. All of the authors reviewed and edited the manuscript.

FUNDING

Ministerio de Economia y Competitividad, Agencia Estatal de Investigación (AEI) and Fondo Europeo de Desarrollo Regional (FEDER), EU Grants SAF2014-58335-P, BFU2017-86579-R, BFU2016-77125-R and Generalitat Valenciana PROMETEO II/2015/016. LM holds a Juan de la Cierva fellowship from the Ministry of Economy, Industry and Competitiveness (IJCI-2015-24482). CIBERDEM is an initiative of the Instituto de Salud Carlos III.

REFERENCES

1. Ingelfinger JR, Jarcho JA. Increase in the incidence of diabetes and its implications. *N Engl J Med.* (2017) 376:1473–4. doi: 10.1056/NEJMe1616575
2. WHO (World Health Organization) (2018). Available online at: http://www.Who.Int/news-room/fact-sheets/detail/diabetes
3. ADA (American Diabetes Association). Classification and diagnosis of diabetes: Standards of medical care in diabetes-2018. *Diab Care* (2018) 41:S13–27. doi: 10.2337/dc18-S002
4. Kahn SE. The importance of beta-cell failure in the development and progression of type 2 diabetes. *J Clin Endocrinol Metab.* (2001) 86:4047–58. doi: 10.1210/jcem.86.9.7713
5. Chatterjee S, Khunti K, Davies MJ. Type 2 diabetes. *Lancet* (2017) 389:2239–51. doi: 10.1016/S0140-6736(17)30058-2
6. Zheng Y, Ley SH, Hu FB. Global aetiology and epidemiology of type 2 diabetes mellitus and its complications. *Nat Rev Endocrinol.* (2018) 14:88–98. doi: 10.1038/nrendo.2017.151
7. Zoeller RT, Brown TR, Doan LL, Gore AC, Skakkebaek NE, Soto AM, et al. Endocrine-disrupting chemicals and public health protection: A statement of principles from the endocrine society. *Endocrinology* (2012) 153:4097–110. doi: 10.1210/en.2012-1422
8. Gore AC, Chappell VA, Fenton SE, Flaws JA, Nadal A, Prins GS, et al. Executive summary to edc-2: the endocrine society's second scientific statement on endocrine-disrupting chemicals. *Endocr. Rev.* (2015) 36:593–602. doi: 10.1210/er.2015-1093
9. Casals-Casas C, Desvergne B. Endocrine disruptors: from endocrine to metabolic disruption. *Annu. Rev. Physiol.* (2011) 73:135–62. doi: 10.1146/annurev-physiol-012110-142200
10. Alonso-Magdalena P, Quesada I, Nadal A. Endocrine disruptors in the etiology of type 2 diabetes mellitus. *Nat. Rev. Endocrinol.* (2011) 7:346–53. doi: 10.1038/nrendo.2011.56
11. Heindel JJ, Blumberg B, Cave M, Machtinger R, Mantovani A, Mendez MA, et al. Metabolism disrupting chemicals and metabolic disorders. *Reprod Toxicol.*(2017) 68:3–33. doi: 10.1016/j.reprotox.2016.10.001

12. Nadal A, Quesada I, Tuduri E, Nogueiras R, Alonso-Magdalena P. Endocrine-disrupting chemicals and the regulation of energy balance. *Nat Rev Endocrinol.* (2017) 13:536–46. doi: 10.1038/nrendo.2017.51
13. Dodds EC, Lawson W. Synthetic estrogenic agents without the phenanthrene nucleus. *Nature* (1936) 137:996. doi: 10.1038/137996a0
14. Lee I, Kim S, Kim KT, Kim S, Park S, Lee H, et al. Bisphenol a exposure through receipt handling and its association with insulin resistance among female cashiers. *Environ Int.* (2018) 117:268–75. doi: 10.1016/j.envint.2018.05.013
15. Calafat AM, Kuklenyik Z, Reidy JA, Caudill SP, Ekong J, Needham LL. Urinary concentrations of bisphenol a and 4-nonylphenol in a human reference population. *Environ Health Perspect.* (2005) 113:391–5. doi: 10.1289/ehp.7534
16. Vandenberg LN, Hauser R, Marcus M, Olea N, Welshons WV. Human exposure to bisphenol a (bpa). *Reprod. Toxicol.* (2007) 24:139–77. doi: 10.1016/j.reprotox.2007.07.010
17. EPA (Environmental Protection Agency). *Bisphenol a. Casrn 80-05-7* (2018) Available online at: https://cfpub.Epa.Gov/ncea/iris2/chemicallanding.Cfm?Substance_nmbr=356
18. vom Saal FS, Hughes C. An extensive new literature concerning low-dose effects of bisphenol a shows the need for a new risk assessment. *Environ Health Perspect.* (2005) 113:926–33. doi: 10.1289/ehp.7713
19. EFSA (European Food Safety Authority). (2018). Available online at: https://www.Efsa.Europa.Eu/en/topics/topic/bisphenol
20. Shelnutt S, Kind J, Allaben W. Bisphenol a: update on newly developed data and how they address ntp's 2008 finding of "some concern". *Food Chem Toxicol.* (2013) 57:284–95. doi: 10.1016/j.fct.2013.03.027
21. Mimoto MS, Nadal A, Sargis RM. Polluted pathways: mechanisms of metabolic disruption by endocrine disrupting chemicals. *Curr Environ Health Reports* (2017) 4:208–22. doi: 10.1007/s40572-017-0137-0
22. Bonefeld-Jorgensen EC, Andersen HR, Rasmussen TH, Vinggaard AM. Effect of highly bioaccumulated polychlorinated biphenyl congeners on estrogen and androgen receptor activity. *Toxicology* (2001) 158:141–53. doi: 10.1016/S0300-483X(00)00368-1
23. Massaad C, Barouki R. An assay for the detection of xenoestrogens based on a promoter containing overlapping eres. *Environ Health Perspect.* (1999) 107:563–6. doi: 10.1289/ehp.99107563
24. Alonso-Magdalena P, Ropero AB, Soriano S, Garcia-Arevalo M, Ripoll C, Fuentes E, et al. Bisphenol-a acts as a potent estrogen via non-classical estrogen triggered pathways. *Mol Cell Endocrinol.* (2012) 355:201–7. doi: 10.1016/j.mce.2011.12.012
25. Nadal A, Fuentes E, Ripoll C, Villar-Pazos S, Castellano-Munoz M, Soriano S, et al. Extranuclear-initiated estrogenic actions of endocrine disrupting chemicals: Is there toxicology beyond paracelsus? *J Steroid Biochem Mol Biol.* (2018) 176:16–22. doi: 10.1016/j.jsbmb.2017.01.014
26. Soriano S, Ripoll C, Alonso-Magdalena P, Fuentes E, Quesada I, Nadal A, et al. Effects of bisphenol a on ion channels: experimental evidence and molecular mechanisms. *Steroids* (2016) 111:12–20. doi: 10.1016/j.steroids.2016.02.020
27. Watson CS, Bulayeva NN, Wozniak AL, Alyea RA. Xenoestrogens are potent activators of nongenomic estrogenic responses. *Steroids* (2007) 72:124–34. doi: 10.1016/j.steroids.2006.11.002
28. Welshons WV, Nagel SC, vom Saal FS. Large effects from small exposures Iii Endocrine mechanisms mediating effects of bisphenol a at levels of human exposure *Endocrinology* (2006) 147:S56–69. doi: 10.1210/en.2005-1159
29. Wozniak AL, Bulayeva NN, Watson CS. Xenoestrogens at picomolar to nanomolar concentrations trigger membrane estrogen receptor-alpha-mediated Ca^{2+} fluxes and prolactin release in gh3/b6 pituitary tumor cells. *Environ Health Perspect.* (2005) 113:431–9. doi: 10.1289/ehp.7505
30. Nadal A, Ropero AB, Laribi O, Maillet M, Fuentes E, Soria B. Nongenomic actions of estrogens and xenoestrogens by binding at a plasma membrane receptor unrelated to estrogen receptor alpha and estrogen receptor beta. *Proc Natl Acad Sci USA.* (2000) 97:11603–8. doi: 10.1073/pnas.97.21.11603
31. Quesada I, Fuentes E, Viso-Leon MC, Soria B, Ripoll C, Nadal A. Low doses of the endocrine disruptor bisphenol-a and the native hormone 17beta-estradiol rapidly activate transcription factor creb. *FASEB J.* (2002) 16:1671–3. doi: 10.1096/fj.02-0313fje
32. Alonso-Magdalena P, Laribi O, Ropero AB, Fuentes E, Ripoll C, Soria B, et al. Low doses of bisphenol a and diethylstilbestrol impair Ca^{2+} signals in pancreatic alpha-cells through a nonclassical membrane estrogen receptor within intact islets of langerhans. *Environ Health Perspect.* (2005) 113:969–77. doi: 10.1289/ehp.8002
33. Alonso-Magdalena P, Morimoto S, Ripoll C, Fuentes E, Nadal A. The estrogenic effect of bisphenol a disrupts pancreatic beta-cell function *in vivo* and induces insulin resistance. *Environ Health Perspect.* (2006) 114:106–12. doi: 10.1289/ehp.8451
34. Yan S, Chen Y, Dong M, Song W, Belcher SM, Wang HS. Bisphenol a and 17beta-estradiol promote arrhythmia in the female heart via alteration of calcium handling. *PLoS ONE* (2011) 6:e25455. doi: 10.1371/journal.pone.0025455
35. Belcher SM, Chen Y, Yan S, Wang HS. Rapid estrogen receptor-mediated mechanisms determine the sexually dimorphic sensitivity of ventricular myocytes to 17beta-estradiol and the environmental endocrine disruptor bisphenol a. *Endocrinology* (2012) 153:712–20. doi: 10.1210/en.2011-1772
36. Liang Q, Gao X, Chen Y, Hong K, Wang HS. Cellular mechanism of the nonmonotonic dose response of bisphenol a in rat cardiac myocytes. *Environ Health Perspect.* (2014) 122:601–8. doi: 10.1289/ehp.1307491
37. Zsarnovszky A, Le HH, Wang HS, Belcher SM. Ontogeny of rapid estrogen-mediated extracellular signal-regulated kinase signaling in the rat cerebellar cortex: Potent nongenomic agonist and endocrine disrupting activity of the xenoestrogen bisphenol a. *Endocrinology* (2005) 146:5388–96. doi: 10.1210/en.2005-0565
38. Alonso-Magdalena P, Ropero AB, Carrera MP, Cederroth CR, Baquie M, Gauthier BR, et al. Pancreatic insulin content regulation by the estrogen receptor er alpha. *PLoS ONE* (2008) 3:e2069. doi: 10.1371/journal.pone.0002069
39. Thomas P, Dong J. Binding and activation of the seven-transmembrane estrogen receptor gpr30 by environmental estrogens: a potential novel mechanism of endocrine disruption. *J Steroid Biochem Mol Biol.* (2006) 102:175–9. doi: 10.1016/j.jsbmb.2006.09.017
40. Chevalier N, Bouskine A, Fenichel P. Bisphenol a promotes testicular seminoma cell proliferation through gper/gpr30. *Int J Cancer* (2012) 130:241–2. doi: 10.1002/ijc.25972
41. Wei J, Ding D, Wang T, Liu Q, Lin Y. Mir-338 controls bpa-triggered pancreatic islet insulin secretory dysfunction from compensation to decompensation by targeting pdx-1. *FASEB J.* (2017) 31:5184–95. doi: 10.1096/fj.201700282R
42. Melnick R, Lucier G, Wolfe M, Hall R, Stancel G, Prins G, et al. Summary of the national toxicology program's report of the endocrine disruptors low-dose peer review. *Environ Health Perspect.* (2002) 110:427–31. doi: 10.1289/ehp.02110427
43. Vandenberg LN, Ehrlich S, Belcher SM, Ben-Jonathan N, Dolinoy DC, Eric R, et al. Low dose effects of bisphenol A. *Endocrine Disrupt.* (2013) 1:e26490. doi: 10.4161/endo.26490
44. Vandenberg LN. Non-monotonic dose responses in studies of endocrine disrupting chemicals: bisphenol a as a case study. *Dose Response* (2014) 12:259–76. doi: 10.2203/dose-response.13-020.Vandenberg
45. Sohoni P, Sumpter JP. Several environmental oestrogens are also anti-androgens. *J Endocrinol.* (1998) 158:327–39. doi: 10.1677/joe.0.1580327
46. Moriyama K, Tagami T, Akamizu T, Usui T, Saijo M, Kanamoto N, et al. Thyroid hormone action is disrupted by bisphenol a as an antagonist. *J Clin Endocrinol Metab.* (2002) 87:5185–90. doi: 10.1210/jc.2002-020209
47. Takayanagi S, Tokunaga T, Liu X, Okada H, Matsushima A, Shimohigashi Y. Endocrine disruptor bisphenol a strongly binds to human estrogen-related receptor gamma (errgamma) with high constitutive activity. *Toxicol Lett.* (2006) 167:95–105. doi: 10.1016/j.toxlet.2006.08.012
48. Sui Y, Ai N, Park SH, Rios-Pilier J, Perkins JT, Welsh WJ, et al. Bisphenol a and its analogues activate human pregnane x receptor. *Environ Health Perspect.* (2012) 120:399–405. doi: 10.1289/ehp.1104426
49. Sargis RM, Johnson DN, Choudhury RA, Brady MJ. Environmental endocrine disruptors promote adipogenesis in the 3t3-l1 cell line through glucocorticoid receptor activation. *Obesity* (2010) 18:1283–8. doi: 10.1038/oby.2009.419
50. Soriano S, Alonso-Magdalena P, Garcia-Arevalo M, Novials A, Muhammed SJ, Salehi A, et al. Rapid insulinotropic action of low doses of bisphenol-a on

mouse and human islets of langerhans: role of estrogen receptor beta. *PLoS ONE* (2012) 7:e31109. doi: 10.1371/journal.pone.0031109

51. Hectors TL, Vanparys C, Pereira-Fernandes A, Martens GA, Blust R. Evaluation of the ins-1 832/13 cell line as a beta-cell based screening system to assess pollutant effects on beta-cell function. *PLoS ONE* (2013) 8:e60030. doi: 10.1371/journal.pone.0060030
52. Makaji E, Raha S, Wade MG, Holloway AC. Effect of environmental contaminants on beta cell function. *Int J Toxicol.* (2011) 30:410–8. doi: 10.1177/1091581811405544
53. Lin Y, Sun X, Qiu L, Wei J, Huang Q, Fang C, et al. Exposure to bisphenol a induces dysfunction of insulin secretion and apoptosis through the damage of mitochondria in rat insulinoma (ins-1) cells. *Cell Death Dis.* (2013) 4:e460. doi: 10.1038/cddis.2012.206
54. Xin F, Jiang L, Liu X, Geng C, Wang W, Zhong L, et al. Bisphenol a induces oxidative stress-associated DNA damage in ins-1 cells. *Mutat Res Genet Toxicol Environ Mutagen* (2014) 769:29–33. doi: 10.1016/j.mrgentox.2014.04.019
55. Dai YE, Chen W, Qi H, Liu QQ. Effect of bisphenol a on socs-3 and insulin signaling transduction in 3t3-l1 adipocytes. *Mol Med Rep.* (2016) 14:331–6. doi: 10.3892/mmr.2016.5224
56. Valentino R, D'Esposito V, Passaretti F, Liotti A, Cabaro S, Longo M, et al. Bisphenol-a impairs insulin action and up-regulates inflammatory pathways in human subcutaneous adipocytes and 3t3-l1 cells. *PLoS ONE* (2013) 8:e82099. doi: 10.1371/journal.pone.0082099
57. Ariemma F, D'Esposito V, Liguoro D, Oriente F, Cabaro S, Liotti A, et al. Low-dose bisphenol-a impairs adipogenesis and generates dysfunctional 3t3-l1 adipocytes. *PLoS ONE* (2016) 11:e0150762. doi: 10.1371/journal.pone.0150762
58. Boucher JG, Boudreau A, Ahmed S, Atlas E. *In vitro* effects of bisphenol a beta-d-glucuronide (bpa-g) on adipogenesis in human and murine preadipocytes. *Environ. Health Perspect.* (2015) 123:1287–93. doi: 10.1289/ehp.1409143
59. Ohlstein JF, Strong AL, McLachlan JA, Gimble JM, Burow ME, Bunnell BA. Bisphenol a enhances adipogenic differentiation of human adipose stromal/stem cells. *J Mol Endocrinol.* (2014) 53:345–53. doi: 10.1530/JME-14-0052
60. Grasselli E, Cortese K, Voci A, Vergani L, Fabbri R, Barmo C, et al. Direct effects of bisphenol a on lipid homeostasis in rat hepatoma cells. *Chemosphere* (2013) 91:1123–9. doi: 10.1016/j.chemosphere.2013.01.016
61. Barker DJ. The fetal and infant origins of disease. *Eur J Clin Invest.* (1995) 25:457–63. doi: 10.1111/j.1365-2362.1995.tb01730.x
62. Barker DJ, Martyn CN. The fetal origins of hypertension. *Adv Nephrol Necker Hosp.* (1997) 26:65–72.
63. Hales CN, Barker DJ. Type 2 (non-insulin-dependent) diabetes mellitus: the thrifty phenotype hypothesis. *Diabetologia* (1992) 35:595–601. doi: 10.1007/BF00400248
64. Gluckman PD, Hanson MA. Living with the past: evolution, development, and patterns of disease. *Science* (2004) 305:1733–6. doi: 10.1126/science.1095292
65. Heindel JJ, Vandenberg LN. Developmental origins of health and disease: a paradigm for understanding disease cause and prevention. *Curr Opin Pediatr.* (2015) 27:248–53. doi: 10.1097/MOP.0000000000000191
66. Alavian-Ghavanini A, Ruegg J. Understanding epigenetic effects of endocrine disrupting chemicals: from mechanisms to novel test methods. *Basic Clin Pharmacol Toxicol.* (2018) 122:38–45. doi: 10.1111/bcpt.12878
67. Feil R, Fraga MF. Epigenetics and the environment: emerging patterns and implications. *Nat Rev Genet.* (2012) 13:97–109. doi: 10.1038/nrg3142
68. Skinner MK, Manikkam M, Guerrero-Bosagna C. Epigenetic transgenerational actions of environmental factors in disease etiology. *Trends Endocrinol. Metab.* (2010) 21:214–22. doi: 10.1016/j.tem.2009.12.007
69. Teperek-Tkacz M, Pasque V, Gentsch G, Ferguson-Smith AC. Epigenetic reprogramming: is deamination key to active DNA demethylation? *Reproduction* (2011) 142:621–32. doi: 10.1530/REP-11-0148
70. Alonso-Magdalena P, Vieira E, Soriano S, Menes L, Burks D, Quesada I, et al. Bisphenol a exposure during pregnancy disrupts glucose homeostasis in mothers and adult male offspring. *Environ. Health Perspect.* (2010) 118:1243–50. doi: 10.1289/ehp.1001993
71. Angle BM, Do RP, Ponzi D, Stahlhut RW, Drury BE, Nagel SC, et al. Metabolic disruption in male mice due to fetal exposure to low but not high doses of bisphenol a (bpa): evidence for effects on body weight, food intake, adipocytes, leptin, adiponectin, insulin and glucose regulation. *Reproduct Toxicol.* (2013) 42:256–68. doi: 10.1016/j.reprotox.2013.07.017
72. Liu J, Yu P, Qian W, Li Y, Zhao J, Huan F, et al. Perinatal bisphenol a exposure and adult glucose homeostasis: identifying critical windows of exposure. *PLoS ONE* (2013) 8:e64143. doi: 10.1371/journal.pone.0064143
73. Fang F, Gao Y, Wang T, Chen D, Liu J, Qian W, et al. Insulin signaling disruption in male mice due to perinatal bisphenol a exposure: role of insulin signaling in the brain. *Toxicol Lett.* (2016) 245:59–67. doi: 10.1016/j.toxlet.2016.01.007
74. Mackay H, Patterson ZR, Khazall R, Patel S, Tsirlin D, Abizaid A. Organizational effects of perinatal exposure to bisphenol-a and diethylstilbestrol on arcuate nucleus circuitry controlling food intake and energy expenditure in male and female cd-1 mice. *Endocrinology* (2013) 154:1465–75. doi: 10.1210/en.2012-2044
75. MacKay H, Patterson ZR, Abizaid A. Perinatal exposure to low-dose bisphenol-a disrupts the structural and functional development of the hypothalamic feeding circuitry. *Endocrinology* (2017) 158:768–77. doi: 10.1210/en.2016-1718
76. Song S, Zhang L, Zhang H, Wei W, Jia L. Perinatal bpa exposure induces hyperglycemia, oxidative stress and decreased adiponectin production in later life of male rat offspring. *Int J Environ Res Public Health* (2014) 11:3728–42. doi: 10.3390/ijerph110403728
77. Veiga-Lopez A, Moeller J, Sreedharan R, Singer K, Lumeng C, Ye W, et al. Developmental programming: Interaction between prenatal bpa exposure and postnatal adiposity on metabolic variables in female sheep. *Am J Physiol Endocrinol Metab.* (2016) 310:E238–47. doi: 10.1152/ajpendo.00425.2015
78. Ryan KK, Haller AM, Sorrell JE, Woods SC, Jandacek RJ, Seeley RJ. Perinatal exposure to bisphenol-a and the development of metabolic syndrome in cd-1 mice. *Endocrinology* (2010) 151:2603–12. doi: 10.1210/en.2009-1218
79. van Esterik JC, Dolle ME, Lamoree MH, van Leeuwen SP, Hamers T, Legler J, et al. Programming of metabolic effects in c57bl/6jxfvb mice by exposure to bisphenol a during gestation and lactation. *Toxicology* (2014) 321:40–52. doi: 10.1016/j.tox.2014.04.001
80. van Esterik JC, Vitins AP, Hodemaekers HM, Kamstra JH, Legler J, Pennings JL, et al. Liver DNA methylation analysis in adult female c57bl/6jxfvb mice following perinatal exposure to bisphenol a. *Toxicol Lett.* (2015) 232:293 300. doi: 10.1016/j.toxlet.2014.10.021
81. Garcia-Arevalo M, Alonso-Magdalena P, Servitja JM, Boronat-Belda T, Merino B, Villar-Pazos S, et al. Maternal exposure to bisphenol-a during pregnancy increases pancreatic beta-cell growth during early life in male mice offspring. *Endocrinology* (2016) 157:4158–71. doi: 10.1210/en.2016-1390
82. Whitehead R, Guan H, Arany E, Cernea M, Yang K. Prenatal exposure to bisphenol a alters mouse fetal pancreatic morphology and islet composition. *Horm Mol Biol Clin Investig.* (2016) 25:171–9. doi: 10.1515/hmbci-2015-0052
83. Wei J, Lin Y, Li Y, Ying C, Chen J, Song L, et al. Perinatal exposure to bisphenol a at reference dose predisposes offspring to metabolic syndrome in adult rats on a high-fat diet. *Endocrinology* (2011) 152:3049–61. doi: 10.1210/en.2011-0045
84. Garcia-Arevalo M, Alonso-Magdalena P, Rebelo Dos Santos J, Quesada I, Carneiro EM, Nadal A. Exposure to bisphenol-a during pregnancy partially mimics the effects of a high-fat diet altering glucose homeostasis and gene expression in adult male mice. *PLoS ONE* (2014) 9:e100214. doi: 10.1371/journal.pone.0100214
85. Cabaton NJ, Canlet C, Wadia PR, Tremblay-Franco M, Gautier R, Molina J, et al. Effects of low doses of bisphenol a on the metabolome of perinatally exposed cd-1 mice. *Environ Health Perspect.* (2013) 121:586–93. doi: 10.1289/ehp.1205588
86. Tremblay-Franco M, Cabaton NJ, Canlet C, Gautier R, Schaeberle CM, Jourdan F, et al. Dynamic metabolic disruption in rats perinatally exposed to low doses of bisphenol-a. *PLoS ONE* (2015) 10:e0141698. doi: 10.1371/journal.pone.0141698
87. Ma Y, Xia W, Wang DQ, Wan YJ, Xu B, Chen X, et al. Hepatic DNA methylation modifications in early development of rats resulting from

perinatal bpa exposure contribute to insulin resistance in adulthood. *Diabetologia* (2013) 56:2059–67. doi: 10.1007/s00125-013-2944-7
88. Li G, Chang H, Xia W, Mao Z, Li Y, Xu S. F0 maternal bpa exposure induced glucose intolerance of f2 generation through DNA methylation change in gck. *Toxicol Lett.* (2014) 228:192–9. doi: 10.1016/j.toxlet.2014.04.012
89. Susiarjo M, Xin F, Bansal A, Stefaniak M, Li C, Simmons RA, et al. Bisphenol a exposure disrupts metabolic health across multiple generations in the mouse. *Endocrinology* (2015) 156:2049–58. doi: 10.1210/en.2014-2027
90. Mao Z, Xia W, Chang H, Huo W, Li Y, Xu S. Paternal bpa exposure in early life alters igf2 epigenetic status in sperm and induces pancreatic impairment in rat offspring. *Toxicol Lett.* (2015) 238:30–8. doi: 10.1016/j.toxlet.2015.08.009
91. Bansal A, Rashid C, Xin F, Li C, Polyak E, Duemler A, et al. Sex- and dose-specific effects of maternal bisphenol a exposure on pancreatic islets of first- and second-generation adult mice offspring. *Environ Health Perspect.* (2017) 125:097022. doi: 10.1289/EHP1674
92. Manikkam M, Guerrero-Bosagna C, Tracey R, Haque MM, Skinner MK. Transgenerational actions of environmental compounds on reproductive disease and identification of epigenetic biomarkers of ancestral exposures. *PLoS ONE* (2012) 7:e31901. doi: 10.1371/journal.pone.0031901
93. Manikkam M, Tracey R, Guerrero-Bosagna C, Skinner MK. Plastics derived endocrine disruptors (bpa, dehp and dbp) induce epigenetic transgenerational inheritance of obesity, reproductive disease and sperm epimutations. *PLoS ONE* (2013) 8:e55387. doi: 10.1371/journal.pone.0055387
94. Bodin J, Bolling AK, Becher R, Kuper F, Lovik M, Nygaard UC. Transmaternal bisphenol a exposure accelerates diabetes type 1 development in nod mice. *Toxicol Sci.* (2014) 137:311–23. doi: 10.1093/toxsci/kft242
95. Malaise Y, Menard S, Cartier C, Gaultier E, Lasserre F, Lencina C, et al. Gut dysbiosis and impairment of immune system homeostasis in perinatally-exposed mice to bisphenol a precede obese phenotype development. *Sci Rep.* (2017) 7:14472. doi: 10.1038/s41598-017-15196-w
96. Batista TM, Alonso-Magdalena P, Vieira E, Amaral ME, Cederroth CR, Nef S, et al. Short-term treatment with bisphenol-a leads to metabolic abnormalities in adult male mice. *PLoS ONE* (2012) 7:e33814. doi: 10.1371/journal.pone.0033814
97. Jayashree S, Indumathi D, Akilavalli N, Sathish S, Selvaraj J, Balasubramanian K. Effect of bisphenol-a on insulin signal transduction and glucose oxidation in liver of adult male albino rat. *Environ Toxicol Pharmacol.* (2013) 35:300–10. doi: 10.1016/j.etap.2012.12.016
98. Kang HS, Yang H, Ahn C, Kang HY, Hong EJ, Jaung EB. Effects of xenoestrogens on streptozotocin-induced diabetic mice. *J Physiol Pharmacol.* (2014) 65:273–82.
99. Marmugi A, Ducheix S, Lasserre F, Polizzi A, Paris A, Priymenko N, et al. Low doses of bisphenol a induce gene expression related to lipid synthesis and trigger triglyceride accumulation in adult mouse liver. *Hepatology* (2012) 55:395–407. doi: 10.1002/hep.24685
100. Corkey BE. Banting lecture 2011: Hyperinsulinemia: cause or consequence? *Diabetes* (2012) 61:4–13. doi: 10.2337/db11-1483
101. Ahangarpour A, Afshari G, Mard SA, Khodadadi A, Hashemitabar M. Preventive effects of procyanidin a2 on glucose homeostasis, pancreatic and duodenal homebox 1, and glucose transporter 2 gene expression disturbance induced by bisphenol a in male mice. *J Physiol Pharmacol.* (2016) 67:243–52.
102. Veissi M, Jafarirad S, Ahangarpour A, Mohaghegh SM, Malehi AS. Co-exposure to endocrine disruptors: effect of bisphenol a and soy extract on glucose homeostasis and related metabolic disorders in male mice. *Endocr Regul.* (2018) 52:76–84. doi: 10.2478/enr-2018-0009
103. Marmugi A, Lasserre F, Beuzelin D, Ducheix S, Huc L, Polizzi A, et al. Adverse effects of long-term exposure to bisphenol a during adulthood leading to hyperglycaemia and hypercholesterolemia in mice. *Toxicology* (2014) 325:133–43. doi: 10.1016/j.tox.2014.08.006
104. Moon MK, Jeong IK, Jung Oh T, Ahn HY, Kim HH, Park YJ, et al. Long-term oral exposure to bisphenol a induces glucose intolerance and insulin resistance. *J Endocrinol.* (2015) 226:35–42. doi: 10.1530/JOE-14-0714
105. Perreault L, McCurdy C, Kerege AA, Houck J, Faerch K, Bergman BC. Bisphenol a impairs hepatic glucose sensing in c57bl/6 male mice. *PLoS ONE* (2013) 8:e69991. doi: 10.1371/journal.pone.0069991
106. Moghaddam HS, Samarghandian S, Farkhondeh T. Effect of bisphenol a on blood glucose, lipid profile and oxidative stress indices in adult male mice. *Toxicol Mech Methods* (2015) 25:507–13. doi: 10.3109/15376516.2015.1056395
107. Bodin J, Bolling AK, Samuelsen M, Becher R, Lovik M, Nygaard UC. Long-term bisphenol a exposure accelerates insulitis development in diabetes-prone nod mice. *Immunopharmacol Immunotoxicol.* (2013) 35:349–58. doi: 10.3109/08923973.2013.772195
108. Bodin J, Kocbach Bolling A, Wendt A, Eliasson L, Becher R, Kuper F, et al. Exposure to bisphenol a, but not phthalates, increases spontaneous diabetes type 1 development in nod mice. *Toxicol Reports* (2015) 2:99–110. doi: 10.1016/j.toxrep.2015.02.010
109. Cetkovic-Cvrlje M, Thinamany S, Bruner KA. Bisphenol a (bpa) aggravates multiple low-dose streptozotocin-induced type 1 diabetes in c57bl/6 mice. *J Immunotoxicol.* (2017) 14:160–8. doi: 10.1080/1547691X.2017.1334722
110. Newbold R. Cellular and molecular effects of developmental exposure to diethylstilbestrol: implications for other environmental estrogens. *Environ Health Perspect.* (1995) 103 (Suppl 7):83–7.
111. Newbold RR, Jefferson WN, Grissom SF, Padilla-Banks E, Snyder RJ, Lobenhofer EK. Developmental exposure to diethylstilbestrol alters uterine gene expression that may be associated with uterine neoplasia later in life. *Mol Carcinog.* (2007) 46:783–96. doi: 10.1002/mc.20308
112. Reed CE, Fenton SE. Exposure to diethylstilbestrol during sensitive life stages: a legacy of heritable health effects. *Birth Defects Res C Embryo Tod.* (2013) 99:134–46. doi: 10.1002/bdrc.21035
113. Vandenberg LN, Colborn T, Hayes TB, Heindel JJ, Jacobs DRJr, Lee DH, et al. Hormones and endocrine-disrupting chemicals: Low-dose effects and nonmonotonic dose responses. *Endocr Rev.* (2012) 33:378–455. doi: 10.1210/er.2011-1050
114. Alonso-Magdalena P, Garcia-Arevalo M, Quesada I, Nadal A. Bisphenol-a treatment during pregnancy in mice: a new window of susceptibility for the development of diabetes in mothers later in life. *Endocrinology* (2015) 156:1659–70. doi: 10.1210/en.2014-1952
115. Susiarjo M, Xin F, Stefaniak M, Mesaros C, Simmons RA, Bartolomei MS. Bile acids and tryptophan metabolism are novel pathways involved in metabolic abnormalities in bpa-exposed pregnant mice and male offspring. *Endocrinology* (2017) 158:2533–42. doi: 10.1210/en.2017-00046

3

Developmental Exposure to Endocrine Disrupting Chemicals and Type 1 Diabetes Mellitus

*Sarah G. Howard**

Diabetes and Environment Program, Commonweal, Bolinas, CA, United States

***Correspondence:**
Sarah G. Howard
sarhow@gmail.com

Exposure to endocrine disrupting chemicals (EDCs) may have implications for the development of type 1 diabetes mellitus (T1DM), especially if exposure occurs during development. Exposure to EDCs during fetal or early life can disrupt the development of both the immune system and the pancreatic beta cells, potentially increasing susceptibility to T1DM later in life. Developmental exposure to some EDCs can cause immune system dysfunction, increasing the risk of autoimmunity. In addition, developmental exposure to some EDCs can affect beta cell development and function, influencing insulin secretion. These changes may increase stress on the beta cells, and identify them as a target to the immune system. Developmental exposure to EDCs that disrupt metabolism by increasing insulin resistance or obesity may also stress the beta cells. Exposure to these EDCs during development may play a role in the pathogenesis of T1DM, and requires further research.

Keywords: type 1 diabetes, endocrine disruptors, arsenic, BPA, phthalates, persistent organic pollutants, air pollution, DOHaD

INTRODUCTION

Type 1 diabetes mellitus (T1DM) is an autoimmune disease characterized by inadequate insulin secretion, in which the insulin-producing pancreatic beta cells are targeted and destroyed by the immune system. In children, the incidence of T1DM began increasing in the mid-Twentieth century simultaneously in numerous industrialized countries, and continued to increase over the following decades (1). This increase has been especially rapid in children under 5 years of age, with an additional trend of diagnosis at earlier ages in life (1, 2). The increase appears to have affected those at moderate genetic risk, as the proportion of children with T1DM who are at high genetic risk has not changed in recent decades (2). The cause of the increase remains unexplained (2).

The development of autoimmunity precedes T1DM, and markers of autoimmunity can appear very early in life, suggesting that environmental exposures in early life play a role in triggering T1DM (2). The autoantibodies associated with T1DM may appear before 6 months of age, and the majority of children who develop T1DM before puberty test positive for autoantibodies before age four (3). Other immunological markers that are associated with the later development of T1DM in children may be present at birth or during mid-gestation, illustrating that even prenatal exposures may play a role in the development of T1DM (4, 5).

The idea that exposure to environmental factors during susceptible developmental periods can affect health later in life is known as the Developmental Origins of Health and Disease (DOHaD) hypothesis. This hypothesis applies to a variety of environmental factors, including exposure to endocrine disrupting chemicals (EDCs). Exposure to EDCs is widespread, and in some cases ubiquitous. Pregnant women are exposed to numerous EDCs, which can cross the placenta, and enter the fetus (6). The developing fetus is particularly vulnerable to these exposures, because bodily systems such as the immune system are developing rapidly in the periods before and after birth (7). Exposures that occur during development may affect the growing fetus and infant in ways that would not occur in adults, and these effects are more persistent (7).

The changes that result from EDC exposures during development may have lifelong ramifications. These changes may be relevant for the development of T1DM later in life. It is hormones that guide development of endocrine glands such as the pancreas (8). Exposure to EDCs during development are linked not only to later-life changes to the immune system, including autoimmunity (7), but also to effects on the developing pancreas, as well as changes in metabolism, including type 2 diabetes mellitus (T2DM), insulin resistance, and obesity (8).

Exposure to some EDCs has been associated with the development of T1DM (9, 10). Yet most studies on T1DM and EDCs do not address exposures during prenatal or early life. Because these developmental exposures can affect the immune system, the pancreatic beta cells, and metabolism, exposure to EDCs during development may play a role in the development of T1DM.

DEVELOPMENTAL EXPOSURE TO EDCS AND T1DM

Very few epidemiological studies have directly examined prenatal exposure to EDCs and later-life T1DM. For example, a study from Sweden found that maternal exposure to higher levels of air pollution during pregnancy was associated with a higher risk of T1DM in the offspring (11). Additional studies on air pollution—which can contain EDCs—have also found links between early childhood exposures and later T1DM (12, 13). However, another study, also from Sweden, found no association between *in utero* levels of two persistent organic pollutants (POPs) and T1DM in childhood (14). In fact, the trend was in the opposite direction, showing a possible protective effect. This finding might be explained by the higher fish intake in Swedes with higher levels of POPs, since the omega three fatty acids found in fish may protect against T1DM. A number of studies have linked T1DM development to exposure to nitrates and related compounds, some with developmental, or childhood exposures (9). Thus, while contradictory, there is some preliminary epidemiological evidence that developmental exposure to some EDCs may affect the later-life risk of T1DM, although more research is clearly needed.

Abbreviations: BPA, bisphenol A; DOHaD, Developmental Origins of Health and Disease; DEHP, di(2-ethylhexyl) phthalate; EDC, endocrine disrupting chemical; MEHP, mono(2-ethylhexyl) phthalate; NOD, non-obese diabetic; PCB, polychlorinated biphenyl; POP, persistent organic pollutant; PFC, perfluorinated chemical; PFOS, perfluorooctanesulfonic acid; PFUnDA, perfluoroundecanoic acid; T1DM, type 1 diabetes mellitus; T2DM, type 2 diabetes mellitus; TCDD, 2,3,7,8-tetrachlorodibenzo-*p*-dioxin.

Similar to the epidemiological evidence, there are also only a handful of experimental studies directly evaluating developmental exposure to EDCs and later T1DM. Some of these studies have used non-obese diabetic (NOD) mice as an animal model of T1DM. For example, maternal exposure to bisphenol A (BPA), used in a wide variety of consumer products, accelerated insulitis, and diabetes development in NOD mice offspring, although only at high exposure levels (15). At lower, environmentally relevant exposure levels, when the exposure occurred from conception throughout life, BPA also accelerated diabetes development in NOD mice (16). A mixture of phthalate plasticizers with BPA, however, seemed to counteract the acceleration of diabetes caused by BPA in these mice, although did not dampen the development of insulitis (16). Developmental exposure to perfluoroundecanoic acid (PFUnDA), a replacement for other perfluorinated chemicals (PFCs), also accelerated the development of insulitis in NOD mice (17). Interestingly, additional studies found that environmental chemicals did not accelerate insulitis or diabetes in NOD mice, and while I questioned whether these mice were appropriate for use in testing chemicals in relation to T1DM (10), the differing results may instead be due to the timing of exposure, with developmental exposures showing different effects than adult exposures. Using anotheranimal model, juvenile alligators exposed to tank water with high levels of nitrate (a possible EDC) after hatching developed biomarkers consistent with T1DM, beginning early in life and becoming stronger later in life (18). Thus some laboratory studies show that developmental exposure to EDCs may influence the development of T1DM in animal models, but very few chemicals have been evaluated.

Due to the lack of direct research on developmental exposure to EDCs and T1DM, additional research on endpoints related to T1DM are illuminating, and suggest that indeed these exposures could be important for T1DM. The endpoints of autoimmunity, pancreatic beta cell development, and metabolism may shed additional light on how developmental EDC exposures could contribute to T1DM.

DEVELOPMENTAL EXPOSURE TO EDCS AND THE IMMUNE SYSTEM

Exposure to EDCs during development are associated with immune system changes in humans. For example, a number of epidemiological studies found that *in utero* exposure to the EDC arsenic, a common drinking water contaminant, is associated with immunological changes in newborns. Some of these changes are in turn linked to markers that may be relevant for T1DM. For example, prenatal exposure to arsenic is associated with populations of cord blood immune cells linked to the development of autoimmunity, and with epigenetic changes in newborns, some involved in pathways relevant for T1DM and T2DM (19–22). We do not yet know if these immunological changes found at birth are persistent or will have later-life health effects, but numerous epidemiological studies have linked chronic arsenic exposure to the development of T2DM, and arsenic metabolism is associated with T1DM (23).

Experimental studies show that developmental exposure to additional EDCs is linked to the development of autoimmunity in particular. For example, prenatal exposure to 2,3,7,8-tetrachlorodibenzo-*p*-dioxin (TCDD), a POP, promoted later-life autoimmunity in mice (24). Developmental exposure to BPA is linked to various immune system diseases, including autoimmune diseases (25). In fact, BPA can impact essentially all the major cells of the immune system, and can cause a number of effects that are linked to autoimmunity triggers (26). The adult offspring of pregnant rats exposed to low levels of the plasticizer di(2-ethylhexyl) phthalate (DEHP) had epigenetic changes to genes that control the immune response. Interestingly, these changes did not occur when adults were exposed (27). Taken together, these studies illustrate that developmental exposure to various EDCs can affect the development of the immune system in ways that may promote autoimmunity. Some also illustrate that the effects of developmental exposures may be different than those of adult exposures.

DEVELOPMENTAL EXPOSURE TO EDCS AND THE PANCREAS

Autoimmunity is not the only contributor to the development of T1DM. Some environmental factors are suspected to contribute to T1DM by overloading the pancreatic beta cells. According to the "overload hypothesis," any environmental factor that stresses or overloads the beta cells may sensitize these cells to damage from the immune system and accelerate their demise (28). Interestingly, beta cell stress could perhaps even act a trigger that initiates beta cell autoimmunity. In fact, recent research has found a potential biological mechanism linking beta cell stress to autoimmunity—the discovery of peptides produced by stressed beta cells that can initiate beta cell specific autoimmunity (29). Whether or not beta cell stress plays a role before or after the development of autoimmunity, environmental factors that stress beta cells may play a role in the development of T1DM.

A number of environmental factors can cause beta cell stress, including excess weight, rapid growth, infection, physical or psychological stress or trauma, inflammation, puberty, pregnancy, and insulin resistance. Many of these factors are linked to T2DM or gestational diabetes, and many are also linked to T1DM. An additional, often unrecognized cause of beta cell stress is developmental exposure to EDCs.

Developmental exposure to EDCs can affect the development of the pancreas, the pancreatic islets, and beta cells, leading to changes in insulin secretion. Longitudinal epidemiological studies have found that perinatal EDC exposures are associated with changes in insulin levels in infants, children, or adolescents (30–33). Exposure to EDCs during childhood is also associated with changes to insulin levels or to beta cell function in childhood (33–35). While the specific findings of these studies vary by chemical, sex, timing of exposure, and even pubertal status, they illustrate that both prenatal and early childhood chemical exposures are associated with changes in insulin secretion from beta cells later in life.

While some of these epidemiological studies found that EDC exposure was associated with decreased insulin secretion (30, 31, 33–35), others found exposure associated with increased insulin secretion (30, 32, 33). Both increased and decreased insulin secretion may be important in the development of diabetes. Decreased insulin secretion is characteristic of T1DM, and indicates toxicity to beta cells. Increased insulin secretion is characteristic of early T2DM, and in itself can contribute to the development of insulin resistance and glucose intolerance (36). Both increased and decreased insulin secretion can therefore cause stress on the beta cells.

Experimental studies in rodents show that developmental exposure to numerous chemicals can affect the development of the pancreas and beta cells. For example, exposure to low levels of arsenic throughout life damaged pancreatic beta cells and caused impaired glucose metabolism in adult rats (37). Developmental exposure to air pollutants caused beta cell dysfunction, reduced islet and beta cell size, lowered insulin secretion, and impaired glucose tolerance in adult male mice (38). Developmental exposure to DEHP impaired the pancreas in early life and led to glucose intolerance in adult rat offspring, at exposure levels relevant to high-level human exposures. Laboratory studies therefore show that developmental exposure to EDCs can affect the pancreas in adulthood.

The effects of developmental exposure to EDCs on the pancreas can begin earlier than adulthood, however. In mice, *in utero* exposure to BPA altered islet cell development in the fetal pancreas (39). After birth, *in utero* exposure to environmentally relevant doses of BPA at first led to increased beta cell mass and insulin levels, but later in life led to the same or lower beta cell mass (36). At the time of weaning, developmental exposure to environmentally relevant levels of DEHP led to reduced beta cell mass, lower pancreatic insulin content, and alterations in the expression of genes involved in pancreas development and beta cell function in offspring. In adulthood, exposed female offspring had higher blood glucose levels, impaired glucose tolerance, lower insulin secretion, and lower insulin levels than controls, while males had higher insulin levels (40). Prenatal exposure to DEHP resulted in higher blood glucose levels, impaired insulin and glucose tolerance, impaired insulin secretion and decreased pancreatic insulin content in young rats. Epigenetic mechanisms appeared to play a role, as DEHP exposed offspring also had down-regulated expression of genes involved in the development and function of beta cells (41). These studies illustrate that developmental exposure to various EDCs can affect pancreatic development beginning in the womb and into adulthood.

Interestingly, maternal folate supplementation during pregnancy counteracted the pancreatic effects of BPA (which included disrupted insulin secretion, impaired beta cell morphology, and glucose intolerance) in adult rat offspring (42). In fact, the association between arsenic metabolism and T1DM in humans also depended on folate levels (23), thus illustrating that nutritional status may interact with EDCs to influence their effects.

In addition to these rodent studies, experimental studies on zebrafish embryos, another animal model used to evaluate the effects of EDCs, also show that developmental exposure to numerous chemicals affect the development of the pancreas and beta cells *in utero*. Developmental exposure to a number of chemicals, including arsenic, phthalates, the POPs polychlorinated biphenyls (PCBs), and perfluorooctanesulfonic acid (PFOS) (a PFC), affected the pancreatic development of zebrafish embryos, resulting in flawed development of the islets and beta cells (43–46). For example, exposure to a dioxin-like PCB resulted in inappropriate development of the pancreatic islets and beta cells in zebrafish embryos (46). Exposure to PFOS led to decreased pancreatic islet size and changes in islet morphology in embryos (45). Mono(2-ethylhexyl) phthalate (MEHP), a metabolite of DEHP, affected pancreatic development, reducing beta cell area, and affected gene expression in embryos as well (43). In sum, these experimental studies illustrate that developmental exposure to numerous EDCs can affect the development of the pancreas and specifically the beta cells *in utero*.

Alarmingly, some of the pancreatic effects of chemical exposure during development can be passed down to subsequent generations. In rats, prenatal exposure to DDE (at levels similar to those found in highly exposed humans) led to pancreatic effects not only in the offspring of exposed pregnant mothers, but also in two subsequent generations. These effects included impaired glucose tolerance, abnormal insulin secretion, beta cell dysfunction, and reduced beta cell area, and were transferred through the male germ line (47). Male mice offspring perinatally exposed to environmentally relevant levels of BPA had lower insulin secretion as adults, as well as islet inflammation that persisted into the next generation. The effects of the BPA exposure varied by sex, as well as by exposure level. Mice exposed to the lower exposure level had reduced beta cell mass and increased beta cell death, while those exposed to higher levels had impaired mitochondrial function in beta cells (48). Another study also found that perinatal exposure to low levels of BPA caused beta cell dysfunction and lower insulin secretion in two generations of adult male rat offspring (49). These studies raise the possibility that developmental exposures to EDCs can have effects on the pancreas that persist not only into adulthood, but into subsequent generations. Whether developmental EDC exposures in prior generations can affect the risk of diabetes in humans is unknown, although there is human evidence that developmental exposure to famine can increase the risk of hyperglycemia in subsequent generations (50).

Experimental studies thus show that developmental exposure to EDCs can affect the development of the pancreas and beta cells, influencing insulin secretion, beginning in the womb and continuing into adulthood. These laboratory results are supported by epidemiological studies showing associations between developmental exposure to EDCs and insulin secretion later in life. As beta cell stress is a potential contributor to T1DM, exposure to EDCs in prenatal and early life should be thoroughly analyzed in relation to the development of T1DM.

DEVELOPMENTAL EXPOSURE TO EDCS AND ADDITIONAL EFFECTS

In addition to autoimmunity and pancreatic development, developmental exposure to EDCs can have additional effects that may be related to T1DM. For example, EDCs can affect the permeability, inflammation, and microbiota of the intestine (51), which in turn are linked to T1DM (2). EDCs are also linked to an increased risk of vitamin D deficiency (52), a risk factor also associated with T1DM development (2).

Exposure to EDCs is strongly linked to the development of T2DM, insulin resistance, and obesity, in both experimental and epidemiological studies (8). In humans, developmental exposures to numerous EDCs are linked to metabolic changes in infants and children, including insulin resistance and obesity-related outcomes (53). While insulin resistance and obesity are clearly important in the development of T2DM, there is some evidence that these metabolic factors may also play a role in the development of T1DM. For example, insulin resistance, and obesity may contribute to the development of T1DM by stressing the pancreatic beta cells and accelerating their loss (2).

CONCLUSION

As early signs of T1DM may be apparent in early childhood, or even before birth, prenatal and early life exposures likely play a role in the development of T1DM, supporting the DOHaD hypothesis. Pregnant women are exposed to multiple EDCs, and these chemicals can cross the placenta and enter the fetus, potentially affecting the later risk of disease in the offspring (6). Developmental exposure to EDCs is under-researched in T1DM. Only a small number of studies have addressed the potential role of developmental exposure to EDCs in T1DM, and only a small number of chemicals have been analyzed—almost none in long-term prospective studies (9, 10). These exposures, however, should be a prime candidate for consideration in the pathogenesis of T1DM. Developmental exposure to EDCs can have effects that could be important in the development of T1DM, including promoting autoimmunity, affecting the development of the pancreas and beta cells specifically, influencing insulin secretion, and disrupting metabolism. Experimental studies show that these effects can appear as early as in the womb, last into adulthood, and sometimes even be passed on to subsequent generations. Certain chemicals, including for example arsenic, BPA, and DEHP, are linked to changes in the development of both the immune system and the pancreas, and should be of prime interest in additional research. The role of developmental exposure to EDCs as contributors to the development of T1DM should be an urgent focus of research, and may help provide an eventual pathway for prevention.

AUTHOR CONTRIBUTIONS

The author confirms being the sole contributor of this work and approved it for publication.

ACKNOWLEDGMENTS

The author would like to thank colleagues who contributed to the development of these ideas.

REFERENCES

1. Gale EA. The rise of childhood type 1 diabetes in the 20th century. *Diabetes* (2002) 51:3353–61. doi: 10.2337/diabetes.51.12.3353
2. Vehik K, Dabelea D. The changing epidemiology of type 1 diabetes: why is it going through the roof? *Diabetes Metab Res Rev.* (2011) 27:3–13. doi: 10.1002/dmrr.1141
3. Knip M, Luopajarvi K, Harkonen T. Early life origin of type 1 diabetes. *Semin Immunopathol.* (2017) 39:653–67. doi: 10.1007/s00281-017-0665-6
4. Thorsen SU, Pipper CB, Eising S, Skogstrand K, Hougaard DM, Svensson J, et al. Neonatal levels of adiponectin, interleukin-10 and interleukin-12 are associated with the risk of developing type 1 diabetes in childhood and adolescence: a nationwide Danish case-control study. *Clin Immunol.* (2016) 174:18–23. doi: 10.1016/j.clim.2016.11.007
5. Vistnes M, Tapia G, Marild K, Midttun O, Ueland PM, Viken MK, et al. Plasma immunological markers in pregnancy and cord blood: a possible link between macrophage chemo-attractants and risk of childhood type 1 diabetes. *Am J Reprod Immunol.* (2018) 79:e12802. doi: 10.1111/aji.12802
6. Woodruff TJ, Zota AR, Schwartz JM. Environmental chemicals in pregnant women in the United States: NHANES 2003-2004. *Environ Health Perspect.* (2011) 119:878–85. doi: 10.1289/ehp.1002727
7. Dietert RR, Piepenbrink MS. Perinatal immunotoxicity: why adult exposure assessment fails to predict risk. *Environ Health Perspect.* (2006) 114:477–83. doi: 10.1289/ehp.8566
8. Gore AC, Chappell VA, Fenton SE, Flaws JA, Nadal A, Prins GS, et al. EDC-2: the endocrine society's second scientific statement on endocrine-disrupting chemicals. *Endocr Rev.* (2015) 36:E1–150. doi: 10.1210/er.2015-1010
9. Bodin J, Stene LC, Nygaard UC. Can exposure to environmental chemicals increase the risk of diabetes type 1 development? *Biomed Res Int.* (2015) 2015:208947. doi: 10.1155/2015/208947
10. Howard SG, Lee DH. What is the role of human contamination by environmental chemicals in the development of type 1 diabetes? *J Epidemiol Community Health* (2012) 66:479–81. doi: 10.1136/jech.2011.133694
11. Malmqvist E, Larsson HE, Jonsson I, Rignell-Hydbom A, Ivarsson SA, Tinnerberg H, et al. Maternal exposure to air pollution and type 1 diabetes-accounting for genetic factors. *Environ Res.* (2015) 140:268–74. doi: 10.1016/j.envres.2015.03.024
12. Beyerlein A, Krasmann M, Thiering E, Kusian D, Markevych I, D'Orlando O, et al. Ambient air pollution and early manifestation of type 1 diabetes. *Epidemiology* (2015) 26:e31–2. doi: 10.1097/EDE.0000000000000254
13. Hathout EH, Beeson WL, Ischander M, Rao R, Mace JW. Air pollution and type 1 diabetes in children. *Pediatr Diabetes* (2006) 7:81–7. doi: 10.1111/j.1399-543X.2006.00150.x
14. Rignell-Hydbom A, Elfving M, Ivarsson SA, Lindh C, Jonsson BA, Olofsson P, et al. A nested case-control study of intrauterine exposure to persistent organochlorine pollutants in relation to risk of type 1 diabetes. *PLoS ONE* (2010) 5:e11281. doi: 10.1371/journal.pone.0011281
15. Bodin J, Bolling AK, Becher R, Kuper F, Lovik M, Nygaard UC. Transmaternal bisphenol A exposure accelerates diabetes type 1 development in NOD mice. *Toxicol Sci.* (2014) 137:311–23. doi: 10.1093/toxsci/kft242
16. Bodin J, Kocbach BA, Wendt A, Eliasson L, Becher R, Kuper F, et al. Exposure to bisphenol A, but not phthalates, increases spontaneous diabetes type 1 development in NOD mice. *Toxicol Rep.* (2015) 2:99–110. doi: 10.1016/j.toxrep.2015.02.010
17. Bodin J, Groeng EC, Andreassen M, Dirven H, Nygaard UC. Exposure to perfluoroundecanoic acid (PFUnDA) accelerates insulitis development in a mouse model of type 1 diabetes. *Toxicol Rep.* (2016) 3:664–72. doi: 10.1016/j.toxrep.2016.08.009
18. Edwards TM, Hamlin HJ, Freymiller H, Green S, Thurman J, Guillette LJ Jr. Nitrate induces a type 1 diabetic profile in alligator hatchlings. *Ecotoxicol Environ Saf.* (2017) 147:767–75. doi: 10.1016/j.ecoenv.2017.09.052
19. Kaushal A, Zhang H, Karmaus WJJ, Everson TM, Marsit CJ, Karagas MR, et al. Genome-wide DNA methylation at birth in relation to in utero arsenic exposure and the associated health in later life. *Environ Health* (2017) 16:50. doi: 10.1186/s12940-017-0262-0
20. Kile ML, Houseman EA, Baccarelli AA, Quamruzzaman Q, Rahman M, Mostofa G, et al. Effect of prenatal arsenic exposure on DNA methylation and leukocyte subpopulations in cord blood. *Epigenetics* (2014) 9:774–82. doi: 10.4161/epi.28153
21. Koestler DC, Avissar-Whiting M, Houseman EA, Karagas MR, Marsit CJ. Differential DNA methylation in umbilical cord blood of infants exposed to low levels of arsenic in utero. *Environ Health Perspect.* (2013) 121:971–7. doi: 10.1289/ehp.1205925
22. Rager JE, Bailey KA, Smeester L, Miller SK, Parker JS, Laine JE, et al. Prenatal arsenic exposure and the epigenome: altered microRNAs associated with innate and adaptive immune signaling in newborn cord blood. *Environ Mol Mutagen.* (2014) 55:196–208. doi: 10.1002/em.21842
23. Grau-Perez M, Kuo CC, Spratlen M, Thayer KA, Mendez MA, Hamman RF, et al. The association of arsenic exposure and metabolism with Type 1 and Type 2 diabetes in youth: the SEARCH case-control study. *Diabetes Care* (2017) 40:46–53. doi: 10.2337/dc16-0810
24. Holladay SD, Mustafa A, Gogal RM Jr. Prenatal TCDD in mice increases adult autoimmunity. *Reprod Toxicol.* (2011) 31:312–8. doi: 10.1016/j.reprotox.2010.08.001
25. Xu J, Huang G, Guo TL. Developmental bisphenol A exposure modulates immune-related diseases. *Toxics* (2016) 4:E23. doi: 10.3390/toxics4040023
26. Kharrazian D. The potential roles of Bisphenol A (BPA) pathogenesis in autoimmunity. *Autoimmune Dis.* (2014) 2014:743616. doi: 10.1155/2014/743616
27. Martinez-Arguelles DB, Papadopoulos V. Identification of hot spots of DNA methylation in the adult male adrenal in response to in utero exposure to the ubiquitous endocrine disruptor plasticizer di-(2-ethylhexyl) phthalate. *Endocrinology* (2015) 156:124–33. doi: 10.1210/en.2014-1436
28. Dahlquist G. Can we slow the rising incidence of childhood-onset autoimmune diabetes? The overload hypothesis. *Diabetologia* (2006) 49:20–4. doi: 10.1007/s00125-005-0076-4
29. Rewers M, Ludvigsson J. Environmental risk factors for type 1 diabetes. *Lancet* (2016) 387:2340–8. doi: 10.1016/S0140-6736(16)30507-4
30. Debost-Legrand A, Warembourg C, Massart C, Chevrier C, Bonvallot N, Monfort C, et al. Prenatal exposure to persistent organic pollutants and organophosphate pesticides, and markers of glucose metabolism at birth. *Environ Res.* (2016) 146:207–17. doi: 10.1016/j.envres.2016.01.005
31. Leijs MM, Koppe JG, Vulsma T, Olie K, van Aalderen WMC, de VP, et al. Alterations in the programming of energy metabolism in adolescents with background exposure to dioxins, dl-PCBs and PBDEs. *PLoS ONE* (2017) 12:e0184006. doi: 10.1371/journal.pone.0184006
32. Tang-Peronard JL, Heitmann BL, Jensen TK, Vinggaard AM, Madsbad S, Steuerwald U, et al. Prenatal exposure to persistent organochlorine pollutants is associated with high insulin levels in 5-year-old girls. *Environ Res.* (2015) 142:407–13. doi: 10.1016/j.envres.2015.07.009
33. Watkins DJ, Peterson KE, Ferguson KK, Mercado-Garcia A, Tamayo YO, Cantoral A, et al. Relating phthalate and BPA exposure to metabolism in peripubescence: the role of exposure timing, sex, and puberty. *J Clin Endocrinol Metab.* (2016) 101:79–88. doi: 10.1210/jc.2015-2706
34. Jensen TK, Timmermann AG, Rossing LI, Ried-Larsen M, Grontved A, Andersen LB, et al. Polychlorinated biphenyl exposure and glucose metabolism in 9-year-old Danish children. *J Clin Endocrinol Metab.* (2014) 99:E2643–51. doi: 10.1210/jc.2014-1683
35. Park SH, Ha E, Hong YS, Park H. Serum Levels of persistent organic pollutants and insulin secretion among children age 7-9 years: a prospective cohort study. *Environ Health Perspect.* (2016) 124:1924–30. doi: 10.1289/EHP147

36. Garcia-Arevalo M, Alonso-Magdalena P, Servitja JM, Boronat-Belda T, Merino B, Villar-Pazos S, et al. Maternal exposure to Bisphenol-A during pregnancy increases pancreatic beta-cell growth during early life in male mice offspring. *Endocrinology* (2016) 157:4158–71. doi: 10.1210/en.2016-1390
37. Davila-Esqueda ME, Morales JM, Jimenez-Capdeville ME, De la CE, Falcon-Escobedo R, Chi-Ahumada E, et al. Low-level subchronic arsenic exposure from prenatal developmental stages to adult life results in an impaired glucose homeostasis. *Exp Clin Endocrinol Diabetes* (2011) 119:613–7. doi: 10.1055/s-0031-1287782
38. Chen M, Liang S, Qin X, Zhang L, Qiu L, Chen S, et al. Prenatal exposure to diesel exhaust PM2.5 causes offspring beta cell dysfunction in adulthood. *Am J Physiol Endocrinol Metab.* (2017) 315:E72–80. doi: 10.1152/ajpendo.00336.2017
39. Whitehead R, Guan H, Arany E, Cernea M, Yang K. Prenatal exposure to bisphenol A alters mouse fetal pancreatic morphology and islet composition. *Horm Mol Biol Clin Investig.* (2016) 25:171–9. doi: 10.1515/hmbci-2015-0052
40. Lin Y, Wei J, Li Y, Chen J, Zhou Z, Song L, et al. Developmental exposure to di(2-ethylhexyl) phthalate impairs endocrine pancreas and leads to long-term adverse effects on glucose homeostasis in the rat. *Am J Physiol Endocrinol Metab.* (2011) 301:E527–38. doi: 10.1152/ajpendo.00233.2011
41. Rajesh P, Balasubramanian K. Gestational exposure to di(2-ethylhexyl) phthalate (DEHP) impairs pancreatic beta-cell function in F1 rat offspring. *Toxicol Lett.* (2015) 232:46–57. doi: 10.1016/j.toxlet.2014.09.025
42. Mao Z, Xia W, Huo W, Zheng T, Bassig BA, Chang H, et al. Pancreatic impairment and Igf2 hypermethylation induced by developmental exposure to bisphenol A can be counteracted by maternal folate supplementation. *J Appl Toxicol.* (2017) 37:825–35. doi: 10.1002/jat.3430
43. Jacobs HM, Sant KE, Basnet A, Williams LM, Moss JB, Timme-Laragy AR. Embryonic exposure to Mono(2-ethylhexyl) phthalate (MEHP) disrupts pancreatic organogenesis in zebrafish (*Danio rerio*). *Chemosphere* (2018) 195:498–507. doi: 10.1016/j.chemosphere.2017.12.094
44. Sant KE, Jacobs HM, Xu J, Borofski KA, Moss LG, Moss JB, et al. Assessment of toxicological perturbations and variants of pancreatic islet development in the zebrafish model. *Toxics* (2016) 4:20. doi: 10.3390/toxics4030020
45. Sant KE, Jacobs HM, Borofski KA, Moss JB, Timme-Laragy AR. Embryonic exposures to perfluorooctanesulfonic acid (PFOS) disrupt pancreatic organogenesis in the zebrafish, *Danio rerio*. *Environ Pollut.* (2017) 220(Pt B):807–17. doi: 10.1016/j.envpol.2016.10.057
46. Timme-Laragy AR, Sant KE, Rousseau ME, diIorio PJ. Deviant development of pancreatic beta cells from embryonic exposure to PCB-126 in zebrafish. *Comp Biochem Physiol C Toxicol Pharmacol.* (2015) 178:25–32. doi: 10.1016/j.cbpc.2015.08.012
47. Song Y, Yang L. Transgenerational pancreatic impairment with Igf2/H19 epigenetic alteration induced by p,p'-DDE exposure in early life. *Toxicol Lett.* (2017) 280:222–31. doi: 10.1016/j.toxlet.2017.08.083
48. Bansal A, Rashid C, Xin F, Li C, Polyak E, Duemler A, et al. Sex- and dose-specific effects of maternal Bisphenol A exposure on pancreatic islets of first- and second-generation adult mice offspring. *Environ Health Perspect.* (2017) 125:097022. doi: 10.1289/EHP1674
49. Mao Z, Xia W, Chang H, Huo W, Li Y, Xu S. Paternal BPA exposure in early life alters Igf2 epigenetic status in sperm and induces pancreatic impairment in rat offspring. *Toxicol Lett.* (2015) 238:30–8. doi: 10.1016/j.toxlet.2015.08.009
50. Li J, Liu S, Li S, Feng R, Na L, Chu X, et al. Prenatal exposure to famine and the development of hyperglycemia and type 2 diabetes in adulthood across consecutive generations: a population-based cohort study of families in Suihua, China. *Am J Clin Nutr.* (2017) 105:221–7. doi: 10.3945/ajcn.116.138792
51. Rosenfeld CS. Gut dysbiosis in animals due to environmental chemical exposures. *Front Cell Infect Microbiol.* (2017) 7:396. doi: 10.3389/fcimb.2017.00396
52. Johns LE, Ferguson KK, Cantonwine DE, McElrath TF, Mukherjee B, Meeker JD. Urinary BPA and phthalate metabolite concentrations and plasma vitamin D levels in pregnant women: a repeated measures analysis. *Environ Health Perspect.* (2017) 125:087026. doi: 10.1289/EHP1178
53. Russ K, Howard S. Developmental exposure to environmental chemicals and metabolic changes in children. *Curr Probl Pediatr Adolesc Health Care* (2016) 46:255–85. doi: 10.1016/j.cppeds.2016.06.001

4

Developmental Exposure to a Mixture of Unconventional Oil and Gas Chemicals Increased Risk-Taking Behavior, Activity and Energy Expenditure in Aged Female Mice After a Metabolic Challenge

Victoria D. Balise[1,2], Jennifer N. Cornelius-Green[1], Brittany Parmenter[1], Sierra Baxter[1], Christopher D. Kassotis[3], R. Scott Rector[4,5,6], John P. Thyfault[7,8], Silvia Paterlini[9], Paola Palanza[9], Daniel Ruiz[10], Robert Sargis[10] and Susan C. Nagel[1,2]*

[1] Department of Obstetrics, Gynecology and Women's Health, University of Missouri, Columbia, MO, United States, [2] Department of Biological Sciences, University of Missouri, Columbia, MO, United States, [3] Nicholas School of the Environment, Duke University, Durham, NC, United States, [4] Department of Nutrition and Health Exercise Physiology, University of Missouri, Columbia, MO, United States, [5] Division of Gastroenterology and Hepatology, School of Medicine, University of Missouri, Columbia, MO, United States, [6] Research Service, Harry S. Truman Memorial Veterans Medical Center, Columbia, MO, United States, [7] Department of Molecular and Integrative Physiology, University of Kansas Medical Center, Kansas City, KS, United States, [8] Kansas City VA Medical Center, Research Service, Kansas City, MO, United States, [9] Unit of Neuroscience, Department of Medicine and Surgery, University of Parma, Parma, Italy, [10] Department of Medicine, University of Illinois at Chicago, Chicago, IL, United States

***Correspondence:**
Susan C. Nagel
nagels@health.missouri.edu

Chemicals used in unconventional oil and gas (UOG) operations can act as endocrine disrupting chemicals and metabolic disruptors. Our lab has reported altered energy expenditure and activity in C57BL/6J mice that were preconceptionally, gestationally, and lactationally exposed via maternal drinking water to a laboratory-created mixture of 23 UOG chemicals from gestational day 1 to postnatal day 21 in 7-month-old female mice with no change in body composition. We hypothesized that allowing the mice to age and exposing them to a high fat, high sugar diet might reveal underlying changes in energy balance. To investigate whether aging and metabolic challenge would exacerbate this phenotype, these mice were aged to 12 months and given a high fat, high sugar diet (HFHSD) challenge. The short 3-day HFHSD challenge increased body weight and fasting blood glucose in all mice. Developmental exposure to the 23 UOG mixture was associated with increased activity and non-resting energy expenditure in the light cycle, increased exploratory behavior in the elevated plus maze test, and decreased sleep in 12 month female mice. Each of these effects was seen in the light cycle when mice are normally less active. Further studies are needed to better understand the behavioral changes observed after developmental exposure to UOG chemicals.

Keywords: unconventional oil and gas, energy expenditure, endocrine disrupting chemicals, activity, hydraulic fracturing, metabolic

INTRODUCTION

Endocrine-disrupting chemicals (EDCs) are chemicals capable of disrupting normal hormone action and can be found in food, consumer products, and our environment (1). EDCs have been linked to health problems including obesity, diabetes, reproduction, cancers, and neurodevelopmental problems (2). EDCs that can alter the predisposition to obesity and metabolic disease are now termed metabolic-disrupting chemicals (MDCs); these chemicals can promote metabolic changes that can result in type 2 diabetes, fatty liver, and/or obesity (3, 4).

We have previously reported that chemicals used in unconventional oil and gas (UOG) operations can act as EDCs. UOG operations use directional drilling and hydraulic fracturing to release natural gas and oil that were previously inaccessible via traditional drilling methods. While only a few dozen chemicals may be used in a single well in this process, over 1,000 different chemicals are used industrywide. We have previously shown that 23 commonly-utilized UOG chemicals tested could disrupt five nuclear hormone receptors [estrogen (ER), androgen (AR), progesterone (PR), glucocorticoid (GR), and thyroid (TR)] (5).

Wastewater from UOG processes can contaminate surface and ground water. UOG activities and processes, such as transportation, well casing failure, wastewater spills, and direct injection have been linked to drinking water contamination (6–10). We have reported that surface water downstream of an injection well disposal site had higher antagonistic activity for ER, AR, PR, GR, and TR compared to surface water upstream of the site (11).

Exposure to MDCs during susceptible windows of development may result in adverse health outcomes (12–14). In a systematic review by Elliot et al., 41 UOG chemicals were identified as being linked to developmental toxicity (15). We recently demonstrated that UOG chemicals and wastewater can act as metabolic disruptors, promoting lipid accumulation and stimulating adipocyte differentiation as well as promoting the proliferation of pre-adipocytes, via activation of peroxisome proliferator activated receptor gamma (PPARγ) or other mechanisms (16). We also found that female mice prenatally exposed to a mixture of these 23 UOG chemicals (which exhibited antagonistic activity for ER, AR, PR, GR, and TR) from gestation day 11 through 19 had altered organ weights, reproductive endpoints, and increased body weights at postnatal days 7, 13, and 21 (5). There is accumulating evidence that UOG chemicals and wastewater are associated with developmental programming of metabolism.

In a recent study, we extended this line of research to encompass a longer exposure window from gestation day 1 to postnatal day 21. Interestingly, we found an opposite effect on female body weight with the longer developmental exposure: female mice exposed to the 23 UOG chemical mixture weighed less on postnatal day 7 and 21, as opposed to mice exposed from PND 11-18, who weighed more than vehicle controls (17). These female offspring were followed into adulthood, and showed no changes in body composition (body weight, fat mass, or lean mass) at 7 months of age, but exhibited a decrease in resting energy expenditure and activity in the dark cycle compared to vehicle-treated controls (17).

Developmental exposure to metabolic disrupting chemicals can be subtle and an absence of altered body composition at one adult age does not necessarily mean an absence of altered metabolism throughout adulthood (18). The endocrine system maintains homeostasis and utilizes many compensatory mechanisms, such as feedback loops. To discern underlying developmental programming, a "second hit" is often needed to challenge the system beyond compensation (3). Common challenges include stressors such as changes in activity, light exposure, or diet. A high fat, high sugar diet (HFHSD) is often-employed as a metabolic challenge to induce obesity or metabolic dysfunction. Since we previously observed altered resting energy expenditure in female mice exposed to the 23 UOG mixture at 7 months of age, but no change in body composition, we hypothesized that allowing the mice to age and exposing them to a HFHSD might reveal underlying metabolic disruption.

MATERIALS AND METHODS

Animals

This study was carried out in accordance with the recommendations National Research Council's Guide for the Care and Use of Laboratory Animals. The protocol was approved by the University of Missouri Animal Care and Use Committee.

Chemical Mixture and Treatment

Female C57BL/6J mice (purchased from Jackson Laboratories) were mated at 9 months of age. It should be noted that these dams were used in a previous study by our lab, in which they were also mated and exposed to the same mixture of 23 UOG chemicals used in the present study. Offspring outcomes from the first experiment were reported previously (5, 19). These females received the same concentrations of chemical mixtures that were randomly assigned in the previous study (5). Dams (n = 14, 9, 11, 8, and 10) were exposed to the chemical mixture at concentrations of 0, 0.01, 0.10, 1.0, or 10 μg/mL, respectively, for 5 weeks prior to mating. Chemical exposure was paused while females were mated in order to bypass the window of fertilization, and to avoid consumption of treatment chemicals by the males. Treatment was resumed at gestational day one (1 day after presence of copulatory plug) and continued through weaning of the F1 generation at PND 21. As reported in Balise et al. (17), dams had no differences in body weight or water consumption (**Supplementary Figure 1**). Also, there were no differences reported in either litter size or sex ratio (**Supplementary Figure 1**) (17).

From birth to 6 months of age, F1 mice were housed in a barrier facility where both feed (LabDiet 5053: 13% kcal fat, 3.25% kcal sucrose) and acidified water were sterilized and provided *ad libitum*. Glass bottles and polysulfone cages were used for all animals. After the F1 generation reached 6 months of age, they were transferred to a conventional facility where the metabolic instrumentation was located. In this facility, they received non-sterilized feed (LabDiet 5053: 13% kcal fat, 3.25% kcal sucrose) and non-acidified, non-sterilized water. Both facilities were temperature controlled and kept on a 12 h light/dark cycle.

The 23 chemicals were mixed equimass in 200 proof ethanol and added to drinking water such that each individual chemical was present at a concentration of 0.01, 0.10, 1.0, or 10 μg/mL in a 0.2% ethanol vehicle in acidified drinking water. Water bottles were changed twice per week to ensure consistent chemical concentrations throughout the dosing period. Water consumption was calculated as the difference in the weight of the water bottle before and after use every time the bottle was changed. Dosages based on weight of the dam and the amount of water consumed were calculated as 1.5, 15, 150, and 1,500 μg/kg/day. Offspring in litters that had less than one male or female per litter were excluded from analysis. After application of inclusion criteria, 0, 1.5, 15, 150, and 1,500 μg/kg/day treatment groups included $n = 9, 11, 9, 10$, and 10 total individual animals, and $n = 6, 4, 5, 4$, and 4 pups from unique litters, respectively (**Supplementary Table 1**).

Elevated Plus Maze Behavioral Test

An elevated plus maze (EPM) test was conducted at 11 months of age. Tests were started in the light cycle, 3 h before the initiation of the dark cycle. Mice were placed gently into the maze facing an open arm and were video-recorded for a period of 5 minutes. Time spent in open arms, closed arms, and center were reported as a percentage of the five-min recording (20).

Time Line of High Fat and High Sugar Diet (HFHSD) Challenge and Necropsy

Mice were given two high fat, high sugar diet (HFHSD) challenges. Two separate challenges were needed since GTT could not be performed while mice were in metabolic cages (**Figure 1**). F1 females were given a HFHSD for 6 days. The high fat, high sugar diet (HFHSD) metabolic challenge contained 45% kcal fat and 17% kcal sucrose; Research Diet D12451). The first HFHSD challenge was given at 11 months of age to perform glucose tolerance tests (GTT). GTT was assessed before and 3 days after the HFHSD challenge (**Figure 1A**). The second HFHSD challenge was given at 12 months of age, to assess energy expenditure and activity in the metabolic cages (**Figure 1B**). Mice were given the HFHSD challenge for 3 days and placed into indirect calorimetry cages on Day 4 for 3 additional days, and necropsy was performed on day 7. Necropsy was performed by carbon dioxide asphyxiation followed by cervical dislocation.

Indirect Calorimetry

Energy expenditure, activity, food and water intake, and behavior were assessed via indirect calorimetry using the Promethion from Sable Systems Int., (Las Vegas, NV). Mice were individually housed in the cages for 72 h. The first 24 h were used as an acclimation period, and the last 48 h were used for analysis. The 12 h light cycles and 12 h dark cycles were separately analyzed. Outcomes were calculated with macros provided by the manufacturer (21).

Energy expenditure was obtained from measured oxygen consumption. Total energy expenditure was calculated using the Weir equation in kilocalories and was the overall energy expenditure for a 12 h cycle. Resting energy expenditure was extrapolated from the lowest average energy expenditure in a 30 min window within a 12 h cycle. Non-resting energy expenditure was calculated for each 12 h cycle by subtracting resting energy expenditure from total energy expenditure. Active energy expenditure was extrapolated from the highest average energy expenditure for 15 min within a 12 h cycle.

Activity and meters traveled were measured by infrared beams that track movement in horizontal (X and Y plane) and vertical directions (Z plane). Spontaneous activity was activity in the X, Y, and Z direction, ambulatory activity in the X and Y directions and rearing activity in the Z direction. Meters traveled counted all meters in the X, Y, and Z direction, while pedestrian meters measured meters in the X and Y directions only. Food consumption and food bouts (number of times the animal made contact with the food hopper) were also measured.

Body Composition

At 12 months of age, body weight, fat mass, and lean mass were measured just prior to starting the HFHSD metabolic challenge on Day 1, and on Day 4 and 7. Fat and lean mass were measured using the EchoMRI-900 (EchoMRI, Houston, TX) (17). Fat and lean percentages were calculated by dividing fat or lean mass by total body weight.

Glucose Tolerance Test

Glucose tolerance tests were performed in mice at 11 months of age before and after HFHSD on Day 0 and Day 4, respectively. Sixteen mice from all treatment groups were randomized to be tested per day over the course of 1 week. Mice were weighed at 1000 h and fasted from 1000 to 1600 h. A baseline (0 min) blood sample was collected via tail snip at 1600-1630 hrs, and blood glucose was determined using a glucose monitor (Accu-Chek Aviva Plus). Immediately after the baseline measurement was taken, 250 mg/mL glucose was injected intraperitoneally at 1 gram of glucose per kg of lean mass (22, 23). Blood glucose concentrations were measured at 30, 60, and 120 min after injection (24).

Liver Triacylglycerol Concentration

At necropsy, livers were collected and stored at −80°C. Liver triacylglycerol concentration was determined as previously described using a commercially available kit (F6428, Sigma, St. Louis, MO) (25).

Serum Insulin Concentration

Blood was collected at time of necropsy by cardiac puncture and stored on ice. Centrifugation was performed to separate serum, and samples were stored at −80°C. Serum insulin concentrations were measured using a commercially available mouse insulin ELISA kit according to manufacturer's instructions (Alpco Diagnostics, cataolog #80-INSMSU-E01, Salem, MA).

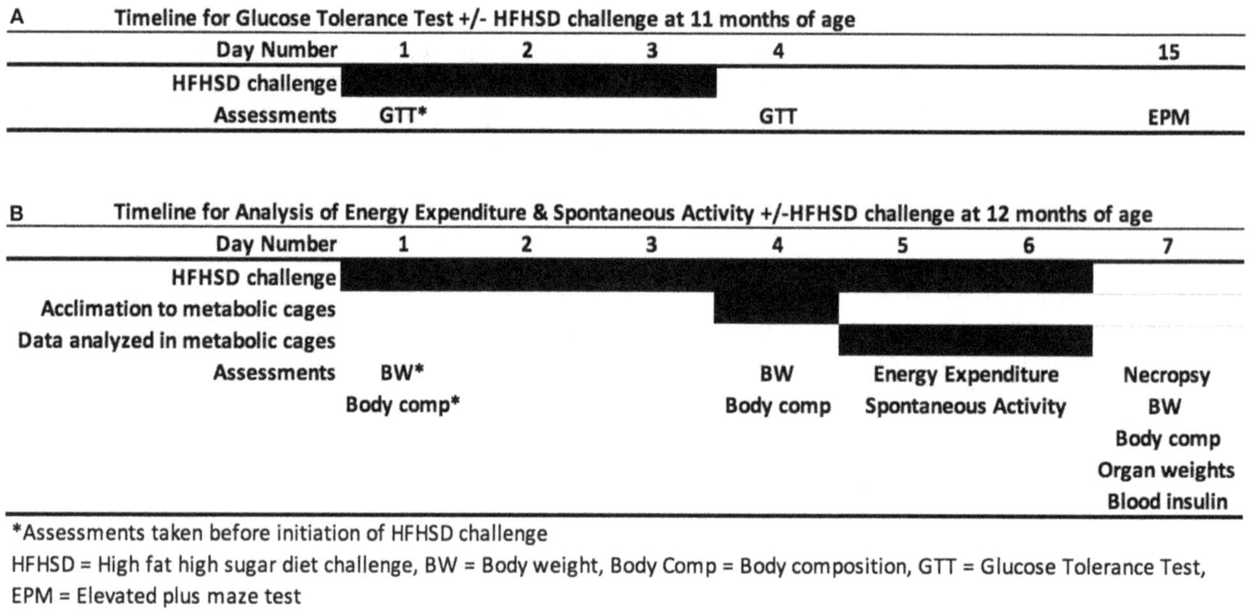

FIGURE 1 | Metabolic challenge. Female mice were given a high fat high sugar diet (HFHSD) at 11 months **(A)** and 12 months of age **(B)**. After 3 days, either a glucose tolerance test (GTT) was performed at 11 months of age **(A)** or mice were placed in metabolic cages for indirect calorimetry for 3 days **(B)**. Mice were allowed to acclimate to the new cage environment on first day (Day 4) of indirect calorimetry and Days 5 and 6 were used for data analysis.

Pancreas Analysis

Pancreatic Histology and Immunohistochemistry (IHC)

At the time of necropsy, pancreata were dissected and fixed in 4% paraformaldehyde overnight and paraffin-embedded. Tissue sections (5 μm in thickness) were immunostained with the following primary antibodies (all at 1:500 dilution): polyclonal guinea pig anti-porcine insulin (DAKO, Carpinteria, CA), mouse monoclonal anti-human glucagon (Sigma-Aldrich, St. Louis, MO), polyclonal goat anti-somatostatin (Santa Cruz, Santa Cruz, CA), and DAPI (Invitrogen, Carlsbad, CA). The primary antibodies were detected using a combination of DyLight 488, 549, and 649-conjugated secondary antibodies (1:200, Jackson Immuno Research Laboratory, West Grove, PA).

Image Capture and Islet Quantification

As previously described (26, 27), microscopic images of pancreatic sections were taken with an Olympus IX8 DSU spinning disk confocal microscope (Melville, NY) with Stereo Investigator imaging software (SI, Micro Bright Field, Williston, VT). A modified method of "virtual slice capture" was utilized. Quantification of cellular composition (i.e., each area of β-, α-, and δ-cell populations, and islet area by automated contouring of each islet) was carried out using custom-written scripts for Fiji/ImageJ (http://rsbweb.nih.gov/ij/). MATLAB (MathWorks, Natick, MA) was used for mathematical analyses (26, 27).

Vaginal Cytology and Estrus Cycle Analysis

Vaginal smears were taken daily for 14 days between 9 and 10 months of age. The vaginal cells of each female were washed out the day before smears were performed and collected in a 96 well plate. Vaginal cytology was assessed and estrus cycle stage given based on proportion of cell types, as previously reported (28).

Mice were in metabolic cages for 3 days immediately preceding necropsy, so estrus cyclicity could not be monitored as mice could not be removed from the metabolic cages. Vaginal cytology was assessed on the day of necropsy. The first single smear contains a mixture of the preceding days vaginal cells. On the day of necropsy, smears contained only cornified epithelium and did not contain white blood cells and were thus concluded to be in persistent estrus at 12 months of age.

Statistics

Data were analyzed with a linear mixed model using SPSS version 32. This model was selected so that litter could be incorporated as a random effect. Treatment group and dates of measurement were included as fixed effects for body weight, fat mass, lean mass, fat percent, lean percent, food consumption, and activity. For analyses of body weight, litter size was included as a fixed effect. For analysis of energy expenditure, body weight was included as a fixed effect.

Data that were not normally distributed were transformed to achieve normality. Results are displayed in all figures as the estimated marginal means, back transformed for presentation if transformation was necessary. Differences between vehicle and treatment groups were analyzed using Fisher's Least Significant Difference tests with 95% confidence intervals. Elevated plus maze decision making was analyzed using Fisher's exact test. All treatment groups were compared to vehicle only.

RESULTS

Exploratory Behavior

Mice were introduced to an elevated plus maze for 5 min at the end of the light cycle at 11 months of age (**Figure 1**). Time spent in center, open and closed arms was measured to assess exploratory behavior. Exploratory activity (defined as the amount of time spent in open areas of the maze) was altered by developmental exposure to the UOG chemical mixture. Animals spent 400, 490, 290% more time in the open arms in the 1.5, 15, and 150 μg/kg/day groups, respectively, relative to vehicle control (**Figure 2A**). Treatment 150 μg/kg/day also spent 115% more time in the center and 20% less time in closed arms relative to vehicle (**Figures 2B,C**). Additionally, 100% of mice in the 15 and 150 μg/kg/day groups chose to enter open arms vs. 43% in the vehicle control group (**Figure 2D**).

Response to the High Fat High Sugar Diet (HFHSD)

Mice were given a HFHSD challenge for a total of 3 days at 11 months of age (**Figure 1A**). Three days on the HFHSD resulted in increase in body weight and a 13–36% increase in fasting blood glucose (**Figure 3**). Mice were given a second metabolic challenge at 12 months of age for a total of 6 days (**Figure 1B**) to examine energy expenditure and activity (below). Between days 0 and 3 on the HFHSD body weight and fat mass increased 9–11% (**Table 1**). Between days 3 and 6 mice lost weight. This was likely due to the stress and novelty of being placed in the metabolic cages (**Table 1**).

Spontaneous Activity

At 12 months of age, mice were placed in metabolic cages on Day 4 of the HFHSD challenge. Spontaneous activity was measured over the last 48 h (Days 5–6), and each parameter was analyzed as an average of two 12 h light or dark cycles (**Figure 1B**). Endpoints that were measured included spontaneous activity (movement in the x, y, and z directions), ambulatory activity (movement in the x and y directions), rearing activity (z direction only), and total meters traveled (meters moved in x, y, and z directions) in the 12 h light or 12 h dark cycles).

Developmental exposure to UOG chemical mixture after a HFHSD metabolic challenge was associated with increased activity during the light cycle. Spontaneous activity was 30–40% and ambulatory activity was 44–78% higher in all treatment groups relative to vehicle (**Figures 4A,B**). Total meters traveled was 50–111% higher in the 1.5, 150, and 1500 μg/kg/day groups relative to vehicle (**Figure 4C**). The difference in meters traveled was not restricted to a certain time of the light cycle but was continuous throughout the light cycle (**Supplementary Figure 2**). Rearing activity did not differ relative to vehicle control within the light cycle (data not shown). Spontaneous activity, ambulatory activity, rearing activity, and meters traveled did not differ in treatment groups relative to vehicle during the dark cycle.

Energy Expenditure

Mice were placed in metabolic cages on Day 4, which was 3 days after the HFHSD metabolic challenge began (**Figure 1B**). The HFHSD continued for 3 days (Days 4–6) and energy expenditure was measured over the last 48 h (Days 5–6). Each parameter was analyzed as an average of two 12 h light or dark cycles (**Figure 1**). Developmental exposure to UOG chemical mixture after a HFHSD metabolic challenge was associated with altered non-resting energy expenditure in the light cycle. Total energy expenditure was 13% lower in the 1,500 μg/kg/day treatment group relative to vehicle during the light cycle (**Figure 5A**). No differences in resting energy expenditures were observed in any of the treatment groups relative to vehicle (**Figure 5B**), but non-resting energy expenditure was 74, 69, 51, and 77% higher in the 1.5, 15, 150, and 1,500 μg/kg/day treatment groups, respectively, in the light cycle (**Figure 5C**). Total energy expenditure, resting energy expenditure, and non-resting energy expenditure did not differ in any treatment group when compared to vehicle in the dark cycle. Respiratory quotient was not different between vehicle and treatment groups in either the light or dark cycles (**Supplementary Figure 3**).

Body Weight and Composition

Developmental exposure to UOG chemical mixture altered body weight at 12 months of age. Before, during, and after the HFHSD challenge, body weight was 10% lower in the 1,500 μg/kg/day group (**Figure 6A**). There were no differences in fat mass or lean mass between treatment groups (**Figures 6B,C**). Body length (nose to rump) at necropsy was not altered in any treatment group, in comparison to vehicle (**Table 1**).

Adipose Tissue and Organ Weights

After 6 days of the HFHSD metabolic challenge, mice were euthanized, and organs and tissues were collected and weighed. Periuterine adipose tissue weight was 35-38% less in the 1.5, 15, and 1,500 μg/kg/day groups compared to vehicle (**Figure 7A**). Brown adipose weight did not differ; however, the 1500 μg/kg/day group demonstrated a 55% increase in brown adipose weight compared to vehicle, when adjusted for body weight (**Figures 7B,C**). Kidney, heart, spleen, uterus, ovary, and liver weights, and liver triglycerides did not differ between treatment groups (**Table 2**).

Food Consumption and Glucose Homeostasis

Glucose tolerance tests were performed prior to initiation of the HFHSD and after 3 days on the HFHSD (**Figure 1A**) at 11 months of age. Serum glucose concentration did not differ before or after HFHSD metabolic challenge relative to vehicle control whether calculated at individual time points, in area under the curve, or relative to basal glucose levels (**Supplementary Figure 4**).

Food consumption and food bouts were measured on days 5-6 of HFHSD challenge at 12 months on age (**Figure 1B**). Total food consumption and food bouts did not differ

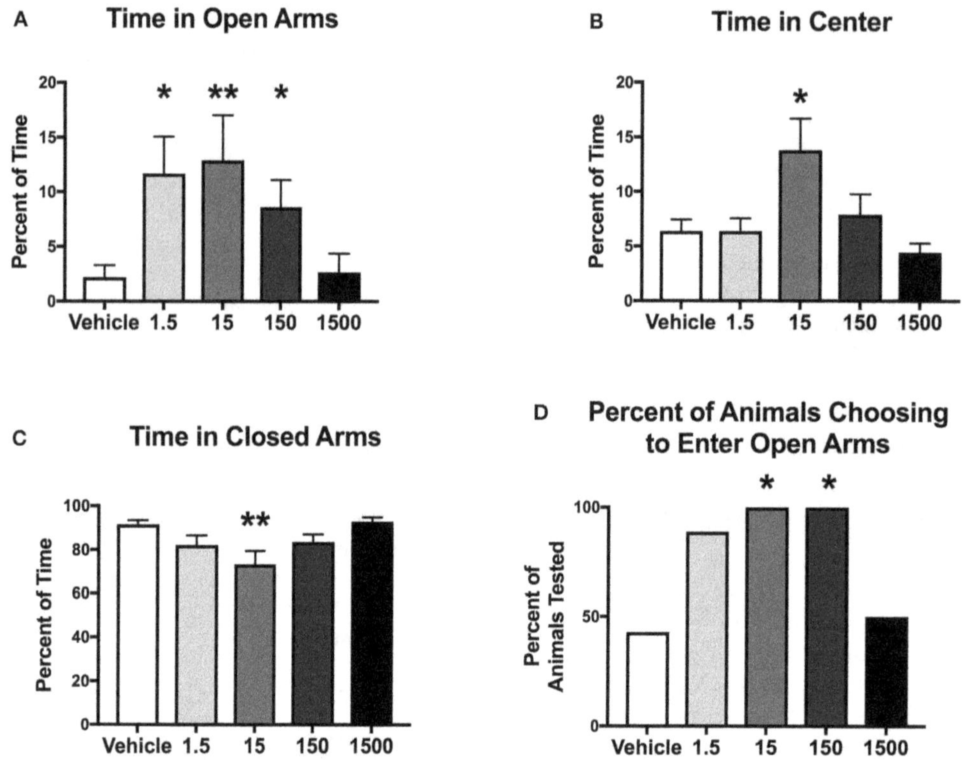

FIGURE 2 | Exploratory activity of female mice at 11 months of age. Estimated marginal means (±SEM) of exploratory activity 3 h before initiation of the dark cycle. Percentage of time spent in the elevated plus maze in open arms **(A)**, center of the maze **(B)**, and closed arms **(C)**. Percent of animals within treatment group choosing to enter open arms **(D)** (n = 7, 9, 7, 6, 6, respectively, for vehicle, 1.5, 15, 150, and 1500 μg/kg/day treatment groups). $^*p < 0.05$ and $^{**}p < 0.0125$ relative to vehicle. Model included covariates: litter and assessment date.

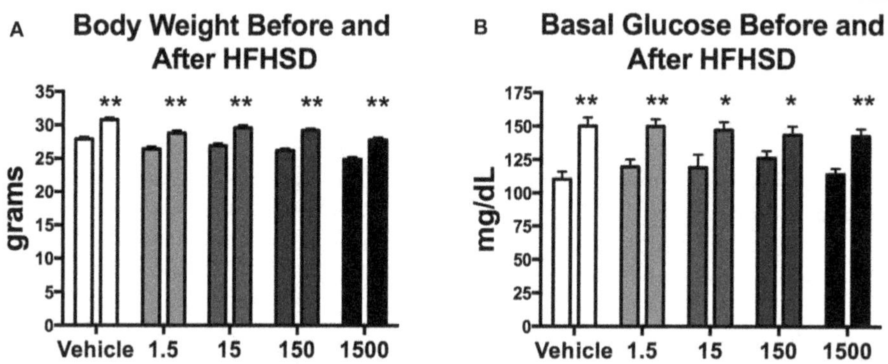

FIGURE 3 | Body weight and basal glucose levels before and after high fat high sugar diet (HFHSD) at 11 months of age. Estimated marginal means (±SEM) of body weight before and after 3 days on HFHSD **(A)**, and basal blood glucose levels before and after 3 days on HFHSD **(B)**. For body weight n = 10, 8, 9, 10, 9, respectively, for vehicle, 1.5, 15, 150, and 1,500 μg/kg/day treatment groups. For basal glucose levels before HFHSD n = 9, 9, 8, 9, 8, and after HFHSD n = 10, 11, 9, 10, 10, respectively for vehicle, 1.5, 15, 150, and 1,500 μg/kg/day treatment groups. Two way ANOVA comparing within group before and after HFHSD $^*p < 0.05$, and $^{**}p < 0.0125$.

between treatment groups in either the light or dark cycle (**Supplementary Figure 5**).

Serum insulin concentrations were measured from blood collected at necropsy, which occurred during the first 4 h of the light cycle after 6 days on the HFHSD challenge at 12 months of age. No differences were detected in insulin concentrations between vehicle and treatment groups (**Supplementary Figure 6**). Total islet cell number and proportion of cells types were quantified in one dose group. Pancreata were collected at necropsy, after 6 days on the HFHSD. The area of pancreas occupied by alpha, beta, and delta cells, and total islet area was quantified using immunohistochemistry

TABLE 1 | Body composition of female mice at 12 months of age: Estimated marginal means (± SEM)** of body weight, fat mass, and lean mass.

	Body weight (g)			Lean mass (g)			Fat mass (g)		
Days on HFHSD	0	3	6	0	3	6	0	3	6
Vehicle	27.9 (1.1)	30.8 (1.1)	29.0 (1.2)	20.0 (0.3)	20.5 (0.3)	19.6 (0.4)	6.7 (0.7)	9.0 (0.8)	8.1 (0.9)
1.5 μg/kg/day	26.4 (1.1)	28.8 (1.1)	27.1 (1.2)	19. 6 (0.3)	19.9 (0.3)	19.2 (0.3)	5.5 (0.7)	7.6 (0.8)	6.4 (0.9)
15 μg/kg/day	26.9 (1.2)	29.6 (1.2)	28.3 (1.3)	19.5 (0.3)	19.8 (0.4)	19.2 (0.4)	6.1 (0.8)	8.2 (0.9)	7.5 (1.0)
150 μg/kg/day	26.2 (0.9)	29.2 (1.0)	27.8 (1.0)	19.5 (0.3)	20.1 (0.3)	19.3 (0.3)	5.6 (0.6)	7.8 (0.7)	7.2 (0.8)
1,500 μg/kg/day	**24.9 (1.0)***	**27.8 (1.1)***	**25.9 (1.1)***	19.1 (0.3)	19.6 (0.3)	18.8 (0.3)	4.8 (0.7)	6.9 (0.8)	6.1 (0.8)

n = 10, 8, 9, 10, 9 respectively, for vehicle, 1.5, 15, 150, and 1,500 μg/kg/day treatment groups.
*Bold represents *p< 0.05 relative to vehicle.*
***Models included covariates: litter, date of body weight assessment, and litter size.*

did not differ between the 1,500 μg/kg/day group and vehicle (**Supplementary Figure 6**).

Estrus Cyclicity

Estrus cyclicity was monitored for 2 weeks at 9.5 months of age. Overall mice tended to have irregular cycles or be in persistent estrus. Within each treatment group 90, 63, 89, 100, and 89% of mice in vehicle, 1.5, 15, 150, and 1,500 ug/kg/day, respectively, spent ≥50% of days in estrus and this did not differ relative to vehicle control. All mice appeared to be in persistent estrus at necropsy as vaginal smears contained only cornified epithelium and no white blood cells.

DISCUSSION

Our findings are the first to report that developmental exposure (GD1-PND21) to a mixture of 23 oil and gas chemicals increased exploratory and risk-taking activity with a subsequent increase in energy expenditure in female C57Bl/6 mice. All UOG exposure groups also had a decrease in peri-uterine fad pad weight, which may have been a consequence of increased activity and energy expenditure. Overall, treatments largely did not affect other aspects of body composition, although mice in the highest treatment group, 1,500 μg/kg/day, had some unique impacts on body composition. The HFHSD metabolic challenge caused all animals to have an increase in body weight, fat mass and higher fasting blood glucose, and did not differ between vehicle and treatment groups.

Female mice developmentally exposed to the 23 UOG mixture had an increase in exploratory activity and spontaneous activity in the light cycle. We assessed exploratory behavior using the elevated plus maze (EPM) test, and found mice developmentally exposed to the 1.5, 15, and 150 μg/kg/day UOG groups spent dramatically more time in the open arms compared to vehicle (400, 490, 290%, respectively). Since mice tend to spend more time in enclosed and protected areas for safety (29), such a robust increase in the amount of time in open arms indicates that UOG exposed mice display lower anxiety-like behavior and are more prone to risk-taking behavior in response to novel and potentially risky environment. Furthermore, when exposed to the HFHSD, these female mice that were developmentally exposed to the 23 UOG mixture, showed increased locomotor activity in the light cycle compared to vehicle mice. Mice are nocturnal and habitually rest and avoid activity in the light, a likely adaptation to evade predators. Increased activity in the light cycle could be either an indication of disturbance of circadian rhythms and sleep disorders or of hyperactive behavior. We cannot determine here if the increased light-related activity in exposed mice was already expressed as a baseline or it was induced by the diet switch or by the hypercaloric diet intake. Diets high in fat or sugar can indeed alter circadian rhythms in mammals (30). Female mice, however, have been reported to be more resistant to the disruption of daily activity rhythms during high fat feeding compared to males because of protective effects of circulating ovarian hormones (31). The 23 UOG mixture exposed female mice could thus be more sensitive to the effects of novelty or of high calories intake on activity. Taken together, increased time spent in open arms in the EPM test and increased spontaneous activity in the light cycle suggest that developmental exposure to the UOG mixture led to an enhanced response to novel stimuli (environment and food) in developmentally exposed females that may be related to high risk-taking behavior.

While determining the exact mechanisms mediating altered behavior is complex, several nuclear receptors have been shown to modulate time spent in open arms in the EPM test and the nuclear receptor antagonist activity in the UOG mixture is a likely candidate. Estrogen and androgen receptor agonists have generally been shown to decrease time spent in open arms, which is generally associated with anxiety. Postnatal exposure to DHT in Long-Evans and Wistar rats, as well as C57Bl/6 mice, resulted in less time in open arms of the EPM and less activity (32–34); this was mirrored in a joint gestational/postnatal DEHP exposure, where female offspring also spent less time in the open arms and made fewer entries into them (35). Gestational exposure to testosterone was associated with less time spent in the open arms in Wistar rats. This behavior was reversed by co-administration with the anti-androgen flutamide or the antiestrogen tamoxifen, indicating that both androgens and estrogens can regulate this behavior (36). Similarly, BPA exposure from either GD-1 to PND1 or PND1-PND8 resulted in females that spent less time in open arms in the EPM test and more anxious behavior in open field test, and a novelty test in CD-1 mice (37). As agonist activity for the

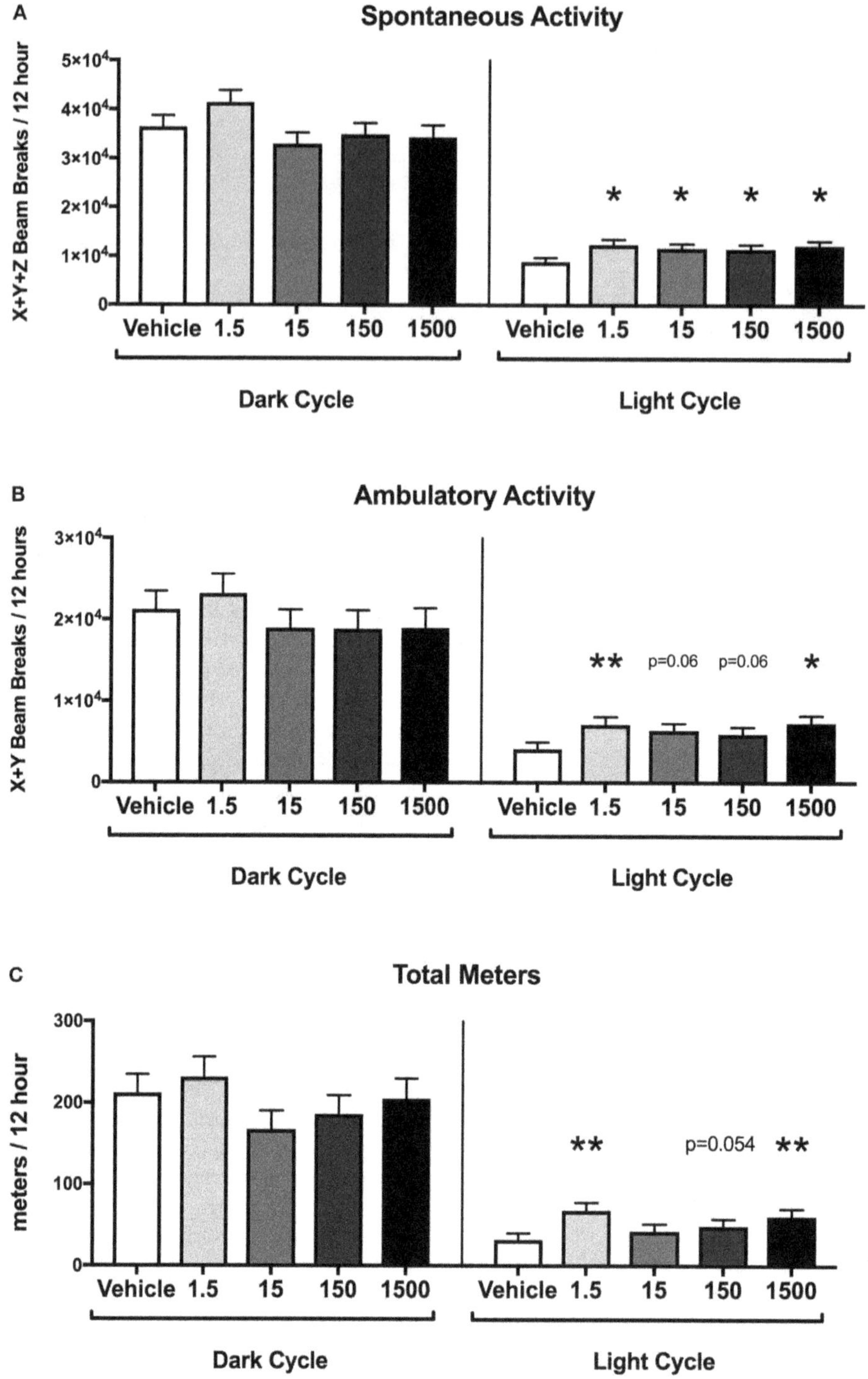

FIGURE 4 | Activity of female mice at 12 months of age on a HFHSD. Estimated marginal means (±SEM) in 12 h increments of: total spontaneous activity **(A)**, ambulatory activity **(B)**, and meters traveled **(C)**. $n = 10, 8, 9, 9$, respectively for vehicle, 1.5, 15, 150, and 1,500 μg/kg/day treatment groups. $^{*}p < 0.05$ and $^{**}p < 0.0125$ relative to vehicle. Model included covariates: litter and assessment date.

androgen and estrogen receptors causes an increase in anxious behavior and a decrease in risk-taking behavior, it is possible that antagonist activity for these receptors might increase risk-taking behavior. In support of this as a possible contributory mechanism, we previously reported that 21 of the chemicals in the 23 UOG mix can antagonize the estrogen and/or androgen receptors with IC50 concentrations of approximately 1 and 5 μM, respectively (5).

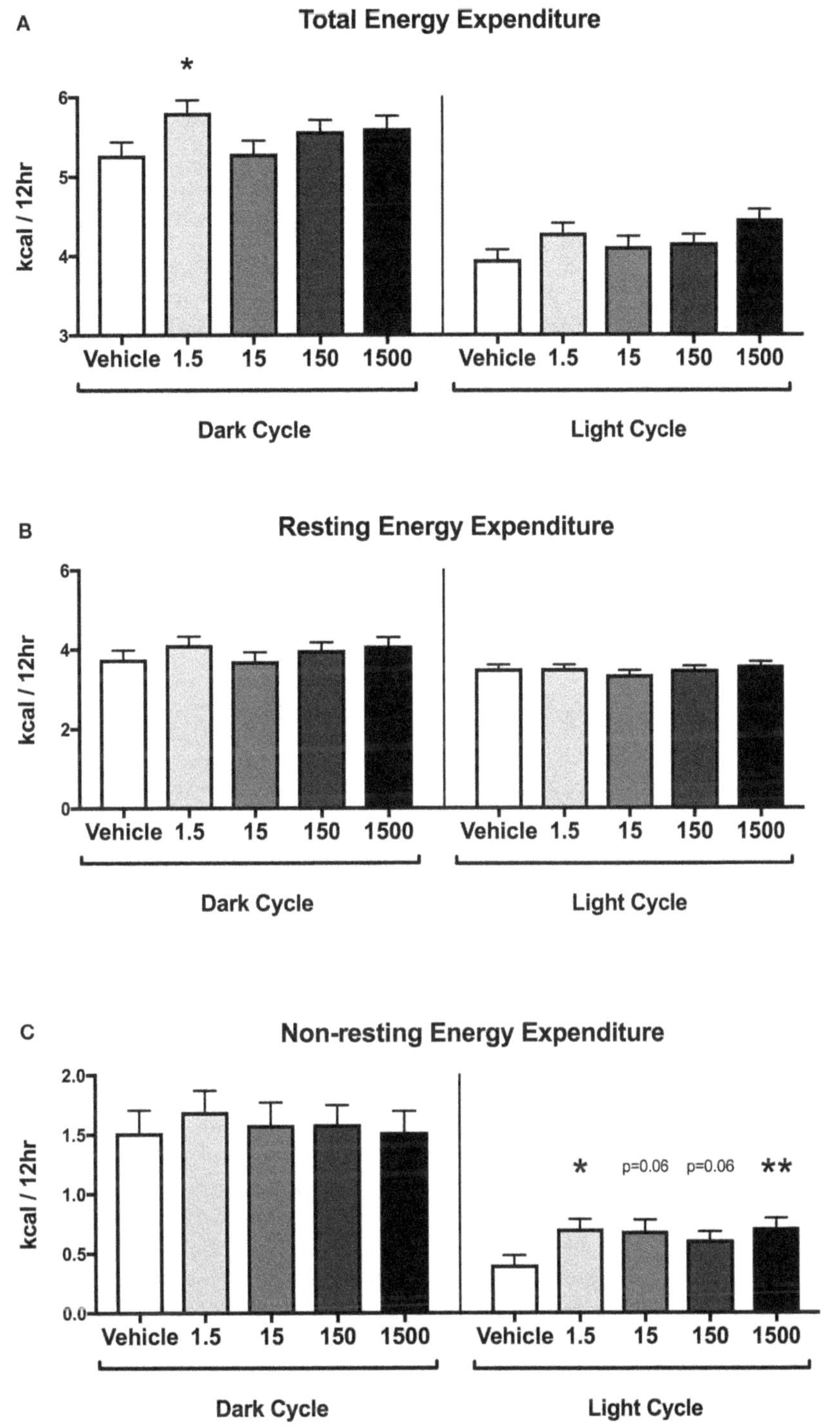

FIGURE 5 | Energy expenditure in female mice at 12 months of age on HFHSD. Estimated marginal means (±SEM) in 12 h increments of: total energy expenditure **(A)**, resting energy expenditure **(B)**, non-resting expenditure **(C)**. $n = 10, 8, 9, 9, 8$, respectively for vehicle, 1.5, 15, 150, and 1,500 µg/kg/day treatment groups. $^{*}p < 0.05$ and $^{**}p < 0.0125$ relative to vehicle. Model included covariates: litter, assessment date, litter size, and body weight.

We previously reported that ten chemicals in the 23 UOG mix antagonized the glucocorticoid receptor *in vitro* (5), suggesting this is a possible mechanism. Exposure to increased stress from GD3-20 in Wistar rats resulted in offspring that displayed anxious behavior: decreased time in open arms of the EPM, decreased time in the light side of the light-dark box, and decreased mobility in the forced swim test (38). However, experimentally increasing or decreasing

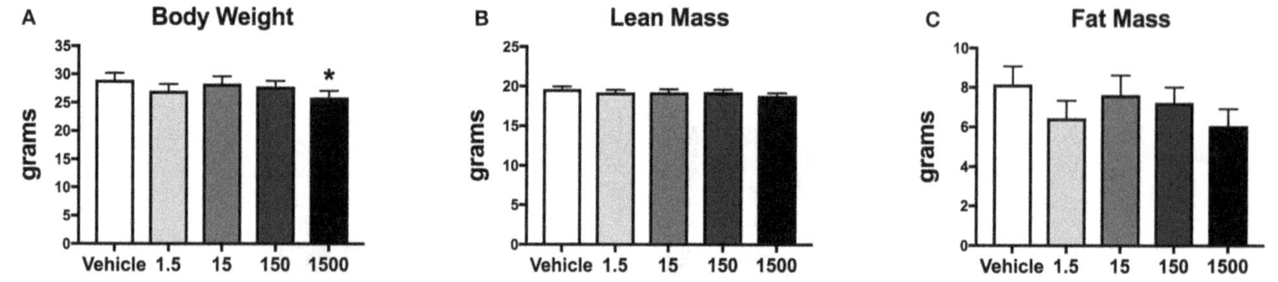

FIGURE 6 | Body composition of female mice at 12 months of age after 6 days on a HFHSD after metabolic cage testing. Collapsed data from days 0, 3, and 6 of a HFHSD metabolic challenge. Estimated marginal means (±SEM) of: body weight **(A)**, nose to rump length at necropsy **(B)**, fat mass **(C)**, and lean mass. $^*p < 0.05$ relative to vehicle. $n = 10, 8, 9, 10, 9$, respectively for vehicle, 1.5, 15, 150, and 1,500 μg/kg/day treatment groups. Models included covariates: litter, date of body weight assessment, and litter size.

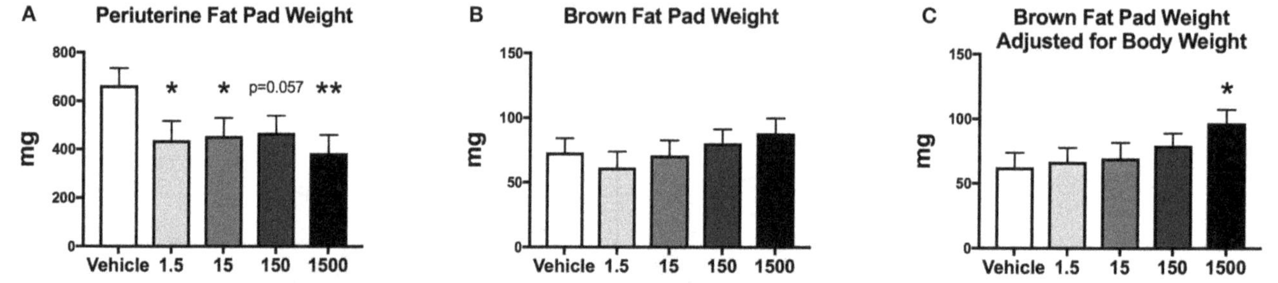

FIGURE 7 | Fat pad weights of female mice at 12 months of age after HFHSD. Estimated marginal means (±SEM) of periuterine fat pad weight **(A)**, brown fat pad weight **(B)**, and brown fat weight adjusted for body weight **(C)**, $^*p < 0.05$ relative to vehicle **($n = 10, 8, 9, 10, 9$ respectively for vehicle, 1.5, 15, 150, and 1,500 μg/kg/day treatment groups). Model included covariates: litter, date.

prenatal cortisol levels exogenously with dexamethasone, betamethasone, or hydrocortisone did not lead to alterations in anxiety-like behavior in the EPM (39–41). As excess cortisol induced anxiety-like behavior in some studies, antagonistic activity could promote the opposite: an increase in risk-taking behavior.

The UOG mix also antagonizes progesterone and thyroid hormone receptors, however, these are less likely to be targets mediating the altered behavior observed in the current study. Progesterone receptor knockout mice supplemented with progesterone spent more time in the open arms of the EPM (42). Exposure to a thyroid antagonist during gestation did not impact alter time spent in open arms in the EPM test in either sex in Wistar rats (43). Given that we reported anti-thyroid and anti-progesterone activity in the UOG chemicals *in vitro,* we do not suspect these are causative mechanisms herein.

The current study involves a complex paradigm with endocrine disrupting chemical mixture exposure during development in addition to aging mice and a diet challenge, it is difficult to dissect the underlying mechanisms by which developmental UOG chemical exposure altered activity and energy expenditure in aging female mice. However, there is evidence that antagonist activity to the glucocorticoid, androgen, and estrogen receptors could be possible underlying mechanisms. These mechanisms should be substantiated through the use of targeted receptor ligand controls in future studies to assess their potential contributory roles in these effects.

While on the HFHSD, all treatment groups showed an increase in spontaneous activity and increased non-resting energy expenditure within the light cycle. Despite this increase, body weight and overall fat mass were not significantly different, though this did appear to contribute to a significant reduction in peri-uterine fat pad mass in the developmentally exposed animals. However, a limitation of the metabolic cages is that energy expenditure is only taken at one time point and cannot reflect the metabolism of an animal throughout its lifespan. While mice were allowed 24 h to acclimate to the cages, they did lose weight across the 3 days spent in the metabolic cages, so it is possible that stress is a complicating factor in the results of the current study.

In the current study, four different doses of the same treatment mixture spanned three orders of magnitude. Doses were selected to include environmentally relevant concentrations to mimic chemical concentrations found to be reported in UOG drilling regions. The concentrations in the drinking water of the 1,500 μg/kg/day group mimic those reported in industry wastewater samples, the 150 μg/kg/day group mimic those reported in surface and groundwater at sites of UOG fluid spills, and the 1.5 and 15 μg/kg/day groups mimic concentrations reported in surface

TABLE 2 | Organ and tissue weights: Estimated marginal means (±SEM) of wet organ and tissue weights.

	Length	Kidney	Heart	Spleen	Uterus	Ovaries	Liver	TAG
Vehicle	9.8 (0.1)	174.0 (4.9)	119.1 (4.3)	89.4 (6.3)	128.2 (13.2)	5.6 (0.5)	1247.5 (74.6)	23.4 (2.7)
1.5 μg/kg/day	9.8 (0.1)	177.6 (4.6)	123.6 (4.2)	90.0 (6.1)	126.1 (12.8)	5.9 (0.5)	1154.7 (81.6)	17.4 (3.0)
15 μg/kg/day	9.9 (0.1)	172.1 (5.3)	114.9 (4.6)	79.9 (6.8)	112.2 (14.2)	6.2 (0.6)	1321.8 (89.1)	17.4 (2.8)
150 μg/kg/day	9.9 (0.1)	171.6 (4.0)	118.2 (3.6)	95.3 (5.3)	129.9 (11.1)	6.1 (0.4)	1274.0 (54.9)	17.7 (2.7)
1,500 μg/kg/day	9.9 (0.1)	168.6 (4.5)	120.0 (4.1)	83.3 (5.9)	133.4 (12.5)	5.3 (0.5)	1243.4 (59.0)	19.7 (2.8)

n = 10, 8, 9, 10, 9 respectively, for vehicle, 1.5, 15, 150, and 1500 μg/kg/day treatment groups.
Length = nose to rump length in cm.
Kidney, heart, liver, spleen, uterus, and ovary weights expressed as mg and included body weight as a covariate.
TAG = liver triacylglycerol mmol/kg wet weight.

and groundwater UOG regions without reported spills (44–46). The lower dose groups are potentially within the range of current human exposures for those living in UOG drilling dense areas.

Given the broad dose response and the known EDC antagonist activity of the UOG mixes, we anticipated and found quantitatively and qualitatively different effects at low vs. high doses across the broad dose response following developmental exposure (47). For example, the 1500 μg/kg/day UOG chemical dose group was unique. These animals exhibited a significant decrease in body weight. Energy expenditure and activity were similar to other dose groups that did not share this body weight difference, though these animals did also have a significant increase in brown adipose, which may have impacted metabolic health. The 1,500 μg/kg/day group also did not show an increase in time spent in open arms in the EPM test as observed in other treatment groups, suggesting differing mechanisms promoting these effects. Future studies directed at this treatment group should include looking further into thermogenic factors of brown adipose, for example, expression of Prdm16, UCP-1 or PGC-1α.

Many developmental programming phenotypes need a secondary adult challenge to be revealed. At seven months of age, these mice exhibited decreased resting energy expenditure and activity (17). To investigate whether aging and a metabolic challenge would exacerbate this phenotype, these mice were aged to 12 months and given a HFHS diet challenge (current study). This led to an overall increase in energy expenditure and activity in treatment groups compared to vehicle. While we did not see an exacerbation of the effects seen at 7 months, age plus a HFHS diet was associated with increased spontaneous activity in treatment groups in the light cycle. Both age and the HFHSD can alter behavior and metabolism and it is possible that the combination could result in unanticipated opposing actions. Future studies are needed to separately examine these two variables to completely understand how age and diet interact with developmental exposure to the UOG mix to modulate activity and energy expenditure in adulthood.

Further research is needed to more conclusively determine the mechanisms driving these effects and substantiate these findings as the current study has limitations. The dams utilized herein were exposed twice to the same concentration of UOG mix for two sets of experiments during pregnancy; we cannot rule out that this double exposure in part contributed to the observed effects. While further research utilizing a single exposure should be performed to substantiate these findings, the current experimental paradigm is completely relevant to women who have more than one child while living in UOG areas. We also evaluated only female mice, and further investigation of males should be explored in future work to assess impacts on male offspring and potential sex differences in these effects. We have previously reported that a prenatal only exposure to the highest doses altered testosterone concentrations in adult males (5); it also altered some pituitary hormones, but did not alter estradiol concentrations in adult females (19). Future studies should evaluate these hormones and others, like cortisol, in F0 and F1 mice. Lastly, we assessed potential effects after a short diet challenge, which has been previously shown to disrupt metabolic health; however, chronic exposure to a HFHSD would more closely mirror a western diet.

Taken together, developmental exposure to the 23 UOG mixture was associated with increased activity and non-resting energy expenditure in the light cycle, increased exploratory behavior in the EPM test, and decreased sleep and fat pad weight in 12 month female mice. All of these effects were seen in the light cycle when mice are normally less active, suggesting potential adverse effects. Increased risk-taking behavior and decreased sleep could be factors associated with attention deficit and hyperactivity disorders, along with major depressive disorders (48). Interestingly in humans, an association between living close to an unconventional natural gas development and symptoms of depression has been reported (49). Further studies are needed to better understand the behavioral changes observed after developmental exposure to UOG chemicals.

ETHICS STATEMENT

This study was carried out in accordance with the recommendations National Research Council's Guide for the Care and Use of Laboratory Animals. The protocol was approved by the University of Missouri Animal Care and Use Committee.

AUTHOR CONTRIBUTIONS

VB and JC-G performed animal experiments. VB analyzed the data. DR and RR provided pancreas analysis. All authors have contributed to the design of experiments and interpretation of the data.

FUNDING

Funding was received from NIH R21ES026395 (SN), R01ES021394-04S1 (SN and VB), and from the department of Obstetrics, Gynecology and Women's Health, University of Missouri (SN and VB), VA-Merit Grant I01BX003271-01 (RR) and NIH DK088940 (JT), VA Merit Award 1I01BX002567-01 (JT), American Diabetes Association 17-JDF-033 (RS); R01ES028879 (RS); and P30ES027792 (RS).

ACKNOWLEDGMENTS

Thank you to Andrew Wolfe for performing insulin analysis in serum and to the Nagel lab members helping with animal maintenance and necropsy: Angela Meng, Rana Kennedy, Chiamaka Isiguzo, BP, Katelyn Cinnamon, Leighton McCabe, Kara Klemp, Michelle Williams, Naziha Elhassan, and Anne Maas. This work was supported with in part with resources and the use of facilities at the Harry S. Truman Memorial Veterans Hospital in Columbia, MO.

REFERENCES

1. Diamanti-Kandarakis E, Bourguignon JP, Giudice LC, Hauser R, Prins GS, Soto AM, et al. Endocrine-disrupting chemicals: an Endocrine Society scientific statement. *Endocr Rev.* (2009) 30:293–342. doi: 10.1210/er.2009-0002
2. Gore AC, Chappell VA, Fenton SE, Flaws JA, Nadal A, Prins GS, et al. EDC-2: the endocrine society's second scientific statement on endocrine-disrupting chemicals. *Endocr Rev.* (2015) 36:E1–50. doi: 10.1210/er.2015-1010
3. Heindel JJ, Blumberg B, Cave M, Machtinger R, Mantovani A, Mendez MA, et al. Metabolism disrupting chemicals and metabolic disorders. *Reprod Toxicol.* (2017) 68:3–33. doi: 10.1016/j.reprotox.2016.10.001
4. Heindel JJ, Newbold R, Schug TT. Endocrine disruptors and obesity. *Nat Rev Endocrinol.* (2015) 11:653–61. doi: 10.1038/nrendo.2015.163
5. Kassotis CD, Klemp KC, Vu DC, Lin CH, Meng CX, Besch-Williford CL, et al. Endocrine-disrupting activity of hydraulic fracturing chemicals and adverse health outcomes after prenatal exposure in male mice. *Endocrinology.* (2015) 156:4458–73. doi: 10.1210/en.2015-1375
6. Burton GA Jr, Basu N, Ellis BR, Kapo KE, Entrekin S, Nadelhoffer K. Hydraulic "fracking": are surface water impacts an ecological concern? *Environ Toxicol Chem.* (2014) 33:1679–89. doi: 10.1002/etc.2619
7. Ingraffea AR, Wells MT, Santoro RL, Shonkoff SB. Assessment and risk analysis of casing and cement impairment in oil and gas wells in Pennsylvania, 2000-2012. *Proc Natl Acad Sci USA.* (2014) 111:10955–60. doi: 10.1073/pnas.1323422111
8. Kassotis CD, Tillitt DE, Lin CH, McElroy JA, Nagel SC. Endocrine-disrupting chemicals and oil and natural gas operations: potential environmental contamination and recommendations to assess complex environmental mixtures. *Environ Health Perspect.* (2016) 124:256–64. doi: 10.1289/ehp.1409535
9. Mauter MS, Alvarez PJ, Burton A, Cafaro DC, Chen W, Gregory KB, et al. Regional variation in water-related impacts of shale gas development and implications for emerging international plays. *Environ Sci Technol.* (2014) 48:8298–306. doi: 10.1021/es405432k
10. Rozell DJ, Reaven SJ. Water pollution risk associated with natural gas extraction from the Marcellus Shale. *Risk Anal.* (2012) 32:1382–93. doi: 10.1111/j.1539-6924.2011.01757.x
11. Kassotis CD, Iwanowicz LR, Akob DM, Cozzarelli IM, Mumford AC, Orem WH, et al. Endocrine disrupting activities of surface water associated with a West Virginia oil and gas industry wastewater disposal site. *Sci Total Environ.* (2016) 557-8:901–10. doi: 10.1016/j.scitotenv.2016.03.113
12. Kavlock RJ, Daston GP, DeRosa C, Fenner-Crisp P, Gray LE, Kaattari S, et al. Research needs for the risk assessment of health and environmental effects of endocrine disruptors: a report of the U.S. EPA-sponsored workshop. *Environ Health Perspect.* (1996) 104(Suppl. 4):715–40. doi: 10.1289/ehp.96104s4715
13. Schug TT, Janesick A, Blumberg B, Heindel JJ, Endocrine disrupting chemicals and disease susceptibility. *J Steroid Biochem Mol Biol.* (2011) 127:204–15. doi: 10.1016/j.jsbmb.2011.08.007
14. Zoeller RT, Brown TR, Doan LL, Gore AC, Skakkebaek NE, Soto AM, et al. Endocrine-disrupting chemicals and public health protection: a statement of principles from the endocrine society. *Endocrinology.* (2012) 153:4097–110. doi: 10.1210/en.2012-1422
15. Elliott EG, Ettinger AS, Leaderer BP, Bracken MB, Deziel NC. A systematic evaluation of chemicals in hydraulic-fracturing fluids and wastewater for reproductive and developmental toxicity. *J Expo Sci Environ Epidemiol.* (2017) 27:90–9. doi: 10.1038/jes.2015.81
16. Kassotis CD, Nagel SC, Stapleton HM. Unconventional oil and gas chemicals and wastewater-impacted water samples promote adipogenesis via PPARgamma-dependent and independent mechanisms in 3T3-L1 cells. *Sci Total Environ.* (2018) 640-1:1601–10. doi: 10.1016/j.scitotenv.2018.05.030
17. Balise V, Cornelius-Green JN, Kassotis CD, Rector S, Thyfault JP. Preconceptional, gestational, and lactational exposure to an unconventional oil and gas chemical mixture alters energy expenditure in adult female mice. *Front Endocrinol.* (2019) 10:323. doi: 10.3389/fendo.2019.00323
18. Johnson SA, Painter MS, Javurek AB, Ellersieck MR, Wiedmeyer CE, Thyfault JP, et al. Sex-dependent effects of developmental exposure to bisphenol A and ethinyl estradiol on metabolic parameters and voluntary physical activity. *J Dev Orig Health Dis.* (2015) 6:539–52. doi: 10.1017/S2040174415001488
19. Kassotis CD, Bromfield JJ, Klemp KC, Meng CX, Wolfe A, Zoeller RT, et al. Adverse reproductive and developmental health outcomes following prenatal exposure to a hydraulic fracturing chemical mixture in female C57Bl/6 mice. *Endocrinology.* (2016) 157:3469–81. doi: 10.1210/en.2016-1242
20. Gioiosa L, Fissore E, Ghirardelli G, Parmigiani S, Palanza P. Developmental exposure to low-dose estrogenic endocrine disruptors alters sex differences in exploration and emotional responses in mice. *Horm Behav.* (2007) 52:307–16. doi: 10.1016/j.yhbeh.2007.05.006
21. Park YM, Kanaley JA, Padilla J, Zidon T, Welly RJ, Will MJ, et al. Effects of intrinsic aerobic capacity and ovariectomy on voluntary wheel running and nucleus accumbens dopamine receptor gene expression. *Physiol Behav.* (2016) 164:383–9. doi: 10.1016/j.physbeh.2016.06.006
22. Kowalski GM, Nicholls HT, Risis S, Watson NK, Kanellakis P, Bruce CR, et al. Deficiency of haematopoietic-cell-derived IL-10 does not exacerbate high-fat-diet-induced inflammation or insulin resistance in mice. *Diabetologia.* (2011) 54:888–99. doi: 10.1007/s00125-010-2020-5
23. McGuinness OP, Ayala JE, Laughlin MR, Wasserman DH, NIH experiment in centralized mouse phenotyping: the Vanderbilt experience and recommendations for evaluating glucose homeostasis in the mouse. *Am J Physiol Endocrinol Metab.* (2009) 297:E849–55. doi: 10.1152/ajpendo.90996.2008
24. Angle BM, Do RP, Ponzi D, Stahlhut RW, Drury BE, Nagel SC, et al. Metabolic disruption in male mice due to fetal exposure to low but not

high doses of bisphenol A (BPA): evidence for effects on body weight, food intake, adipocytes, leptin, adiponectin, insulin and glucose regulation. *Reprod Toxicol.* (2013) 42:256–68. doi: 10.1016/j.reprotox.2013.07.017
25. Thyfault JP, Rector RS, Uptergrove GM, Borengasser SJ, Morris EM, Wei Y, et al. Rats selectively bred for low aerobic capacity have reduced hepatic mitochondrial oxidative capacity and susceptibility to hepatic steatosis and injury. *J Physiol.* (2009) 587:1805–16. doi: 10.1113/jphysiol.2009.169060
26. Poudel A, Savari O, Striegel DA, Periwal V, Taxy J, Millis JM, et al. Beta-cell destruction and preservation in childhood and adult onset type 1 diabetes. *Endocrine.* (2015) 49:693–702. doi: 10.1007/s12020-015-0534-9
27. Poudel A, Fowler JL, Zielinski MC, Kilimnik G, Hara M. Stereological analyses of the whole human pancreas. *Sci Rep.* (2016) 6:34049. doi: 10.1038/srep34049
28. Byers SL, Wiles MV, Dunn SL, Taft RA. Mouse estrous cycle identification tool and images. *PLoS ONE.* (2012) 7:e35538. doi: 10.1371/journal.pone.0035538
29. Walf AA, Frye CA, The use of the elevated plus maze as an assay of anxiety-related behavior in rodents. *Nat Protoc.* (2007) 2:322–8. doi: 10.1038/nprot.2007.44
30. Oosterman JE, Kalsbeek A, la Fleur SE, Belsham DD. Impact of nutrients on circadian rhythmicity. *Am J Physiol Regul Integr Comp Physiol.* (2015) 308:R337–50. doi: 10.1152/ajpregu.00322.2014
31. Palmisano BT, Stafford JM, Pendergast JS. High-fat feeding does not disrupt daily rhythms in female mice because of protection by ovarian hormones. *Front Endocrinol.* (2017) 8:44. doi: 10.3389/fendo.2017.00044
32. Ressler IB, Grayson BE, Ulrich-Lai YM, Seeley RJ. Diet-induced obesity exacerbates metabolic and behavioral effects of polycystic ovary syndrome in a rodent model. *Am J Physiol Endocrinol Metab.* (2015) 308:E1076–84. doi: 10.1152/ajpendo.00182.2014
33. Feng Y, Shao R, Weijdegard B, Wang T, Johansson J, Sun S, et al. Effects of androgen and leptin on behavioral and cellular responses in female rats. *Horm Behav.* (2011) 60:427–38. doi: 10.1016/j.yhbeh.2011.07.012
34. Manti M, Fornes R, Qi X, Folmerz E, Linden Hirschberg A, de Castro Barbosa T, et al. Maternal androgen excess and obesity induce sexually dimorphic anxiety-like behavior in the offspring. *FASEB J.* (2018) 32:4158–71. doi: 10.1096/fj.201701263RR
35. Xu X, Yang Y, Wang R, Wang Y, Ruan Q, Lu Y. Perinatal exposure to di-(2-ethylhexyl) phthalate affects anxiety- and depression-like behaviors in mice. *Chemosphere.* (2015) 124:22–31. doi: 10.1016/j.chemosphere.2014.10.056
36. Hu M, Richard JE, Maliqueo M, Kokosar M, Fornes R, Benrick A, et al. Maternal testosterone exposure increases anxiety-like behavior and impacts the limbic system in the offspring. *Proc Natl Acad Sci USA.* (2015) 112:14348–53. doi: 10.1073/pnas.1507514112
37. Gioiosa L, Parmigiani S, Vom Saal FS, Palanza P. The effects of bisphenol A on emotional behavior depend upon the timing of exposure, age and gender in mice. *Horm Behav.* (2013) 63:598–605. doi: 10.1016/j.yhbeh.2013.02.016
38. Soares-Cunha C, Coimbra B, Borges S, Domingues AV, Silva D, Sousa N, et al. Mild prenatal stress causes emotional and brain structural modifications in rats of both sexes. *Front Behav Neurosci.* (2018) 12:129. doi: 10.3389/fnbeh.2018.00129
39. Zeng Y, Brydges NM, Wood ER, Drake AJ, Hall J. Prenatal glucocorticoid exposure in rats: programming effects on stressreactivity and cognition in adult offspring. *Stress.* (2015) 18:353–61. doi: 10.3109/10253890.2015.1055725
40. Velisek L. Prenatal corticosteroid exposure alters early developmental seizures and behavior. *Epilepsy Res.* (2011) 95:9–19. doi: 10.1016/j.eplepsyres.2011.01.019
41. Rayburn WF, Christensen HD, Gonzalez CL, Rayburn LA, Stewart JD. Effect of in utero exposure to betamethasone on motivation/anxiety testing in mice offspring. *Neurotoxicol Teratol.* (1998) 20:475–81. doi: 10.1016/S0892-0362(97)00131-1
42. Reddy DS, O'Malley BW, Rogawski MA. Anxiolytic activity of progesterone in progesterone receptor knockout mice. *Neuropharmacology.* (2005) 48:14–24. doi: 10.1016/j.neuropharm.2004.09.002
43. Melancia F, Servadio M, Schiavi S, Campolongo P, Giusti-Paiva A, Trezza V. Testing the correlation between experimentally-induced hypothyroidism during pregnancy and autistic-like symptoms in the rat offspring. *Behav Brain Res.* (2017) 321:113–22. doi: 10.1016/j.bbr.2016.12.032
44. Gross SA, Avens HJ, Banducci AM, Sahmel J, Panko JM, Tvermoes BE. Analysis of BTEX groundwater concentrations from surface spills associated with hydraulic fracturing operations. *J Air Waste Manag Assoc.* (2013) 63:424–32. doi: 10.1080/10962247.2012.759166
45. Orem W, Tatu C, Varonka M, Lerch H, Bates A, Engle M, et al. Organic substances in produced and formation water from unconventional natural gas extraction in coal and shale. *Int J Coal Geol.* (2014) 126:20–31. doi: 10.1016/j.coal.2014.01.003
46. US. EPA. *Assessment of the Potential Impacts of Hydraulic Fracturing for Oil and Gas on Drinking Water Resources (External Review Draft).* Washington, DC: US Environmental Protection Agency, EPA/600/R-15/047 (2015).
47. vom Saal FS, Welshons WV. Large effects from small exposures. II. The importance of positive controls in low-dose research on bisphenol A. *Environ Res.* (2006) 100:50–76. doi: 10.1016/j.envres.2005.09.001
48. Martel MM, Klump K, Nigg JT, Breedlove SM, Sisk CL. Potential hormonal mechanisms of attention-deficit/hyperactivity disorder and major depressive disorder: a new perspective. *Horm Behav.* (2009) 55:465–79. doi: 10.1016/j.yhbeh.2009.02.004
49. Casey JA, Wilcox HC, Hirsch AG, Pollak J, Schwartz BS. Associations of unconventional natural gas development with depression symptoms and disordered sleep in Pennsylvania. *Sci Rep.* (2018) 8:11375. doi: 10.1038/s41598-018-29747-2

5

Current Research Approaches and Challenges in the Obesogen Field

Raquel Chamorro-Garcia [1] *and Bruce Blumberg* [1,2,3*]

[1] *Department of Developmental and Cell Biology, University of California, Irvine, Irvine, CA, United States,* [2] *Department of Pharmaceutical Sciences, University of California, Irvine, Irvine, CA, United States,* [3] *Department of Biomedical Engineering, University of California, Irvine, Irvine, CA, United States*

Correspondence:
Bruce Blumberg
blumberg@uci.edu

Obesity is a worldwide pandemic that also contributes to the increased incidence of other diseases such as type 2 diabetes. Increased obesity is generally ascribed to positive energy balance. However, recent findings suggest that exposure to endocrine-disrupting chemicals such as obesogens during critical windows of development, may play an important role in the current obesity trends. Several experimental approaches, from *in vitro* cell cultures to transgenerational *in vivo* studies, are used to better understand the mechanisms of action of obesogens, each of which contributes to answer different questions. In this review, we discuss current knowledge in the obesogen field and the existing tools developed in research laboratories using tributyltin as a model obesogen. By understanding the advantages and limitations of each of these tools, we will better focus and design experimental approaches that will help expanding the obesogen field with the objective of finding potential therapeutic targets in human populations.

Keywords: obesogens, obesity, MSCs, 3T3-L1, transgeneration, isoDMBs, tributyltin, metabolism

In the last 40 years obesity rates have dramatically increased worldwide both in adults and in youth (1). A recent report on obesity trends in the U.S. estimated that 39.8% of adults are clinically obese (BMI > 30) (1). Importantly, obesity is a risk factor for other metabolic disorders such as type 2 diabetes whose prevalence has increased in parallel with obesity and which is predicted to affect 642 million people worldwide by 2040 (2, 3). The health costs associated with obesity were estimated at over $275 annually in the U.S alone (4). Although the major driving factor in obesity is usually considered to be a simple function of energy balance (calorie consumption higher than calorie expenditure) (5), recent reports showing the increasing trends of obesity in children under 1 year of age and in animal populations suggest that other factors may be playing important roles in obesity (6, 7). Understanding those factors, the windows of susceptibility and the mechanisms through which they to alter human metabolism and promote obesity will aid treating and preventing the increasing rates of obesity and related disorders worldwide.

Obesity is sexually dimorphic (8). Overall, females accumulate more fat than males, and it tends to be located subcutaneously, while in males, adipose tissue tends to accumulate in the visceral cavity. Subcutaneous adipose tissue is generally associated with healthier fat since it is involved in regulating thermogenesis while visceral adipose tissue is associated with increased risk of cardiovascular disease (9). Adipose tissue is now known not only for its ability to store lipids, but also for its contribution to metabolic homeostasis by secreting hormones (e.g., leptin and adiponectin) and other signaling molecules involved in the regulation of appetite and fat mobilization. This suggests that maintaining a healthy and functional adipose tissue improves the overall metabolic state of the individual (9). The sexually dimorphic content and distribution of fat is highly influenced by steroid hormones such as testosterone and estrogens (8). Therefore, alterations of the endocrine system may contribute to disturbances in the regulation of adipose tissue formation and maintenance.

Endocrine disrupting chemicals (EDCs) are exogenous chemicals that alter the natural function of hormones (10). Several human and animal studies have found associations between exposure to EDCs and increased adiposity (11–16). However, the effects of EDCs that may lead to obesity might not be linked exclusively to life style or environmental exposures during adulthood. Epidemiological studies have shown that the environment during *in utero* development may affect the prevalence of non-communicable diseases, including metabolic disorders, later in life (13–21). Notably, the nutritional state of the mother is strongly linked to body weight of the offspring at birth and later in life (22–26) suggesting that suboptimal environments during development may contribute to permanent alterations in the individual that will counteract any lifestyle actions to ameliorate weight gain, thereby increasing susceptibility to obesity (22, 27).

A large body of evidence shows that exposure to environmental pollutants during *in utero* development and early life may contribute to obesity later in life (11). Studies performed using both *in vitro* and *in vivo* models showed that a subset of endocrine disrupting chemicals, called obesogens, can have important effects on the development of adipose tissue. Obesogens are exogenous chemicals that inappropriately stimulate adipogenesis and fat storage, can disturb adipose tissue homeostasis and affect metabolic rates and/or the regulation of appetite and satiety (28). Our recent findings suggested that one consequence of these disturbances is the alteration of the metabolic setpoint of the individual, that is, the capability of the body maintain a particular weight regardless of the lifestyle changes taken to increase or reduce that weight (29). These results are supported by human studies showing an association between higher levels of perfluoroalkyl compounds in plasma and a more rapid weight regain after diet-induced weight loss plan (12). Moreover, individuals with the highest levels of perfluoroaklyl compounds has the lowest resting metabolic rate (12). Despite numerous studies demonstrating the existence and effects of obesogens, a longstanding debate about the mechanisms through which obesogens exert their obesogenic effects still persists. In this review, we discuss the current experimental approaches to study the mechanisms of function of obesogens from *in vitro* analysis to transgenerational *in vivo* studies.

IN VITRO APPROACHES

The prototypical obesogen tributyltin (TBT) is known to activate two nuclear receptors critical for adipogenesis. These are the peroxisome proliferator-activated receptor gamma (PPARγ)(30–33), which is considered to be the master regulator of adipogenesis (34), and its heterodimeric partner the retinoid X receptor (RXR)(30), which we recently showed to be an important regulator of adipocyte commitment (35). Adipogenic commitment is the process through which multipotent mesenchymal stem cells (MSC) lose their multipotency and become irreversibly destined to the adipocyte lineage, in part via the expression of PPARγ2. Activation of PPARγ2 elicits terminal differentiation into white adipose tissue (36). Other already characterized obesogens such as fludioxonil, quinoxyfen, dibutyltin or triphenyltin, also activate PPARγ and/or RXR (37, 38), suggesting that these nuclear receptors are common targets for EDCs. However, nuclear receptors other than PPARγ2 and RXR have been shown to play important roles in adipogenesis, including the glucocorticoid receptor (GR) (39), estrogen receptor (ER) (40) and androgen receptor (AR) (41) and obesogens such as tolylfluanid, bisphenol A (BPA) or dichlorodiphenyltrichloroethane (DDT) have been shown to act through them (42–44). The fact that estrogen and androgen receptors are also involved in regulation of adipogenesis and fat storage, may explain, at least in part, the sexually dimorphic distribution of the fat in individuals from different genders. Therefore, assessing the capability of a candidate obesogen to induce adipogenic commitment, its ability to promote final adipocyte differentiation, and the mechanisms through which these processes occur requires the use of an array of assays that tests the various potential paths used by obesogens to promote fat storage.

One frequently used tool to screen for new obesogens is the murine pre-adipocyte cell line 3T3-L1 (45). This immortalized cell line has some beneficial aspects that include the short length of the assay and the amenability of cell lines to high throughput screening approaches. However, one key limitation of 3T3-L1 cells is that, since they are already pre-adipocytes, they are not useful for examining mechanisms, including screening for chemicals that may be involved in adipocyte commitment. It was recently suggested that the commercial source of the cell line (e.g., ATCC or Zenbio), the type of plates used, as well as the number of passages the cells have experienced play a critical role in the process of cell differentiation (46). 3T3-L1 cells from different commercial sources showed different expression of nuclear receptors such as PPARγ, RXRβ, and ERβ, and variable capability to differentiate into adipocytes using well-established adipogenic positive controls such as rosiglitazone (PPARγ activator) or TBT (46). These findings highlight some of the limitations of using 3T3-L1 cells as an adipogenic model when the goal is to hypothesize about *in vivo* outcomes after exposure to obesogens. Screening of new obesogens using this model will depend critically on poorly controlled variables such as the source and number of passages of the cells, bovine sera, inconsistencies in coatings on tissue culture plates and other culture conditions which can confound reproducibility of the results.

In contrast, assays performed with uncommitted cells such as MSCs (47), allow analyses with a broader scope. We recently described for the first time the role of RXR in adipogenic commitment using MSCs as a cell model, revealing that this phase of adipogenesis can be targeted by obesogens (35). Others have used murine cell lines such as C3H/10T1/2 which resemble MSCs in some properties (but contain a karyotype of 80 chromosomes), or BMS2 to screen for new obesogens or to dive into adipogenic mechanisms through which obesogens may act. Although both cell types are accepted adipogenic models (48, 49), they are both immortalized cell lines that do not fully recapitulate the behavior of uncommitted precursors *in vivo*. Both are also murine cells which can somewhat limit the extrapolation of results to other species. Therefore, conclusions and inferences made from the use of these cells should account for such limitations. One advantage of using MSCs is that they can be isolated as primary cells from different individuals in a variety of species allowing a more extensive analysis. The use of human MSCs can also allow researchers to assess the variability that exists in human populations, which would contribute to a deeper understanding of the role obesogens may play in the current obesity pandemic.

IN VIVO APPROACHES

TBT has been shown to act as an obesogen in multiple organisms including mice (30–32, 50–52) rats (53), goldfish (54), and zebrafish (55) which supports the hypothesis that obesogens are largely not species specific. However, although there are several *in vitro* models available to study the molecular underpinnings of obesogen exposure, the mechanisms through which obesogens contribute to obesity in animal models are likely to be more complex than those described for cell cultures. Experiments performed in adult rodents exposed to TBT showed alterations of the hypothalamic-pituitary-gonadal axis (56) as well as non-alcoholic fatty liver (52) supporting the current knowledge that the regulation of metabolism requires coordination between different organs including fat tissue, liver, muscle, pancreas, or brain.

Another source of discussion in the obesogen field is related to the functionality of the adipocytes produced after exposure to obesogens (57). As mentioned above, the adipose tissue has an important role to play in maintaining an overall healthy metabolic state (58). Interestingly, white fat cells produced by TBT exposure lack some beneficial properties of normal white adipocytes since the former show reduced levels of the antidiabetic hormone adiponectin, reduced glucose uptake capability, impaired ability to develop into thermogenic beige/brite adipocytes and increased expression of pro-inflammatory and pro-fibrotic genes (57, 59, 60). These results suggest that TBT promotes the development of dysfunctional adipocytes (57, 59, 60). Understanding which obesogens produce adipocytes of normal function and which elicit the production of dysfunctional adipocytes may also contribute to a better understanding of the potential mechanistic differences between different obesogens.

TRANSGENERATIONAL APPROACHES

It has been shown that some obesogens including TBT, DDT, and BPA, are able to induce heritable changes that are propagated through multiple generations without any further exposure (29, 61–64). The non-Mendelian transmission of these alterations suggests that epigenetic mechanisms are involved in this process. This raises yet another challenge for the obesogen field: what are the mechanisms underlying transgenerational inheritance?

The field of environmental epigenetics studies the epigenetic alterations introduced by environmental factors that contribute to phenotypic variation and/or disease (65). Studies performed in animal models showed that exposure to obesogens during development increased predisposition to obesity not only in the directly exposed F1 and F2 generations (F2 are exposed as germ cells inside the F1 fetus) but also in subsequent F3 and F4 generations (and beyond) which are not exposed (29, 61–64, 66, 67). These studies showed alterations of epigenetic factors such as DNA methylation and post-translational histone modifications in somatic tissues and/or germ cells (29, 61–64, 66–68). However, there are key knowledge gaps in this transgenerational puzzle, including the characterization of the molecular mechanisms that occur in the directly exposed stages that trigger the transgenerational phenotype, and the molecular mechanisms by which these alterations are transmitted through multiple generations.

There is extensive epigenetic reprogramming at different stages of mammalian development. Shortly after fertilization, the first erasure of epigenetic marks (DNA methylation) occurs from the zygote to the blastocyst during maternal-to-zygotic transition in a sex-specific manner (69). Between E 6.5 and E 13.5, after somatic and germ lines separate, the primordial germ cells (PGCs) undergo another round of DNA methylation erasure while they travel to the genital ridge where they will mature into sex-specific germ cells (70). Considering that from the moment of fertilization until birth there is an extensive epigenetic reprogramming of various epigenetic marks, the presence of agents that may disturb these processes, such as obesogens and other EDCs, at any of the stages may contribute to alterations in the newly determined epigenetic landscape. Since this reprogramming occurs in every generation, it is critical to determine which alterations are introduced by environmental factors and how many of these epigenomic changes can be propagated to subsequent generations in order to better understand mechanisms of transgenerational inheritance. This is currently a very controversial topic in the field (63, 65, 68, 71–73).

We recently proposed a new mechanism for the transmission of epigenetic information. In our transgenerational paradigm, we exposed pregnant F0 female mice to environmentally relevant doses of the obesogen TBT throughout pregnancy (61) or throughout pregnancy and lactation (29). Following either approach, we consistently found increased adiposity in F3 and F4 males, but not females (29, 61). Interestingly, the differences in fat storage between controls and ancestrally-TBT treated animals was exacerbated when the diet of the animals was switched from a standard diet to a diet with higher fat content (29). This supports the hypothesis that ancestral exposure to TBT alters the metabolic set point of these animals multiple generations after exposure has ceased (29). Integrative methylome and transcriptome analyses of fat tissue isolated from obese F4 males did not reveal any direct associations between changes in mRNA expression levels of genes whose promoter was either hypermethylated or hypomethylated. In contrast, we found a significant number of differentially methylated regions (DMR) located in intergenic regions. We re-analyzed the data, focusing on large blocks of the genome where the alteration in DNA methylation was in the same direction (hypo- or hyper-methylated) and denoted these as **iso**directional, **d**ifferentially **m**ethylated **b**locks (isoDMBs). IsoDMBs spanned large regions of the genome and we found a strong association between hypomethylated isoDMBs and over-expressed genes and between hypermethylated isoDMBs and under-expressed genes (29). Additionally, analysis of chromatin accessibility in sperm samples from F3 and F4 mice showed significant overlaps in accessibility between sperm samples in both generations (**Figure 1A**), suggesting that there is a conservation of the differentially accessible regions across generations. We also found an intriguing association between chromatin accessibility in sperm and isoDMBs in white adipose tissue of F4 male mice (**Figure 1B**). Regions that were inaccessible in sperm were hypomethylated in fat and regions that were accessible in sperm were hypermethylated in fat. We inferred that altered chromatin accessibility in the germ cells may promote or permit differential DNA methylation, epigenetic marks and gene expression in somatic tissues of the next generation (**Figure 1C**) (29).

We also noted that hypomethylated isoDMBs tend to be located in areas of the genome with high GC content, whereas hypermethylated isoDMBs are located in areas of the genome with low GC content (**Figure 1D**). In other words, rather than being located randomly distributed throughout the genome, changes in methylation were enriched in regions with specific base composition (GC content) (29). Others have shown that there is an association between base composition and higher order chromatin organization in the nucleus (74). This led us to hypothesize that *in utero* exposure to TBT causes heritable alterations in chromatin architecture that will contribute to changes in the epigenetic landscape that are reflected in the transcriptome (29). This new model provides a potential molecular mechanism that embraces previously described results showing alterations of epigenetic marks, such as DNA methylation, histone modification and expression of small non-coding RNAs in germ cells and somatic cells after ancestral exposure to EDCs such obesogens (62–64, 66, 67).

WINDOWS OF SUSCEPTIBILITY

There are different windows of susceptibility to obesity after obesogen exposure. Rodents exposed to obesogens such as TBT or nonylphenol during early adulthood showed increased ectopic lipid storage in liver elevated body weight, and altered levels of metabolic hormones (52, 75). BPA or tolylfluanid exposure led to alterations in glucose metabolism and adiposity in adult mice (76, 77). Some of the metabolic alterations are only observed when the animals are exposed to high fat diets or high fat/high sugar diets (75, 77), suggesting that obesogen exposure may be increasing susceptibility to obesity in the presence of other metabolic challenges. This has important implications for the human obesity pandemic.

Exposures during *in utero* development have the potential to affect critical developmental steps that may have dramatic effects not only in the offspring, but in subsequent generations. Two different approaches have been used to study the effects of obesogens within early developmental windows: exposure of females throughout pregnancy (from fertilization to birth) (29, 37, 61) and exposure at discrete embryonic stages (E8–E14) (62–64, 67). The objective of the latter is to expose the embryos only

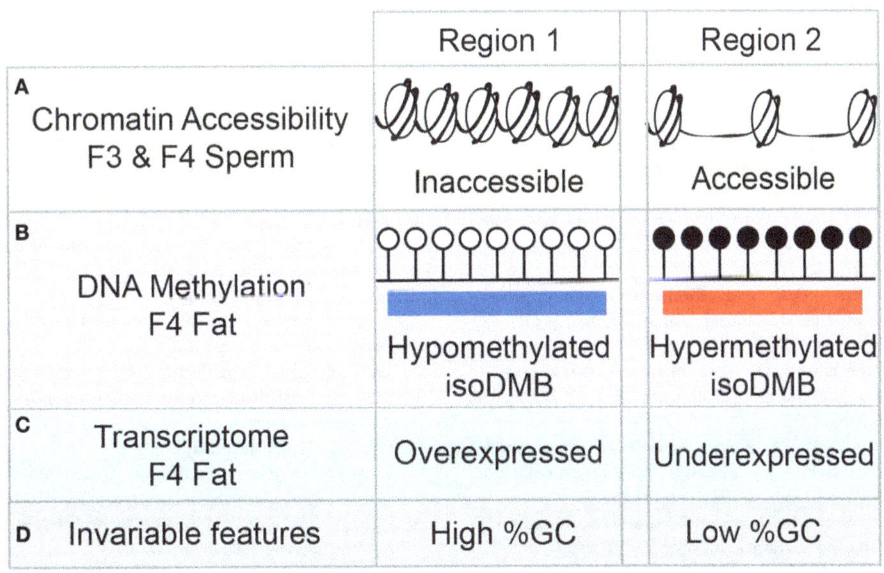

FIGURE 1 | Schematic summary of the results from (29). Region 1 represents that genomic areas inaccessible in sperm samples of F3 and F4 mice **(A)** are hypomethylated in fat tissue of F4 males **(B)**, and the genes contained in those regions tend to be overexpressed **(C)**. Opposite trends are found in genomic areas represented by Region 2, with high accessibility in F3 and F4 sperm samples, and hypermethylation and underexpression in fat tissue. Genomic areas depicted by Region 1 have content of GCs, whereas genomic areas depicted by Region 2 have low GC content **(D)**.

during the time the primordial germ cells (PGCs) are traveling to the genital ridge, and during which DNA methylation is largely erased (70). However, the benefit of studying the former approach is that it allows the exposure to obesogens throughout the different phases of embryonic development, all of which may be important for obesity in later generations.

Another important factor that must be considered when assessing the effect of environmental pollutants using animal models is the concentration the animals are receiving. In order to be able to extrapolate the information obtained from animal studies to humans, it is necessary to work with concentrations of EDCs that are in the realm of what human exposure is measured or estimated to be. Typically, the chemical doses at which the endocrine system is altered are significantly lower than the concentrations that induce toxic effects in the body (44).

SUMMARY AND FUTURE DIRECTIONS

Since the obesogen hypothesis was first proposed, studies in many laboratories have supported the existence and effects of obesogens (78). The list of *bona fide* obesogens (those shown to influence obesity, *in vivo*) continues to grow and mechanisms through which these chemicals act to promote obesity are emerging. Experimental approaches to study these mechanisms are improving. *In vitro* studies continue to provide a strong foundation to evaluate the effects of obesogens in cells, particularly as more investigators adopt stem cell models, over the limited studies possible in 3T3-L1 preadipocytes. These cell culture-based studies offer the possibility to increase the numbers of chemicals screened and may reveal new mechanisms or hypotheses about the effects of these chemicals using *in vivo* animal models. Current technology based on deep sequencing in bulk or in single cells will allow extensive whole-genome analyses that can provide information critical to understanding the epigenomic and transcriptomal state of the cells in different tissues and life stages. A major challenge in this area will be to integrate and interpret these large, multi-omic data sets to provide the most useful information.

Another major obstacle in understanding the effects of EDCs and obesogens in humans is the paucity of exposure data, particularly data from longitudinal prospective cohort studies. In addition, humans are exposed to mixtures of EDCs throughout the life course. Fortunately, experimental researchers and epidemiologists are teaming up and the advent of "exposome" studies that assess and analyze levels of exposure to obesogens together with a multitude of other chemicals, including EDCs, will enable strong mechanistic links to be made between chemical exposure and human disease (79). This will inform and guide future laboratory and epidemiological approaches that will overcome the current limitations. In turn, this will allow us to assess the costs to society of EDC and obesogen exposure more accurately. In an optimistic view, this information might influence policy makers to take appropriate steps to protect the public health.

AUTHOR CONTRIBUTIONS

RC-G and BB participated in the discussion of and wrote the ideas reflected in this review.

ACKNOWLEDGMENTS

This work was supported by awards from the National Institutes of Health (ES023316, ES021832) to BB. BB is a named inventor on patents related to nuclear receptors some of which have been licensed to for profit entities.

REFERENCES

1. Hales C, Carroll M, Fryar CD, Ogden CL. *Prevalence of Obesity Among Adults and Youth: United States, 2015–2016, NCHS Data Brief.*, Hyattsville, MD: U.S. Department of Health & Human Services (2017).
2. Menke A, Casagrande S, Geiss L, Cowie CC. Prevalence of and trends in diabetes among adults in the United States, 1988-2012. *JAMA.* (2015) 314:1021–9. doi: 10.1001/jama.2015.10029
3. Kahn SE, Hull RL, Utzschneider KM. Mechanisms linking obesity to insulin resistance and type 2 diabetes. *Nature.* (2006) 444:840–6. doi: 10.1038/nature05482
4. Biener A, Cawley J, Meyerhoefer C. The high and rising costs of obesity to the US health care system. *J Gen Intern Med.* (2017) 32:6–8. doi: 10.1007/s11606-016-3968-8
5. Hall KD, Heymsfield SB, Kemnitz JW, Klein S, Schoeller DA, Speakman JR. Energy balance and its components: implications for body weight regulation. *Am J Clin Nutr.* (2012) 95:989–94. doi: 10.3945/ajcn.112.036350
6. Ng M, Fleming T, Robinson M, Thomson B, Graetz N, Margono C. et al., Global, regional, and national prevalence of overweight and obesity in children and adults during 1980-2013: a systematic analysis for the Global Burden of Disease Study 2013. *Lancet.* (2014) 384:766–81. doi: 10.1016/S0140-6736(14)60460-8
7. Klimentidis YC, Beasley TM, Lin HY, Murati G, Glass GE, Guyton M. et al. Canaries in the coal mine: a cross-species analysis of the plurality of obesity epidemics. *Proc Biol Sci.* (2011) 278:1626–32. doi: 10.1098/rspb.2010.1890
8. Palmer BF, Clegg DJ. The sexual dimorphism of obesity. *Mol Cell Endocrinol.* (2015) 402:113–9. doi: 10.1016/j.mce.2014.11.029
9. Trayhurn P. Endocrine and signalling role of adipose tissue: new perspectives on fat. *Acta Physiol Scand.* (2005) 184:285–93. doi: 10.1111/j.1365-201X.2005.01468.x
10. Zoeller RT, Brown TR, Doan LL, Gore AC, Skakkebaek NE, Soto AM, et al. Endocrine-disrupting chemicals and public health protection: a statement of principles from the endocrine society. *Endocrinology.* (2012) 153:4097–110. doi: 10.1210/en.2012-1422
11. Darbre PD. Endocrine disruptors and obesity. *Curr Obes Rep.* (2017) 6:18–27. doi: 10.1007/s13679-017-0240-4
12. Liu G, Dhana K, Furtado JD, Rood J, Zong G, Liang L, et al. Perfluoroalkyl substances and changes in body weight and resting metabolic rate in response to weight-loss diets: a prospective study. *PLoS Med.* (2018) 15:e1002502. doi: 10.1371/journal.pmed.1002502
13. Mendez MA, Garcia-Esteban R, Guxens M, Vrijheid M, Kogevinas M, Goni F, et al. Prenatal organochlorine compound exposure, rapid weight gain, and overweight in infancy. *Environ Health Perspect.* (2011) 119:272–8. doi: 10.1289/ehp.1002169
14. Valvi D, Mendez MA, Garcia-Esteban R, Ballester F, Ibarluzea J, Goni F, et al. Prenatal exposure to persistent organic pollutants and rapid weight gain and overweight in infancy. *Obesity (Silver Spring).* (2014) 22:488–96. doi: 10.1002/oby.20603
15. Valvi D, Mendez MA, Martinez D, Grimalt JO, Torrent M, Sunyer J, et al. Prenatal concentrations of polychlorinated biphenyls, DDE, and DDT and

overweight in children: a prospective birth cohort study. *Environ Health Perspect.* (2012) 120:451–7. doi: 10.1289/ehp.1103862
16. Erkin-Cakmak A, Harley KG, Chevrier J, Bradman A, Kogut K, Huen K, et al. In utero and childhood polybrominated diphenyl ether exposures and body mass at age 7 years: the CHAMACOS study. *Environ Health Perspect.* (2015) 123:636–42. doi: 10.1289/ehp.1408417
17. Hanson MA, Gluckman PD. Early developmental conditioning of later health and disease: physiology or pathophysiology? *Physiol Rev.* (2014) 94:1027–76. doi: 10.1152/physrev.00029.2013
18. Stein Z. *Famine and Human Development : The Dutch Hunger Winter of 1944-1945*, New York, NY: Oxford University Press (1975).
19. Barker DJ, Bull AR, Osmond C, Simmonds SJ. Fetal and placental size and risk of hypertension in adult life. *BMJ.* (1990) 301:259–62. doi: 10.1136/bmj.301.6746.259
20. Barker DJ, Winter PD, Osmond C, Margetts B, Simmonds SJ. Weight in infancy and death from ischaemic heart disease. *Lancet.* (1989) 2:577–80. doi: 10.1016/S0140-6736(89)90710-1
21. Hales CN, Barker DJ, Clark PM, Cox LJ, Fall C, Osmond C, et al. Fetal and infant growth and impaired glucose tolerance at age 64. *BMJ.* (1991) 303:1019–22. doi: 10.1136/bmj.303.6809.1019
22. Gluckman PD, Hanson M, Zimmet P, Forrester T. Losing the war against obesity: the need for a developmental perspective. *Sci Transl Med.* (2011) 3:93cm19. doi: 10.1126/scitranslmed.3002554
23. Godfrey KM, Reynolds RM, Prescott SL, Nyirenda M, Jaddoe VW, Eriksson JG, et al. of maternal obesity on the long-term health of offspring. *Lancet Diabetes Endocrinol.* (2017) 5:53–64. doi: 10.1016/S2213-8587(16)30107-3
24. Forsen T, Eriksson JG, Tuomilehto J, Teramo K, Osmond C, Barker DJ. Mother's weight in pregnancy and coronary heart disease in a cohort of Finnish men: follow up study. *BMJ.* (1997) 315:837–40. doi: 10.1136/bmj.315.7112.837
25. Lawlor DA, Relton C, Sattar N, Nelson SM. Maternal adiposity–a determinant of perinatal and offspring outcomes? *Nat Rev Endocrinol.* (2012) 8:679–88. doi: 10.1038/nrendo.2012.176
26. Desai M, Hales CN. Role of fetal and infant growth in programming metabolism in later life. *Biol Rev Camb Philos Soc.* (1997) 72:329–48. doi: 10.1017/S0006323196005026
27. Lin XY, Lim IY, Wu YH, Teh AL, Chen L, Aris IM, et al. Developmental pathways to adiposity begin before birth and are influenced by genotype, prenatal environment and epigenome. *BMC Med.* (2017) 15:50. doi: 10.1186/s12916-017-0800-1
28. Janesick AS, Blumberg B. Obesogens: an emerging threat to public health. *Am J Obstet Gynecol.* (2016) 214:559–65. doi: 10.1016/j.ajog.2016.01.182
29. Chamorro-Garcia R, Diaz-Castillo C, Shoucri BM, Kach H, Leavitt R, Shioda T, et al. Ancestral perinatal obesogen exposure results in a transgenerational thrifty phenotype in mice. *Nat Commun.* (2017) 8:2012. doi: 10.1038/s41467-017-01944-z
30. Grun F, Watanabe H, Zamanian Z, Maeda L, Arima K, Cubacha R, et al. Endocrine-disrupting organotin compounds are potent inducers of adipogenesis in vertebrates. *Mol Endocrinol.* (2006) 20:2141–55. doi: 10.1210/me.2005-0367
31. Kirchner S, Kieu T, Chow C, Casey S, Blumberg B. Prenatal exposure to the environmental obesogen tributyltin predisposes multipotent stem cells to become adipocytes. *Mol Endocrinol.* (2010) 24:526–39. doi: 10.1210/me.2009-0261
32. Li X, Ycaza J, Blumberg B. The environmental obesogen tributyltin chloride acts via peroxisome proliferator activated receptor gamma to induce adipogenesis in murine 3T3-L1 preadipocytes. *J Steroid Biochem Mol Biol.* (2011) 127:9–15. doi: 10.1016/j.jsbmb.2011.03.012
33. Kanayama T, Kobayashi N, Mamiya S, Nakanishi T, Nishikawa J. Organotin compounds promote adipocyte differentiation as agonists of the peroxisome proliferator-activated receptor gamma/retinoid X receptor pathway. *Mol Pharmacol.* (2005) 67:766–74. doi: 10.1124/mol.104.0 08409
34. Tontonoz P, Spiegelman BM. Fat and beyond: the diverse biology of PPARgamma. *Annu Rev Biochem.* (2008) 77:289–312. doi: 10.1146/annurev.biochem.77.061307.091829
35. Shoucri BM, Martinez ES, Abreo TJ, Hung VT, Moosova Z, Shioda T, et al. Retinoid X receptor activation alters the chromatin landscape to commit mesenchymal stem cells to the adipose lineage. *Endocrinology.* (2017) 158:3109–25. doi: 10.1210/en.2017-00348
36. Cristancho AG, Lazar MA. Forming functional fat: a growing understanding of adipocyte differentiation. *Nat Rev Mol Cell Biol.* (2011) 12:722–34. doi: 10.1038/nrm3198
37. Chamorro-Garcia R, Shoucri BM, Willner S, Kach H, Janesick A, Blumberg B. Effects of perinatal exposure to dibutyltin chloride on fat and glucose metabolism in mice, and molecular mechanisms, in vitro. *Environ Health Perspect.* (2018) 126:057006. doi: 10.1289/EHP3030
38. Janesick AS, Dimastrogiovanni G, Vanek L, Boulos C, Chamorro-Garcia R, Tang W, et al. On the utility of toxcast and toxpi as methods for identifying new obesogens. *Environ Health Perspect.* (2016) 124:1214–26. doi: 10.1289/ehp.1510352
39. Steger DJ, Grant GR, Schupp M, Tomaru T, Lefterova MI, Schug J, et al. Propagation of adipogenic signals through an epigenomic transition state. *Genes Dev.* (2010) 24:1035–44. doi: 10.1101/gad.1907110
40. Cooke PS, Naaz A. Role of estrogens in adipocyte development and function. *Exp Biol Med (Maywood).* (2004) 229:1127–35. doi: 10.1177/153537020422901107
41. Dieudonne MN, Pecquery R, Boumediene A, Leneveu MC, Giudicelli Y. Androgen receptors in human preadipocytes and adipocytes: regional specificities and regulation by sex steroids. *Am J Physiol.* (1998) 274:C1645–52. doi: 10.1152/ajpcell.1998.274.6.C1645
42. Sargis RM, Johnson DN, Choudhury RA, Brady MJ. Environmental endocrine disruptors promote adipogenesis in the 3T3-L1 cell line through glucocorticoid receptor activation. *Obesity (Silver Spring).* (2010) 18:1283–8. doi: 10.1038/oby.2009.419
43. Newbold RR, Padilla-Banks E, Snyder RJ, Jefferson WN. Perinatal exposure to environmental estrogens and the development of obesity. *Mol Nutr Food Res.* (2007) 51:912–7. doi: 10.1002/mnfr.200600259
44. Vandenberg LN, Colborn T, Hayes TB, Heindel JJ, Shioda T, Soto AM, et al. Hormones and endocrine-disrupting chemicals: low-dose effects and nonmonotonic dose responses. *Endocr Rev.* (2012) 33:378–455. doi: 10.1210/er.2011-1050
45. Ruiz-Ojeda FJ, Ruperez AI, Gomez-Llorente C, Gil A, Aguilera CM. Cell models and their application for studying adipogenic differentiation in relation to obesity: a review. *Int J Mol Sci.* (2016) 17:e1040. doi: 10.3390/ijms17071040
46. Kassotis CD, Masse L, Kim S, Schlezinger JJ, Webster TF, Stapleton HM, Characterization of adipogenic chemicals in three different cell culture systems: implications for reproducibility based on cell source and handling. *Sci Rep.* (2017) 7:42104. doi: 10.1038/srep42104
47. Singer NG, Caplan AI. Mesenchymal stem cells: mechanisms of inflammation. *Annu Rev Pathol.* (2011) 6:457–78. doi: 10.1146/annurev-pathol-011110-130230
48. Tang QQ, Otto TC, Lane MD. Commitment of C3H10T1/2 pluripotent stem cells to the adipocyte lineage. *Proc Natl Acad Sci USA.* (2004) 101:9607–11. doi: 10.1073/pnas.0403100101
49. Kelly KA, Tanaka S, Baron R, Gimble JM. Murine bone marrow stromally derived BMS2 adipocytes support differentiation and function of osteoclast-like cells in vitro. *Endocrinology.* (1998) 139:2092–101. doi: 10.1210/endo.139.4.5915
50. Bo E, Viglietti-Panzica C, Panzica GC. Acute exposure to tributyltin induces c-fos activation in the hypothalamic arcuate nucleus of adult male mice. *Neurotoxicology.* (2011) 32:277–80. doi: 10.1016/j.neuro.2010.12.011
51. Penza M, Jeremic M, Marrazzo E, Maggi A, Ciana P, Rando G, et al. The environmental chemical tributyltin chloride (TBT) shows both estrogenic and adipogenic activities in mice which might depend on the exposure dose. *Toxicol Appl Pharmacol.* (2011) 255:65–75. doi: 10.1016/j.taap.2011.05.017
52. Zuo Z, Chen S, Wu T, Zhang J, Su Y, Chen Y, et al. Tributyltin causes obesity and hepatic steatosis in male mice. *Environ Toxicol.* (2011) 26:79–85. doi: 10.1002/tox.20531
53. He K, Zhang J, Chen Z. Effect of tributyltin on the food intake and brain neuropeptide expression in rats. *Endokrynol Pol.* (2014) 65:485–90. doi: 10.5603/EP.2014.0068
54. Zhang J, Sun P, Yang F, Kong T, Zhang R. Tributyltin disrupts feeding and energy metabolism in the goldfish (Carassius auratus). *Chemosphere.* (2016) 152:221–8. doi: 10.1016/j.chemosphere.2016.02.127

55. Tingaud-Sequeira A, Ouadah N, Babin PJ. Zebrafish obesogenic test: a tool for screening molecules that target adiposity. *J Lipid Res.* (2011) 52:1765–72. doi: 10.1194/jlr.D017012
56. Sena GC, Freitas-Lima LC, Merlo E, Podratz PL, de Araujo JF, Brandao PA, et al. Environmental obesogen tributyltin chloride leads to abnormal hypothalamic-pituitary-gonadal axis function by disruption in kisspeptin/leptin signaling in female rats. *Toxicol Appl Pharmacol.* (2017) 319:22–38. doi: 10.1016/j.taap.2017.01.021
57. Regnier SM, El-Hashani E, Kamau W, Zhang X, Massad NL, Sargis RM. Tributyltin differentially promotes development of a phenotypically distinct adipocyte. *Obesity (Silver Spring).* (2015) 23:1864–71. doi: 10.1002/oby.21174
58. Asarian L, Geary N. Sex differences in the physiology of eating. *Am J Physiol Regul Integr Comp Physiol.* (2013) 305:R1215–67. doi: 10.1152/ajpregu.00446.2012
59. Shoucri BM, Hung VT, Chamorro-Garcia R, Shioda T, Blumberg B. Retinoid X receptor activation during adipogenesis of female mesenchymal stem cells programs a dysfunctional adipocyte. *Endocrinology.* (2018) 159:2863–83. doi: 10.1210/en.2018-00056
60. Kim S, Li A, Monti S, Schlezinger JJ. Tributyltin induces a transcriptional response without a brite adipocyte signature in adipocyte models. *Arch Toxicol.* (2018) 92:2859–74. doi: 10.1007/s00204-018-2268-y
61. Chamorro-Garcia R, Sahu M, Abbey RJ, Laude J, Pham N, Blumberg B. Transgenerational inheritance of increased fat depot size, stem cell reprogramming, and hepatic steatosis elicited by prenatal exposure to the obesogen tributyltin in mice. *Environ Health Perspect.* (2013) 121:359–66. doi: 10.1289/ehp.1205701
62. Manikkam M, Tracey R, Guerrero-Bosagna C, Skinner MK, Plastics derived endocrine disruptors (BPA, DEHP and DBP) induce epigenetic transgenerational inheritance of obesity, reproductive disease and sperm epimutations. *PLoS ONE.* (2013) 8:e55387. doi: 10.1371/journal.pone.0055387
63. Skinner MK, Manikkam M, Tracey R, Guerrero-Bosagna C, Haque M, Nilsson EE. Ancestral dichlorodiphenyltrichloroethane (DDT) exposure promotes epigenetic transgenerational inheritance of obesity. *Bmc Med.* (2013) 11:228. doi: 10.1186/1741-7015-11-228
64. Tracey R, Manikkam M, Guerrero-Bosagna C, Skinner MK. Hydrocarbons (jet fuel JP-8) induce epigenetic transgenerational inheritance of obesity, reproductive disease and sperm epimutations. *Reprod Toxicol.* (2013) 36:104–16. doi: 10.1016/j.reprotox.2012.11.011
65. Skinner MK, Environmental epigenetics and a unified theory of the molecular aspects of evolution: a neo-lamarckian concept that facilitates neo-darwinian evolution. *Genome Biol Evol.* (2015) 7:1296–302. doi: 10.1093/gbe/evv073
66. Ben Maamar M, Sadler-Riggleman I, Beck D, McBirney M, Nilsson E, Klukovich R, et al. Alterations in sperm DNA methylation, non-coding RNA expression, and histone retention mediate vinclozolin-induced epigenetic transgenerational inheritance of disease. *Environ Epigenet.* (2018) 4:dvy010. doi: 10.1093/eep/dvy010
67. Skinner MK, Ben Maamar M, Sadler-Riggleman I, Beck D, Nilsson E, McBirney M, et al. Alterations in sperm DNA methylation, non-coding RNA and histone retention associate with DDT-induced epigenetic transgenerational inheritance of disease. *Epigenetics Chromatin.* (2018) 11:8. doi: 10.1186/s13072-018-0178-0
68. Haque MM, Nilsson EE, Holder LB, Skinner MK. Genomic clustering of differential DNA methylated regions (epimutations) associated with the epigenetic transgenerational inheritance of disease and phenotypic variation. *BMC Genomics.* (2016) 17:418. doi: 10.1186/s12864-016-2748-5
69. Eckersley-Maslin MA, Alda-Catalinas C, Reik W. Dynamics of the epigenetic landscape during the maternal-to-zygotic transition. *Nat Rev Mol Cell Biol.* (2018) 19:436–50. doi: 10.1038/s41580-018-0008-z
70. Saitou M, Yamaji M. Primordial germ cells in mice. *Cold Spring Harb Perspect Biol.* (2012) 4:a008375. doi: 10.1101/cshperspect.a008375
71. Iqbal K, Tran DA, Li AX, Warden C, Bai AY, Singh P, et al. Deleterious effects of endocrine disruptors are corrected in the mammalian germline by epigenome reprogramming. *Genome Biol.* (2015) 16:59. doi: 10.1186/s13059-015-0619-z
72. Whitelaw E, Disputing lamarckian epigenetic inheritance in mammals. *Genome Biol.* (2015) 16:60. doi: 10.1186/s13059-015-0626-0
73. Heard E, Martienssen RA. Transgenerational epigenetic inheritance: myths and mechanisms. *Cell.* (2014) 157:95–109. doi: 10.1016/j.cell.2014.02.045
74. Flyamer IM, Gassler J, Imakaev M, Brandao HB, Ulianov SV, Abdennur N, et al. Single-nucleus Hi-C reveals unique chromatin reorganization at oocyte-to-zygote transition. *Nature.* (2017) 544:110–4. doi: 10.1038/nature21711
75. Yu J, Yang X, Yang X, Yang M, Wang P, Yang Y, et al. Nonylphenol aggravates non-alcoholic fatty liver disease in high sucrose-high fat diet-treated rats. *Sci Rep.* (2018) 8:3232. doi: 10.1038/s41598-018-21725-y
76. Batista TM, Alonso-Magdalena P, Vieira E, Amaral ME, Cederroth CR, Nef S, et al. Short-term treatment with bisphenol-A leads to metabolic abnormalities in adult male mice. *PLoS ONE.* (2012) 7:e33814. doi: 10.1371/journal.pone.0033814
77. Regnier SM, Kirkley AG, Ruiz D, Kamau W, Wu Q, Kannan K, et al. Diet-dependence of metabolic perturbations mediated by the endocrine disruptor tolylfluanid. *Endocr Connect.* (2018) 7:159–68. doi: 10.1530/EC-17-0320
78. Heindel JJ, Blumberg B, Cave M, Machtinger R, Mantovani A, Mendez MA, et al. Metabolism disrupting chemicals and metabolic disorders. *Reprod Toxicol.* (2017) 68:3–33. doi: 10.1016/j.reprotox.2016.10.001
79. Rappaport SM, Smith MT. Epidemiology. environment and disease risks. *Science.* (2010) 330:460–1. doi: 10.1126/science.1192603

6

Particulate Matter Air Pollution: Effects on the Cardiovascular System

*Robert B. Hamanaka and Gökhan M. Mutlu**

Section of Pulmonary and Critical Care Medicine, Department of Medicine, The University of Chicago, Chicago, IL, United States

***Correspondence:** Gökhan M. Mutlu gmutlu@medicine.bsd.uchicago.edu*

Air pollution is a complex mixture of gaseous and particulate components, each of which has detrimental effects on human health. While the composition of air pollution varies greatly depending on the source, studies from across the world have consistently shown that air pollution is an important modifiable risk factor for significantly increased morbidity and mortality. Moreover, clinical studies have generally shown a greater impact of particulate matter (PM) air pollution on health than the gaseous components. PM has wide-ranging deleterious effects on human health, particularly on the cardiovascular system. Both acute and chronic exposure to PM air pollution is associated with increased risk of death from cardiovascular diseases including ischemic heart disease, heart failure, and ischemic/thrombotic stroke. Particulate matter has also been shown to be an important endocrine disrupter, contributing to the development of metabolic diseases such as obesity and diabetes mellitus, which themselves are risk factors for cardiovascular disease. While the epidemiological evidence for the deleterious effects of PM air pollution on health is increasingly accepted, newer studies are shedding light on the mechanisms by which PM exerts its toxic effects. A greater understanding of how PM exerts toxic effects on human health is required in order to prevent and minimize the deleterious health effects of this ubiquitous environmental hazard. Air pollution is a growing public health problem and mortality due to air pollution is expected to double by 2050. Here, we review the epidemiological evidence for the cardiovascular effects of PM exposure and discuss current understanding about the biological mechanisms, by which PM exerts toxic effects on cardiovascular system to induce cardiovascular disease.

Keywords: particulate matter, cardiovascular, lung, macrophage, inflammation, interleukin-6, thrombosis, coagulation

INTRODUCTION

Ambient air pollution is a growing global health problem estimated to contribute to as many as 3.1 million all-cause deaths per year (1–3). Exposure to air pollution is the largest environmental health risk and ranks ninth among modifiable disease risk factors, above other common factors such as low physical activity, high cholesterol, and drug use (2). Most of the excess deaths attributable to air pollution exposure are due to acute ischemic/thrombotic cardiovascular events. In addition to excess mortality, air pollution is associated with significant reductions in healthy life years and worker productivity (2, 4). Air pollution may also be an important endocrine disrupter, contributing to the development of metabolic diseases such as obesity and diabetes mellitus (5). While the developing world is most burdened by air pollution-associated health effects, the association between air pollution and mortality is still evident in developed countries where pollution levels are well below target standards (6, 7). The purpose of this article is (1) to introduce the reader to the major studies that have established the link between particulate matter (PM) air pollution and human cardiovascular and metabolic disease and (2) to discuss the mechanisms by which PM mediates its biologic effects. For systematic review of the connection between air pollution and human disease, we refer the reader to several recent systematic reviews and meta-analyses (8–14).

AIR POLLUTION

Air pollution is a complex mixture of gaseous and particulate components, each of which has detrimental effects on cardiovascular and respiratory systems. The composition of air pollution varies greatly, depending on the source, emission rate, and sunlight and wind conditions. Gaseous components of air pollution include nitrogen dioxide (NO_2), nitric oxide (NO), sulfur dioxide (SO_2), ozone (O_3), and carbon monoxide (CO) (2, 15, 16). Particulate matter (PM) components of air pollution consist of carbonaceous particles with associated adsorbed organic chemicals and reactive metals. Common components of PM include nitrates, sulfates, polycyclic aromatic hydrocarbons, endotoxin, and metals such as iron, copper, nickel, zinc, and vanadium (2, 15, 17). PM is subclassified according to particle size into (a) coarse (PM_{10}, diameter <10μm), (b) fine ($PM_{2.5}$, diameter <2.5μm), and (c) ultrafine ($PM_{0.1}$, diameter <0.1μm). Coarse particles derive from numerous natural and industrial sources and generally do not penetrate beyond the upper bronchus. Fine and ultrafine particles are produced through the combustion of fossil fuels and represent a greater threat to health than coarse particles as they penetrate into the small airways and alveoli (16–19). While the organic and metal components of particles vary with location, levels of $PM_{2.5}$ have consistently correlated with negative cardiovascular outcomes regardless of location (15).

EPIDEMIOLOGICAL STUDIES LINKING PM EXPOSURE TO MORBIDITY AND MORTALITY IN HUMANS

The association between high levels of PM air pollution and adverse health outcomes has been known since the first half of the twentieth century. Smog incidents in Meuse Valley, Belgium (1930), Donora, Pennsylvania (1948), and London, UK (1952) acutely caused increased hospitalizations and deaths, particularly in the elderly and those with preexisting cardiac and respiratory diseases. An estimated 4,000 people died as a direct result of the London smog with 100,000 more suffering adverse health effects (20, 21). These incidents resulted in policy changes including the implementation of Clean Air Act in 1970 (22). The reduction in PM levels have led to gradual reduction in PM-associated morbidity and mortality; however, recent epidemiologic studies still consistently show a link between PM exposure and cardiopulmonary mortality.

Short-Term Exposure Studies

The increased deaths due to the smog in Meuse Valley, Donora, and London clearly suggested that acute exposure to air pollution is associated with adverse health outcomes. These classic cases of air pollution-induced mortality represent extreme examples, with the London smog reaching air PM concentrations of 4.5 mg/m^3 (World Health Organization current safety guideline is 25 $\mu g/m^3$) (21). A large number of short-term exposure studies have evaluated the associations between less extreme levels of air pollution and daily changes in mortality (15, 18). A recent meta-analysis of 110 peer-reviewed studies revealed that every 10 $\mu g/cm^3$ increase in $PM_{2.5}$ concentration was associated with a 1.04% (95% CI 0.52%-1.56%) increase in all-cause mortality (10). Hospitalizations and mortality due to cardiovascular and respiratory illnesses were positively correlated with increases in $PM_{2.5}$ concentrations.

Several large, multi-city studies have been conducted in both North America and Europe, the largest being the NMMAPS (National Morbidity, Mortality, and Air Pollution Study) (23–25) and APHEA (Air Pollution and Health: A European Approach) (26, 27) studies. Findings from these studies were remarkably consistent and demonstrated that PM levels are significantly associated with daily all-cause, cardiovascular, and pulmonary mortality. Seasonal and regional variations existed in both studies possibly attributable to different sources of pollutants, meteorological conditions, and population differences. For example, the APHEA study found a stronger effect of PM on daily mortality in cities with a larger contribution of traffic emissions to total PM. This is in agreement with a recent study on triggers of myocardial infarction (MI) in which traffic exposure was found to be as significant of a trigger of MI as physical exertion and alcohol use (28). The NMMAPS study also found that the relationship between PM exposure and mortality was independent of gaseous co-pollutants, including NO_2, CO, and SO_2.

Studies carried out in Asia and the developing world have generally shown smaller effects on daily mortality due to PM than studies from the United States and Europe. A recent meta-analysis of 85 studies from 12 low- and middle-income countries showed a 0.47% (95% CI 0.34-0.61) increase for cardiovascular mortality and 0.57% (95% CI 0.28-0.86) increase for respiratory mortality for every 10 $\mu g/cm^3$ increase in $PM_{2.5}$ concentration (14). The cities covered by this analysis have mean $PM_{2.5}$ levels ranging from 56 to 179 $\mu g/cm^3$, which is significantly higher than the mean the $PM_{2.5}$ levels in cities in the US and Europe. The reduced concentration-response relationship between $PM_{2.5}$ levels and mortality in these countries is likely due to the higher baseline PM level seen in these countries. Indeed, current evidence suggests that the concentration-response relationship between $PM_{2.5}$ levels and mortality is biphasic (29–33). A steep concentration-response function is observed at lower PM concentrations, while the curve flattens at higher concentrations. A recent study from Beijing, China found that while the slope of the concentration-response curve flattened at higher PM concentrations, there was no saturation for increased risk of ischemic heart disease mortality, even at PM concentrations as high as 500 $\mu g/cm^3$ (33).

The biphasic relationship between PM concentration and adverse health outcomes means that the major health benefits from reducing PM levels will occur in countries with already cleaner air and that improvements in cardiovascular health will be more difficult to achieve in countries with higher levels of air pollution unless they can achieve a drastic improvement in PM concentrations. The results of the NMMAPS and APHEA studies suggest that there is no "safe" threshold under which increases in PM are not associated with increased deaths.

Long-Term Exposure Studies

In addition to studies on the acute effects of PM exposure, studies on the effect of chronic exposure to PM have revealed negative effects on long-term health outcomes. The first of these was the Harvard Six Cities study, which prospectively measured the effect of air pollution on mortality in a cohort of 8,111 adults while controlling for individual risk factors, including smoking, body mass index, occupational exposures, hypertension, and diabetes (34). The adjusted mortality rate ratio for the most polluted cities compared with the least polluted cities was 1.26 (95% CI 1.08-1.47). Air pollution, particularly $PM_{2.5}$ and sulfates was positively associated with death from lung cancer and cardiopulmonary diseases.

A larger study, the ACS Cancer Prevention II study linked risk factor data for 552,138 adults with air pollution data and mortality statistics (35, 36). Both $PM_{2.5}$ and SO_2 were positively correlated with all-cause, lung cancer, and cardiopulmonary mortality and every 10 $\mu g/cm^3$ increase in $PM_{2.5}$ was associated with a 4, 6 and 8% increased risk of all-cause, cardiopulmonary, and lung cancer mortality, respectively. Coarse particles and gaseous co-pollutants other than SO_2 were not significantly related to mortality.

A study on 22 European cohorts within the multicenter European Study of Cohorts for Air Pollution Effects (ESCAPE) found an increased hazard ratio for all-cause mortality of 1.07 (95% CI 1.02-1.13) per 5 $\mu g/cm^3$ $PM_{2.5}$ (37). Significant associations persisted even among participants exposed to $PM_{2.5}$ levels below the European annual mean limit value of 25 $\mu g/cm^3$.

Overall, the evidence from both short-term and long-term exposure studies demonstrates a consistent association between increased air pollution exposure and mortality. While the magnitude of this effect is small, the ubiquity of air pollution exposure makes it a significant source of early mortality. A global assessment of mortality attributable to several risk factors, including air pollution was carried out in the Global Burden of Diseases, Injuries, and Risk Factors Study 2015 (GBD 2015) (38). This study estimated that $PM_{2.5}$ is the fifth-ranking mortality risk factor, leading to 4.2 million deaths and 103.1 million disability-adjusted life-years in 2015. The largest number of deaths attributable to air pollution occurred in China with an estimated 1.11 million deaths. These numbers are similar to the findings of a recent study from China that attributed 40.3% of deaths due to stroke, 26.8% of deaths due to ischemic heart disease, 23.9% of deaths due to lung cancer, and 18.7% of deaths due to chronic obstructive pulmonary disease (COPD) to $PM_{2.5}$ exposure (39). According to the GBD 2015 study, these represent the 1st, 2nd, 4th, and 5th leading causes of death in China, respectively (12).

Susceptibility to PM-Induced Morbidity and Mortality

Enhanced risk of cardiovascular death from PM exposure has been linked to old age, low socioeconomic status, preexisting heart and lung disease, and smoking. The APHENA (Air Pollution and Health: A Combined European and North American Approach) study, which analyzed data from the NMMAPS and APHEA studies found that the elderly and unemployed are at higher risk for the deleterious health effects associated with short-term exposure to PM (40). The ACS study found that mortality from ischemic heart disease was positively correlated with chronic $PM_{2.5}$ exposure among never smokers, former smokers, and current smokers (41). However, the risk for death due to arrhythmia, hearth failure, and cardiac arrest was not elevated by $PM_{2.5}$ for never smokers, but significantly elevated for former and current smokers.

Studies have not shown a clear association between race and susceptibility to PM-induced health effects (42–44). However, air pollution in non-white neighborhoods tends to be higher than in majority-white areas, resulting in exposure disparities (45). Indeed, inter-city gradients of PM (i.e., gradients among communities within a city) are associated with larger negative health effects than the average PM measurements within a city (46, 47).

Finally, it has been suggested that women may be more susceptible than men to the PM-induced health effects. Particularly, robust risk estimates have been reported for studies that include only women. The Women's Health Initiative Observational Study found that every 10 $\mu g/cm^3$ increase in $PM_{2.5}$ was associated with a 76% increase in fatal cardiovascular events while the Nurses' Health Study found that every 10 $\mu g/cm^3$ increase in PM_{10} was associated with a 43% increase fatal coronary heart disease (48, 49). More recent large studies have given conflicting results (42, 43). On a global scale, exposure disparities may play a role in increased risk for women as use of biomass fuels for cooking in sub-Saharan Africa and south Asia expose women to disproportionately high levels of indoor air pollution (50).

Interventional Studies

The implementation of the 1970 Clean Air Act and following amendments resulted in a progressive decline in $PM_{2.5}$ levels in the United States. As would be expected from the concentration-response curve of $PM_{2.5}$ vs. mortality, extended analysis of the NMMAPS and Harvard Six Cities Study, among others, have revealed that reductions in $PM_{2.5}$ concentrations over time are associated with reductions in mortality risk (51–53). Pope et al. showed that a reduction of 10 $\mu g/cm^3$ in $PM_{2.5}$ levels increased the life expectancy by 0.61 ± 0.20 years (54). Similar reductions in mortality have been seen after policy changes regulating the use of diesel in Tokyo, Japan and coal in Dublin, Ireland (55, 56).

EXPOSURE TO PM AND CARDIOVASCULAR DISEASE

Deaths due to air pollution exposure result primarily from cardiovascular causes, with stronger associations with adverse effects of PM compared with gaseous co-pollutants (2, 7, 15). Chronic and acute exposure to elevated $PM_{2.5}$ levels is closely associated with elevated risks for ischemic heart disease, heart failure, and cerebrovascular disease. Air pollution exacerbates existing heart conditions and appears to have a role in disease development.

Both long- and short-term studies have associated $PM_{2.5}$ exposure with increased risk of fatal and non-fatal ischemic heart disease (33, 41, 48, 57). Risk of myocardial infarction is also associated with $PM_{2.5}$ exposure (28, 58). The ACS study found increased risk of heart failure with $PM_{2.5}$ exposure, although to a lesser degree than the association with ischemic heart disease. Additional studies and meta-analyses have associated both chronic and acute $PM_{2.5}$ exposure with heart failure (9, 41, 59, 60). Significant associations also exist between $PM_{2.5}$ exposure and cerebrovascular disease (48, 61). Short-term studies have shown that elevations in pollution increase the risk of ischemic, but not hemorrhagic stroke (8, 62).

Subclinical Effects

Exposure to PM air pollution is also correlated with subclinical pathologies underlying cardiovascular disease. These include systemic inflammation and oxidative stress, atherosclerosis, thrombosis, endothelial dysfunction, hypertension, cardiac remodeling, and arrhythmia.

Inflammation, Oxidative Stress, and Atherosclerosis

PM inhalation induces inflammatory responses both within the lung and systemically. Exposure of human volunteers to PM via inhalation for 2 h resulted in increased pulmonary neutrophil numbers (63). Circulating levels of C-reactive protein, fibrinogen, IL-1β (interleukin-1β), IL-6 (interleukin-6), GM-CSF (Granulocyte-Macrophage Colony Stimulating Factor), and TNF-α (Tumor Necrosis Factor-α) have been shown to correlate with environmental PM exposure levels (63–66).

PM exposure is also associated with systemic markers of oxidative stress, including atherogenic precursors such as oxidized lipids (67–70). Using carotid artery intima-media thickness as a surrogate for atherosclerotic progression, several studies, including the Multi-Ethnic Study of Atherosclerosis (MESA) have shown that intima-media thickness correlates positively with long-term exposure to PM (71–74). Other studies have shown that coronary artery calcification correlates with residence in a city center or near a major roadway (75, 76).

Studies in the atherosclerosis model apolipoprotein E (ApoE) knockout mice have shown that exposure to PM results in elevated levels of oxidized low-density lipoproteins, lipid peroxidation, and systemic oxidative stress. This is associated with increased atheroma burden, and increased plaque cellularity and lipid content (77–80).

Hypercoagulability and Thrombosis

Exposure to PM has been shown to induce a prothrombotic state, which may play a role in its ability to cause arterial thrombotic (myocardial infarction, ischemic/thrombotic cerebrovascular events) and venous thrombotic events (deep venous thrombosis) (81, 82). Exposure to PM induces the production of fibrinogen, and other factors that play a role in hemostasis including Von Willebrand factor, sCD62P, and sCD40L (65, 83–85). In addition to prothrombotic pathways, antifibrinolytic pathways are also activated by PM exposure. Plasminogen Activator Inhibitor-1 (PAI1) has been shown to be upregulated by PM exposure and tissue Plasminogen Activator (t-PA) activity is inhibited (85–88). These findings correlate with previous reports of PM-associated increases in plasma viscosity, platelet activation, and *ex vivo* coagulation (89–92).

The 2008 Summer Olympics in Beijing, China offered a unique opportunity to study the effects of PM exposure on cardiovascular biomarkers. As government-mandated restrictions on industrial and vehicular emissions were enacted, particulate and gaseous pollutants decreased. In test subjects, this corresponded with decreases in circulating levels of sCD62P and Von Willebrand factor. When restrictions were eased after the games, levels of these factors increased to pre-Olympic levels (84).

Endothelial Dysfunction, Increased Blood Pressure, and Cardiac Remodeling

Both short- and long-term exposure to PM has been correlated with changes in vascular function. Controlled exposure to diesel exhaust or concentrated ambient particles leads to vascular dysfunction characterized by acute arterial vasoconstriction and inhibition of response to vasodilators (86, 93–96). The MESA study found that chronic exposure to $PM_{2.5}$ correlated with decreased flow-mediated dilation of the brachial artery and retinal arteriolar narrowing (97, 98).

Several studies have reported associations between chronic PM exposure and development of hypertension (99, 100). Controlled-exposure studies using acute exposure of humans to concentrated ambient particles or diesel exhaust have demonstrated rapid increases in systolic blood pressure following exposure (101, 102). Exposure to PM has also been shown to increase the risk of gestational hypertension and pre-eclampsia (11, 103, 104).

Finally, traffic exposure has been associated with both left and right ventricular hypertrophy, suggesting that pollution-associated vasoconstriction and hypertension may exacerbate congestive heart failure (105, 106). Similar results have been found in mice. A 3-month exposure of mice to concentrated ambient particles exacerbates cardiac hypertrophy and fibrosis in response to angiotensin II infusion (107). A longer, 9-month exposure of mice to concentrated ambient particles was sufficient to result in increased ventricular size, systolic and diastolic dysfunction, and myocardial fibrosis (108).

Cardiac Electrical Changes and Irregular Heart Rhythm

In patients with implantable cardioverter defibrillators, positive associations have been made between short-term increases in air pollution and incidence of cardiac arrhythmias including atrial fibrillation, ventricular fibrillation, and ventricular tachycardia (109–112). Exposure to air pollution is also associated with, increased heart rate, electric instability, ectopic beats, ST-segment depression, repolarization irregularities, and changes in heart-rate variability (65, 113–120).

The strongest correlations between arrhythmia and pollution exposure have been found when analysis was restricted to a subgroup of patients with frequent arrhythmias, suggesting that risk of arrhythmia is restricted to the most susceptible individuals (109). Similarly, a murine study found that wild-type mice did not exhibit arrhythmias after exposure to PM; however, significant arrhythmias were seen in mice engineered to exhibit cardiomyopathic changes that closely resemble congestive heart failure (121). In rats, greater effects of PM exposure on arrhythmogenesis were seen in animals previously injected with monocrotaline to induce pulmonary vascular inflammation and hypertension (122).

Metabolic Syndrome and Insulin Resistance

Several clinical studies have linked PM with insulin resistance and type II diabetes mellitus (DM) suggesting PM as a modifiable risk factor for DM, an important risk factor for cardiovascular disease. Significant positive correlations between PM exposure and fasting insulin levels and insulin resistance have been found in both adults and children (123–125). A large study conducted using data from both the United States Centers for Disease Control and Prevention and the Environmental Protection Agency found that diabetes prevalence increases by 1% with each 10 $\mu g/m^3$ $PM_{2.5}$ (126). Another study of over 3,500 individuals in Germany revealed that each 1 $\mu g/m^3$ of traffic-related $PM_{2.5}$ was associated with a relative risk for type II DM of 1.36 (95% CI.97-1.89) after adjusting for variables including age, gender, BMI, and socioeconomic status (127). This effect size was similar to that obtained by comparing individuals living close to a major road with those that live farther than 200 meters from a major road (127). A recent meta-analysis suggests that the correlation of PM with DM is stronger in women (13). How PM-associated insulin resistance and type II DM may interact with other PM-associated health effects to affect cardiovascular system is a complex question. For example, diabetics have been shown to be more susceptible to PM-associated endothelial dysfunction (128).

Animal studies have confirmed the effect of PM exposure on insulin sensitivity. Mice genetically susceptible to type II DM, or mice fed high-fat diet and exposed to PM exhibit increased insulin resistance, glucose intolerance, elevated fasting glucose, and increased visceral adiposity when compared with mice exposed to filtered air (129–131). Interestingly, young mice exposed to PM beginning at 3 weeks of age developed homeostatic insulin resistance after 10 weeks of exposure without additional stress indicating a developmental window of susceptibility to the effects of PM (132).

BIOLOGICAL MECHANISMS

Recent controlled exposure studies in both humans and animals have shed light on the biological mechanisms behind PM-induced cardiovascular disease (**Figure 1**). There are presently three hypotheses on the mechanisms by which PM exposure exerts its biological effect (7, 15, 16, 133). The first hypothesis proposes that PM inhalation activates inflammatory responses in the lung leading to a "spillover" effect and systemic inflammation, which promotes thrombosis, endothelial dysfunction, and atherosclerosis. The second hypothesis suggests that inhaled PM activates sensory receptors in the lung, leading to imbalance of the autonomic nervous system (ANS), favoring sympathetic pathways and leading to alterations in heart rate, vasoconstriction, endothelial dysfunction, and hypertension. The third hypothesis proposes that some particles, particularly ultrafine particles ($PM_{0.1}$) can enter the circulation from the lung and interact directly with target tissues; however, this mechanism remains controversial. Recent evidence suggests that majority of ultrafine particles are cleared from the lung in a similar manner as larger particles (i.e., alveolar macrophage-mediated clearance to the larynx) (134, 135). Nevertheless, soluble material adsorbed to the surface of inhaled particles may pass into the circulation. Further studies will be required to determine whether any portion of inhaled particles is translocated into the bloodstream and if so, whether these translocated particles contribute to PM-associated pathologies. We will discuss the evidence for inflammatory and ANS signaling as regulators of the biologic effects of PM exposure. It should be noted that these pathways are not mutually exclusive. In fact, there is significant evidence that while each plays an important role in mediating the cardiovascular effects of pollution exposure, they may also interact to drive the PM-induced health effects.

Reactive Oxygen Species and Mitochondria

It is widely accepted that PM exerts many of its biologic effects via the generation of reactive oxygen species (ROS) and induction of oxidative stress responses (19, 136). Exposure to air pollution is associated with systemic markers of oxidative stress (67, 69, 70). At the cellular level, many cell types have been shown to respond to *in vitro* PM exposure with elevations in cellular ROS levels and oxidative stress. This includes nasal, airway, and lung epithelial cells (137–141), macrophages (142–144), endothelial cells (145, 146), cardiomyocytes (147, 148), gastrointestinal epithelial cells (149), epidermal keratinocytes (150), and corneal epithelial cells (151). Moreover, elevated ROS levels are required for PM-induced biologic effects as antioxidant treatment or inhibition of oxidant production is sufficient to inhibit downstream pathways including proinflammatory cytokine production and induction of apoptosis (137, 138, 152–155).

While PM-adsorbed chemicals and metals are capable of generating free radicals inside cells, cells can respond to stimuli with generation of ROS as signaling molecules (156). Mitochondrial generation of ROS has been found to be an important signaling regulator of the cellular response to PM. Indeed exposure to PM has been found to alter

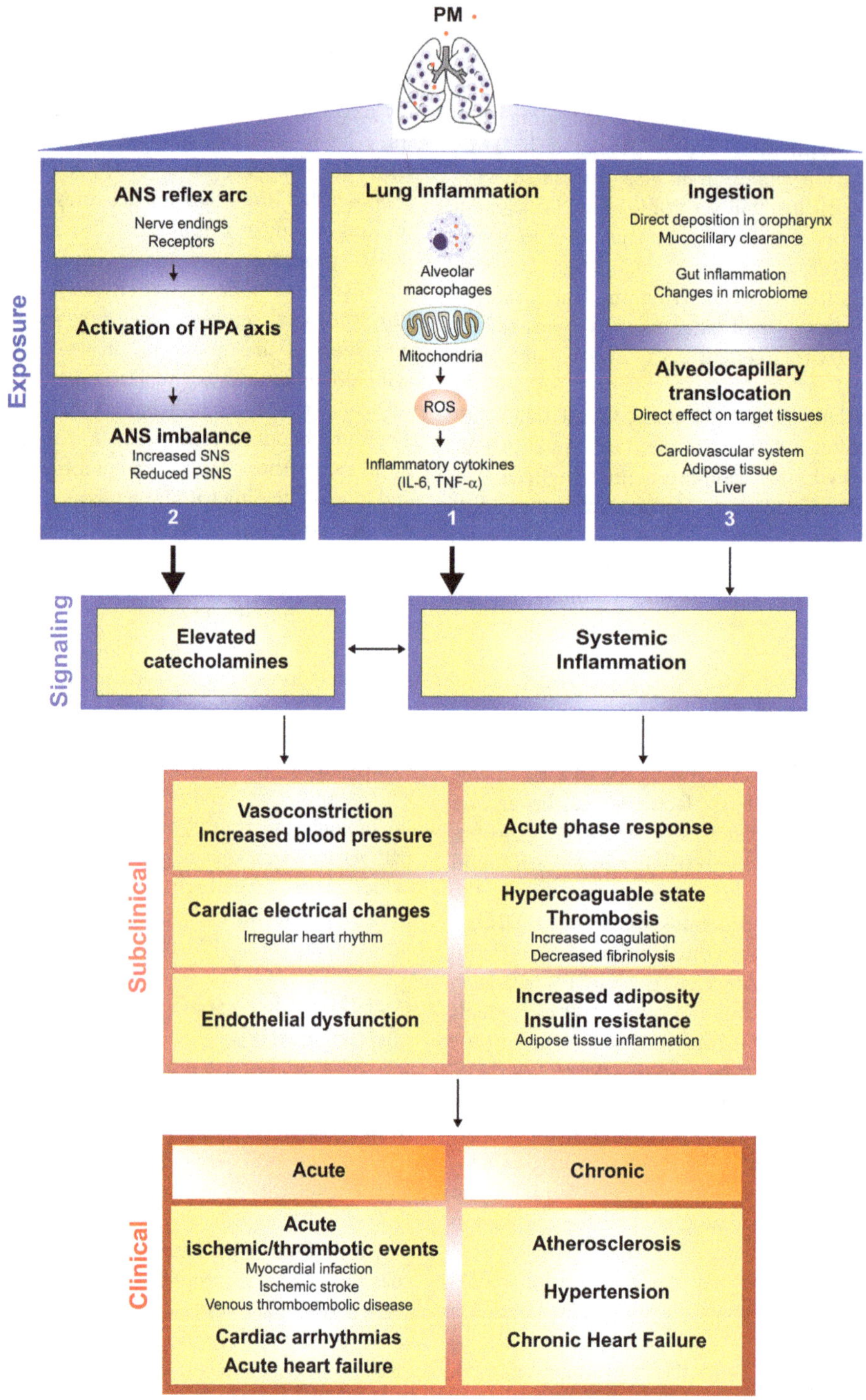

FIGURE 1 | Current evidence for the mechanisms by which particulate matter air pollution causes cardiovascular health effects.
Exposure Level: PM exposure is hypothesized to exert its effects on the cardiovascular system by three routes: (1) PM induces an inflammatory response in the lung. PM acts on the cells of the lung, including alveolar macrophages, leading to mitochondrial reactive oxygen species (mROS)-dependent pro-inflammatory cytokine production. (2) Inhaled PM acts on sensory receptors in the lung, promoting activation of the hypothalamic pituitary adrenal (HPA) axis and sympathetic pathway activation in the autonomic nervous system (ANS). (3) Other effects of PM exposure may be mediated by translocation of particles into the circulatory system, or by particle ingestion, which may promote inflammation in the gut.
Signaling Level: Cytokines produced into the lung "spillover" into the circulation, leading to a systemic state of inflammation. Translocated particles as well as inflammation resulting from particle injection may also contribute to a general state of systemic inflammation. Sympathetic activation leads to elevated levels of circulating catecholamines.

(Continued)

FIGURE 1 | Subclinical Level: Systemic inflammation and elevated catecholamine levels act on target cells leading to acute phase response, hypercoagulable state (activation of coagulation, and suppressed fibrinolysis), vasoconstriction, increased blood pressure, cardiac electrical changes, endothelial dysfunction, and increased adiposity and insulin resistance complicated by adipose tissue inflammation. Elevated catecholamine levels due to ANS imbalance further increase inflammation. Sympathetic activation leads to increased catecholamine production, which increases heart rate and promotes vasoconstriction, endothelial dysfunction, and hypertension.
Clinical Level: The combined effects of systemic inflammation and sympathetic activation on their cellular targets lead to the clinical effects of PM on cardiovascular disease. These effects are seen at both the acute level (acute ischemic/thrombotic events, cardiac arrhythmias, or acute heart failure), or at the chronic level (atherosclerosis, hypertension, and chronic heart failure).

mitochondrial morphology and function (142, 151, 157, 158). PM exposure leads to oxidation of redox probes specifically targeted to mitochondria (149, 159). Furthermore, cells genetically engineered to lack mitochondrial ROS production or cells treated with mitochondria-targeted antioxidants or respiratory chain inhibitors have inhibited responses to PM, strongly supporting the role of mitochondria-derived ROS in PM-induced biologic effects (138, 153, 159–161).

Alveolar Macrophages

Alveolar Macrophages (AMs) reside on the luminal epithelial surface of alveoli and are crucial for lung development, surfactant homeostasis, and immune surveillance (162). These cells also represent a critical signaling node for the effects of PM on target organs such as heart and vasculature. Treatment of AMs *in vitro* with PM elicits a transcriptional upregulation of inflammatory cytokines including TNFα, IL-1β, IL-6, IL-8 and GM-CSF (64, 163). Lung epithelial cells also respond to PM treatment *in vitro* and the interaction between AMs and epithelial cells may regulate their response to PM (164, 165); however, studies in animals suggest that the response of AMs to PM exposure is required and sufficient for downstream cardiovascular effects.

Elimination of AMs in mice using liposomal clodronate inhibits both pulmonary and systemic accumulation of IL-6 or TNFα protein after exposure to PM (166, 167). The prothrombotic and endothelial-activating effects of PM exposure were also inhibited by clodronate, suggesting that the pro-inflammatory responses initiated by AMs in the lung promote the systemic and cardiovascular effects of PM exposure (166, 167). The ability of AMs to influence systemic responses to PM is supported by studies on bone marrow activation in rabbits. Instillation of PM into the lungs of rabbits results in increased release of polymorphonuclear leukocytes from bone marrow, with elevated numbers of circulating band cells, a marker of bone marrow activation (168). Similar responses have been seen in humans (169). Instillation of supernatants from human AMs treated with PM *ex vivo* has a similar ability to activate rabbit bone marrow as instillation of PM suggesting that PM-induced inflammatory responses in AMs regulate the systemic effects of PM on target cells and organs (170).

Pro-inflammatory Cytokines

Interleukin 6

Initially identified as a regulator of T cell activation and B cell differentiation, IL-6 is a pleotropic cytokine with key roles in diverse biological processes such as immune responses, the acute phase response and inflammation, hematopoiesis, vascular function, lipid metabolism, and neuroendocrine regulation (171, 172).

IL-6 is a major regulator of the acute phase response and stimulates hepatocytes to synthesize acute phase proteins, particularly C-reactive protein and coagulation factors (173, 174). IL-6 has been shown to increase the expression of coagulation factors including fibrinogen, tissue factor, Factor VIII and von Willebrand factor, and decrease anticoagulants including protein S and antithrombin (174). Recent reports in IL-6-deficient mice have demonstrated the critical role of IL-6 in promoting thrombotic events downstream of PM exposure. Exposure of wild-type mice to PM led to accelerated blood clotting and vascular thrombosis after $FeCl_3$ application (166, 175). This accelerated clotting was associated with increased platelet count, increased Factor VIII activity, increased plasma thrombin antithrombin complexes, increased lung tissue factor levels, reduced prothrombin time, and reduced activated partial thromboplastin time. In IL-6 deficient mice, no increase in clotting capability was seen after exposure to PM, demonstrating the key role that IL-6 plays in regulating the prothrombotic effects of PM exposure.

Elevations in IL-6 may also promote vascular dysfunction after PM exposure. Administration of IL-6 to mice promotes endothelial dysfunction and impaired endothelium-dependent vasodilation (176). As in humans, exposure of mice to PM impairs vasodilation in response to acetylcholine. No significant change in vascular response was noted in IL-6 deficient mice after exposure to PM (177). Interestingly, in this same report, the authors demonstrated that instillation of recombinant IL-6 into the lungs of IL-6 knockout mice resulted in systemic elevations in IL-6 after endotoxin-mediated lung injury (177). While endotoxin is a stronger inducer of lung injury than PM, this finding provides support for the hypothesis that inflammatory cytokine induction in the lung can spillover into the circulation to promote systemic effects.

Tumor Necrosis Factor-α

TNFα is a pleiotropic cytokine originally identified as an endotoxin-inducible molecule with anti-cancer activity (178). TNFα has since been shown to be a critical regulator of the cytokine cascade in many inflammatory diseases and is a therapeutic target for a number of chronic inflammatory diseases (179, 180). Similar to IL-6, TNFα expression is induced in both AMs and lung epithelial cells after exposure to PM (64, 163, 165). TNFα also accumulates in both the lung and systemically after exposure of mice to PM (167, 175, 181, 182). Elimination of AMs with liposomal clodronate inhibited the accumulation of TNFα in plasma after exposure of mice to PM.

Surprisingly, studies in TNFα-deficient mice demonstrate that PM-mediated recruitment of neutrophils to the lung, as well as induction of cytokines, including IL-6, IL-8, and MCP-1 (monocyte chemoattractant protein 1), are independent of TNFα. (183, 184). This is despite the fact that TNFα is a known regulator of IL-6 expression (185, 186). TNFα was shown to be required for accumulation of PAI1 after exposure of mice to PM; however, TNFα remained dispensable for PM-mediated pro-thrombotic effects (175). More recent studies have shown that pulmonary T-cell recruitment is impaired after PM exposure in TNFα deficient mice (182) and that endothelial activation and impaired cardiac contractile function after PM exposure can be rescued by treatment with a TNFα-neutralizing antibody (167, 181).

Sympathetic Activation and Endogenous Catecholamines

The effects of PM exposure on heart rate variability and blood pressure indicate that air pollution may regulate the balance between the sympathetic and parasympathetic arms of the autonomic nervous system. Indeed, a study of Brazilian sugarcane harvesters found that during harvest time, when ambient PM is high due to sugarcane burning, workers' blood pressure and heart rate variability measurements correlated significantly with sympathetic nerve activity measured by microneurography (187). A more recent study found that elevated exposure to PM was associated with increased serum levels of norepinephrine and epinephrine, among other stress hormones (188).

Increased catecholamine levels have also been found in mice exposed to PM and this sympathetic activation has been shown to augment the inflammatory response and prothrombotic effects downstream of PM exposure (153). Deletion of β-adrenergic receptors either globally or in AMs alone resulted in reduced IL-6 accumulation after PM exposure. Inhibition of β-adrenergic receptors either genetically or pharmacologically prevented the prothrombotic effects of PM exposure while treatment of mice with the β-agonist formoterol further increased IL-6 accumulation and thrombosis after PM exposure (153). These findings from an experimental study have recently been confirmed in humans (188). Collectively, these results suggest that the PM-induced inflammation and modulation of the autonomic nervous system both contribute to the prothrombotic effects of PM exposure.

Increased Adiposity and Adipose Inflammation

Animal studies have shown that long-term PM exposure leads to increased adipocyte size and increased visceral fat mass (129, 189). PM exposure induced genes associated with lipogenesis in adipose tissue, impaired adipose mitochondrial function, and led to changes in circulating levels of leptin and adiponectin (130, 189–191). This increased adiposity was also associated with associated with increased macrophage infiltration into adipose tissue and induction of pro-inflammatory programs (129, 189).

Adipose inflammation is linked with insulin resistance (192). Indeed mice deficient for the NADPH oxidase subunit p47phox exhibited improved adipose inflammation and insulin resistance in response to PM exposure (132). Similar findings were found in mice deficient for the chemokine receptor CCR2 (131)

In humans, living near a major roadway (<60 m) is associated a 0.37 kg/m^2 (95% CI: 0.10 to 0.65 kg/m^2) increase in body mass index (BMI) when compared with those who live over 440 m away from a major road (193). The finding that inflammation is associated with PM-induced insulin resistance in mice is consistent with the findings of the SALIA (Study on the Influence of Air Pollution on Lung Inflammation and Aging), which demonstrated that Complement C3c, a marker of subclinical inflammation, is associated with PM exposure in a cohort of non-diabetic women. Elevated C3c was a strong independent predictor of diabetes development (194).

Animal studies have confirmed the effect of PM exposure on insulin sensitivity. Mice genetically susceptible to type II DM, or mice fed high-fat diet and exposed to PM exhibit increased insulin resistance, glucose intolerance, elevated fasting glucose, and increased visceral adiposity when compared with mice exposed to filtered air (129–131). Interestingly, young mice exposed to PM beginning at 3 weeks of age developed homeostatic insulin resistance after 10 weeks of exposure without additional stress indicating a developmental window of susceptibility to the effects of PM (132).

Epigenetic Changes

How the effects of air pollution exposure may endure after exposure is not clear; however studies from mice suggest that exposure early in life can have long lasting effects. Exposure of pregnant mice to diesel exhaust resulted in an increased susceptibility to pressure overload-induced heart failure in pups raised to adulthood (195). While the mechanisms behind this susceptibility is unknown, a potential mechanism for long-term disease susceptibility may lie in epigenetic changes that occur during exposure.

Epigenetic regulation of gene expression can result in transient, and potentially permanent changes in tissue function. Although studies are limited, air pollution exposure has been shown to affect multiple epigenetic mechanisms, including alterations in DNA methylation and histone modifications. Hypermethylation was observed in the DNA from sperm collected from mice exposed to particulate air pollution for 10 weeks when compared with mice exposed to filtered air (196). These changes were still evident when mice were examined 6 weeks after termination of exposure. In humans, hypomethylation in DNA repetitive elements has been seen in circulating leukocytes after exposure to particles (197, 198). Furthermore hypomethylation of LINE-1 elements correlates with increased risk for ischemic heart disease, stroke, and all-cause mortality (199).

Epigenetic regulation of certain genes by PM has been seen in cultured lung epithelial cells (200, 201); however, a genome-wide assessment of epigenetic changes induced in various tissues by

PM exposure is yet to be carried out. A new large-scale study, sponsored by the National Institute of Environmental Health Sciences seeks to determine the genome-wide epigenetic effects of exposure to various environmental pollutants, including PM, on multiple tissues (202). The data collected by the TaRGET II (Toxicant Exposures and Responses by Genomic and Epigenomic Regulators of Transcription) Consortium will greatly advance the knowledge of the effects of air pollution exposure on the epigenome.

CONCLUSIONS AND FUTURE DIRECTIONS

There is abundant evidence that air pollution is a major contributor to cardiovascular morbidity and mortality. Exposure to pollution is a major modifiable risk factor in the prevention and management of cardiovascular disease; however, the health effects of air pollution are not limited to the cardiovascular system. PM also appears to be an important contributor to development of metabolic diseases including obesity and type II diabetes. Emerging evidence suggests that PM exposure affects timing of puberty and reproductive health in both men and women (203–208). Furthermore, air pollution exposure may affect other systems including the central nervous system as well as the gastrointestinal tract and microbiome. (149, 209, 210). At current projections, premature mortality due to air pollution exposure is expected to double by 2050 (1). Reducing the effect of air pollution on public health will require both policy efforts to reduce production of air pollution as well individual efforts to limit exposure, particularly for those with preexisting susceptibility to cardiovascular disease.

The effects of PM exposure on catecholamine levels, insulin resistance, adiposity, and reproductive health, suggest that PM exposure is an important endocrine disruptor. Mechanistically, little is known about how PM exposure affects the endocrine system. Endocrine disrupting compounds are found in both the gaseous and particulate components of air pollution (211–214), however, further research will be required to determine if these compounds are the specific causes for the adverse health outcomes associated with PM exposure.

The totality of the evidence suggests that there is no "safe" level of PM exposure. Therefore, in addition to efforts to reduce PM production and exposure, future studies should increasingly focus on mechanistic investigations to better understand how PM causes adverse health effects. Further exploration of the signaling mediators and epigenetic regulators of the effects of air pollution on health may lead to pharmacological agents capable of mitigating the detrimental effects of air pollution on health. This effort will require cell-based and animal studies utilizing real-life exposures to PM as well as translational research in humans.

Finally, there should be increased efforts at public education on the harmful effects of air pollution exposure, particularly by physicians with at risk patients. Air pollution exposure should be seen as a major modifiable risk factor for cardiovascular disease. The United States Environmental Protection Agency provides daily ozone and PM level readings for cities in the US, Canada, and Mexico. Greater dissemination of these readings may not only help those at risk for PM-related health effects, but also increase awareness of the impact of PM exposure on health, possibly increasing demand for policy changes to reduce air pollution production.

AUTHOR CONTRIBUTIONS

RBH and GMM contributed equally and wrote the manuscript together.

FUNDING

NIH K01 AR066579 and an ATS Foundation Unrestricted Grant (RBH) and R01 ES015024, U01 ES026718 and P30 ES027792 (GMM).

REFERENCES

1. Lelieveld J, Evans JS, Fnais M, Giannadaki D, Pozzer A. The contribution of outdoor air pollution sources to premature mortality on a global scale. *Nature* (2015) 525:367–71. doi: 10.1038/nature15371
2. Newby DE, Mannucci PM, Tell GS, Baccarelli AA, Brook RD, Donaldson K, et al. Expert position paper on air pollution and cardiovascular disease. *Eur Heart J.* (2015) 36:83–93b. doi: 10.1093/eurheartj/ehu458
3. Brook RD, Newby DE, Rajagopalan S. The global threat of outdoor ambient air pollution to cardiovascular health: time for intervention. *JAMA Cardiol.* (2017) 2:353–4. doi: 10.1001/jamacardio.2017.0032
4. Zivin JG, Neidell M. Air pollution's hidden impacts. *Science* (2018) 359:39–40. doi: 10.1126/science.aap7711
5. Darbre PD. Overview of air pollution and endocrine disorders. *Int J Gen Med.* (2018) 11:191–207. doi: 10.2147/IJGM.S102230
6. Mills NL, Donaldson K, Hadoke PW, Boon NA, MacNee W, Cassee FR, et al. Adverse cardiovascular effects of air pollution. *Nat Clin Pract Cardiovasc Med.* (2009) 6:36–44. doi: 10.1038/ncpcardio1399
7. Cosselman KE, Navas-Acien A, Kaufman JD. Environmental factors in cardiovascular disease. *Nat Rev Cardiol.* (2015) 12:627–42. doi: 10.1038/nrcardio.2015.152
8. Mustafic H, Jabre P, Caussin C, Murad MH, Escolano S, Tafflet M, et al. Main air pollutants and myocardial infarction: a systematic review and meta-analysis. *JAMA* (2012) 307:713–21. doi: 10.1001/jama.2012.126
9. Shah AS, Langrish JP, Nair H, McAllister DA, Hunter AL, Donaldson K, et al. Global association of air pollution and heart failure: a systematic review and meta-analysis. *Lancet* (2013) 382:1039–48. doi: 10.1016/S0140-6736(13)60898-3
10. Atkinson RW, Kang S, Anderson HR, Mills IC, Walton HA. Epidemiological time series studies of PM2.5 and daily mortality and hospital admissions: a systematic review and meta-analysis. *Thorax* (2014) 69:660–5. doi: 10.1136/thoraxjnl-2013-204492
11. Pedersen M, Stayner L, Slama R, Sorensen M, Figueras F, Nieuwenhuijsen MJ, et al. Ambient air pollution and pregnancy-induced hypertensive disorders: a systematic review and meta-analysis. *Hypertension* (2014) 64:494–500. doi: 10.1161/HYPERTENSIONAHA.114.03545
12. Collaborators GBDRF, Forouzanfar MH, Alexander L, Anderson HR, Bachman VF, Biryukov S, et al. Global, regional, and national comparative

risk assessment of 79 behavioural, environmental and occupational, and metabolic risks or clusters of risks in 188 countries, 1990-2013: a systematic analysis for the Global Burden of Disease Study 2013. *Lancet* (2015) 386:2287–323. doi: 10.1016/S0140-6736(15)00128-2

13. Eze IC, Hemkens LG, Bucher HC, Hoffmann B, Schindler C, Kunzli N, et al. Association between ambient air pollution and diabetes mellitus in Europe and North America: systematic review and meta-analysis. *Environ Health Perspect.* (2015) 123:381–9. doi: 10.1289/ehp.1307823
14. Newell K, Kartsonaki C, Lam KBH, Kurmi OP. Cardiorespiratory health effects of particulate ambient air pollution exposure in low-income and middle-income countries: a systematic review and meta-analysis. *Lancet Planet Health* (2017) 1:e368–80. doi: 10.1016/S2542-5196(17)30166-3
15. Brook RD, Rajagopalan S, Pope CA III, Brook JR, Bhatnagar A, Diez-Roux AV, et al. Particulate matter air pollution and cardiovascular disease: an update to the scientific statement from the American Heart Association. *Circulation* (2010) 121:2331–78. doi: 10.1161/CIR.0b013e3181dbece1
16. Chin MT. Basic mechanisms for adverse cardiovascular events associated with air pollution. *Heart* (2015) 101:253–6. doi: 10.1136/heartjnl-2014-306379
17. Brook RD, Franklin B, Cascio W, Hong Y, Howard G, Lipsett M, et al. Air pollution and cardiovascular disease: a statement for healthcare professionals from the Expert panel on population and prevention science of the american heart association. *Circulation* (2004) 109:2655–71. doi: 10.1161/01.CIR.0000128587.30041.C8
18. Pope CA III. Epidemiology of fine particulate air pollution and human health: biologic mechanisms and who's at risk? *Environ Health Perspect* (2000) 108 (Suppl. 4):713–23. doi: 10.1289/ehp.108-1637679
19. Miller MR, Shaw CA, Langrish JP. From particles to patients: oxidative stress and the cardiovascular effects of air pollution. *Future Cardiol.* (2012) 8:577–602. doi: 10.2217/fca.12.43
20. Logan WP. Mortality in the London fog incident, 1952. *Lancet* (1953) 1:336–8.
21. Stanek LW, Brown JS, Stanek J, Gift J, Costa DL. Air pollution toxicology–a brief review of the role of the science in shaping the current understanding of air pollution health risks. *Toxicol Sci.* (2011) 120 (Suppl. 1):S8–27. doi: 10.1093/toxsci/kfq367
22. Berger RE, Ramaswami R, Solomon CG, Drazen JM. Air pollution still kills. *N Engl J Med.* (2017) 376:2591–2. doi: 10.1056/NEJMe1706865
23. Samet JM, Dominici F, Curriero FC, Coursac I, Zeger SL. Fine particulate air pollution and mortality in 20 U.S. cities, 1987-1994. *N Engl J Med.* (2000) 343:1742–9. doi: 10.1056/NEJM200012143432401
24. Peng RD, Dominici F, Pastor-Barriuso R, Zeger SL, Samet JM. Seasonal analyses of air pollution and mortality in 100 US cities. *Am J Epidemiol.* (2005) 161:585–94. doi: 10.1093/aje/kwi075
25. Bell ML, Ebisu K, Peng RD, Walker J, Samet JM, Zeger SL, et al. Seasonal and regional short-term effects of fine particles on hospital admissions in 202 US counties, 1999-2005. *Am J Epidemiol.* (2008) 168:1301–10. doi: 10.1093/aje/kwn252
26. Katsouyanni K, Touloumi G, Spix C, Schwartz J, Balducci F, Medina S, et al. Short-term effects of ambient sulphur dioxide and particulate matter on mortality in 12 European cities: results from time series data from the APHEA project. *Air Pollution and Health* (1997) 314:1658–63.
27. Katsouyanni K, Touloumi G, Samoli E, Gryparis A, Le Tertre A, Monopolis Y, et al. Confounding and effect modification in the short-term effects of ambient particles on total mortality: results from 29 European cities within the APHEA2 project. *Epidemiology* (2001) 12:521–31. doi: 10.1097/00001648-200109000-00011
28. Nawrot TS, Perez L, Kunzli N, Munters E, Nemery B. Public health importance of triggers of myocardial infarction: a comparative risk assessment. *Lancet* (2011) 377:732–40. doi: 10.1016/S0140-6736(10)62 296-9
29. Pope CA III, Burnett RT, Krewski D, Jerrett M, Shi Y, Calle EE, et al. Cardiovascular mortality and exposure to airborne fine particulate matter and cigarette smoke: shape of the exposure-response relationship. *Circulation* (2009) 120:941–8. doi: 10.1161/CIRCULATIONAHA.109.857888
30. Burnett RT, Pope CA III, Ezzati M, Olives C, Lim SS, Mehta S, et al. An integrated risk function for estimating the global burden of disease attributable to ambient fine particulate matter exposure. *Environ Health Perspect.* (2014) 122:397–403. doi: 10.1289/ehp.1307049
31. Apte JS, Marshall JD, Cohen AJ, Brauer M. Addressing global mortality from ambient PM2.5. *Environ Sci Technol.* (2015) 49:8057–66. doi: 10.1021/acs.est.5b01236
32. Shin HH, Cohen AJ, Pope CA III, Ezzati M, Lim SS, Hubbell BJ, et al. Meta-analysis methods to estimate the shape and uncertainty in the association between long-term exposure to ambient fine particulate matter and cause-specific mortality over the global concentration range. *Risk Anal.* (2015) 36:1813–25. doi: 10.1111/risa.12421
33. Xie W, Li G, Zhao D, Xie X, Wei Z, Wang W, et al. Relationship between fine particulate air pollution and ischaemic heart disease morbidity and mortality. *Heart* (2015) 101:257–63. doi: 10.1136/heartjnl-2014-306165
34. Dockery DW, Pope CA III, Xu X, Spengler JD, Ware JH, Fay ME, et al. An association between air pollution and mortality in six U.S. cities. *N Engl J Med.* (1993) 329:1753–9. doi: 10.1056/NEJM199312093292401
35. Pope CA III, Thun MJ, Namboodiri MM, Dockery DW, Evans JS, Speizer FE, et al. Particulate air pollution as a predictor of mortality in a prospective study of U.S. adults. *Am J Respir Crit Care Med.* (1995). 151:669–74. doi: 10.1164/ajrccm/151.3_Pt_1.669
36. Pope CA III, Burnett RT, Thun MJ, Calle EE, Krewski D, Ito K, et al. Lung cancer, cardiopulmonary mortality, and long-term exposure to fine particulate air pollution. *JAMA* (2002) 287:1132–41. doi: 10.1001/jama.287.9.1132
37. Beelen R, Raaschou-Nielsen O, Stafoggia M, Andersen ZJ, Weinmayr G, Hoffmann B, et al. Effects of long-term exposure to air pollution on natural-cause mortality: an analysis of 22 European cohorts within the multicentre ESCAPE project. *Lancet* (2014) 383:785–95. doi: 10.1016/S0140-6736(13)62158-3
38. Cohen AJ, Brauer M, Burnett R, Anderson HR, Frostad J, Estep K, et al. Estimates and 25-year trends of the global burden of disease attributable to ambient air pollution: an analysis of data from the Global Burden of Diseases Study 2015. *Lancet* (2017) 389:1907–18. doi: 10.1016/S0140-6736(17)30505-6
39. Song C, He J, Wu L, Jin T, Chen X, Li R, et al. Health burden attributable to ambient PM2.5 in China. *Environ Pollut.* (2017) 223:575–86. doi: 10.1016/j.envpol.2017.01.060
40. Samoli E, Peng R, Ramsay T, Pipikou M, Touloumi G, Dominici F, et al. Acute effects of ambient particulate matter on mortality in Europe and North America: results from the APHENA study. *Environ Health Perspect.* (2008) 116:1480–6. doi: 10.1289/ehp.11345
41. Pope CA III, Burnett RT, Thurston GD, Thun MJ, Calle EE, Krewski D, et al. Cardiovascular mortality and long-term exposure to particulate air pollution: epidemiological evidence of general pathophysiological pathways of disease. *Circulation* (2004) 109:71–7. doi: 10.1161/01.CIR.0000108927.80044.7F
42. Di Q, Dai L, Wang Y, Zanobetti A, Choirat C, Schwartz JD, et al. Association of short-term exposure to air pollution with mortality in older adults. *JAMA* (2017) 318:2446–56. doi: 10.1001/jama.2017.17923
43. Di Q, Wang Y, Zanobetti A, Wang Y, Koutrakis P, Choirat C, et al. Air pollution and mortality in the medicare population. *N Engl J Med.* (2017) 376:2513–22. doi: 10.1056/NEJMoa1702747
44. Parker JD, Kravets N, Vaidyanathan A. Particulate matter air pollution exposure and heart disease mortality risks by race and ethnicity in the United States: 1997 to 2009 national health interview survey with mortality follow-up through 2011. *Circulation* (2018) 137:1688–97. doi: 10.1161/CIRCULATIONAHA.117.029376
45. Clark LP, Millet DB, Marshall JD. Changes in transportation-related air pollution exposures by race-ethnicity and socioeconomic status: outdoor nitrogen dioxide in the United States in 2000 and 2010. *Environ Health Perspect* (2017) 125:097012. doi: 10.1289/EHP959
46. Hoek G, Brunekreef B, Goldbohm S, Fischer P, van den Brandt PA. Association between mortality and indicators of traffic-related air pollution in the Netherlands: a cohort study. *Lancet* (2002) 360:1203–9. doi: 10.1016/S0140-6736(02)11280-3
47. Jerrett M, Burnett RT, Ma R, Pope CA III, Krewski D, Newbold KB, et al. Spatial analysis of air pollution and mortality in Los Angeles. *Epidemiology* (2005) 16:727–36. doi: 10.1097/01.ede.0000181630.15826.7d

48. Miller KA, Siscovick DS, Sheppard L, Shepherd K, Sullivan JH, Anderson GL, et al. Long-term exposure to air pollution and incidence of cardiovascular events in women. *N Engl J Med.* (2007) 356:447–58. doi: 10.1056/NEJMoa054409
49. Puett RC, Schwartz J, Hart JE, Yanosky JD, Speizer FE, Suh H, et al. Chronic particulate exposure, mortality, and coronary heart disease in the nurses' health study. *Am J Epidemiol.* (2008) 168:1161–8. doi: 10.1093/aje/kwn232
50. Landrigan PJ, Fuller R, Acosta NJR, Adeyi O, Arnold R, Basu NN, et al. The *Lancet* Commission on pollution and health. *Lancet* (2018) 391:462–512. doi: 10.1016/S0140-6736(17)32345-0
51. Laden F, Schwartz J, Speizer FE, Dockery DW. Reduction in fine particulate air pollution and mortality: extended follow-up of the Harvard six cities study. *Am J Respir Crit Care Med.* (2006) 173:667–72. doi: 10.1164/rccm.200503-443OC
52. Dominici F, Peng RD, Zeger SL, White RH, Samet JM. Particulate air pollution and mortality in the United States: did the risks change from 1987 to 2000? *Am J Epidemiol.* (2007) 166:880–8. doi: 10.1093/aje/kwm222
53. Schwartz J, Coull B, Laden F, Ryan L. The effect of dose and timing of dose on the association between airborne particles and survival. *Environ Health Perspect.* (2008) 116:64–9. doi: 10.1289/ehp.9955
54. Pope CA III, Ezzati M, Dockery DW. Fine-particulate air pollution and life expectancy in the United States. *N Engl J Med.* (2009) 360:376–86. doi: 10.1056/NEJMsa0805646
55. Clancy L, Goodman P, Sinclair H, Dockery DW. Effect of air-pollution control on death rates in Dublin, Ireland: an intervention study. *Lancet* (2002) 360:1210–4. doi: 10.1016/S0140-6736(02)11281-5
56. Yorifuji T, Kashima S, Doi H. Fine-particulate air pollution from diesel emission control and mortality rates in Tokyo: a quasi-experimental study. *Epidemiology* (2016) 27:769–78. doi: 10.1097/EDE.0000000000000546
57. Cesaroni G, Forastiere F, Stafoggia M, Andersen ZJ, Badaloni C, Beelen R, et al. Long term exposure to ambient air pollution and incidence of acute coronary events: prospective cohort study and meta-analysis in 11 European cohorts from the ESCAPE Project. *BMJ* (2014) 348:f7412. doi: 10.1136/bmj.f7412
58. Madrigano J, Kloog I, Goldberg R, Coull BA, Mittleman MA, Schwartz J. Long-term exposure to PM2.5 and incidence of acute myocardial infarction. *Environ Health Perspect.* (2013) 121:192–6. doi: 10.1289/ehp.1205284
59. Wellenius GA, Bateson TF, Mittleman MA, Schwartz J. Particulate air pollution and the rate of hospitalization for congestive heart failure among medicare beneficiaries in Pittsburgh, Pennsylvania. *Am J Epidemiol.* (2005) 161:1030–6. doi: 10.1093/aje/kwi135
60. Atkinson RW, Carey IM, Kent AJ, van Staa TP, Anderson HR, Cook DG. Long-term exposure to outdoor air pollution and incidence of cardiovascular diseases. *Epidemiology* (2013) 24:44–53. doi: 10.1097/EDE.0b013e318276ccb8
61. Stafoggia M, Cesaroni G, Peters A, Andersen ZJ, Badaloni C, Beelen R, et al. Long-term exposure to ambient air pollution and incidence of cerebrovascular events: results from 11 European cohorts within the ESCAPE project. *Environ Health Perspect.* (2014) 122:919–25. doi: 10.1289/ehp.1307301
62. Wellenius GA, Burger MR, Coull BA, Schwartz J, Suh HH, Koutrakis P, et al. Ambient air pollution and the risk of acute ischemic stroke. *Arch Intern Med.* (2012) 172:229–34. doi: 10.1001/archinternmed.2011.732
63. Ghio AJ, Kim C, Devlin RB. Concentrated ambient air particles induce mild pulmonary inflammation in healthy human volunteers. *Am J Respir Crit Care Med.* (2000) 162:981–8. doi: 10.1164/ajrccm.162.3.9911115
64. van Eeden SF, Tan WC, Suwa T, Mukae H, Terashima T, Fujii T, et al. Cytokines involved in the systemic inflammatory response induced by exposure to particulate matter air pollutants [PM(10)]. *Am J Respir Crit Care Med.* (2001) 164:826–30. doi: 10.1164/ajrccm.164.5.2010160
65. Riediker M, Cascio WE, Griggs TR, Herbst MC, Bromberg PA, Neas L, et al. Particulate matter exposure in cars is associated with cardiovascular effects in healthy young men. *Am J Respir Crit Care Med.* (2004) 169:934–40. doi: 10.1164/rccm.200310-1463OC
66. Tsai DH, Amyai N, Marques-Vidal P, Wang JL, Riediker M, Mooser V, et al. Effects of particulate matter on inflammatory markers in the general adult population. *Part Fibre Toxicol.* (2012) 9:24. doi: 10.1186/1743-8977-9-24
67. Moller P, Loft S. Oxidative damage to DNA and lipids as biomarkers of exposure to air pollution. *Environ Health Perspect.* (2010) 118:1126–36. doi: 10.1289/ehp.0901725
68. Jacobs L, Emmerechts J, Hoylaerts MF, Mathieu C, Hoet PH, Nemery B, et al. Traffic air pollution and oxidized LDL. *PLoS ONE* (2011) 6:e16200. doi: 10.1371/journal.pone.0016200
69. Huang W, Wang G, Lu SE, Kipen H, Wang Y, Hu M, et al. Inflammatory and oxidative stress responses of healthy young adults to changes in air quality during the Beijing Olympics. *Am J Respir Crit Care Med.* (2012) 186:1150–9. doi: 10.1164/rccm.201205-0850OC
70. Yin F, Lawal A, Ricks J, Fox JR, Larson T, Navab M, et al. Diesel exhaust induces systemic lipid peroxidation and development of dysfunctional pro-oxidant and pro-inflammatory high-density lipoprotein. *Arterioscler Thromb Vasc Biol.* (2013) 33:1153–61. doi: 10.1161/ATVBAHA.112.300552
71. Kunzli N, Jerrett M, Mack WJ, Beckerman B, LaBree L, Gilliland F, et al. Ambient air pollution and atherosclerosis in Los Angeles. *Environ Health Perspect.* (2005) 113:201–6. doi: 10.1289/ehp.7523
72. Diez Roux AV, Auchincloss AH, Franklin TG, Raghunathan T, Barr RG, Kaufman J, et al. Long-term exposure to ambient particulate matter and prevalence of subclinical atherosclerosis in the Multi-Ethnic Study of Atherosclerosis. *Am J Epidemiol.* (2008) 167:667–75. doi: 10.1093/aje/kwm359
73. Bauer M, Moebus S, Mohlenkamp S, Dragano N, Nonnemacher M, Fuchsluger M, et al. Urban particulate matter air pollution is associated with subclinical atherosclerosis: results from the HNR (Heinz Nixdorf Recall) study. *J Am Coll Cardiol.* (2010) 56:1803–8. doi: 10.1016/j.jacc.2010.04.065
74. Adar SD, Sheppard L, Vedal S, Polak JF, Sampson PD, Diez Roux AV, et al. Fine particulate air pollution and the progression of carotid intima-medial thickness: a prospective cohort study from the multi-ethnic study of atherosclerosis and air pollution. *PLoS Med.* (2013) 10:e1001430. doi: 10.1371/journal.pmed.1001430
75. Hoffmann B, Moebus S, Mohlenkamp S, Stang A, Lehmann N, Dragano N, et al. Residential exposure to traffic is associated with coronary atherosclerosis. *Circulation* (2007) 116:489–96. doi: 10.1161/CIRCULATIONAHA.107.693622
76. Lambrechtsen J, Gerke O, Egstrup K, Sand NP, Norgaard BL, Petersen H, et al. The relation between coronary artery calcification in asymptomatic subjects and both traditional risk factors and living in the city centre: a DanRisk substudy. *J Intern Med.* (2012) 271:444–50. doi: 10.1111/j.1365-2796.2011.02486.x
77. Sun Q, Wang A, Jin X, Natanzon A, Duquaine D, Brook RD, et al. Long-term air pollution exposure and acceleration of atherosclerosis and vascular inflammation in an animal model. *JAMA* (2005) 294:3003–10. doi: 10.1001/jama.294.23.3003
78. Araujo JA, Barajas B, Kleinman M, Wang X, Bennett BJ, Gong KW, et al. Ambient particulate pollutants in the ultrafine range promote early atherosclerosis and systemic oxidative stress. *Circ Res.* (2008) 102:589–96. doi: 10.1161/CIRCRESAHA.107.164970
79. Campen MJ, Lund AK, Knuckles TL, Conklin DJ, Bishop B, Young D, et al. Inhaled diesel emissions alter atherosclerotic plaque composition in ApoE(-/-) mice. *Toxicol Appl Pharmacol.* (2010) 242:310–7. doi: 10.1016/j.taap.2009.10.021
80. Bai N, Kido T, Suzuki H, Yang G, Kavanagh TJ, Kaufman JD, et al. Changes in atherosclerotic plaques induced by inhalation of diesel exhaust. *Atherosclerosis* (2011) 216:299–306. doi: 10.1016/j.atherosclerosis.2011.02.019
81. Baccarelli A, Martinelli I, Pegoraro V, Melly S, Grillo P, Zanobetti A, et al. Living near major traffic roads and risk of deep vein thrombosis. *Circulation* (2009) 119:3118–24. doi: 10.1161/CIRCULATIONAHA.108.836163
82. Signorelli SS, Ferrante M, Gaudio A, Fiore V. Deep vein thrombosis related to environment (Review). *Mol Med Rep.* (2017) 15:3445–8. doi: 10.3892/mmr.2017.6395
83. Riediker M, Devlin RB, Griggs TR, Herbst MC, Bromberg PA, Williams RW, et al. Cardiovascular effects in patrol officers are associated with fine particulate matter from brake wear and engine emissions. *Part Fibre Toxicol.* (2004) 1:2. doi: 10.1186/1743-8977-1-2

84. Rich DQ, Kipen HM, Huang W, Wang G, Wang Y, Zhu P, et al. Association between changes in air pollution levels during the Beijing Olympics and biomarkers of inflammation and thrombosis in healthy young adults. *JAMA* (2012) 307:2068–78. doi: 10.1001/jama.2012.3488
85. Liu C, Cai J, Qiao L, Wang H, Xu W, Li H, et al. The acute effects of fine particulate matter constituents on blood inflammation and coagulation. *Environ Sci Technol.* (2017) 51:8128–37. doi: 10.1021/acs.est.7b00312
86. Mills NL, Tornqvist H, Robinson SD, Gonzalez M, Darnley K, MacNee W, et al. Diesel exhaust inhalation causes vascular dysfunction and impaired endogenous fibrinolysis. *Circulation* (2005) 112:3930–6. doi: 10.1161/CIRCULATIONAHA.105.588962
87. Chuang KJ, Chan CC, Su TC, Lee CT, Tang CS. The effect of urban air pollution on inflammation, oxidative stress, coagulation, and autonomic dysfunction in young adults. *Am J Respir Crit Care Med.* (2007) 176:370–6. doi: 10.1164/rccm.200611-1627OC
88. Mills NL, Tornqvist H, Gonzalez MC, Vink E, Robinson SD, Soderberg S, et al. Ischemic and thrombotic effects of dilute diesel-exhaust inhalation in men with coronary heart disease. *N Engl J Med.* (2007) 357:1075–82. doi: 10.1056/NEJMoa066314
89. Peters A, Doring A, Wichmann HE, Koenig W. Increased plasma viscosity during an air pollution episode: a link to mortality? *Lancet* (1997) 349:1582–7. doi: 10.1016/S0140-6736(97)01211-7
90. Lucking AJ, Lundback M, Mills NL, Faratian D, Barath SL, Pourazar J, et al. Diesel exhaust inhalation increases thrombus formation in man. *Eur Heart J.* (2008) 29:3043–51. doi: 10.1093/eurheartj/ehn464
91. Jacobs L, Emmerechts J, Mathieu C, Hoylaerts MF, Fierens F, Hoet PH, et al. Air pollution related prothrombotic changes in persons with diabetes. *Environ Health Perspect.* (2010) 118:191–6. doi: 10.1289/ehp.0900942
92. Lucking AJ, Lundback M, Barath SL, Mills NL, Sidhu MK, Langrish JP, et al. Particle traps prevent adverse vascular and prothrombotic effects of diesel engine exhaust inhalation in men. *Circulation* (2011) 123:1721–8. doi: 10.1161/CIRCULATIONAHA.110.987263
93. Brook RD, Brook JR, Urch B, Vincent R, Rajagopalan S, Silverman F. Inhalation of fine particulate air pollution and ozone causes acute arterial vasoconstriction in healthy adults. *Circulation* (2002) 105:1534–6. doi: 10.1161/01.CIR.0000013838.94747.64
94. Tornqvist H, Mills NL, Gonzalez M, Miller MR, Robinson SD, Megson IL, et al. Persistent endothelial dysfunction in humans after diesel exhaust inhalation. *Am J Respir Crit Care Med.* (2007) 176:395–400. doi: 10.1164/rccm.200606-872OC
95. Peretz A, Sullivan JH, Leotta DF, Trenga CA, Sands FN, Allen J, et al. Diesel exhaust inhalation elicits acute vasoconstriction *in vivo*. *Environ Health Perspect.* (2008) 116:937–42. doi: 10.1289/ehp.11027
96. Barath S, Mills NL, Lundback M, Tornqvist H, Lucking AJ, Langrish JP, et al. Impaired vascular function after exposure to diesel exhaust generated at urban transient running conditions. *Part Fibre Toxicol.* (2010) 7:19. doi: 10.1186/1743-8977-7-19
97. Adar SD, Klein R, Klein BE, Szpiro AA, Cotch MF, Wong TY, et al. Air Pollution and the microvasculature: a cross-sectional assessment of *in vivo* retinal images in the population-based multi-ethnic study of atherosclerosis (MESA). *PLoS Med.* (2010) 7:e1000372. doi: 10.1371/journal.pmed.1000372
98. Krishnan RM, Adar SD, Szpiro AA, Jorgensen NW, Van Hee VC, Barr RG, et al. Vascular responses to long- and short-term exposure to fine particulate matter: MESA Air (Multi-Ethnic Study of Atherosclerosis and Air Pollution). *J Am Coll Cardiol.* (2012) 60:2158–66. doi: 10.1016/j.jacc.2012.08.973
99. Coogan PF, White LF, Jerrett M, Brook RD, Su JG, Seto E, et al. Air pollution and incidence of hypertension and diabetes mellitus in black women living in Los Angeles. *Circulation* (2012) 125:767–72. doi: 10.1161/CIRCULATIONAHA.111.052753
100. Chen H, Burnett RT, Kwong JC, Villeneuve PJ, Goldberg MS, Brook RD, et al. Spatial association between ambient fine particulate matter and incident hypertension. *Circulation* (2014) 129:562–9. doi: 10.1161/CIRCULATIONAHA.113.003532
101. Cosselman KE, Krishnan RM, Oron AP, Jansen K, Peretz A, Sullivan JH, et al. Blood pressure response to controlled diesel exhaust exposure in human subjects. *Hypertension* (2012) 59:943–8. doi: 10.1161/HYPERTENSIONAHA.111.186593
102. Bellavia A, Urch B, Speck M, Brook RD, Scott JA, Albetti B, et al. DNA hypomethylation, ambient particulate matter, and increased blood pressure: findings from controlled human exposure experiments. *J Am Heart Assoc.* (2013) 2:e000212. doi: 10.1161/JAHA.113.000212
103. Vinikoor-Imler LC, Gray SC, Edwards SE, Miranda ML. The effects of exposure to particulate matter and neighbourhood deprivation on gestational hypertension. *Paediatr Perinat Epidemiol.* (2012) 26:91–100. doi: 10.1111/j.1365-3016.2011.01245.x
104. Dadvand P, Ostro B, Amato F, Figueras F, Minguillon MC, Martinez D, et al. Particulate air pollution and preeclampsia: a source-based analysis. *Occup Environ Med.* (2014) 71:570–7. doi: 10.1136/oemed-2013-101693
105. Van Hee VC, Adar SD, Szpiro AA, Barr RG, Bluemke DA, Diez Roux AV, et al. Exposure to traffic and left ventricular mass and function: the Multi-Ethnic Study of Atherosclerosis. *Am J Respir Crit Care Med.* (2009) 179:827–34. doi: 10.1164/rccm.200808-1344OC
106. Leary PJ, Kaufman JD, Barr RG, Bluemke DA, Curl CL, Hough CL, et al. Traffic-related air pollution and the right ventricle. The multi-ethnic study of atherosclerosis. *Am J Respir Crit Care Med.* (2014) 189:1093–100. doi: 10.1164/rccm.201312-2298OC
107. Ying Z, Yue P, Xu X, Zhong M, Sun Q, Mikolaj M, et al. Air pollution and cardiac remodeling: a role for RhoA/Rho-kinase. *Am J Physiol Heart Circ Physiol.* (2009) 296:H1540–1550. doi: 10.1152/ajpheart.01270.2008
108. Wold LE, Ying Z, Hutchinson KR, Velten M, Gorr MW, Velten C, et al. Cardiovascular remodeling in response to long-term exposure to fine particulate matter air pollution. *Circ Heart Fail* (2012) 5:452–61. doi: 10.1161/CIRCHEARTFAILURE.112.966580
109. Dockery DW, Luttmann-Gibson H, Rich DQ, Link MS, Mittleman MA, Gold DR, et al. Association of air pollution with increased incidence of ventricular tachyarrhythmias recorded by implanted cardioverter defibrillators. *Environ Health Perspect.* (2005) 113:670–4. doi: 10.1289/ehp.7767
110. Rich DQ, Mittleman MA, Link MS, Schwartz J, Luttmann-Gibson H, Catalano PJ, et al. Increased risk of paroxysmal atrial fibrillation episodes associated with acute increases in ambient air pollution. *Environ Health Perspect.* (2006) 114:120–3. doi: 10.1289/ehp.8371
111. Link MS, Luttmann-Gibson H, Schwartz J, Mittleman MA, Wessler B, Gold DR, et al. Acute exposure to air pollution triggers atrial fibrillation. *J Am Coll Cardiol.* (2013) 62:816–25. doi: 10.1016/j.jacc.2013.05.043
112. Folino F, Buja G, Zanotto G, Marras E, Allocca G, Vaccari D, et al. Association between air pollution and ventricular arrhythmias in high-risk patients (ARIA study): a multicentre longitudinal study. *Lancet Planet Health* (2017) 1:e58–64. doi: 10.1016/S2542-5196(17)30020-7
113. Pope CA III, Verrier RL, Lovett EG, Larson AC, Raizenne ME, Kanner RE, et al. Heart rate variability associated with particulate air pollution. *Am Heart J.* (1999) 138:890–9.
114. Gold DR, Litonjua A, Schwartz J, Lovett E, Larson A, Nearing B, et al. Ambient pollution and heart rate variability. *Circulation* (2000) 101:1267–73. doi: 10.1161/01.cir.101.11.1267
115. Pekkanen J, Peters A, Hoek G, Tiittanen P, Brunekreef B, de Hartog J, et al. Particulate air pollution and risk of ST-segment depression during repeated submaximal exercise tests among subjects with coronary heart disease: the Exposure and Risk Assessment for Fine and Ultrafine Particles in Ambient Air (ULTRA) study. *Circulation* (2002) 106:933–8. doi: 10.1161/01.CIR.0000027561.41736.3C
116. Henneberger A, Zareba W, Ibald-Mulli A, Ruckerl R, Cyrys J, Couderc JP, et al. Repolarization changes induced by air pollution in ischemic heart disease patients. *Environ Health Perspect.* (2005) 113:440–6. doi: 10.1289/ehp.7579
117. Zanobetti A, Stone PH, Speizer FE, Schwartz JD, Coull BA, Suh HH, et al. T-wave alternans, air pollution and traffic in high-risk subjects. *Am J Cardiol.* (2009) 104:665–70. doi: 10.1016/j.amjcard.2009.04.046
118. Zanobetti A, Gold DR, Stone PH, Suh HH, Schwartz J, Coull BA, et al. Reduction in heart rate variability with traffic and air pollution in patients with coronary artery disease. *Environ Health Perspect.* (2010) 118:324–30. doi: 10.1289/ehp.0901003
119. He F, Shaffer ML, Rodriguez-Colon S, Yanosky JD, Bixler E, Cascio WE, et al. Acute effects of fine particulate air pollution on cardiac arrhythmia: the APACR study. *Environ Health Perspect.* (2011) 119:927–32. doi: 10.1289/ehp.1002640

120. Cakmak S, Dales R, Kauri LM, Mahmud M, Van Ryswyk K, Vanos J, et al. Metal composition of fine particulate air pollution and acute changes in cardiorespiratory physiology. *Environ Pollut.* (2014) 189:208–14. doi: 10.1016/j.envpol.2014.03.004
121. Wang T, Lang GD, Moreno-Vinasco L, Huang Y, Goonewardena SN, Peng YJ, et al. Particulate matter induces cardiac arrhythmias via dysregulation of carotid body sensitivity and cardiac sodium channels. *Am J Respir Cell Mol Biol.* (2012) 46:524–31. doi: 10.1165/rcmb.2011-0213OC
122. Watkinson WP, Campen MJ, Costa DL. Cardiac arrhythmia induction after exposure to residual oil fly ash particles in a rodent model of pulmonary hypertension. *Toxicol Sci.* (1998) 41:209–16. doi: 10.1006/toxs.1997.2406
123. Brook RD, Xu X, Bard RL, Dvonch JT, Morishita M, Kaciroti N, et al. Reduced metabolic insulin sensitivity following sub-acute exposures to low levels of ambient fine particulate matter air pollution. *Sci Total Environ.* (2013) 448:66–71. doi: 10.1016/j.scitotenv.2012.07.034
124. Thiering E, Cyrys J, Kratzsch J, Meisinger C, Hoffmann B, Berdel D, et al. Long-term exposure to traffic-related air pollution and insulin resistance in children: results from the GINIplus and LISAplus birth cohorts. *Diabetologia* (2013) 56:1696–704. doi: 10.1007/s00125-013-2925-x
125. Wolf K, Popp A, Schneider A, Breitner S, Hampel R, Rathmann W, et al. Association between long-term exposure to air pollution and biomarkers related to insulin resistance, subclinical inflammation, and adipokines. *Diabetes* (2016) 65:3314–26. doi: 10.2337/db15-1567
126. Pearson JF, Bachireddy C, Shyamprasad S, Goldfine AB, Brownstein JS. Association between fine particulate matter and diabetes prevalence in the U.S. *Diabetes Care* (2010) 33:2196–201. doi: 10.2337/dc10-0698
127. Weinmayr G, Hennig F, Fuks K, Nonnemacher M, Jakobs H, Mohlenkamp S, et al. Long-term exposure to fine particulate matter and incidence of type 2 diabetes mellitus in a cohort study: effects of total and traffic-specific air pollution. *Environ Health* (2015) 14:53. doi: 10.1186/s12940-015-0031-x
128. O'Neill MS, Veves A, Zanobetti A, Sarnat JA, Gold DR, Economides PA, et al. Diabetes enhances vulnerability to particulate air pollution-associated impairment in vascular reactivity and endothelial function. *Circulation* (2005) 111:2913–20. doi: 10.1161/CIRCULATIONAHA.104.517110
129. Sun Q, Yue P, Deiuliis JA, Lumeng CN, Kampfrath T, Mikolaj MB, et al. Ambient air pollution exaggerates adipose inflammation and insulin resistance in a mouse model of diet-induced obesity. *Circulation* (2009) 119:538–46. doi: 10.1161/CIRCULATIONAHA.108.799015
130. Liu C, Bai Y, Xu X, Sun L, Wang A, Wang TY, et al. Exaggerated effects of particulate matter air pollution in genetic type II diabetes mellitus. *Part Fibre Toxicol.* (2014) 11:27. doi: 10.1186/1743-8977-11-27
131. Liu C, Xu X, Bai Y, Wang TY, Rao X, Wang A, et al. Air pollution-mediated susceptibility to inflammation and insulin resistance: influence of CCR2 pathways in mice. *Environ Health Perspect.* (2014) 122:17–26. doi: 10.1289/ehp.1306841
132. Xu X, Yavar Z, Verdin M, Ying Z, Mihai G, Kampfrath T, et al. Effect of early particulate air pollution exposure on obesity in mice: role of p47phox. *Arterioscler Thromb Vasc Biol.* (2010) 30:2518–27. doi: 10.1161/ATVBAHA.110.215350
133. Franklin BA, Brook R, Arden Pope C III Air pollution and cardiovascular disease. *Curr Probl Cardiol.* (2015) 40:207–38. doi: 10.1016/j.cpcardiol.2015.01.003
134. Semmler M, Seitz J, Erbe F, Mayer P, Heyder J, Oberdorster G, et al. Long-term clearance kinetics of inhaled ultrafine insoluble iridium particles from the rat lung, including transient translocation into secondary organs. *Inhal Toxicol.* (2004) 16:453–9. doi: 10.1080/08958370490439650
135. Semmler-Behnke M, Takenaka S, Fertsch S, Wenk A, Seitz J, Mayer P, et al. Efficient elimination of inhaled nanoparticles from the alveolar region: evidence for interstitial uptake and subsequent reentrainment onto airways epithelium. *Environ Health Perspect.* (2007) 115:728–33. doi: 10.1289/ehp.9685
136. Rao X, Zhong J, Brook RD, Rajagopalan S. Effect of particulate matter air pollution on cardiovascular oxidative stress pathways. *Antioxid Redox Signal* (2018) 28:797–818. doi: 10.1089/ars.2017.7394
137. Mutlu GM, Snyder C, Bellmeyer A, Wang H, Hawkins K, Soberanes S, et al. Airborne particulate matter inhibits alveolar fluid reabsorption in mice via oxidant generation. *Am J Respir Cell Mol Biol.* (2006) 34:670–6. doi: 10.1165/rcmb.2005-0329OC
138. Soberanes S, Panduri V, Mutlu GM, Ghio A, Bundinger GR, Kamp DW. p53 mediates particulate matter-induced alveolar epithelial cell mitochondria-regulated apoptosis. *Am J Respir Crit Care Med.* (2006) 174:1229–38. doi: 10.1164/rccm.200602-203OC
139. Manzo ND, LaGier AJ, Slade R, Ledbetter AD, Richards JH, Dye JA. Nitric oxide and superoxide mediate diesel particle effects in cytokine-treated mice and murine lung epithelial cells–implications for susceptibility to traffic-related air pollution. *Part Fibre Toxicol.* (2012) 9:43. doi: 10.1186/1743-8977-9-43
140. Hong Z, Guo Z, Zhang R, Xu J, Dong W, Zhuang G, et al. Airborne fine particulate matter induces oxidative stress and inflammation in human nasal epithelial cells. *Tohoku J Exp Med.* (2016) 239:117–25. doi: 10.1620/tjem.239.117
141. Wang J, Huang J, Wang L, Chen C, Yang D, Jin M, et al. Urban particulate matter triggers lung inflammation via the ROS-MAPK-NF-kappaB signaling pathway. *J Thorac Dis.* (2017) 9:4398–412. doi: 10.21037/jtd.2017.09.135
142. Li N, Sioutas C, Cho A, Schmitz D, Misra C, Sempf J, et al. Ultrafine particulate pollutants induce oxidative stress and mitochondrial damage. *Environ Health Perspect.* (2003) 111:455–60. doi: 10.1289/ehp.6000
143. Ohyama K, Kubo H, Harada M, Sasahara Y, Nozaki A, Takei N, et al. Comparison of 3 Tesla whole heart coronary MRA (WHCA) with 1.5 Tesla. *Nihon Hoshasen Gijutsu Gakkai Zasshi* (2008) 64:1540–6. doi: 10.6009/jjrt.64.1540
144. Zhao Q, Chen H, Yang T, Rui W, Liu F, Zhang F, et al. Direct effects of airborne PM2.5 exposure on macrophage polarizations. *Biochim Biophys Acta* (2016) 1860:2835–43. doi: 10.1016/j.bbagen.2016.03.033
145. Li R, Ning Z, Cui J, Khalsa B, Ai L, Takabe W, et al. Ultrafine particles from diesel engines induce vascular oxidative stress via JNK activation. *Free Radic Biol Med.* (2009) 46:775–82. doi: 10.1016/j.freeradbiomed.2008.11.025
146. Montiel-Davalos A, Ibarra-Sanchez Mde J, Ventura-Gallegos JL, Alfaro-Moreno E, Lopez-Marure R. Oxidative stress and apoptosis are induced in human endothelial cells exposed to urban particulate matter. *Toxicol In Vitro* (2010) 24:135–41. doi: 10.1016/j.tiv.2009.08.004
147. Cao J, Qin G, Shi R, Bai F, Yang G, Zhang M, et al. Overproduction of reactive oxygen species and activation of MAPKs are involved in apoptosis induced by PM2.5 in rat cardiac H9c2 cells. *J Appl Toxicol.* (2016) 36:609–17. doi: 10.1002/jat.3249
148. Yang X, Feng L, Zhang Y, Hu H, Shi Y, Liang S, et al. Cytotoxicity induced by fine particulate matter (PM2.5) via mitochondria-mediated apoptosis pathway in human cardiomyocytes. *Ecotoxicol Environ Saf.* (2018) 161:198–207. doi: 10.1016/j.ecoenv.2018.05.092
149. Mutlu EA, Engen PA, Soberanes S, Urich D, Forsyth CB, Nigdelioglu R, et al. Particulate matter air pollution causes oxidant-mediated increase in gut permeability in mice. *Part Fibre Toxicol.* (2011) 8:19. doi: 10.1186/1743-8977-8-19
150. Jin SP, Li Z, Choi EK, Lee S, Kim YK, Seo EY, et al. Urban particulate matter in air pollution penetrates into the barrier-disrupted skin and produces ROS-dependent cutaneous inflammatory response *in vivo*. *J Dermatol Sci.* (2018). doi: 10.1016/j.jdermsci.2018.04.015
151. Park EJ, Chae JB, Lyu J, Yoon C, Kim S, Yeom C, et al. Ambient fine particulate matters induce cell death and inflammatory response by influencing mitochondria function in human corneal epithelial cells. *Environ Res.* (2017) 159:595–605. doi: 10.1016/j.envres.2017.08.044
152. Imrich A, Ning Y, Lawrence J, Coull B, Gitin E, Knutson M, et al. Alveolar macrophage cytokine response to air pollution particles: oxidant mechanisms. *Toxicol Appl Pharmacol.* (2007) 218:256–64. doi: 10.1016/j.taap.2006.11.033
153. Chiarella SE, Soberanes S, Urich D, Morales-Nebreda L, Nigdelioglu R, Green D, et al. beta(2)-Adrenergic agonists augment air pollution-induced IL-6 release and thrombosis. *J Clin Invest.* (2014) 124:2935–46. doi: 10.1172/JCI75157
154. Tripathi P, Deng F, Scruggs AM, Chen Y, Huang SK. Variation in doses and duration of particulate matter exposure in bronchial epithelial cells results in upregulation of different genes associated with airway disorders. *Toxicol In Vitro* (2018) 51:95–105. doi: 10.1016/j.tiv.2018.05.004

155. Xu C, Shi Q, Zhang L, Zhao H. High molecular weight hyaluronan attenuates fine particulate matter-induced acute lung injury through inhibition of ROS-ASK1-p38/JNK-mediated epithelial apoptosis. *Environ Toxicol Pharmacol.* (2018) 59:190–8. doi: 10.1016/j.etap.2018.03.020
156. Hamanaka RB, Chandel NS. Mitochondrial reactive oxygen species regulate cellular signaling and dictate biological outcomes. *Trends Biochem Sci.* (2010) 35:505–13. doi: 10.1016/j.tibs.2010.04.002
157. Li R, Kou X, Geng H, Xie J, Yang Z, Zhang Y, et al. Effect of ambient PM(2.5) on lung mitochondrial damage and fusion/fission gene expression in rats. *Chem Res Toxicol.* (2015) 28:408–18. doi: 10.1021/tx5003723
158. Jin X, Xue B, Zhou Q, Su R, Li Z. Mitochondrial damage mediated by ROS incurs bronchial epithelial cell apoptosis upon ambient PM2.5 exposure. *J Toxicol Sci.* (2018) 43:101–11. doi: 10.2131/jts.43.101
159. Soberanes S, Urich D, Baker CM, Burgess Z, Chiarella SE, Bell EL, et al. Mitochondrial complex III-generated oxidants activate ASK1 and JNK to induce alveolar epithelial cell death following exposure to particulate matter air pollution. *J Biol Chem.* (2009) 284:2176–86. doi: 10.1074/jbc.M808844200
160. Huang YC, Soukup J, Harder S, Becker S. Mitochondrial oxidant production by a pollutant dust and NO-mediated apoptosis in human alveolar macrophage. *Am J Physiol Cell Physiol.* (2003) 284:C24–32. doi: 10.1152/ajpcell.00139.2002
161. Soberanes S, Misharin AV, Jairaman A, Morales-Nebreda L, McQuattie-Pimentel AC, Cho T, et al. Metformin targets mitochondrial electron transport to reduce air-pollution-induced thrombosis. *Cell Metab.* (2018). doi: 10.1016/j.cmet.2018.09.019. [Epub ahead of print].
162. Morales-Nebreda L, Misharin AV, Perlman H, Budinger GR. The heterogeneity of lung macrophages in the susceptibility to disease. *Eur Respir Rev.* (2015) 24:505–9. doi: 10.1183/16000617.0031-2015
163. Soukup JM, Becker S. Human alveolar macrophage responses to air pollution particulates are associated with insoluble components of coarse material, including particulate endotoxin. *Toxicol Appl Pharmacol.* (2001) 171:20–6. doi: 10.1006/taap.2000.9096
164. Fujii T, Hayashi S, Hogg JC, Vincent R, Van Eeden SF. Particulate matter induces cytokine expression in human bronchial epithelial cells. *Am J Respir Cell Mol Biol.* (2001) 25:265–71. doi: 10.1165/ajrcmb.25.3.4445
165. Fujii T, Hayashi S, Hogg JC, Mukae H, Suwa T, Goto Y, et al. Interaction of alveolar macrophages and airway epithelial cells following exposure to particulate matter produces mediators that stimulate the bone marrow. *Am J Respir Cell Mol Biol.* (2002) 27:34–41. doi: 10.1165/ajrcmb.27.1.4787
166. Mutlu GM, Green D, Bellmeyer A, Baker CM, Burgess Z, Rajamannan N, et al. Ambient particulate matter accelerates coagulation via an IL-6-dependent pathway. *J Clin Invest.* (2007) 117:2952–61. doi: 10.1172/JCI30639
167. Marchini T, Wolf D, Michel NA, Mauler M, Dufner B, Hoppe N, et al. Acute exposure to air pollution particulate matter aggravates experimental myocardial infarction in mice by potentiating cytokine secretion from lung macrophages. *Basic Res Cardiol.* (2016) 111:44. doi: 10.1007/s00395-016-0562-5
168. Mukae H, Vincent R, Quinlan K, English D, Hards J, Hogg JC, et al. The effect of repeated exposure to particulate air pollution (PM10) on the bone marrow. *Am J Respir Crit Care Med.* (2001) 163:201–9. doi: 10.1164/ajrccm.163.1.2002039
169. Tan WC, Qiu D, Liam BL, Ng TP, Lee SH, van Eeden SF, et al. The human bone marrow response to acute air pollution caused by forest fires. *Am J Respir Crit Care Med.* (2000) 161:1213–7. doi: 10.1164/ajrccm.161.4.s9904084
170. Goto Y, Ishii H, Hogg JC, Shih CH, Yatera K, Vincent R, et al. Particulate matter air pollution stimulates monocyte release from the bone marrow. *Am J Respir Crit Care Med.* (2004) 170:891–7. doi: 10.1164/rccm.200402-235OC
171. Mihara M, Hashizume M, Yoshida H, Suzuki M, Shiina M. IL-6/IL-6 receptor system and its role in physiological and pathological conditions. *Clin Sci.* (2012) 122:143–59. doi: 10.1042/CS20110340
172. Hunter CA, Jones SA. IL-6 as a keystone cytokine in health and disease. *Nat Immunol.* (2015) 16:448–57. doi: 10.1038/ni.3153
173. Heinrich PC, Castell JV, Andus T. Interleukin-6 and the acute phase response. *Biochem J.* (1990) 265:621–36.
174. Kerr R, Stirling D, Ludlam CA. Interleukin 6 and haemostasis. *Br J Haematol.* (2001) 115:3–12. doi: 10.1046/j.1365-2141.2001.03061.x
175. Budinger GR, McKell JL, Urich D, Foiles N, Weiss I, Chiarella SE, et al. Particulate matter-induced lung inflammation increases systemic levels of PAI-1 and activates coagulation through distinct mechanisms. *PLoS ONE* (2011) 6:e18525. doi: 10.1371/journal.pone.0018525
176. Wassmann S, Stumpf M, Strehlow K, Schmid A, Schieffer B, Bohm M, et al. Interleukin-6 induces oxidative stress and endothelial dysfunction by overexpression of the angiotensin II type 1 receptor. *Circ Res.* (2004) 94:534–41. doi: 10.1161/01.RES.0000115557.25127.8D
177. Kido T, Tamagawa E, Bai N, Suda K, Yang HH, Li Y, et al. Particulate matter induces translocation of IL-6 from the lung to the systemic circulation. *Am J Respir Cell Mol Biol.* (2011) 44:197–204. doi: 10.1165/rcmb.2009-0427OC
178. Carswell EA, Old LJ, Kassel RL, Green S, Fiore N, Williamson B. An endotoxin-induced serum factor that causes necrosis of tumors. *Proc Natl Acad Sci USA* (1975) 72:3666–70.
179. Sedger LM, McDermott MF. TNF and TNF-receptors: from mediators of cell death and inflammation to therapeutic giants - past, present and future. *Cytokine Growth Factor Rev.* (2014) 25:453–72. doi: 10.1016/j.cytogfr.2014.07.016
180. Kalliolias GD, Ivashkiv LB. TNF biology, pathogenic mechanisms and emerging therapeutic strategies. *Nat Rev Rheumatol.* (2016) 12:49–62. doi: 10.1038/nrrheum.2015.169
181. Marchini T, D'Annunzio V, Paz ML, Caceres L, Garces M, Perez V, et al. Selective TNF-alpha targeting with infliximab attenuates impaired oxygen metabolism and contractile function induced by an acute exposure to air particulate matter. *Am J Physiol Heart Circ Physiol.* (2015) 309:H1621–1628. doi: 10.1152/ajpheart.00359.2015
182. Kumar S, Joos G, Boon L, Tournoy K, Provoost S, Maes T. Role of tumor necrosis factor-alpha and its receptors in diesel exhaust particle-induced pulmonary inflammation. *Sci Rep.* (2017) 7:11508. doi: 10.1038/s41598-017-11991-7
183. Saber AT, Bornholdt J, Dybdahl M, Sharma AK, Loft S, Vogel U, et al. Tumor necrosis factor is not required for particle-induced genotoxicity and pulmonary inflammation. *Arch Toxicol.* (2005) 79:177–82. doi: 10.1007/s00204-004-0613-9
184. Saber AT, Jacobsen NR, Bornholdt J, Kjaer SL, Dybdahl M, Risom L, et al. Cytokine expression in mice exposed to diesel exhaust particles by inhalation. Role of tumor necrosis factor. *Part Fibre Toxicol.* (2006) 3:4. doi: 10.1186/1743-8977-3-4
185. Kohase M, Henriksen-DeStefano D, May LT, Vilcek J, Sehgal PB. Induction of beta 2-interferon by tumor necrosis factor: a homeostatic mechanism in the control of cell proliferation. *Cell* (1986) 45:659–66.
186. Shalaby MR, Waage A, Aarden L, Espevik T. Endotoxin, tumor necrosis factor-alpha and interleukin 1 induce interleukin 6 production *in vivo*. *Clin Immunol Immunopathol.* (1989) 53:488–98.
187. Barbosa CM, Terra-Filho M, de Albuquerque AL, Di Giorgi D, Grupi C, Negrao CE, et al. Burnt sugarcane harvesting - cardiovascular effects on a group of healthy workers, Brazil. *PLoS ONE* (2012) 7:e46142. doi: 10.1371/journal.pone.0046142
188. Li H, Cai J, Chen R, Zhao Z, Ying Z, Wang L, et al. Particulate matter exposure and stress hormone levels: a randomized, double-blind, crossover trial of air purification. *Circulation* (2017) 136:618–27. doi: 10.1161/CIRCULATIONAHA.116.026796
189. Mendez R, Zheng Z, Fan Z, Rajagopalan S, Sun Q, Zhang K. Exposure to fine airborne particulate matter induces macrophage infiltration, unfolded protein response, and lipid deposition in white adipose tissue. *Am J Transl Res.* (2013) 5:224–34.
190. Xu X, Liu C, Xu Z, Tzan K, Zhong M, Wang A, et al. Long-term exposure to ambient fine particulate pollution induces insulin resistance and mitochondrial alteration in adipose tissue. *Toxicol Sci.* (2011) 124:88–98. doi: 10.1093/toxsci/kfr211
191. Xu Z, Xu X, Zhong M, Hotchkiss IP, Lewandowski RP, Wagner JG, et al. Ambient particulate air pollution induces oxidative stress and alterations of mitochondria and gene expression in brown and white adipose tissues. *Part Fibre Toxicol.* (2011) 8:20. doi: 10.1186/1743-8977-8-20
192. Shoelson SE, Lee J, Goldfine AB. Inflammation and insulin resistance. *J Clin Invest.* (2006) 116:1793–801. doi: 10.1172/JCI29069

193. Li W, Dorans KS, Wilker EH, Rice MB, Schwartz J, Coull BA, et al. Residential proximity to major roadways, fine particulate matter, and adiposity: the framingham heart study. *Obesity* (2016) 24:2593–9. doi: 10.1002/oby.21630
194. Kramer U, Herder C, Sugiri D, Strassburger K, Schikowski T, Ranft U, et al. Traffic-related air pollution and incident type 2 diabetes: results from the SALIA cohort study. *Environ Health Perspect.* (2010) 118:1273–9. doi: 10.1289/ehp.0901689
195. Weldy CS, Liu Y, Liggitt HD, Chin MT. *In utero* exposure to diesel exhaust air pollution promotes adverse intrauterine conditions, resulting in weight gain, altered blood pressure, and increased susceptibility to heart failure in adult mice. *PLoS ONE* (2014) 9:e88582. doi: 10.1371/journal.pone.0088582
196. Yauk C, Polyzos A, Rowan-Carroll A, Somers CM, Godschalk RW, Van Schooten FJ, et al. Germ-line mutations, DNA damage, and global hypermethylation in mice exposed to particulate air pollution in an urban/industrial location. *Proc Natl Acad Sci USA* (2008) 105:605–10. doi: 10.1073/pnas.0705896105
197. Baccarelli A, Wright RO, Bollati V, Tarantini L, Litonjua AA, Suh HH, et al. Rapid DNA methylation changes after exposure to traffic particles. *Am J Respir Crit Care Med.* (2009) 179:572–8. doi: 10.1164/rccm.200807-1097OC
198. Madrigano J, Baccarelli A, Mittleman MA, Wright RO, Sparrow D, Vokonas PS, et al. Prolonged exposure to particulate pollution, genes associated with glutathione pathways, and DNA methylation in a cohort of older men. *Environ Health Perspect.* (2011) 119:977–82. doi: 10.1289/ehp.1002773
199. Baccarelli A, Wright R, Bollati V, Litonjua A, Zanobetti A, Tarantini L, et al. Ischemic heart disease and stroke in relation to blood DNA methylation. *Epidemiology* (2010) 21:819–28. doi: 10.1097/EDE.0b013e3181f20457
200. Gilmour PS, Rahman I, Donaldson K, MacNee W. Histone acetylation regulates epithelial IL-8 release mediated by oxidative stress from environmental particles. *Am J Physiol Lung Cell Mol Physiol.* (2003) 284:L533–540. doi: 10.1152/ajplung.00277.2002
201. Soberanes S, Gonzalez A, Urich D, Chiarella SE, Radigan KA, Osornio-Vargas A, et al. Particulate matter air pollution induces hypermethylation of the p16 promoter Via a mitochondrial ROS-JNK-DNMT1 pathway. *Sci Rep.* (2012) 2:275. doi: 10.1038/srep00275
202. Wang T, Pehrsson EC, Purushotham D, Li D, Zhuo X, Zhang B, et al. The NIEHS TaRGET II Consortium and environmental epigenomics. *Nat Biotechnol.* (2018) 36:225–7. doi: 10.1038/nbt.4099
203. Dejmek J, Selevan SG, Benes I, Solansky I, Sram RJ. Fetal growth and maternal exposure to particulate matter during pregnancy. *Environ Health Perspect.* (1999) 107:475–80.
204. Selevan SG, Borkovec L, Slott VL, Zudova Z, Rubes J, Evenson DP, et al. Semen quality and reproductive health of young Czech men exposed to seasonal air pollution. *Environ Health Perspect.* (2000) 108:887–94. doi: 10.1289/ehp.00108887
205. Pedersen M, Giorgis-Allemand L, Bernard C, Aguilera I, Andersen AM, Ballester F, et al. Ambient air pollution and low birthweight: a European cohort study (ESCAPE). *Lancet Respir Med.* (2013) 1:695–704. doi: 10.1016/S2213-2600(13)70192-9
206. Slama R, Bottagisi S, Solansky I, Lepeule J, Giorgis-Allemand L, Sram R. Short-term impact of atmospheric pollution on fecundability. *Epidemiology* (2013) 24:871–9. doi: 10.1097/EDE.0b013e3182a702c5
207. Huang JV, Leung GM, Schooling CM. The association of air pollution with pubertal development: evidence from hong kong's "children of 1997" birth cohort. *Am J Epidemiol.* (2017) 185:914–23. doi: 10.1093/aje/kww200
208. Janssen BG, Saenen ND, Roels HA, Madhloum N, Gyselaers W, Lefebvre W, et al. Fetal thyroid function, birth weight, and in utero exposure to fine particle air pollution: a birth cohort study. *Environ Health Perspect.* (2017) 125:699–705. doi: 10.1289/EHP508
209. Block ML, Calderon-Garciduenas L. Air pollution: mechanisms of neuroinflammation and CNS disease. *Trends Neurosci.* (2009) 32:506–16. doi: 10.1016/j.tins.2009.05.009
210. Mutlu EA, Comba IY, Cho T, Engen PA, Yazici C, Soberanes S, et al. Inhalational exposure to particulate matter air pollution alters the composition of the gut microbiome. *Environ Pollut.* (2018) 240:817–30. doi: 10.1016/j.envpol.2018.04.130
211. Takeda K, Tsukue N, Yoshida S. Endocrine-disrupting activity of chemicals in diesel exhaust and diesel exhaust particles. *Environ Sci.* (2004) 11:33–45.
212. Oh SM, Ryu BT, Chung KH. Identification of estrogenic and antiestrogenic activities of respirable diesel exhaust particles by bioassay-directed fractionation. *Arch Pharm Res.* (2008) 31:75–82. doi: 10.1007/s12272-008-1123-8
213. Novak J, Jalova V, Giesy JP, Hilscherova K. Pollutants in particulate and gaseous fractions of ambient air interfere with multiple signaling pathways *in vitro*. *Environ Int* (2009) 35:43–9. doi: 10.1016/j.envint.2008.06.006
214. Wenger D, Gerecke AC, Heeb NV, Schmid P, Hueglin C, Naegeli H, et al. *In vitro* estrogenicity of ambient particulate matter: contribution of hydroxylated polycyclic aromatic hydrocarbons. *J Appl Toxicol.* (2009) 29:223–32. doi: 10.1002/jat.1400

7

Braving the Element: Pancreatic β-Cell Dysfunction and Adaptation in Response to Arsenic Exposure

Christopher M. Carmean [1,2*] *and Susumu Seino* [1*]

[1] *Division of Molecular and Metabolic Medicine, Department of Physiology and Cell Biology, Kobe University Graduate School of Medicine, Kobe, Japan,* [2] *Division of Endocrinology, Diabetes, and Metabolism, Department of Medicine, University of Illinois at Chicago, Chicago, IL, United States*

Correspondence:
Christopher M. Carmean
christopher.carmean@gmail.com
Susumu Seino
seino@med.kobe-u.ac.jp

Type 2 diabetes mellitus (T2DM) is a serious global health problem, currently affecting an estimated 451 million people worldwide. T2DM is characterized by hyperglycemia and low insulin relative to the metabolic demand. The precise contributing factors for a given individual vary, but generally include a combination of insulin resistance and insufficient insulin secretion. Ultimately, the progression to diabetes occurs only after β-cells fail to meet the needs of the individual. The stresses placed upon β-cells in this context manifest as increased oxidative damage, local inflammation, and ER stress, often inciting a destructive spiral of β-cell death, increased metabolic stress due to further insufficiency, and additional β-cell death. Several pathways controlling insulin resistance and β-cell adaptation/survival are affected by a class of exogenous bioactive compounds deemed endocrine disrupting chemicals (EDCs). Epidemiological studies have shown that, in several regions throughout the world, exposure to the EDC inorganic arsenic (iAs) correlates significantly with T2DM. It has been proposed that a lifetime of exposure to iAs may exacerbate problems with both insulin sensitivity as well as β-cell function/survival, promoting the development of T2DM. This review focuses on the mechanisms of iAs action as they relate to known adaptive and maladaptive pathways in pancreatic β-cells.

Keywords: arsenic, diabetes, pancreas, β-cells, reactive oxygen species, glucose tolerance, endocrine disrupters, insulin secretion

INTRODUCTION

An estimated 451 million people worldwide have type 2 diabetes (T2DM), with as many as 693 million expected to be affected by the disease in 2045 (1). T2DM is characterized by insufficient insulin production relative to metabolic demand resulting in poor glycemic control. In normal glucose homeostasis, a postprandial increase in circulating glucose concentration initiates a spike in insulin secretion from pancreatic β-cells (2, 3). This circulating insulin then binds to its cognate receptor on muscle, liver, and adipose tissues (among others), inducing glucose uptake to lower the concentration of glucose in the bloodstream. In many cases of T2DM, muscle and liver cells (the major sites of glucose disposal in the body) become insulin resistant, which induces β-cells to compensate by secreting more insulin. As insulin resistance becomes more severe, greater stresses are placed on the β-cells to increase their insulin output. Years of this chronic stress on β-cells eventually causes β-cell dysfunction and/or death. With fewer functional β-cells secreting insulin in the context of severe insulin resistance, an inability to properly maintain glucose homeostasis ensues, manifesting as T2DM (4).

Though there are many factors that contribute to the progression of diabetes, it is important to recognize that ultimately a failure of β-cells to secrete sufficient amounts of insulin is what results in hyperglycemia and the diagnosis of T2DM (5). While tremendous stress may be placed on β-cells from a metabolic standpoint, they also face other insults from environmental factors such as endocrine-disrupting chemicals (EDCs). EDCs may work alone or synergistically to derange the normal compensatory mechanisms enabling β-cells to promote glucose tolerance in insulin-resistant individuals (6). In this sense, EDCs may act as drivers of diabetes risk, becoming more deleterious as they compound with lifestyle factors and genetic susceptibilities. It is therefore especially important to consider that EDCs may impair the functionality of β-cells or increase their susceptibility to the chronic metabolic stressors associated with insulin resistance. The purpose of this review will be to explore the β-cell-specific effects of one such EDC, arsenic, as it poses a substantial and ongoing threat to public health.

Arsenic is widely recognized as a carcinogen and oxidizing agent that damages neuronal, hepatic, cardiovascular, integumentary, and renal organ systems (7). Its health effects vary depending on valence, mixture with other toxins, dosage, route of exposure, and length of exposure. Capable of causing death within 24 h, the acute lethal dose in humans is estimated to be 0.6 mg/kg/day (8). Common routes of exposure include the skin, lungs, and digestive tract. Though inhalation of iAs is a concern during hazardous occupational work and traditional coal-based food preservation practices (9), the greatest number of individuals are at risk of exposure to unsafe levels of iAs from contaminated groundwater (10–12). The most prevalent species of arsenic found naturally in drinking water are inorganic arsenic (iAs) in its trivalent (As^{III}) or pentavalent (As^{V}) forms (13). Organic arsenicals can be found in the food chain as arsenobetaine, arsenocholine, and arsenolipids, and are generally considered relatively non-toxic (14).

Inorganic arsenic is estimated to naturally contaminate the shallow groundwater underneath 140 million people worldwide (12). Among these people at risk, the number actually exposed to iAs is believed to be lower, as not all contaminated groundwater sources are utilized and excellent remediation methods are available in developed countries (12). Despite this fact, the problem of chronic iAs exposure through shallow groundwater consumption persists on an immense scale. As of 2007, an estimated 20 million people in Bangladesh alone were still served by wells naturally contaminated with iAs at a concentration more than 5x higher than the WHO safe limit of 10 μg/L (15). In these areas, where exposure has been pervasive in communities since the digging of shallow groundwater wells in the mid-1900s, it has been estimated that ~21% of all-cause mortality is attributable to iAs exposure (16). The lasting effects of this contamination may represent one of the greatest failures of public health management in recent history.

One observation from this unintended mass-poisoning and other cases of natural exposure is a potential relationship between iAs exposure and diabetes (11). In addition to its role in increasing the risk of several cancers, peripheral neuropathy, and keratinosis, iAs exposure correlates with glucose intolerance or diabetes prevalence in areas with relatively high exposure levels (17–20). The epidemiological analysis regarding the relationship between iAs exposure and diabetes have been reviewed in detail elsewhere (11). For the purposes of this review, an examination of the specific effects of iAs on β-cells will be undertaken, including the evidence from pancreatic endpoints in animal models and mechanistic insights gained from *ex vivo* and/or interventional studies.

ACUTE vs. CHRONIC iAs EXPOSURE

The effects of iAs can be conceptualized on a sliding scale of dosage and time. A single large dose of iAs can cause nausea, vomiting, abdominal pain, diarrhea, and even death (8, 21). Chronic ingestion of lower doses of iAs can occur without any immediate sensory feedback, and yet the ensuing damage over several years may span most organ systems, increasing an individual's risk of cancer, peripheral neuropathy, cardiovascular disease, diabetes, and a multitude of skin problems (7). In trying to better understand the relationship between iAs exposure and diabetes, the effects of chronic, sub-toxic exposure are of the greatest concern and should be delineated from acute toxic effects.

The National Toxicology Program Workshop Review's assessment in 2012 suggested that cell-culture studies utilizing iAs concentrations ≥ 1 mM can be considered acute stress-response studies rather than functional studies of β-cells' role in iAs-associated diabetes, even in cases where physiologically-relevant model systems or physiological endpoints were utilized (11). Given that the highest circulating plasma concentration of iAs ever recorded in a human population drinking iAs-contaminated water was 0.6 μM, and clear evidence of reduced cell growth or survival *ex vivo* has been reported for iAs exposures ≥5 μM (22, 23), 1 mM appears to be a generous and appropriate cutoff (24, 25).

Although studies have repeatedly shown that exposure to ≤1 μM iAs significantly decreases glucose-induced insulin secretion in clonal β-cells, it should be noted that the use of somewhat higher concentrations for short periods has spurned fruitful follow-up at lower, more physiological concentrations of iAs. For instance, Pi et al reported that 5 μM iAs significantly induced antioxidant gene expression (26), eventually leading to deeper investigation of the role of nuclear factor (erythroid-derived)-like 2 (Nrf2), a major antioxidant-regulating transcription factor, in the adaptive response to iAs. This launched a series of investigations that expanded our understanding of iAs's mechanism(s) of action (27, 28). Given the fine line between the concentration of iAs capable of inhibiting insulin secretion and cytotoxicity or the induction of apoptosis, this course of studies might be taken as an excellent example of how to successfully exploit shorter time courses and higher dosages to generate novel, environmentally-relevant findings.

PANCREATIC iAs ACCUMULATION, SPECIATION, DISPOSAL

IAs undergoes several stages of metabolism once ingested (29). IAs enters cells via ion transporters, including aquaporin proteins 3, 7, and 9 and glucose transporter 1 (30–33). Although a reduction of these transporters protects cell lines against iAs toxicity (34), efficient cellular import of arsenicals is critical for normal *in vivo* iAs detoxification and urinary excretion (35). A single sub-lethal bolus of iAs (1 mg/kg) administered intraperitoneally to rats, mice, hamsters, and guinea pigs, can be cleared from the bloodstream in ~24 h (36). Once inside the cell, iAs may be conjugated to glutathione or methylated multiple times (37, 38). Once modified, methylated or glutathione-conjugated arsenicals are exported from the cell by ABC transporters, including multidrug resistance-associated proteins 1a, 1b, and 2 (39, 40), enabling more efficient renal excretion and minimizing internal exposure. Arsenical efflux activity partially determines an organism's sensitivity to iAs, as the activities and expression levels of these ABC transporters are critical for adaptation to iAs (31).

IAs is taken up by pancreatic tissue and β-cells dose-dependently (41). Of the *in vivo* rodent studies utilizing chronic iAs exposure considered here, several studies specifically measured iAs accumulation in the pancreas (**Table 1**). In all these cases except one, iAs accumulated significantly in the pancreas (41, 43, 44, 46, 57–60, 64, 74). In the one exception, with low levels of iAs used in a cocktail of other dilute toxins, no appreciable pancreatic iAs accumulation was observed (77). The concentration of iAs used in this study by Radike et al was lower than the World Health Organization's safe limit of 10 μg/L.

Chronic administration of iAs in drinking water results in iAs accumulation as both iAs and methylated arsenicals in the pancreas, with the majority stored as monomethyl arsenous acid (MMA) or dimethylarsenous acid (DMA) (43, 44, 57, 60, 64). Isolated islet and β-cell cell line studies have demonstrated the ability of β-cells to methylate iAs intracellularly (78, 79). The physiological effects of these methylated arsenicals appear to be different from those of iAs. MMA can inhibit mitochondrial function and decrease glucose-induced insulin secretion, even at 5-fold lower concentrations than other arsenicals (80). Since MMA is necessarily created prior to repeated bouts of methylation resulting in dimethylation and trimethylation, it is noteworthy that this intermediate may be more toxic than its precursor or end-products.

The relationship between exposure and tissue-level accumulation as well as the propensity to induce DNA damage vary across organ systems. One study measured iAs accumulation and cytosine methylation in several tissues following 24 weeks of iAs administration (41). Relative to the lung, kidney, heart, and spleen, the pancreas accumulated less iAs as a function of exposure level and displayed a resistance to the iAs-induced 5-hydroxymethylation events observed in these other tissues. Despite this apparent resistance, the pancreas itself was smaller after adjusting for body weight in iAs-exposed mice, a phenomenon also observed by other groups (50, 52), raising the possibility that the organ may possess a unique resistance to iAs accumulation, but also a unique susceptibility to the effects of iAs exposure.

MODEL SYSTEM EVIDENCE FOR PANCREATIC β-CELL INVOLVEMENT

The data are mixed in animal models of iAs-induced metabolic dysfunction regarding the relative contributions of insulin-secretory vs. insulin-sensitivity factors in the development of glucose intolerance (**Table 1**). Impairments in pancreatic (41, 50–52, 54–56, 68, 69) and hepatic (48, 55, 59, 61–63, 66) function have been implicated. Insulin sensitivity, however, has been reported to increase (44), decrease (43, 47, 49, 53), or remain unchanged (44, 47, 50) in sex-specific or diet-specific manners, making the integration of this particular endpoint across studies more difficult. It is worth noting, however, that where insulin sensitivity was reported to increase, this was on a background of already-impaired diet-induced glucose intolerance in which Paul et al also reported both lower circulating insulin, lower adiposity, and lower HOMA-IR in the high-fat diet, iAs-treated group vs. high-fat diet controls. In this study as well as others, a reduction in circulating insulin was reported either following fasting or during a glucose tolerance test (44, 46, 50, 57–60, 64, 74, 77–80). In consideration of the studies examined here, it appears that a primary defect in β-cell function precedes the development of glucose intolerance, which may or may not include a component of insulin resistance. IAs may be protective against insulin resistance in diet-induced obesity while simultaneously impairing pancreatic β-cells, a model that deviates from the canonical type I, type II, or gestational forms of diabetes (81). Replication will be critical for reconciling the differences between insulin sensitivity outcomes in these recent animal models of iAs exposure.

In β-cell lines there is a consistently observed reduction in GIIS associated with chronic, sub-toxic iAs exposure (**Table 2**), although there is some disagreement in the literature about whether basal insulin secretion is altered by iAs exposure (23, 28, 42, 82, 83). Some of these differences may be related to the model systems employed. It is notable that, in cell line studies, the dosages and times used to study the effects of iAs exposure have varied dramatically. Timeframes utilized for studying the effects of GIIS have ranged from 1 to 144 h, with higher concentrations evaluated on shorter time courses, such as 5 mM iAs exposure for 60 min (22) or over 100 μM for 90 min (86, 87), and lower doses for longer time courses, such as 50 nM for 96 h (28). The lowest concentration thus far reported to significantly affect GIIS in cell culture studies is 0.1 μM (23).

Significant effects of iAs on insulin gene expression and transcription factor activities have also been reported. A decrease of MafA transcriptional activity regulated by miR-149 may contribute to the iAs-induced impairment of β-cell function (72). Such decreases in *MafA*, *Pdx1*, or *Nkx6.1* are generally considered indications of β-cell failure or de-differentiation (91). Other model systems of iAs exposure, in which gene expression levels of these transcription factors were measured, did not report such a de-differentiation phenotype (23). One study even observed an increase in nuclear PDX1 following exposure to iAs, suggestive of increased insulin gene expression (88). DNA binding of the β-cell specific transcription factor UIF1, which promotes insulin

TABLE 1 | Rodent models of iAs exposure with pancreatic endpoints.

Animal model	As species	Dose (route)	Time	Pancreatic As Accumulation	Glucose tolerance effects	Insulin effects	Pancreatic endpoints	General findings	References
Wistar rat (m)	As_2O_3	17.75–100 mg/L (dw)	8 wk	NR	OGTT glucose clearance delayed OGTT AUC lower	Fasting blood insulin ϕ	NR	Oxidative stress induces mito dysfunction	(42)
Wistar rat (m)	As^{III}	1.7 mg/kg (og)	2x daily 90 d	Yes	Fasting glucose ↑ HOMA-IR ↑	Fasting insulin ↑ Glucose:insulin ratio ↓	Glucagon staining ↓ Insulin IHC signal ↓	Serum glucagon ↓	(43)
C57BL/6 mouse (m)	As^{III}	25–50 ppm (og)	20 wk	Yes	FBG in HFD + iAs group was lower than HFD controls. OGTT AUC for iAs exposed mice in high fat diet group ϕ HOMA-IR in HFD + iAs group was lower than HFD controls	Insulin during first 15 min of OGTT in high-fat diet group iAs exposed mice ↓	NR	Water intake ↓ HFD iAs adiposity was lower than HFD controls	(44)
LM/Bc/Fnn mouse (gf)	Na_2HAsO_4	9.6 mg/kg (ip)	2 doses (G7.5 and G8.5)	NR	FPG ↑ Glucose tolerance ↓ (IPGTT) RPG ↑	Fasting insulin ϕ IPGTT insulin at 30 min ↑	NR	NAC, methionine, sodium selenate,	(45)
ICR mouse (m)	As_2O_3	5 ppm (dw)	6 wk	Yes	FPG ϕ Glucose tolerance (ogtt) ↓	Fasting insulin ↓	Markers of β-cell apoptosis ↑	NAC co-improved glucose tolerance	(46)
Sprague-Dawley rat (mf)	Mix As + Pb*	30 ppb As, 53 ppb Pb (dw)	3 mo	NR	f rat FPG ↓ m insulin resistance ↑ f insulin sensitivity ↑ mf glucose intolerant (OGTT)	f OGTT insulin ϕ m OGTT insulin ↑	NR	NR	(47)
C57/BLKS/J db/m and C57BKS/Lepr^{db} (db/db) mouse (m)	As^{III}	3 mg/L (dw)	16 wk	NR	HOMA-IR ϕ Normal mice glucose tolerance ϕ (OGTT) Db/db mice glucose tolerance ↓	FBI ↑ db/db mice HOMA-β ↓ db/db mice FBI ↓	Normal mice HOMA-β ↑ As worsened inflammation	Daily food intake altered Daily water intake ϕ Hepatic gluconeogenesis ↑	(48)
Sprague Dawley rat (gf, o)	As^{III}	5–50 mg/L (dw)	8 wk + gestation from day 1	NR	Gestational BG IPGTT ↓ HOMA-IR ϕ Gestational FPG ϕ	Gestational circulating insulin IPGTT ↓m and f offspring insulin AUC IPGTT ↓	Gestational panc insulin ↑	Daily water consumption ϕ Maternal weight gain ↓	(49)
Sprague Dawley rat (mf)	As^{III}	5–50 mg/L (o)	8 wk + gestation from day 1	NR	mf FPG ϕ f BG IPGTT ↓ f HOMA-IR ↑ m HOMA-IR ↓ m BG IPGTT ϕ	Mf insulin IPGTT ↓	NR	Body weight ↓ Hepatic GSH ↑ Hepatic MDA ↑	(49)
C57BL/6J mouse (m)	As^{III}	50 mg/L (dw)	8 wk	NR	Glucose tolerance (IPGTT) ↓ HOMA-IR ↓	IPGTT 1st phase Insulin vs. glucose ↓	Pancreas mass ↓	Water intake ↓ Circadian feeding pattern disrupted	(50)
C57BL/6J mouse (m)	As_2O_3	1–4 mg/L (dw)	12 wk	NR	NR	Harvested islet GIIS ↓	ER stress ↑ Autophagy ↑	NR	(51)
NMRI mouse (m)	As^{III}	25–50 ppm (dw)	20 wk	NR	HFD-fed mice + As FPG ↓ HFD-fed mice + As HFD + As HOMA-IR ↓ Glucose tolerance in HFD + As group vs. HFD only (OGTT) ↓	HFD + As FPI ↓	Pancreas mass ↓ HFD + As islet diameter ↓	Water consumption ↓	(52)
C57BL/6J mouse (mf)	As^{III}	100–1000 ppb (dw)	1 wk before and 1st wk of pregnancy	NR	Male prenatal As exposure adulthood FPG ↑ Male prenatal As exposure adulthood HOMA-IR ϕ	FPI ϕ	NR	Male prenatal 1 ppm body fat % ↑ HOMA-IR in males at 100 ppb ↑	(53)

(Continued)

TABLE 1 | Continued

Animal model	As species	Dose (route)	Time	Pancreatic As Accumulation	Glucose tolerance effects	Insulin effects	Pancreatic endpoints	General findings	References
Albino rat (m)	As_2O_3	3 mg/kg (og)	Daily, 30 days	NR	NR	NR	Islet size ↓ Markers of ROS ↑ NO ↑	Folic acid intervention	(54)
Albino Wistar rat (m)	As^{III}	1.5 or 5 mg/kg (og)	5 wk	NR	≥ 1.5 mg/kg FBG ↑ ≥ 1.5 mg/kg HbA1C ↑ OGTT glucose ↑	NR	Antioxidant activities ↑ Oxidative stress ↑	Zn and Cu ↓	(55)
Wistar rat (gf, o)	As_2O_3	2–8 mg/kg (og)	G6 to postnatal day 42	NR	NR	NR	Islet size ↓ autophagosomes ↑ LC3-II ↑ Nrf2, Trx ↓	Taurine intervention	(56)
C57BL/6 mouse (m)	As^{III}	10, 25, 50 ppm (dw)	8 wk	Yes	FPG ϕ 50 ppm OGTT blood glucose ↑	NR	NR	NR	(57)
C57BL/6 mouse (m)	MMA	2.5, 5 ppm (dw)	8 wk	Yes	FPG ϕ OGTT blood glucose ϕ	NR	NR	NR	(57)
C57BL/6 mouse (mf)	As^{III}	10 mg/kg (ip)	Bolus	NR	Fasting glucose ↓	NR	NR	Some mice died after 1 day	(21)
Wistar rat (m)	Diphenylarsinic acid (DPAA)	5 mg As/kg (og)	Bolus	Yes	NR	NR	NR	Highest DPAA accumulation in brain	(58)
Swiss albino mouse (NR)	As^{III}	3 mg/kg (og)	Daily for 12 wk	Yes	FPG ↑	NR	NR	(6)-gingerol intervention	(59)
Sprague Dawley rat (m)	$NaAsO_2$	0.5–10 ppm (dw)	8 wk	Yes	NR	NR	Pancreas mass ↓	As accumulated in every organ examined	(41)
C57BL/6J mouse (m)	As^{III}	15–50 mg/L (dw)	4 wk	Yes	NR	NR	NR	As3mt-KO mice + As water intake ↓	(60)
CD rat (m)	As^{III}	5–10 mg/kg (ip)	Bolus or daily for 7 d	NR	Single dose or 7d iAs, fasting blood glucose ↑ Single dose or 7d iAs, OGTT blood glucose ↑	NR	NR	Adrenalectomy partially prevented glucose intolerance after iAs	(61)
SD rat (m)	As^{III}	0.1–1 mg/kg (ip)	Bolus	NR	FBG ϕ	NR	NR	Kidney PDH activity ↓	(36)
B6C3F1 mouse (m)	As^{III}	0.1–1 mg/kg (ip)	Bolus	NR	FBG ϕ	NR	NR	Kidney PDH activity ↓	(36)
Golden-Syrian hamster (m)	As^{III}	0.1–1 mg/kg (ip)	Bolus	NR	FBG ϕ	NR	NR	Kidney PDH activity ↓	(36)
Hartley guinea pig (m)	As^{III}	1 mg/kg (ip)	Bolus	NR	FBG ↑	NR	NR	Kidney PDH activity ↓	(36)
Wistar rat (m)	As^{III}	5.55 mg/kg (ip)	Daily for 21 d	NR	FPG ↓ (rats were hypogycemic)	NR	NR	Liver glycogen ↓ Methionine intervention	(62)
Wistar rat (m)	As^{III}	5.55 mg/kg (ip)	Daily for 30 d	NR	FPG ↓ (rats were hypogycemic)	NR	NR	Oral NAC intervention	(63)
C57BL/6 mouse (m)	As^{III}	25–50 ppm (dw)	8 wk	Yes	FPG ϕ IPGTT glucose ↑	NR	NR	Water consumption ↓	(64)
Wistar rat (m)	As^{III}	5 mg/kg (og)	Daily for 30 d	NR	FPG ↑	NR	NR	Curcumin intervention	(65)
ICR mouse (f)	As_2O_3	0.05–0.5 mg/kg (dw)	2–6 wk	NR	As only group became glucose intolerant Ovariectomized + As had worst Ovariectomized + As + estrogen restored glucose tolerance	0.05, 0.5 μM AS, 2, 4, 6 wk FPI ↓ 2 4, 6, wk, 0.05, 0.5 μM AS, ovariectomized mice + iAs ↑ 2 4, 6, wk ovariectomized mice + iAs + estradiol ϕ	NR	Liver glycogen ↓ Body fat % ϕ Estradiol intervention	(66)

(Continued)

TABLE 1 | Continued

Animal model	As species	Dose (route)	Time	Pancreatic As Accumulation	Glucose tolerance effects	Insulin effects	Pancreatic endpoints	General findings	References
Sprague-Dawley rat (m)	As^{III}	8 mg/kg (ip)	1 dose	NR	IPGTT BG ↑	NR	NR	NAC improved glucose tolerance	(67)
Sprague-Dawley rat (m)	As^{III}	20–200 ppm (dw)	20 wk	NR	FBG ϕ IPGTT BG ϕ	NR	NR	NR	(67)
CD-1 ICR mouse (m)	As_2O_3	10 mg/L (dw)	3–12 wk	NR	NR	5–12 wk FPI ↓	5 wk inflammatory cells ↑ and acinar cells ↓	Humic acid also decreases FPI	(68)
B6C3F1 mouse (mf)	MMA	10–400 ppm (food)	2 yr	NR	FBG ϕ	NR	Adenoma/carcinoma ϕ	Water consumption ↑	(69)
Fischer F344 rat (mf)	MMA	50–1,300 ppm (food)	2 yr	NR	FBG ϕ	NR	Adenoma ↑	Water consumption ↑	(69)
Wistar rat (mf)	As_2O_3	2–8 mg/kg (og)	Daily for 56 d	NR	NR	NR	ROS ↑ Mitophagy ↓	Taurine restored mitophagy	(70)
Wistar rat (mf)	As_2O_3	2–8 mg/kg (og) (gf)	Daily post-weaning for 14 d	NR	NR	NR	Irregular structures Inflammasome ↑	Taurine restored structure and reduced inflammation	(71)
CD1 mouse (m)	As^{III}	20–40 ppm (dw)	52 wk (dw)	NR	OGTT glucose AUC ↑	Fasting insulin ↓ OGTT insulin fold-change ↓ Islet GIIS ↓ Islet Insulin content ↓	mafA mRNA ↓ mir-149, mir-153 ↑	NR	(72)
ICR mouse (m)	As^{III}	10 ppb	G10–G18	NR	IPGTT ϕ	NR	NR	BPA + iAs IPGTT AUC ↓	(73)
Balb/C mouse (m)	As^{III}	5 μM	6 wk (dw)	Yes	FPG ↑	NR	Pancreas morphology ϕ Pancreas miR-2909 ↓	NR	(74)
C57BL/6J mouse	As^{III}	100 ppb	6–37 wk (dw)	NR	FBG ϕ Insulin tolerance ϕ	FPI ϕ	NR	Sex-specific enhanced iAs metabolism with folate sufficiency	(75)
NMRI mouse (m)	As^{III}	50 ppm	20 wk	NR	HFD FBG ↓ HFD HOMA-IR ↓	NC and HFD FSI ↓ NC and HFD HOMA-β ↓	NR	Liver ROS ↑ Liver lipid peroxidation ↑	(76)

m, male; f, female; gf, gravid female; ip, intraperitoneal injection; og, oral gavage; dw, drinking water; NR, not reported; d, days; wk, weeks; yr, year; G, gestational day; FBG, fasting blood glucose; FPG, fasting plasma glucose; RPG, random plasma glucose; FSI, fasting plasma insulin; o, offspring exposed to iAs during gestation; OGTT, oral glucose tolerance test; IPGTT, intraperitoneal tolerance test; MMA, monomethylarsenous acid; DMA, dimethylarsenous acid.

**Chemical identities of iAs were not described and samples were directly taken from a drinking water source.*

gene expression, has also been observed to increase in response to iAs, suggesting a mechanism by which iAs may affect insulin content (89). Additional replication may therefore be warranted to identify which features of transcription factor activities are robust and translatable to human exposure.

INFLAMMATION AND REACTIVE-OXYGEN SPECIES (ROS)

ROS accumulation is a hallmark of iAs toxicity. There is strong evidence from both *in vivo* and *in vitro* studies suggesting that iAs damages pancreatic tissue, observed as elevated pro-inflammatory genes (48), pancreatic nitric oxide (54, 55) glutathione levels (43, 55), endoplasmic reticulum stress (51), and autophagy (51, 56). More severe phenotypes have been observed with increased apoptosis (46), decreased islet size (54), accumulation of pro-inflammatory cells (68), and detection of pancreatic adenomas (69). The generalized cellular responses to iAs-induced ROS have been reviewed in detail elsewhere (92). Markers of ROS have been observed at the lowest concentrations that also affect GIIS (28). Interestingly, arsenic trioxide (As_2O_3) appears to increase ROS production, apoptosis, and TUNEL staining while decreasing PPARγ in the INS-1 cell line. Restoration of normal ROS production by taurine administration or

TABLE 2 | *Ex vivo* models of iAs exposure.

Model	Tissue type	As species	Dosage	Time	Insulin content	Insulin secretion	General findings	References
Wistar rat (m)	Islets	As_2O_3	NR	NR	NR	Basal ↑ GIIS ↓	O_2 consumption ↓	(42)
rat	INS-1	As^{III}	0.05–0.5 μM	96 h	Insulin mRNA ↑ Insulin ↑	Basal ↑ GIIS ↓ KIIS ↑	H_2O_2 scavenging ↑ Nrf2-regulated gene mRNA ↑ Mito mass ↑	(28)
C57BL/6J mouse (m)	Islets	As^{III}	0.1–2 μM	48 h	0.1–2 μM ϕ	2 μM GIIS ↓ 2 μM KIIS ↓	iAs^{III} accumulated in islets after 48 h exposure	(78)
rat	INS-1	MAs^{III}	0.1–2 μM	2–24 h	NR	4+ h, 2 μM GIIS ↓ 24 h, 0.375 μM GIIS ↓	≥ 0.2 μM Mito respiration impaired	(80)
IT6 mouse	MIN6-K8	As^{III}	0.1–2 μM	72 h	NR	Basal ϕ GIIS ↓	O_2 consumption ϕ Dependent on intact 5HT metabolism 5-HT disposal ↑ *Ugt1a6a* mRNA ↑ Supplementation with 5HTP recovered GIIS	(23)
C57BL/6J mouse (m)	Islets	As^{III}	2 μM	48 h	NR	Basal ϕ GIIS ↓	*Ugt1a6a* mRNA ↑	(23)
human	Islets	As^{III}	1–2 μM	72 h	NR	Basal ϕ GIIS ↓	*UGT1A6* mRNA ↑	(23)
rat	RINm5F	As^{III}	0.5–5 μM	72 h	0.5–5 μM insulin ϕ	1, 2 μM Basal ↓ 2 μM GIIS ↓	Glucose-induced Ca2+ ↓ Glucose-induced SNAP-25 proteolysis ↓ Cell cycle arrested	(82)
Wistar rat (m)	1° β-cells	As^{III}	0.5–10 μM	72–144 h	1 μM ϕ 5 μM ↓ 5 μM insulin mRNA ↓	Basal ϕ 1, 5 μM GIIS ↓	5 μM Insulin mRNA ↓	(83)
rat	RINm5F	As_2O_3	0.5–10 μM	4–8 h	NR	2 μM, 5 μM, 24 h GIIS ↓	Calpain activity ↑ ROS ↑ Supplementation with NAC decreased apoptosis	(46)
IT6 mouse	MIN6	As^{III}	1–20 μM	2–24 h	NR	NR	iAs accumulates as iAs and MMA Antioxidant gene mRNA ↑	(79)
129S1/Svlmj mouse (NR)	Islets	As^{III}	1–10 μM	7–15 h	NR	Basal ϕ 1 μM, 15 h GIIS ↓	ROS-scavenging genes and protein ↑	(26)
Hamster	HIT-T15 β-cells	As_2O_3	1 μM–25 μM	2–24 h	4 h, ≤ 2 μM ϕ 4 h, 5 μM ↓	NR	≥ 2.5 μM, 2, 8 or 24 h ATP ↓ LD_{50} = 2.5 μM 5–20 μM 2, 4 h ROS ↑	(68)
Rat	INS-1	As^{III}	5–50 μM	6–24 h	NR	5 μM, 6 h GIIS ↓	Glucose-induced H_2O_2 ↓	(26)
	Islets	As^{III}	1 μM	15 h	NR	Basal ϕ GIIS ↓	Basal H_2O_2 ↑ Glucose-stimulated H_2O_2 ↓	(26)
Rat	INS-1	As^{III}	1–10 μM	2–24 h	NR	6 h, 10 μM GIIS ↓ 24 h 2 μM GIIS ↓	2 μM OCR ↓	(80)
Rat	INS-1	As^{III}	1–4 μM	24 h	NR	NR	≥ 2 μM Viability ↓ ≥ 2 μM Autophagosomes ↑ ≥1 μM LC3II protein ↑ NAC intervention	(84)
Rat	INS-1	$DMAs^{III}$	2–10 μM	2–24 h	NR	2+ h, 10 μM GIIS ↓ 24 h, ≤ 2 μM GIIS ϕ	≤2 μM Mito respiration ϕ	(80)
rat	INS-1	As^{III}	2.5 μM–160 μM	12–72 h	NR	NR	≥ 2.5 μM AS is cytotoxic ≥ 2.5 μM AS causes L3/CytC apoptosis	(85)

(Continued)

TABLE 2 | Continued

Model	Tissue type	As species	Dosage	Time	Insulin content	Insulin secretion	General findings	References
rat	INS-1	As^{III}	4 μM	3–24 h	NR	NR	12, 24 h LC3-II protein ↑ 24 h p62 protein ↓ 6–24 h ER stress ↑	(51)
rat	INS-1	As^{III}	5 μM	6–15 h	NR	Basal ϕ GIIS ↓	Nrf2 activation ↑ Antioxidant activity ↑ Antioxidant gene + protein expression ↑ H_2O_2 accumulation ↓	(26)
Swiss Albino mouse	1° β-cells	As^{III}	10 μM	72 h	NR	NR	72 h, 10 μM ROS ↑	(59)
NMRI mouse (m)	Islets	As^{III}	20–200 μM	90 min	NR	≥ 100 μM GIIS ↓	≥ 50 μM viability ↓ ≥ 100 μM ROS ↑	(86)
NMRI mouse (m)	Islets	As^{III}	100 μM	90 min	NR	GIIS ↓	Metformin pre-treatment protected GIIS	(87)
Human	Islets	As^{III}	1 mM	30 min	NR	NR	Nuclear PDX1 ↑	(88)
Human	Islets	As^{III}	1 mM	15–30 min	NR	NR	UIF1 DNA binding ↑	(89)
IT6 mouse	MIN6	As^{III}	1 mM	5–20 min	NR	NR	MAPKAP-K2 activity ↑	(89)
Ob/Ob mouse (m)	Islets	As^{V}	5 mM	60 min	NR	Basal ϕ GIIS ↓	Glucose-stimulated O_2 consumption ↓	(22)
Rat	INS-1	As_2O_3	1–4 μM	24 h	NR	NR	Apoptosis ↑ PPARγ ↓ Taurine decreased apoptosis	(70)
rat	INS-1	As_2O_3	1–64 μM	24 h	NR	4 μM As_2O_3 + LPS Basal ↓ 4 μM As_2O_3 + LPS GIIS ↓	As_2O_3 + LPS Pyroptosis ↑ As_2O_3 + LPS GIIS ↓ Taurine partially restored GIIS Inflammasome inhibitors partially restored GIIS ↓	(71)
IT6 mouse	MIN6	As^{III}	1–5 μM	6–48 h	≥2 μM ≥24 h insulin content ↓	2 μM ≥12 h GIIS ↓	2 μM 48 h mir-149 ↑ Mir-149 knockdown restored GIIS through mafA Mir-149 knockdown restored insulin content	(72)
IT6 mouse	MIN6	As^{III}	2 μM	24 h	NR	2 μM 24 h Basal ϕ	2 μM 24 h miR-2909 ↑ 2 μM 24 h MafA mRNA ↓ 2 μM 24 h MafA protein ↓ 2 μM 24 h PDX1, C-Jun, UCP2 protein ↑	(74)
rat	INS-1 832/13	As^{III}	1–2 μM	24 h	NR	≥1 μM 24 h GIIS ↓	≥1 μM 24 h XTT viability ↓ 2 μM 24 h basal and glucose-stimulated OCR ↓ ≥1 μM 24 h maximal OCR ↓	(90)

NR, not reported; m, male; f, female; MMA, monomethylarsenous acid; DMA, dimethylarsenous acid; GIIS, glucose-induced insulin secretion; KIIS, potassium-induced insulin secretion; OCR, oxygen consumption rate.

rescue of PPARγ expression ameliorates the apoptotic and DNA-damaging effects of As_2O_3 exposure (70). This is in line with similar observations for liver cells lines by the same group (93).

The ROS produced as a result of iAs exposure induce a compensatory increase in gene expression levels for genes regulated by antioxidant response elements (26–28, 94). These genes, which include catalase, superoxide dismutase 1, and superoxide dismutase 2, are critical for reducing otherwise toxic accumulation of ROS, and are positively regulated at the level of transcription by Nrf2 (94, 95). In β-cells specifically, induction of the Nrf2-mediated antioxidant-response program has been shown to protect against iAs-induced toxicity (94). Deletion of the major transcription factor regulating this pathway, Nrf2, in β-cells has been shown to enhance susceptibility to iAs toxicity (79). In the context of β-cell function, this antioxidant activity may actually suppress the normal physiological changes in ROS that β-cells depend on to induce insulin secretion in response to a rise in extracellular glucose (26). In this way, a tradeoff may occur in which β-cells' survival improves by adaptive upregulation of antioxidant activity, while at the same time glucose-induce insulin secretion is suppressed by the same mechanism (96). That several interventional studies focused on suppressing the antioxidant response successfully ameliorated some of the effects of iAs supports the hypothesis that ROS may be one of the salient, translatable, and addressable features of low-dose, chronic iAs exposure (**Table 3**) (45, 46, 53, 59, 63, 65, 67, 71, 75, 84, 97).

TABLE 3 | *In vivo* interventional studies.

Biological and Exposure Model	Intervention (substance/dose)	Effects/proposed mechanism	References
Wistar rats, 5.55 mg/kg/day As^{III} (ip) for 30 days	N-acetylcysteine, 1 mmol/kg/day (og)for final 7 days of As^{III} exposure	Nacetylcysteine's anti-oxidant properties reversed iAs-induced hepatic ROS-mediated toxicity, restored lower liver glycogen levels, and reversed hypoglycemia	(63)
Wistar rats, 5.55 mg/kg/day As^{III} (ip) for 30 days	Melatonin, 10 mg/kg/day (og) for final 5 days of As^{III} exposure	Melatonin's anti-oxidant properties reversed iAs-induced reductions in superoxide dismutase and catalase activities in the liver and kidney.	(97)
Wistar rats, 5.55 mg/kg/day As^{III} (ip) for 21 days	Methionine, 0.8% of food supplement for final 5 days of As^{III} exposure	Methionine treatment may have enhanced methylation of iAs reduced its toxicity, reversed hypoglycemia, reversed the iAs-induced reduction in liver pyruvic acid, and partially reversed the reduction in liver glycogen levels.	(62)
Swiss-albino mice, 3 mg/kg/day As^{III} (og) for 12 weeks	(6)-gingerol, 50–75 mg/kg body weight/day (og) for 3 weeks after As^{III} exposure	(6)-gingerol administration restored iAs-induced hyperglycemia to normoglycemia, decreased iAs deposition in the pancreas and liver, and restored liver antioxidant activities.	(59)
Wistar rats, 8 mg/kg/day As_2O_3 (og) from GD 6 to postnatal day 42	Taurine, 150 mg/kg/day (og) from GD 6 to postnatal day 42	Taurine reversed iAs-induced autophagosome formation, iAs-induced decrease in Nrf2 protein levels, and iAs-induced ROS accumulation in the pancreas.	(56)
Wistar rats, 8 mg/kg/day As_2O_3 (og) from GD 6 to postnatal day 42	Taurine, 150 mg/kg/day (og) from GD 6 to postnatal day 42	Taurine reversed iAs-induced TNF-α expression and markers of pyroptosis and inflammation in the pancreas.	(71)
Pregnant LM/Bc/Fnn mice, 9.6 mg/kg As^{III} (ip), at GD 7.5 and GD 8.5	Sodium selenate, 0.5 mg/kg (og) daily from GD 0.5 to GD 10.5	Sodium selenite decreased the number of fetuses with neural tube defects.	(45)
Pregnant LM/Bc/Fnn mice, 9.6 mg/kg As^{III} (ip), at GD 7.5 and GD 8.5	L-Methionine, 70 mg/kg (og) daily from GD 0.5 to GD 10.5	L-Methionine decreased the number of fetuses with neural tube defects.	(45)
Pregnant LM/Bc/Fnn mice, 9.6 mg/kg As^{III} (ip), at GD 7.5 and GD 8.5	N-acetylsysteine, 200 mg/kg (og) daily from GD 0.5 to GD 10.5	N-acetylsysteine decreased the number of fetuses with neural tube defects but did not affect FPG or maternal circulating insulin	(45)
Pregnant LM/Bc/Fnn mice, 9.6 mg/kg As^{III} (ip), at GD 7.5 and GD 8.5	N-tert-Butyl-α-phenylnitrone,40 mg/kg (ip) on GD 7.5 and GD 8.5	N-tert-Butyl-α-phenylnitrone decreased the number of fetuses with neural tube defects and significantly increased the rate of fetal resorption	(45)
Pregnant LM/Bc/Fnn mice, 9.6 mg/kg As^{III} (ip), at GD 7.5 and GD 8.5	LinBit insulin pellet implanted from GD 2.5–3.5	LinBit decreased the number of fetuses with neural tube defects, decreased FPG, and increased matermal circulating insulin	(45)
C57BL/6J mice, 100 ppb As^{III} (dw) for 24 weeks	Folate, 10 mg/kg of food supplement for 24 weeks	High folate supplementation improved iAs-induced insulin resistance and stimulated iAs metabolism in females.	(75)
Wistar rats, 5 mg/kg/day (og), for 30 days	Curcumin, 15 mg/kg/day (og), 30 days	Curcumin supplementation prevented iAs-induced changes in serum markers of hepatic and renal function.	(65)

Although oxidative damage is a common observation following iAs exposure in many different tissues, the implications for ROS accumulation in β-cells may be unique. For instance, a recent meta-analysis of iAs-exposure studies in mice and rats indicated that iAs tends to decrease expression levels of key antioxidant genes (92). These include superoxide dismutase, catalase, and glutathione-peroxidase, among others. This is inverted compared to the response to iAs in β-cells, which manifests as increased expression of antioxidant genes, presumably to limit changes to the cellular redox state (27). This may be because glucose-induced insulin secretion in β-cells is partly mediated by relatively small changes in redox status (26). These cells are so sensitive to ROS that incubation with just 1 μM H_2O_2 affects basal insulin secretion (26), and just 100 μM H_2O_2 significantly decreases viability (98). In stark contrast, 250 μM H_2O_2 is used as a moderate positive control to quantify accumulation of ROS in liver cell lines (99). Thus, this unique sensitivity highlights the need to study the effects of iAs on β-cells directly, and not to rely too heavily on studies in other tissues.

CYTOTOXICITY, AUTOPHAGY, AND THE CELL CYCLE

Indications of cytotoxicity, disrupted autophagy, or apoptosis have been observed in β-cell lines using concentrations of iAs as low as 1 μM, although the minimum threshold for toxic effects vary with cell line and duration of exposure (46, 70,

84). Reduced viability as measured by reducing potential has been observed in the MIN6 cell line following 24 h exposure to $\geq 1\,\mu M$ arsenite (although reducing potential may also be affected by changes to cellular energetics independent of toxicity), with a 50% reduction in viability at approximately $5\,\mu M$ and activation of the antioxidant-response gene expression program (79). The INS-1 line exposed to iAs for just 24 h showed significantly decreased proliferation at $\geq 2.5\,\mu M$, with decreased mitochondrial membrane potential and increased cytoplasmic cytochrome c, indicative of autophagy (85). This cell line at 1–$2\,\mu M$ iAs exposure also exhibits reduced oxygen consumption capacity and viability (90). Pan et al estimated the IC50 for INS-1 cells to be about $30\,\mu M$ (85). By comparison, isolated islets exposed to 20–$50\,\mu M$ iAs for 24 h exhibited >50% islet destruction, suggesting that islets, INS-1 cells, and MIN6 cells may be similarly sensitive to the cytotoxic effects of iAs (100).

There is substantial evidence that chronic *in vivo* iAs exposure disrupts autophagy in other tissues. In one such study, 20 weeks of exposure to 50 ppm iAs in drinking water during high-fat diet administration significantly induced hepatic expression of 17 out of 21 autophagy-related genes examined, with the remaining 4 genes trending toward an increase. This was also accompanied by a significant increase in hepatic lipid peroxidation and ROS accumulation (76). In β-cell lines as well, investigators have observed iAs-induced changes in autophagy (51, 56, 84), often noting enhanced levels of the autophagy marker LC3-II.

There is some debate about whether autophagy induced by iAs in β-cells is mediated by ROS. Some investigators have found that iAs induces autophagy in an ROS-dependent fashion (84). Other groups using non-β-cell lines have shown that autophagy can be activated in the absence of excessive ROS generation, and have therefore concluded that iAs-induced autophagy is ROS-independent (99). That autophagy induction occurs at comparable doses of iAs in other tissues without significant ROS accumulation suggests that perhaps β-cells, while susceptible to ROS, may also be affected by parallel, ROS-independent iAs-induced autophagy. This may be considered an unresolved topic in the field and additional mechanistic investigations at environmentally-relevant concentrations of iAs are warranted.

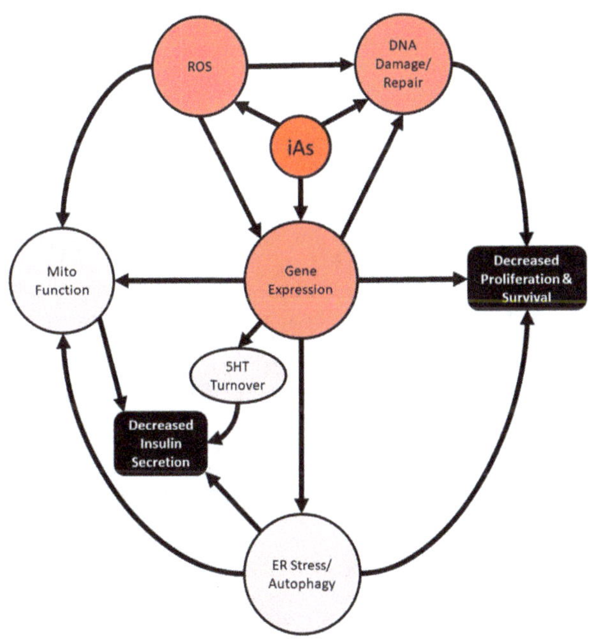

FIGURE 1 | Summary of routes to iAs-induced toxicity and insulin-secretory effects.

SEROTONIN METABOLISM

In mouse β-cells and islets, and to a lesser extent in human islets, serotonin regulates glucose-induced insulin secretion and proliferation (101, 102). Several parameters determine the concentration and effects of serotonin in β-cells, including serotonin production, serotonin disposal, and the specific distribution of serotonin receptors (103, 104). IAs exposure was recently observed to enhance serotonin disposal in the MIN6-K8 line by upregulation of the serotonin disposal gene *Ugt1a6a*. The upregulation phenomenon in response to iAs exposure was replicated in mouse islets, and the same pattern was observed for the human homolog of this gene, *UGT1A6*, in human islets upon chronic exposure to iAs (23). It is not clear what pathways are responsible for induction of *Ugt1a6a*, however *Ugt1a6a* expression is known in other tissues to be regulated by Nrf2 and the aryl hydrocarbon receptor. As *Ugt1a6a* was previously unappreciated as a regulator of β-cell function, this study highlights how EDCs such as iAs can be utilized to identify novel regulators of glucose-induced insulin secretion. Further study is warranted to evaluate the translatability of this work to animal models and cases of human exposure.

CONSIDERATIONS AND FUTURE DIRECTIONS

Importantly, these studies intersect two major public health crises: chronic arsenic exposure and diabetes. In the past 20 years, substantial supporting evidence for the involvement of disrupted autophagy and oxidative damage as the major mediators of iAs-induced pancreatic β-cell dysfunction, manifesting as altered cell survival and impaired insulin secretion, has been reported both *in vivo* and *in vitro* (**Figure 1**). In more recent years, the concentrations used to study the phenomenon have decreased dramatically, and the lengths of exposure time have increased. These are positive trends for the field and are largely possible as a result of more sensitive analytical methods that are now more widespread. The use of these techniques has enabled the relatively recent discovery that MMA and DMA have different activities in β-cells and should be further explored. Now that human pancreatic islets are more widely available for research purposes throughout the world, replication of animal model findings in human islets is a more practical and reasonable option.

With the largest population-scale exposures of arsenic ongoing in developing or impoverished nations, it is less likely that synthetic therapeutic interventions targeting β-cells (without broader applicability to arsenic-independent β-cell function) may find traction at the levels of commercial development and clinical use. Appropriately, interventional studies aimed at improving β-cell resistance to arsenic exposure appear designed in consideration of this fact, mostly utilizing relatively inexpensive nutritional supplementation that may also have more systemic benefits to arsenic-exposed individuals (**Table 3**). Thus, the model system research presented here provide evidence that optimal nutrition rich in natural antioxidants may improve β-cells' resistance to chronic arsenic exposure *in vivo*.

The problem of arsenic exposure through contaminated drinking water is ultimately addressable at the level of public policy. Though diabetes itself may feel less immediate than acutely-life-threatening afflictions associated with arsenic exposure (such as cancer, cardiovascular disease, and nephropathy), highlighting the diabetes link provides yet another mechanism by which the scientific community can provide lawmakers and policy officials with justification to prioritize access to clean and safe water. That population-level arsenic exposure has been a known problem for more than 30 years in Bangladesh alone, with other pockets of exposure around the globe, reveals a global failure of institutions to address the needs of the impoverished and exposed. As water treatment technology and infrastructure are developed to address the pressing dangers of arsenic exposure, they will undoubtedly reduce economic and inertial barriers to the further improvement of water quality. Future studies and research communications might emphasize the preventability of chronic arsenic exposure as a point of discussion in the hopes that the issue can be continually brought to the forefront of public concern.

AUTHOR CONTRIBUTIONS

CC and SS conceived, authored, revised, and approved the manuscript and take responsibility for its publication.

FUNDING

CC received financial support from the Japan Society for the Promotion of Science Standard Term Postdoctoral Fellowship for Overseas Researchers. SS received financial support from the Japan Society for the Promotion of Science Grant-in-Aid for Scientific Research (S) 24229007 and MSD K.K. Japan.

ACKNOWLEDGMENTS

The authors would like to thank Robert M. Sargis and Daniel Ruiz for their productive feedback and insights.

REFERENCES

1. Cho NH, Shaw JE, Karuranga S, Huang Y, da Rocha Fernandes JD, Ohlrogge AW, et al. IDF diabetes atlas: global estimates of diabetes prevalence for 2017 and projections for 2045. *Diabetes Res Clin Pract.* (2018) 138:271–81. doi: 10.1016/j.diabres.2018.02.023
2. Seino S, Shibasaki T, Minami K. Pancreatic beta-cell signaling: toward better understanding of diabetes and its treatment. *Proc Jpn Acad Ser B Phys Biol Sci.* (2010) 86:563–77. doi: 10.2183/pjab.86.563
3. Henquin JC. Regulation of insulin secretion: a matter of phase control and amplitude modulation. *Diabetologia.* (2009) 52:739–51. doi: 10.1007/s00125-009-1314-y
4. Halban PA, Polonsky KS, Bowden DW, Hawkins MA, Ling C, Mather KJ, et al. β-cell failure in type 2 diabetes: postulated mechanisms and prospects for prevention and treatment. *Diabetes Care.* (2014) 37:1751–8. doi: 10.2337/dc14-0396
5. Seino S, Shibasaki T, Minami K. Dynamics of insulin secretion and the clinical implications for obesity and diabetes. *J Clin Invest.* (2011) 121:2118–25. doi: 10.1172/JCI45680
6. Bonini MG, Sargis RM. Environmental toxicant exposures and type 2 diabetes mellitus: two interrelated public health problems on the rise. *Curr Opin Toxicol.* (2018) 7:52–9. doi: 10.1016/j.cotox.2017.09.003
7. Singh AP, Goel RK, Kaur T. Mechanisms pertaining to arsenic toxicity. *Toxicol Int.* (2011) 18:87–93. doi: 10.4103/0971-6580.84258
8. Ratnaike RN. Acute and chronic arsenic toxicity. *Postgrad Med J.* (2003) 79:391–6. doi: 10.1136/pmj.79.933.391
9. Finkelman RB, Belkin HE, Zheng B. Health impacts of domestic coal use in China. *Proc Natl Acad Sci USA.* (1999) 96:3427–31. doi: 10.1073/pnas.96.7.3427
10. Naujokas MF, Anderson B, Ahsan H, Aposhian HV, Graziano JH, Thompson C, et al. The broad scope of health effects from chronic arsenic exposure: update on a worldwide public health problem. *Environ Health Perspect.* (2013) 121:295–302. doi: 10.1289/ehp.1205875
11. Maull EA, Ahsan H, Edwards J, Longnecker MP, Navas-Acien A, Pi J, et al. Evaluation of the association between arsenic and diabetes: a National Toxicology Program workshop review. *Environ Health Perspect.* (2012) 120:1658–70. doi: 10.1289/ehp.1104579
12. Ravenscroft P, Brammer H, Richards K. *Arsenic Pollution: A Global Synthesis.* Wiley-Blackwell (2009).
13. Frumkin H. *Toxicological Profile for Arsenic.* Agency for Toxic Substances and Disease Registry, Agency for Toxic Substances and Disease Registry (2007).
14. Navas-Acien A, Francesconi KA, Silbergeld EK, Guallar E. Seafood intake and urine concentrations of total arsenic, dimethylarsinate and arsenobetaine in the US population. *Environ Res.* (2011) 111:110–8. doi: 10.1016/j.envres.2010.10.009
15. Johnston RB, Sarker MH. Arsenic mitigation in Bangladesh: national screening data and case studies in three upazilas. *J Environ Sci Health A Tox Hazard Subst Environ Eng.* (2007) 42:1889–96. doi: 10.1080/10934520701567155
16. Karagas MR. Arsenic-related mortality in Bangladesh. *Lancet.* (2010) 376:213–4. doi: 10.1016/S0140-6736(10)61002-1
17. Tseng CH, Tai TY, Chong CK, Tseng CP, Lai MS, Lin BJ, et al. Long-term arsenic exposure and incidence of non-insulin-dependent diabetes mellitus: a cohort study in arseniasis-hyperendemic villages in Taiwan. *Environ Health Perspect.* (2000) 108:847–51. doi: 10.1289/ehp.00108847
18. Lai M-S, Hsueh Y-M, Chen C-J, Shyu M-P, Chen S-Y, Kuo T-L, et al. Ingested inorganic arsenic and prevalence of diabetes mellitus. *Am J Epidemiol.* (1994) 139:484–92. doi: 10.1093/oxfordjournals.aje.a117031
19. Pan WC, Seow WJ, Kile ML, Hoffman EB, Quamruzzaman Q, Rahman M, et al. Association of low to moderate levels of arsenic exposure with risk of type 2 diabetes in Bangladesh. *Am J Epidemiol.* (2013) 178:1563–70. doi: 10.1093/aje/kwt195
20. Wang SL, Chiou JM, Chen CJ, Tseng CH, Chou WL, Wang CC, et al. Prevalence of non-insulin-dependent diabetes mellitus and related vascular diseases in southwestern arseniasis-endemic and nonendemic areas in Taiwan. *Environ Health Perspect.* (2003) 111:155–9. doi: 10.1289/ehp.5457
21. Boquist L, Boquist S, Ericsson I. Structural beta-cell changes and transient hyperglycemia in mice treated with compounds inducing inhibited citric acid cycle enzyme activity. *Diabetes.* (1988) 37:89–98. doi: 10.2337/diabetes.37.1.89

22. Ortsäter H, Liss P, Akerman KE, Bergsten P. Contribution of glycolytic and mitochondrial pathways in glucose-induced changes in islet respiration and insulin secretion. *Pflugers Arch.* (2002) 444:506–12. doi: 10.1007/s00424-002-0842-9
23. Carmean CM, Yokoi N, Takahashi H, Oduori OS, Kang C, Kanagawa A, et al. Arsenic modifies serotonin metabolism through glucuronidation in pancreatic β-cells. *Am J Physiol Endocrinol Metab.* (2019) 316:E464–74. doi: 10.1152/ajpendo.00302.2018
24. C.-Tseng H, The potential biological mechanisms of arsenic-induced diabetes mellitus. *Toxicol Appl Pharmacol.* (2004) 197:67–83. doi: 10.1016/j.taap.2004.02.009
25. Wu MM, Chiou HY, Ho IC, Chen CJ, Lee TC. Gene expression of inflammatory molecules in circulating lymphocytes from arsenic-exposed human subjects. *Environ Health Perspect.* (2003) 111:1429–38. doi: 10.1289/ehp.6396
26. Pi J, Bai Y, Zhang Q, Wong V, Floering LM, Daniel K, et al. Reactive oxygen species as a signal in glucose-stimulated insulin secretion. *Diabetes.* (2007) 56:1783–91. doi: 10.2337/db06-1601
27. Pi J, Zhang Q, Fu J, Woods CG, Hou Y, Corkey BE, et al. ROS signaling, oxidative stress and Nrf2 in pancreatic beta-cell function. *Toxicol Appl Pharmacol.* (2010) 244:77–83. doi: 10.1016/j.taap.2009.05.025
28. Fu J, Woods CG, Yehuda-Shnaidman E, Zhang Q, Wong V, Collins S, et al. Low-level arsenic impairs glucose-stimulated insulin secretion in pancreatic beta cells: involvement of cellular adaptive response to oxidative stress. *Environ Health Perspect.* (2010) 118:864–70. doi: 10.1289/ehp.0901608
29. Thomas DJ. Molecular processes in cellular arsenic metabolism. *Toxicol Appl Pharmacol.* (2007) 222:365–73. doi: 10.1016/j.taap.2007.02.007
30. Liu Z, Shen J, Carbrey JM, Mukhopadhyay R, Agre P, Rosen BP. Arsenite transport by mammalian aquaglyceroporins AQP7 and AQP9. *Proc Natl Acad Sci USA.* (2002) 99:6053–8. doi: 10.1073/pnas.092131899
31. Lee TC, Ho IC, Lu WJ, Huang JD. Enhanced expression of multidrug resistance-associated protein 2 and reduced expression of aquaglyceroporin 3 in an arsenic-resistant human cell line. *J Biol Chem.* (2006) 281:18401–7. doi: 10.1074/jbc.M601266200
32. Liu Z, Sanchez MA, Jiang X, Boles E, Landfear SM, Rosen BP. Mammalian glucose permease GLUT1 facilitates transport of arsenic trioxide and methylarsonous acid. *Biochem Biophys Res Commun.* (2006) 351:424–30. doi: 10.1016/j.bbrc.2006.10.054
33. Shinkai Y, Sumi D, Toyama T, Kaji T, Kumagai Y. Role of aquaporin 9 in cellular accumulation of arsenic and its cytotoxicity in primary mouse hepatocytes. *Toxicol Appl Pharmacol.* (2009) 237:232–6. doi: 10.1016/j.taap.2009.03.014
34. Leung J, Pang A, Yuen WH, Kwong YL, Tse EW. Relationship of expression of aquaglyceroporin 9 with arsenic uptake and sensitivity in leukemia cells. *Blood.* (2007) 109:740–6. doi: 10.1182/blood-2006-04-019588
35. Carbrey JM, Song L, Zhou Y, Yoshinaga M, Rojek A, Wang Y, et al. Reduced arsenic clearance and increased toxicity in aquaglyceroporin-9-null mice. *Proc Natl Acad Sci USA.* (2009) 106:15956–60. doi: 10.1073/pnas.0908108106
36. Mitchell RD, Ayala-Fierro F, Carter DE. Systemic indicators of inorganic arsenic toxicity in four animal species. *J Toxicol Environ Health A.* (2000) 59:119–34. doi: 10.1080/009841000157014
37. Drobna Z, Styblo M, Thomas DJ. An overview of arsenic metabolism and toxicity. *Curr Protoc Toxicol.* (2009) 42:4.31.1–6. doi: 10.1002/0471140856.tx0431s42
38. Watanabe T, Hirano S. Metabolism of arsenic and its toxicological relevance. *Arch Toxicol.* (2013) 87:969–79. doi: 10.1007/s00204-012-0904-5
39. Kala SV, Neely MW, Kala G, Prater CI, Atwood DW, Rice JS, et al. The MRP2/cMOAT transporter and arsenic-glutathione complex formation are required for biliary excretion of arsenic. *J Biol Chem.* (2000) 275:33404–8. doi: 10.1074/jbc.M007030200
40. Kala SV, Kala G, Prater CI, Sartorelli AC, Lieberman MW. Formation and urinary excretion of arsenic triglutathione and methylarsenic diglutathione. *Chem Res Toxicol.* (2004) 17:243–9. doi: 10.1021/tx0342060
41. Zhang J, Mu X, Xu W, Martin FL, Alamdar A, Liu L, et al. Exposure to arsenic via drinking water induces 5-hydroxymethylcytosine alteration in rat. *Sci Total Environ.* (2014) 497–8:618–25. doi: 10.1016/j.scitotenv.2014.08.009
42. Cobo JM, Castiñeira M. Oxidative stress, mitochondrial respiration, and glycemic control: clues from chronic supplementation with Cr3+ or As3+ to male Wistar rats. *Nutrition.* (1997) 13:965–70. doi: 10.1016/S0899-9007(97)00338-9
43. Izquierdo-Vega JA, Soto CA, Sanchez-Peña LC, De Vizcaya-Ruiz A, Del Razo LM. Diabetogenic effects and pancreatic oxidative damage in rats subchronically exposed to arsenite. *Toxicol Lett.* (2006) 160:135–42. doi: 10.1016/j.toxlet.2005.06.018
44. Paul DS, Walton FS, Saunders RJ, Stýblo M. Characterization of the impaired glucose homeostasis produced in C57BL/6 mice by chronic exposure to arsenic and high-fat diet. *Environ Health Perspect.* (2011) 119:1104–9. doi: 10.1289/ehp.1003324
45. Hill DS, Wlodarczyk BJ, Mitchell LE, Finnell RH. Arsenate-induced maternal glucose intolerance and neural tube defects in a mouse model. *Toxicol Appl Pharmacol.* (2009) 239:29–36. doi: 10.1016/j.taap.2009.05.009
46. Lu TH, Su CC, Chen YW, Yang CY, Wu CC, Hung DZ, et al. Arsenic induces pancreatic β-cell apoptosis via the oxidative stress-regulated mitochondria-dependent and endoplasmic reticulum stress-triggered signaling pathways. *Toxicol Lett.* (2011) 201:15–26. doi: 10.1016/j.toxlet.2010.11.019
47. Palacios J, Roman D, Cifuentes F. Exposure to low level of arsenic and lead in drinking water from Antofagasta city induces gender differences in glucose homeostasis in rats. *Biol Trace Elem Res.* (2012) 148:224–31. doi: 10.1007/s12011-012-9355-3
48. Liu S, Guo X, Wu B, Yu H, Zhang X, Li M. Arsenic induces diabetic effects through beta-cell dysfunction and increased gluconeogenesis in mice. *Sci Rep.* (2014) 4:6894. doi: 10.1038/srep06894
49. Bonaventura MM, Bourguignon NS, Bizzozzero M, Rodriguez D, Ventura C, Cocca C, et al. Arsenite in drinking water produces glucose intolerance in pregnant rats and their female offspring. *Food Chem Toxicol.* (2017) 100:207–16. doi: 10.1016/j.fct.2016.12.025
50. Kirkley AG, Carmean CM, Ruiz D, Ye H, Regnier SM, Poudel A, et al. Arsenic exposure induces glucose intolerance and alters global energy metabolism. *Am J Physiol Regul Integr Comp Physiol.* (2017). doi: 10.1152/ajpregu.00522.2016
51. Wu W, Yao X, Jiang L, Zhang Q, Bai J, Qiu T, et al. Pancreatic islet-autonomous effect of arsenic on insulin secretion through endoplasmic reticulum stress-autophagy pathway. *Food Chem Toxicol.* (2018) 111:19–26. doi: 10.1016/j.fct.2017.10.043
52. Ahangarpour A, Alboghobeish S, Rezaei M, Khodayar MJ, Oroojan AA, Zainvand M. Evaluation of diabetogenic mechanism of high fat diet in combination with arsenic exposure in male mice. *Iran J Pharm Res.* (2018) 17:164–83.
53. Huang MC, Douillet C, Dover EN, Stýblo M. Prenatal arsenic exposure and dietary folate and methylcobalamin supplementation alter the metabolic phenotype of C57BL/6J mice in a sex-specific manner. *Arch Toxicol.* (2018) 92:1925–37. doi: 10.1007/s00204-018-2206-z
54. Mukherjee S, Das D, Mukherjee M, Das AS, Mitra C. Synergistic effect of folic acid and vitamin B12 in ameliorating arsenic-induced oxidative damage in pancreatic tissue of rat. *J Nutr Biochem.* (2006) 17:319–27. doi: 10.1016/j.jnutbio.2005.08.003
55. Patel HV, Kalia K. Role of hepatic and pancreatic oxidative stress in arsenic induced diabetic condition in Wistar rats. *J Environ Biol.* (2013) 34:231–6.
56. Bai J, Yao X, Jiang L, Qiu T, Liu S, Qi B, et al. Taurine protects against As2O3-induced autophagy in pancreas of rat offsprings through Nrf2/Trx pathway. *Biochimie.* (2016) 123:1–6. doi: 10.1016/j.biochi.2016.01.002
57. Paul DS, Devesa V, Hernandez-Zavala A, Adair BM, Walton FS, Drobnâ Z, et al. Environmental arsenic as a disruptor of insulin signaling. *Met Ions Biol Med.* (2008) 10:1–7.
58. Naranmandura H, Suzuki N, Takano J, McKnight-Whitford T, Ogra Y, Suzuki KT, et al. Systemic distribution and speciation of diphenylarsinic acid fed to rats. *Toxicol Appl Pharmacol.* (2009) 237:214–20. doi: 10.1016/j.taap.2009.03.023
59. Chakraborty D, Mukherjee A, Sikdar S, Paul A, Ghosh S, Khuda-Bukhsh AR. [6]-Gingerol isolated from ginger attenuates sodium arsenite induced oxidative stress and plays a corrective role in improving insulin signaling in mice. *Toxicol Lett.* (2012) 210:34–43. doi: 10.1016/j.toxlet.2012.01.002
60. Currier JM, Douillet C, Drobná Z, Stýblo M. Oxidation state specific analysis of arsenic species in tissues of wild-type and arsenic (+3 oxidation

state) methyltransferase-knockout mice. *J Environ Sci.* (2016) 49:104–12. doi: 10.1016/j.jes.2016.06.018

61. Ghafghazi T, Ridlington JW, Fowler BA. The effects of acute and subacute sodium arsenite administration on carbohydrate metabolism. *Toxicol Appl Pharmacol.* (1980) 55:126–30. doi: 10.1016/0041-008X(80)90228-8
62. Pal S, Chatterjee AK. Protective effect of methionine supplementation on arsenic-induced alteration of glucose homeostasis. *Food Chem Toxicol.* (2004) 42:737–42. doi: 10.1016/j.fct.2003.12.009
63. Pal S, Chatterjee AK. Protective effect of N-acetylcysteine against arsenic-induced depletion *in vivo* of carbohydrate. *Drug Chem Toxicol.* (2004) 27:179–89. doi: 10.1081/DCT-120037501
64. Paul DS, Hernández-Zavala A, Walton FS, Adair BM, Dedina J, Matousek T, et al. Examination of the effects of arsenic on glucose homeostasis in cell culture and animal studies: development of a mouse model for arsenic-induced diabetes. *Toxicol Appl Pharmacol.* (2007) 222:305–14. doi: 10.1016/j.taap.2007.01.010
65. Yousef MI, El-Demerdash FM, Radwan FM. Sodium arsenite induced biochemical perturbations in rats: ameliorating effect of curcumin. *Food Chem Toxicol.* (2008) 46:3506–11. doi: 10.1016/j.fct.2008.08.031
66. Huang CF, Yang CY, Chan DC, Wang CC, Huang KH, Wu CC, et al. Arsenic exposure and glucose intolerance/insulin resistance in estrogen-deficient female mice. *Environ Health Perspect.* (2015) 123:1138–44. doi: 10.1289/ehp.1408663
67. Rezaei M, Khodayar MJ, Seydi E, Soheila A, Parsi IK. Acute, but not chronic, exposure to arsenic provokes glucose intolerance in rats: possible roles for oxidative stress and the adrenergic pathway. *Can J Diabetes.* (2017) 41:273–80. doi: 10.1016/j.jcjd.2016.10.008
68. Yen CC, Lu FJ, Huang CF, Chen WK, Liu SH, Lin-Shiau SY. The diabetogenic effects of the combination of humic acid and arsenic: *in vitro* and *in vivo* studies. *Toxicol Lett.* (2007) 172:91–105. doi: 10.1016/j.toxlet.2007.05.008
69. Arnold LL, Eldan M, van Gemert M, Capen CC, Cohen SM. Chronic studies evaluating the carcinogenicity of monomethylarsonic acid in rats and mice. *Toxicology.* (2003) 190:197–219. doi: 10.1016/S0300-483X(03)00165-3
70. Zhang Q, Bai J, Yao X, Jiang L, Wu W, Yang L, et al. Taurine rescues the arsenic-induced injury in the pancreas of rat offsprings and in the INS-1 cells. *Biomed Pharmacother.* (2019) 109:815–22. doi: 10.1016/j.biopha.2018.10.134
71. Pei P, Yao X, Jiang L, Qiu T, Wang N, Yang L, et al. Inorganic arsenic induces pyroptosis and pancreatic β cells dysfunction through stimulating the IRE1α/TNF-α pathway and protective effect of taurine. *Food Chem Toxicol.* (2019) 125:392–402. doi: 10.1016/j.fct.2019.01.015
72. Sun Q, Yang Q, Xu H, Xue J, Chen C, Yang X, et al. miR-149 negative regulation of mafA is involved in the arsenite-induced dysfunction of insulin synthesis and secretion in pancreatic beta cells. *Toxicol Sci.* (2019) 167:116–25. doi: 10.1093/toxsci/kfy150
73. Wang D, Zhu W, Yan S, Meng Z, Yan J, Teng M, et al. Impaired lipid and glucose homeostasis in male mice offspring after combined exposure to low-dose bisphenol A and arsenic during the second half of gestation. *Chemosphere.* (2018) 210:998–1005. doi: 10.1016/j.chemosphere.2018.07.094
74. Ramdas M, Sharma S, Kaul D, Bhatia A. Possible role of miR-2909 RNomics in arsenic mediated pancreatic β-cell dysfunction. *J Trace Elem Med Biol.* (2018) 50:263–7. doi: 10.1016/j.jtemb.2018.07.006
75. Huang MC, Douillet C, Dover EN, Zhang C, Beck R, Tejan-Sie A, et al. Metabolic phenotype of wild-type and As3mt-knockout C57BL/6J mice exposed to inorganic arsenic: the role of dietary fat and folate intake. *Environ Health Perspect.* (2018) 126:127003. doi: 10.1289/EHP3951
76. Zeinvand-Lorestani M, Kalantari H, Khodayar MJ, Teimoori A, Saki N, Ahangarpour A, et al. Autophagy upregulation as a possible mechanism of arsenic induced diabetes. *Sci Rep.* (2018) 8:11960. doi: 10.1038/s41598-018-30439-0
77. Radike M, Warshawsky D, Caruso J, Goth-Goldstein R, Reilman R, Collins T, et al. Distribution and accumulation of a mixture of arsenic, cadmium, chromium, nickel, and vanadium in mouse small intestine, kidneys, pancreas, and femur following oral administration in water or feed. *J Toxicol Environ Health A.* (2002) 65:2029–52. doi: 10.1080/00984100290071324
78. Douillet C, Currier J, Saunders J, Bodnar WM, Matoušek T, Stýblo M. Methylated trivalent arsenicals are potent inhibitors of glucose stimulated insulin secretion by murine pancreatic islets. *Toxicol Appl Pharmacol.* (2013) 267:11–5. doi: 10.1016/j.taap.2012.12.007
79. Cui Q, Fu J, Hu Y, Li Y, Yang B, Li L, et al. Deficiency of long isoforms of Nfe2l1 sensitizes MIN6 pancreatic β cells to arsenite-induced cytotoxicity. *Toxicol Appl Pharmacol.* (2017) 329:67–74. doi: 10.1016/j.taap.2017.05.013
80. Dover EN, Beck R, Huang MC, Douillet C, Wang Z, Klett EL, et al. Arsenite and methylarsonite inhibit mitochondrial metabolism and glucose-stimulated insulin secretion in INS-1 832/13 β cells. *Arch Toxicol.* (2018) 92:693–704. doi: 10.1007/s00204-017-2074-y
81. DeFronzo RA, Ferrannini E, Groop L, Henry RR, Herman WH, Holst JJ, et al. Type 2 diabetes mellitus. *Nat Rev Dis Primers.* (2015) 1:15019. doi: 10.1038/nrdp.2015.19
82. Díaz-Villaseñor A, Burns AL, Salazar AM, Sordo M, Hiriart M, Cebrián ME, et al. Arsenite reduces insulin secretion in rat pancreatic beta-cells by decreasing the calcium-dependent calpain-10 proteolysis of SNAP-25. *Toxicol Appl Pharmacol.* (2008) 231:291–9. doi: 10.1016/j.taap.2008.05.018
83. Díaz-Villaseñor A, Sánchez-Soto MC, Cebrián ME, Ostrosky-Wegman P, Hiriart M. Sodium arsenite impairs insulin secretion and transcription in pancreatic beta-cells. *Toxicol Appl Pharmacol.* (2006) 214:30–4. doi: 10.1016/j.taap.2005.11.015
84. Zhu XX, Yao XF, Jiang LP, Geng CY, Zhong LF, Yang G, et al. Sodium arsenite induces ROS-dependent autophagic cell death in pancreatic β-cells. *Food Chem Toxicol.* (2014) 70:144–50. doi: 10.1016/j.fct.2014.05.006
85. Pan X, Jiang L, Zhong L, Geng C, Jia L, Liu S, et al. Arsenic induces apoptosis by the lysosomal-mitochondrial pathway in INS-1 cells. *Environ Toxicol.* (2016) 31:133–41. doi: 10.1002/tox.22027
86. Ahangarpour A, Oroojan AA, Rezae M, Khodayar MJ, Alboghobeish S, Zeinvand M. Effects of butyric acid and arsenic on isolated pancreatic islets and liver mitochondria of male mouse. *Gastroenterol Hepatol Bed Bench.* (2017) 10:44–53.
87. Ahangarpour A, Zeidooni L, Rezaei M, Alboghobeish S, Samimi A, Oroojan AA. Protective effect of metformin on toxicity of butyric acid and arsenic in isolated liver mitochondria and langerhans islets in male mice: an *in vitro* study. *Iran J Basic Med Sci.* (2017) 20:1297–305. doi: 10.22038/IJBMS.2017.9567
88. Macfarlane WM, McKinnon CM, Felton-Edkins ZA, Cragg H, James RF, Docherty K. Glucose stimulates translocation of the homeodomain transcription factor PDX1 from the cytoplasm to the nucleus in pancreatic beta-cells. *J Biol Chem.* (1999) 274:1011–6. doi: 10.1074/jbc.274.2.1011
89. Macfarlane WM, Smith SB, James RF, Clifton AD, Doza YN, Cohen P, et al. The p38/reactivating kinase mitogen-activated protein kinase cascade mediates the activation of the transcription factor insulin upstream factor 1 and insulin gene transcription by high glucose in pancreatic beta-cells. *J Biol Chem.* (1997) 272:20936–44. doi: 10.1074/jbc.272.33.20936
90. Dover EN, Patel NY, Stýblo M. Impact of *in vitro* heavy metal exposure on pancreatic β-cell function. *Toxicol Lett.* (2018) 299:137–44. doi: 10.1016/j.toxlet.2018.09.015
91. Shirakawa J, Terauchi Y. Selective and sequential loss of transcriptional factors: a hallmark of β-cell failure in type 2 diabetes? *J Diabetes Investig.* (2014) 5:359–61. doi: 10.1111/jdi.12212
92. Xu M, Rui D, Yan Y, Xu S, Niu Q, Feng G, et al. Oxidative damage induced by arsenic in mice or rats: a systematic review and meta-analysis. *Biol Trace Elem Res.* (2017) 176:154–75. doi: 10.1007/s12011-016-0810-4
93. Bai J, Yao X, Jiang L, Zhang Q, Guan H, Liu S, et al. Taurine protects against As2O3-induced autophagy in livers of rat offsprings through PPARγ pathway. *Sci Rep.* (2016) 6:27733. doi: 10.1038/srep27733
94. Fu J, Zheng H, Wang H, Yang B, Zhao R, Lu C, et al. Protective role of nuclear factor E2-related factor 2 against acute oxidative stress-induced pancreatic β -cell damage. *Oxid Med Cell Longev.* (2015) 2015:639191. doi: 10.1155/2015/639191
95. Wang H, Zhu J, Li L, Li Y, Lv H, Xu Y, et al. Effects of Nrf2 deficiency on arsenic metabolism in mice. *Toxicol Appl Pharmacol.* (2017) 337:111–9. doi: 10.1016/j.taap.2017.11.001
96. Fu J, Hou Y, Xue P, Wang H, Xu Y, Qu W, et al. Nrf2 in type 2 diabetes and diabetic complications: Yin and Yang. *Curr Opin Toxicol.* (2016) 1:9–19. doi: 10.1016/j.cotox.2016.08.001
97. Pal S, Chatterjee AK. Possible beneficial effects of melatonin supplementation on arsenic-induced oxidative stress in Wistar rats. *Drug Chem Toxicol.* (2006) 29:423–33. doi: 10.1080/01480540600837993

98. Meares GP, Fontanilla D, Broniowska KA, Andreone T, Lancaster JR, Corbett JA. Differential responses of pancreatic β-cells to ROS and RNS. *Am J Physiol Endocrinol Metab.* (2013) 304:E614–22. doi: 10.1152/ajpendo.00424.2012
99. Dodson M, de la Vega MR, Harder B, Castro-Portuguez R, Rodrigues SD, Wong PK, et al. Low-level arsenic causes proteotoxic stress and not oxidative stress. *Toxicol Appl Pharmacol.* (2018) 341:106–13. doi: 10.1016/j.taap.2018.01.014
100. Yang B, Fu J, Zheng H, Xue P, Yarborough K, Woods CG, et al. Deficiency in the nuclear factor E2-related factor 2 renders pancreatic β-cells vulnerable to arsenic-induced cell damage. *Toxicol Appl Pharmacol.* (2012) 264:315–23. doi: 10.1016/j.taap.2012.09.012
101. Ohta Y, Kosaka Y, Kishimoto N, Wang J, Smith SB, Honig G, et al. Convergence of the insulin and serotonin programs in the pancreatic β-cell. *Diabetes.* (2011) 60:3208–16. doi: 10.2337/db10-1192
102. Ohara-Imaizumi M, Kim H, Yoshida M, Fujiwara T, Aoyagi K, Toyofuku Y, et al. Serotonin regulates glucose-stimulated insulin secretion from pancreatic β cells during pregnancy. *Proc Natl Acad Sci USA.* (2013) 110:19420–5. doi: 10.1073/pnas.1310953110
103. Almaça J, Molina J, Menegaz D, Pronin AN, Tamayo A, Slepak V, et al. Human beta cells produce and release serotonin to inhibit glucagon secretion from alpha cells. *Cell Rep.* (2016) 17:3281–91. doi: 10.1016/j.celrep.2016.11.072
104. Kim H, Toyofuku Y, Lynn FC, Chak E, Uchida T, Mizukami H, et al. Serotonin regulates pancreatic beta cell mass during pregnancy. *Nat Med.* (2010) 16:804–8. doi: 10.1038/nm.2173

8

Developmental Exposure to 2,2′,4,4′-Tetrabromodiphenyl Ether Permanently Alters Blood-Liver Balance of Lipids in Male Mice

Ahmed Khalil[1,2]*, Sebnem E. Cevik*[1]*, Stephanie Hung*[1]*, Sridurgadevi Kolla*[1]*, Monika A. Roy*[1] *and Alexander Suvorov*[1*]

[1] *Department of Environmental Health Sciences, University of Massachusetts Amherst, Amherst, MA, United States,*
[2] *Medical Biotechnology Department, Genetic Engineering & Biotechnology Research Institute, City of Scientific Research & Technological Applications, Alexandria, Egypt*

Correspondence:
Alexander Suvorov
asuvorov@umass.edu

Polybrominated diphenyl ethers (PBDEs) were used as flame-retardant additives starting 1965 and were recently withdrawn from commerce in North America and Europe. Approximately 1/5 of the total U.S. population were born when environmental concentrations of PBDE plateaued at their maximum. Accumulating evidence suggests that developmental exposures to PBDE may result in long-lasting programming of liver metabolism. In this study, CD-1 mice were exposed prenatally or neonatally to 1 mg/kg body weight of 2,2′,4,4′-tetrabromodiphenyl ether (BDE-47), and changes in liver histology, transcriptome, and liver-blood balance of triglycerides were analyzed in 10 months old male offspring. In both exposure groups, long-term reprogramming of lipid metabolism was observed, including increased liver triglycerides and decreased blood triglycerides, and altered expression of metabolic genes in the liver. Significant upregulation of lipid influx transporter *Cd36* 2.3- and 5.7-fold in pre- and neonatal exposure groups, respectively was identified as a potential mechanism of blood/liver imbalance of triglycerides. Analysis of our and previously published all-genome gene expression data identified changes in expression of ribosomal protein genes as a transcriptomic signature of PBDE exposure. Further comparison of our new data and published data demonstrate that low doses (0.2 mg/kg body weight) of PBDE induce long-lasting up-regulation of ribosomal genes, suppression of *Cd36* in liver and increase circulating triglycerides in blood, while moderated doses ($\geq$1 mg/kg body weight) produce opposite long-lasting effects. To conclude, this study shows that an environmentally relevant developmental exposures to BDE-47 permanently alter lipid uptake and accumulation in the liver, with low and moderate doses having opposite effect on liver transcriptomics and triglyceride balance. Similar effects of pre- and neonatal exposures point at hepatocyte maturation as a sensitive window of the liver metabolism programming. These results suggest that PBDE exposure may be an important factor increasing risks of cardio-vascular disease and non-alcoholic fatty liver disease via modulation of liver/blood balance of lipids. The translational relevance of these findings for human remain to be studied.

Keywords: polybrominated diphenyl ether, *Cd36*, fatty acid, triglyceride, metabolism, rodent, ribosome, NAFLD

INTRODUCTION

Polybrominated diphenyl ethers (PBDEs) are a group of ubiquitous and persistent chemical compounds that include 209 congeners. PBDEs are highly lipophilic xenobiotics (1, 2) with a half-life of 1.8–6.5 years in human tissues (3). PBDEs persist in the environment due to pollution by industrial chemicals and biosynthesis in natural ecosystems. The manufacturing of commercial products containing PBDEs began in 1965 (4) and synthetic PBDEs were widely used as flame-retardant additives in a range of products, including building materials, electronics, furnishings, motor vehicles, airplanes, plastics, polyurethane foams, and baby pajamas. Production of PBDEs was banned in Europe in 2003 because of concerning toxicological evidence (5). In the US PBDEs were voluntarily withdrawn from commercial use by industry by 2013 (6). Before these decisions were made PBDEs increased exponentially in human blood, breast milk and tissues (7), including fetal tissues (8) over a 30 years period. In Europe, the discontinued use of PBDEs led to a decrease in environmental concentrations in the recent years. However, an epidemiological study of 1,253 women in California suggests that PBDE concentrations continue to rise in North America (9). This on-going persistence of PBDE exposure in humans can be attributed to many factors, including, the prevalence of PBDE in waste and recycling sites, indoor use of products containing PBDEs (10), global circulation of PBDE toward the Northern Hemisphere, biosynthesis of PBDE by microflora of the marine environment including γ-proteobacteria (11), and endosymbiotic microflora of benthic sponges (12–15) and high bioaccumulation and bioconcentration of PBDEs in food chains (16). Younger generations of Americans that were exposed *in utero* and during early postnatal life to the highest environmental doses of PBDE account for approximately one-fifth of the US population (17, 18). The long term consequences of developmental exposures to PBDE for this population are not well-understood.

In the general population, exposures to highly lipophilic environmental xenobiotics usually peak during fetal and early postnatal development, due to the active transfer of lipophilic compounds from the mothers' storage depots through cord blood and breast milk (19, 20). Additional factors that lead to an increased exposure during the early postnatal period are the ingestion of PBDE-containing household dust by toddlers (21) and high food intake per kilogram of body weight by toddlers (22). As a result, breastfeeding toddlers have several-fold higher plasma levels of PBDEs than their mothers (23). Thus, PBDE exposure is highest during early stages of development (*in utero* and early postnatal) when biological plasticity is high and even modest exposures to environmental stressors may result in dramatic and long-term health effects (24–26).

The ability of chemical compounds to disrupt lipid metabolism in liver has been known for many years (27). The term "metabolic disruptor" was suggested recently by a group of experts to characterize the growing list of environmental compounds that are able to alter metabolism in the mammalian organism (26). Another term, "toxicant-associated steatohepatitis" (TASH) was coined (28) to characterize cases of fatty-liver disease in highly exposed chemical workers. The ability of chemical compounds to produce long lasting changes in lipid metabolism following developmental short-term exposures is poorly understood, although this type of exposure is relevant for many lipophilic environmental xenobiotics. In our recent study, we reported that mice exposed to 0.2 mg/kg body weight of 2,2′,4,4′-tetrabromodiphenyl ether (BDE-47), the most prevalent PBDE congener in human samples, from gestation day 8 (GD8) till postnatal day 21 (PND21), develop long lasting suppression of fatty acid (FA) translocase *Cd36* in hepatocytes (18), a membrane receptor responsible for FA uptake. Changes in expression of this gene were concordant with increased blood triglycerides in exposed animals (18). Increased level of blood lipids is the primary risk factor for heart attack, which is the most common cause of mortality in the developed world, with more than 700,000 deaths attributed to the disease in the US annually (29). Exposure of significant part of the general population to PBDE during early stages of development together with the ability of PBDE to program lipid metabolism in a mammalian organism by early life exposures raises significant concerns about metabolic health of young Americans and suggests a need for additional studies, to examine the relations between early life PBDE exposures and permanent changes in liver metabolism.

In this study we analyze developmental windows sensitive to liver metabolism programming by PBDE using a mouse model. We report that exposures to 1 mg/kg body weight of BDE-47 during prenatal or neonatal windows produce similar changes in 10 months old mice. These changes include altered liver transcriptome, including increased expression of *Cd36*, altered balance of triglycerides between blood and liver and hepatic steatosis-like phenotype. All these effects are opposite in direction in comparison with effects observed in our previous study (18), where mice were exposed to 0.2 mg/kg body weight of BDE-47 perinatally, suggesting complex dose-response relationships for developmental programming of liver metabolism by PBDEs.

MATERIALS AND METHODS

Animals and Treatment

Timed pregnant CD-1 mice were obtained from Charles River Laboratories (Kingston, NY, USA) at pregnancy day 6 and housed in a temperature (23 ± 2°C)- and humidity (40 ± 10%)-controlled environment, with a 12-h light/dark cycle, and food and water available *ad libitum*. The dams were assigned to one of three treatment groups ($n = 10$ per group) based on weight match. The control group was exposed to vehicle—tocopherol-stripped corn oil (MP Biomedicals, Solon, OH) from pregnancy day 8 till postpartum day 21. The prenatal exposure group received 1 mg/ml solution of BDE-47 (AccuStandard, Inc., New Haven, CT; 100% purity) in tocopherol-stripped corn oil from pregnancy day 8 through delivery and then vehicle only from the day of delivery till postpartum day 21. Neonatal exposure group received only vehicle from gestational day 8 till delivery and was then exposed to 1 mg/ml solution of BDE-47 in tocopherol-stripped corn oil through postpartum day 21. Either vehicle or BDE-47 solution was orally administered daily via micropipette in a volume of 1 μl/gram body weight (BW) resulting in exposures to 1 mg/kg BW/day during pre- or neonatal periods. This method of exposure is routinely used in our laboratory as a substitution of oral gavage, which induces a significant stress response by the endocrine system, which may interfere with the evaluation of endpoints of interest (30). The dams delivered naturally, and the litters were not culled to maintain consistency of nutrient distribution among the same number of fetuses/pups at pre- and postnatal periods, and to avoid catch-up growth (31). The dams and pups were kept together until weaning on postnatal day (PND) 21, when the male and female pups were separated. One randomly selected male pup per litter was euthanized using cervical dislocation on PND300 between 9 and 11 a.m. following 2 h of fasting. Tissue samples were collected immediately upon euthanasia. Blood samples were centrifuged at 3,000 g for 10 min and serum was collected and stored at -80°C. Liver was snap-frozen in liquid nitrogen and stored at -80°C. Only male pups were used for further analysis to avoid the interaction of measured health outcomes with hormonal fluctuations due to estrus cycle. Other male and female pups were used in a different study. All procedures met the guidelines of the National Institutes of Health Guide for the Care and Use of Laboratory Animals and this study was approved by the Institutional Animal Care and Use Committee at University of Massachusetts, Amherst.

RNA Extraction and Sequencing

Total RNA was isolated from liver samples using TRIzol reagent (Invitrogen) and quantified using a NanoDrop 1000 instrument (Thermo Fisher Scientific, Wilmington, DE). RNA quality was assessed using Agilent 2100 Bioanalyzer (Agilent Technologies, Santa Clara, CA). Samples of RNA isolated from liver tissue with integrity values >9 were used for library preparation. RS-122-2101-TruSeq® Stranded mRNA LT-SetA kit (Illumina, San-Diego, CA) was used to isolate intact poly(A)+ RNA from 4 μg of total RNA and to construct strand-specific libraries with multiplexing indexes. The quality and purity of the libraries were assessed using the Agilent 2100 Bioanalyzer. The concentration of the libraries was measured using Qubit 3.0 fluorometer (Life Technologies, Carlsbad, CA). High-throughput sequencing was performed using NextSeq500 sequencing system (Illumina, San-Diego, CA) in the Genomic Resource Laboratory of the University of Massachusetts, Amherst. cDNA libraries were single-end sequenced in 76 cycles using a NextSeq 500 Kit v2 (FC-404-2005, Illumina, San-Diego, CA) in one multiplex run (3–4 samples per exposure group). All sequencing data were uploaded to the GEO public repository and GEO were assigned series accession number GSE115143.

Analysis of Mouse RNA-seq Data

Read filtering, trimming and de-multiplexing were performed using the BaseSpace cloud computing service supported by Illumina (https://basespace.illumina.com/home/index). Furthermore, the preprocessed reads were mapped to the reference mouse genome (MM10) using TopHat 2 aligner (32). Aligned reads were then used for assembly of novel transcripts with Cufflinks 2.1.1 and differential expression of novel and reference transcripts with Cuffdiff 2.1.1 (33). Differential expression datasets were further used for gene set enrichment analysis (GSEA, www.broadinstitute.org/gsea). This approach is particularly effective for the identification of biologically significant changes in gene expression that are associated with relatively small effects across multiple members of a gene set (34). The details of the method and statistical approaches used by GSEA are described elsewhere (35, 36). We used GSEA against the Hallmark, KEGG and Reactome collections of datasets. Short-lists of significantly differentially expressed genes were identified by applying thresholds of 2-fold differential expression and false discovery rate (FDR) $q \leq 0.05$. These lists were analyzed using DAVID Functional Annotation Clustering tool (37) and Disease and BioFunctions tool of Ingenuity Pathway Analysis (38) with default settings. To explore further liver lipid metabolism mechanisms affected by BDE-47 we inspected changes in expression of genes, that encode key enzymes of lipid trafficking, de-novo synthesis and/or disposal (39, 40). The following genes were selected for analysis (see **Supplemental File 1**): fatty acid uptake proteins—fatty acid translocase (FAT; gene *Cd36*) and fatty acid uptake proteins (FATP; *Slc27a* genes); de-novo synthesis of fatty acids—acetyl-CoA carboxylase (ACC; genes *Acaca* and *Acacb*) and fatty acid synthase (FAS; gene *Fasn*); synthesis of triglycerides—glycerol-3-phosphate acyltransferase (GPAT; gene *Gpam*), 1-acylglycerol-3-phosphate O-acyltransferase (AGPAT; *Agpat* genes), diacylglycerol O-acyltransferase (DGAT; *Dgat* genes), lipin (LIPIN; *Lpin* genes), mannoside acetylglucosaminyltransferase (MGAT; *Mgat1* genes), and adiponutrin (gene *Pnpla3*); oxidation of fatty acids—acyl-CoA synthetase (ACS; *Acsl, Acsm,* and *Acss* genes), carnitine palmitoyltransferase (CPT; genes *Cpt1a, Cpt1b, Cpt1c, Cpt2*), adipose triglyceride lipase (ATGL, gene *Pnpla2*), and 3-hydroxy-3-methylglutaryl-coenzyme A synthase (HMG-CoA; *Hmgcs* genes); very low density lipoprotein (VLDL) secretion—apolipoprotein B (gene *Apob*), microsomal triglyceride transfer protein (MTP, gene *Mttp*), carboxylesterase (CES; genes *Ces1d, Ces1g,* and *Ces3a*), and cell death-inducing DFF-45-like effector B (gene *Cideb*).

RT-qPCR

The RNA-seq results were validated using RT-qPCR for selected genes: *Cd36, Abcd2, Prelid2, Apoa4, Fabp4, Fgl1, Gdpd3,* and *Hao2.* These gene were selected based on the following criteria (1) they were significantly regulated in both exposure groups based on RNA-seq results and (2) they encode proteins important for liver metabolic function. RT-qPCR was done using independent set of samples, six per exposure group. Total RNA was purified of genomic DNA contamination using DNase (RQ1 RNAse-free DNAse, Cat. # M610A, Promega, Madison, WI), and reverse transcribed using the High Capacity cDNA Reverse Transcription Kit (Cat.# 4368814, Applied Biosystems, Vilnus, Lithuania). Using free online software Primer3Plus (http://primer3plus.com/cgi-bin/dev/primer3plus.cgi), forward and reverse primers were designed to anneal different exons spanning long intron (**Table 1**). The housekeeping gene (*B2m*) was selected from genes that were not regulated in our RNA-seq dataset, with the consideration of its ubiquitous presence in

TABLE 1 | Quantitative reverse transcription polymerase chain reaction (RT-qPCR) validation of RNA-seq genes for selected differentially expressed genes.

Gene	qPCR primers	Fold change			
		Prenatal exposure		Postnatal exposure	
		RNA-seq	qPCR	RNA-seq	qPCR
Cd36	TGTGTTTGGAGGCATTCTCA TTTGAAAGCAGTGGTTCCTTC	2.25	2.01	5.58	4.99
Abcd2	TGTGGAGCAGCTGTGGACTA CATAGCCTGCTTTGGACCAT	11.00	9.76	5.90	5.37
Prelid2	TGTTCCAGTACCCCTTCGAG TTCCACAGTTTTTACAGAGATGACA	−5.28	−6.11	−5.13	−6.20
Apoa4	AGTGAGGAGCCCAGGATGTT CACCTGGTCCGAAGTGACCT	−3.48	−2.98	−3.81	−3.45
Fabp4	AATGTGTGATGCCTTTGTGG CACTTTCCTTGTGGCAAAGC	−6.68	−5.34	−6.06	−7.01
Fgl1	GTGGATGGACTGAGCCTAGC TTCCCATTCTTCCCACTGAG	−2.41	−2.55	−6.59	−5.17
Gdpd3	CCTTTTGTCTCCATCCCTGA CCACAGCGAAATGGGAAGTA	16.91	11.39	6.23	5.86
Hao2	GAGGCAGCTTGATGAGGTTC CCCACCATCCATGTACACTTC	4.86	5.12	7.73	6.03
B2m	CCGGCCTGTATGCTATCCAG TGTTCGGCTTCCCATTCTCC				Housekeeping gene

different cell types. A triplicate of 5 μl real-time PCR reactions, each containing iTaq Universal SYBR Green Supermix (Cat 172-5124, BioRad), primers, and cDNA template were loaded onto a 384-well plate and run through 40 cycles on a CFX384 real time cycler (Bio-Rad Laboratories, Inc). The data were analyzed using the manufacturer's CFX manager software, version 3.1. Relative quantification was determined using the ΔΔCq method (41).

Protein Expression of Cd36

Expression of Cd36 was analyzed by western blotting in liver samples of male offspring euthanized on PND300. Liver samples were lysed in T-PER tissue protein extraction buffer (ThermoFisher Scientific, Cat. # 78510) containing protease and phosphatase inhibitors cocktail (ThermoFisher Scientific, Cat. # 78442). A microplate-based BCA Protein Assay Kit (ThermoFisher Scientific, Cat. # 23227) was then used to determine protein concentrations. Western blot analyses were performed after separating the proteins on 4–20% SDS-PAGE gels (Bio-Rad, Cat. # 456-1094) and transferring them onto a PVDF membrane (0.2 μm) under wet conditions using a Biorad mini trans-blot cell. Anti-Cd36 (1:2000, Cell Signaling, Cat. #14347) and anti-Actin (1:2000, Cell Signaling, Cat. # 4970) primary antibodies were used at indicated dilutions. Proteins were visualized using secondary antibody conjugated with HRP (1:5000, Abcam, Cat. # ab6721), and Pierce ECL enhanced chemiluminesence reagent (ThermoFisher Scientific, Cat. # 32106). Western blot densitometry was quantified using Image Studio Lite Ver 5.2 software.

Histological Analysis

Oil Red O staining was performed in accordance with the protocol for frozen tissue described elsewhere [IHS (42)]. Liver samples were sectioned at 10 μm for lipid staining. Sections were fixed in 10% neutral buffered formalin for 10 min, rinsed with water, and immersed in 100% propylene glycol for 5 min. Slides were stained with Oil Red O solution (Sigma) for 10 min at 60°C, and placed in 85% propylene glycol for 5 min followed by a rinse in distilled water. Slides were counterstained with Harris' hematoxylin for 30 sec, washed in running tap water and coverslipped using Kaiser's Glycerin Jelly. Sections were imaged through a Zeiss Axio Observer Z1 inverted light microscope with ZEN imaging software, at ×10 and ×40 magnification. Images were captured at 88,000 dpi using the AxioCam 506 color digital camera.

Triglycerides in Blood and Liver

To quantify changes in triglycerides concentrations were measured in blood and liver samples of 10 months old mice using a Triglyceride Colorimetric Assay Kit (Cat. # 10010303, Cayman Chemical, Ann Arbor MI). Ten biological replicates (one pup per litter) were analyzed per exposure group. Each biological replicate was analyzed in triplicate.

Reanalysis of Published Transcriptional Datasets

Changes in liver gene expression for many individual genes, as well as for groups of metabolic genes, which were observed in this current study were opposite in direction to the changes reported in our previous study (18). We hypothesize that differences in exposure protocols may have been responsible for the opposite effects in the direction of change of the gene expression in livers of exposed animals. To test this hypothesis we analyzed changes in expression of ribosomal genes, a group of genes that is most sensitive to PBDE exposure according to our current and previously published data (18), in transcriptomic datasets obtained from toxicological experiments with PBDE. The search for transcriptomic datasets was completed on June 1, 2017. Specifically, we searched Gene Expression Omnibus (GEO, http://www.ncbi.nlm.nih.gov/geo/) and ArrayExpress (https://www.ebi.ac.uk/arrayexpress/) genomic data depositories using the following key words: *PBDE, BDE, polybrominated, diphenyl ether, and flame retardant.* We also ran a search in the PubMed (http://www.ncbi.nlm.nih.gov/pubmedn) using a combination of the words *PBDE, BDE, and polybrominated diphenyl ether* with one of the following: *gene expression, transcriptome, microarray, RNA-seq, and genomic.* All selected papers were then checked for the presence of all-genome gene expression analysis and, if positive, for links to the original gene expression data. As a result of this search, we identified transcriptomic datasets produced by our research group (18, 43, 44) and another research group (45). Experimental designs of these studies are summarized in **Table 2**. To address changes in expression of ribosomal genes we used GSEA with the "KEGG Ribosome" gene set. This gene set includes 88 human genes of ribosomal proteins and RNA, and is curated by Kyoto Encyclopedia of Genes and Genomes (KEGG, http://www.genome.jp/kegg/).

Statistical Analysis

All statistical analyses were performed using SPSS Statistics 22 software. ANOVA with subsequent Dunnett's test were used to compare body weights and triglyceride values in blood and liver between exposed and control groups. *T*-test was used to compare western blot densitometry for CD36 protein expression between control and each exposed group. Correlation coefficient was calculated to determine reproducibility of RNA-seq results using RT-qPCR for selected genes and to compare effects of pre- and neonatal exposures on gene expression.

RESULTS

We found no significant relationship between litter size and exposure to BDE-47, with the number of pups varying from 9 to 15 per litter. On PND300, body weights of male animals were 58.5 ± 1.9 g in the control group, 52.5 ± 1.4 g in the prenatally exposed group ($p = 0.02$), and 56.6 ± 1.9 g in the neonatally exposed group ($p = 0.09$). All data are mean ± SE and p-values are for comparison with controls.

Pre-and Neonatal Exposures to BDE-47 Induce Similar Transcriptomic Changes in Livers of 10 Months Old Mice

We analyzed using an RNA-seq approach transcriptional changes in liver tissue of 10 months old male mice. Sequencing was completed with an average of 45 million reads per sample and more than 90% of the reads aligned to the reference genome. After filtering out transcripts that did not correspond to any of known identifiers (genes, non-coding RNAs) and those that had LogFPKM ≤ 0 in both conditions (control and exposed), lists of genes with differential expression values were generated for both exposure groups. These lists consisted of 10,962 transcripts for the prenatal exposure group and 11,035 transcripts for the neonatal exposure group. Short lists of the

TABLE 2 | Gene set enrichment analysis (GSEA) of ribosome dataset in transcriptomic studies of PBDE effect in rodents and details of experimental design of these studies.

Model	Sex	Tissue	Exposure chemical	Daily dose, mg/kg/ body weight	Exposure duration (ED–embryonic day, (PND–postnatal day)	PND for outcome	Gene expression analysis approach	Normalized enrichment score/Nominal p-value KEGG* ribosome	Source
Rat	Male	liver	DE-71**	50	ED6-PND22	22	Affymetrix Rat Genome 230 2.0 Array	−2.14/0.000	(45)
Rat	Female	liver	DE-71**	50	ED6-PND22	22	Affymetrix Rat Genome 230 2.0 Array	−1.98/0.000	(45)
Rat	Male	liver	DE-71**	50	ED6-PND91	91	Affymetrix Rat Genome 230 2.0 Array	−1.97/0.000	(45)
Rat	Male	liver	BDE-47	0.2	ED15-PND21	27	Illumina BeadChips RatRef-12	1.39/0.034	(43)
Rat	Female	brain frontal lobes	BDE-47	0.2	ED15-PND21	41	Illumina BeadChips RatRef-12	1.40/0.033	(44)
CD1 mice	Male	liver	BDE-47	0.2	ED8-PND21	21	Illumina TruSeq RNA-Seq	1.60/0.006	(18)
CD1 mice	Male	liver	BDE-47	0.2	ED8-PND21	140	Illumina TruSeq RNA-Seq	3.21/0.000	(18)
CD1 mice	Male	liver	BDE-47	1	ED8-ED21	300	Illumina TruSeq RNA-Seq	−2.49/0.000	Current study
CD1 mice	Male	liver	BDE-47	1	PND1-PND21	300	Illumina TruSeq RNA-Seq	−1.59/0.019	Current study

**KEGG, Kyoto Encyclopedia of Genes and Genomes. **DE-71 is a commercial mix of PBDE, which includes primarily the tetra- through penta-PBDEs and a small component of hexa-BDE.*

significantly differentially expressed genes were generated using cut-off thresholds of 2-fold change in expression and a false discovery rate (FDR) $q \leq 0.05$. RNA-seq results were confirmed by RT-qPCR for select genes (**Table 1**). Correlation coefficients between values of gene expression change measured by RNA-seq and RT-qPCR were 0.98 in both exposure groups. Short lists of genes that were differentially expressed following prenatal or neonatal exposure consisted of 176 and 191 genes, respectively. These lists overlapped for 88 genes (**Figure 1A**). Correlation coefficient between values of gene expression change in the merged list of 279 genes significantly altered in either exposure group was 0.87. Most of these genes that did not overlap were still altered in the same direction in both exposure groups although with lower significance and fold change (**Figures 1B,C**). In fact only 10 out of 191 non-overlapping genes were altered in different directions and correlation coefficient was 0.52 for the merged list of non-overlapping genes between exposure groups.

Developmental Exposure to BDE-47 Alters Blood/Liver Balance of Triglycerides and Leads to Lipid Accumulation in Livers of 10 Months Old Mice

We analyzed concentrations of triglycerides in serum and in livers of exposed and control animals. We also used Oil Red O staining of liver sections to visualize triglyceride droplets. In both exposed groups, liver tissue had a higher number of lipid droplets in hepatocytes (**Figures 2A,B**). Triglycerides concentrations in serum were decreased in both exposure groups compared to the control group (2.81 ± 0.32 mg/ml in the control group; 1.87 ± 0.15 mg/ml, $p = 0.019$ in the prenatal exposure group; and 2.18 ± 0.21 mg/ml, $p = 0.131$ in the neonatal exposure group)—**Figure 2D**. Concentrations of triglycerides in the liver were increased in both exposure groups (8.23 ± 0.88 mg/g in the control group; 10.31 ± 0.79 mg/g, $p = 0.102$ in the prenatal exposure group; and 13.18 ± 1.46 mg/g, $p = 0.015$ in the neonatal exposure group)—**Figure 2E**. The ratio of liver to serum triglyceride concentrations was significantly higher in both exposed groups (2.94 ± 0.12 in the control group; 5.57 ± 0.27, $p = 3.3E\text{-}07$ in the prenatal exposure group; and 5.99 ± 0.23, $p = 1.3E\text{-}08$ in the neonatal exposure group)—**Figure 2F**. All data shown are mean ± SE and p-values are for comparison with controls.

Pre-and Neonatal Exposures to BDE-47 Alters Expression of Genes Responsible for Lipid Metabolism and Protein Biosynthesis in Livers of 10 Months Old Mice

Gene sets enriched with Normalized Enrichment Score >1.6, nominal $p \leq 0.05$ and FDR $q \leq 0.2$ were selected for further analysis. Thus, we used a more stringent criteria than that

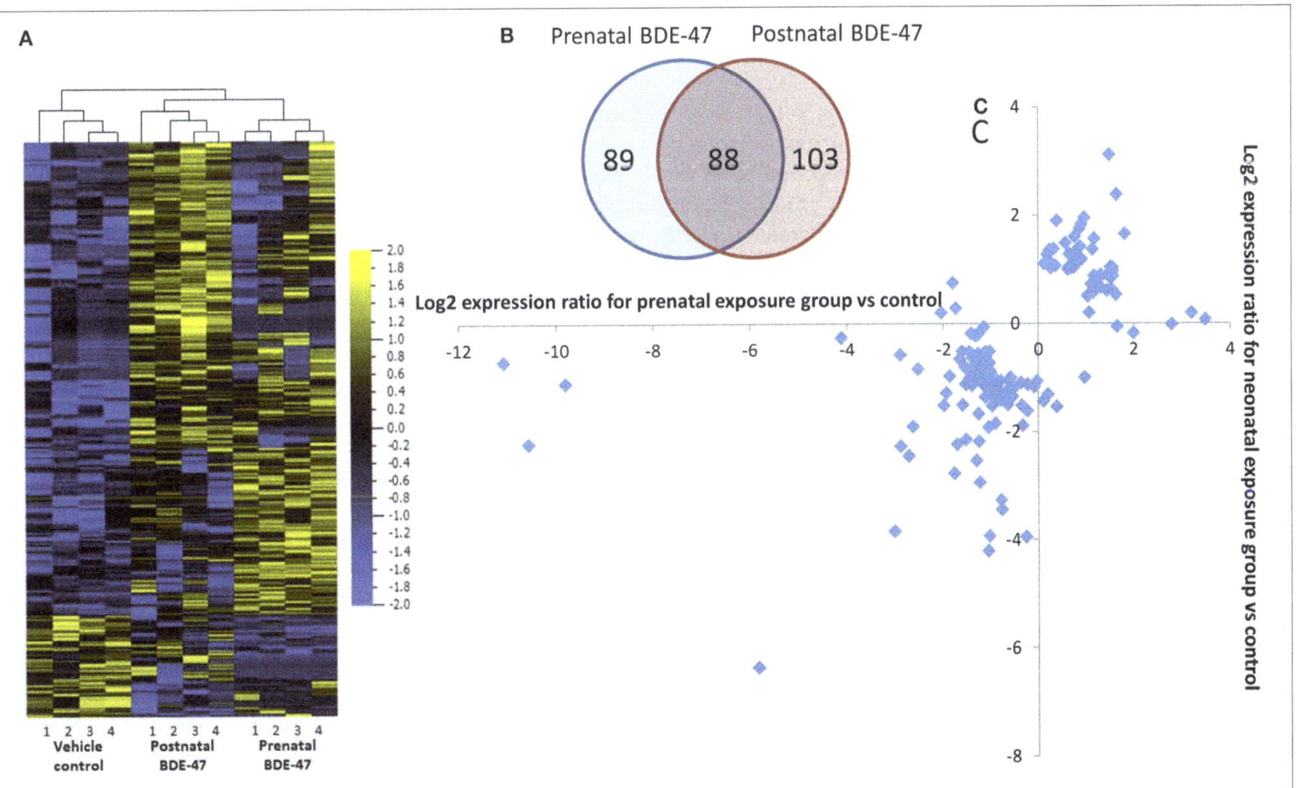

FIGURE 1 | Changes in liver gene expression in 10 months old mice are highly overlapping in groups exposed prenatally only and neonatally only to 1 mg/kg/body weight BDE-47: **(A)**–overlap in lists of significantly (FDR $q \leq 0.05$) 2-fold differentially expressed genes; **(B)**–heat-map and unsupervised hierarchical clustering based on merged list 280 genes significantly (FDR $q \leq 0.05$) 2-fold differentially expressed in pre- and/or postnatally exposed groups; **(C)**–changes in expression of non-overlapping genes (89 + 103 genes) in pre- and neonatal exposure groups, for majority of genes direction of change is the same in both groups.

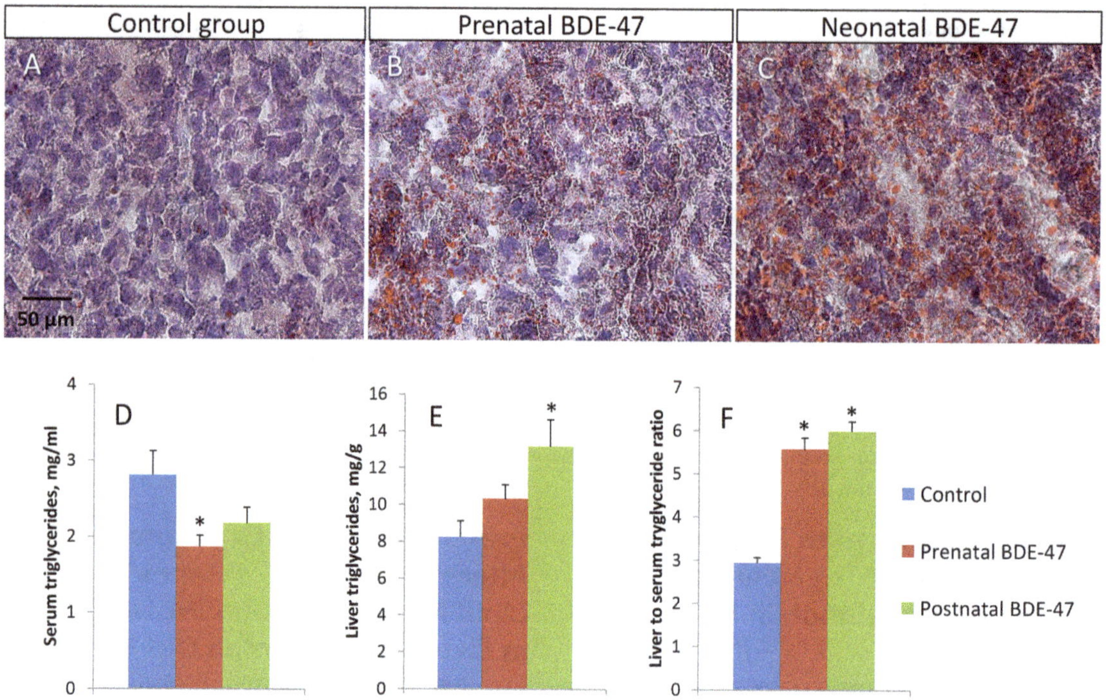

FIGURE 2 | Developmental exposure to BDE-47 results in altered triglyceride concentrations in hepatocytes and blood of 10 months old mice. **(A–C)**–representative liver tissue sections stained with Oil Red O and Harris' hematoxylin (×400): **(A)**–control group, **(B)**–prenatal exposure group, **(C)**–neonatal exposure group. Lipid droplets are stained in orange. **(D,E)**–triglyceride concentrations in blood and liver, respectively. **(F)**–liver to serum triglyceride ratio. All data are Mean ± SE, n = 10/exposure group, ANOVA followed by Dunnett's test, $^*p < 0.05$ when compared with control group.

recommended by GSEA developers (FDR $q \leq 0.25$, http://software.broadinstitute.org/gsea/doc/) for a more exclusive focus on significantly altered biological processes. Gene sets that satisfy these criteria in at least one exposure group (prenatal or neonatal) are shown in **Table 3** and **Supplemental File 2**. All negatively enriched gene-sets from KEGG and Reactome collections and a few from the Hallmark collection point to a suppression of mRNA processing, translation and post-translational processing of protein, such as: KEGG: Ribosome (**Figure 3A**) and Spliceosome; Reactome: Translation, Peptide Chain Elongation, Protein Metabolism, mRNA Metabolism and Protein Folding; Hallmark: Protein Secretion and others. The gene set of an mTORC1 pathway, which is a major pathway of protein synthesis control, was also negatively enriched (Hallmark: mTORC1 Signaling). Gene sets from Hallmark also include negatively enriched gene-sets that are related to cellular stress (Unfolded Protein Response, DNA Repair), cell cycle progression, apoptosis and cellular transformation (MYC Targets V1 and V2), and immune response (Interferon Gamma and Interferon Alpha Response). Significant Hallmark gene-sets relevant for lipid metabolism include negatively enriched Cholesterol Homeostasis gene set and positively enriched Bile Acid Metabolism gene set. Cholesterol Homeostasis gene set was negatively enriched partly due to decreased expression of genes encoding proteins responsible for lipid transport into cells (*Plscr1, Fabp5, Lpl*) and genes encoding enzymes of cholesterol biosynthesis (*Sqle, Hmgcs1, Idi1, Mvd*). Some of the latter genes encode for rate-limiting enzymes of different stages of cholesterol synthesis (*Sqle, Hmgcs1*). The positively enriched Bile Acid Metabolism gene set was due to the increased expression of many genes participating in bile acid biosynthesis, including many key enzymes of the pathway (*Cyp7a1, Cyp46a1, Cyp27a1, Cyp8b1, Akr1d1, Slc27a2, Slc27a5, Amacr, Hsd17b4*).

DAVID Functional Annotation Clustering analysis was done separately for upregulated and downregulated genes from the shortlists of significantly altered genes in the prenatally and postnatally exposed groups. The most enriched clusters are shown in the **Table 4**. The "*Cytochrome P450*" cluster was positively enriched in the postnatal exposure group due to the upregulation of cytochrome genes, largely in family 2. The "*Transmembrane and transmembrane transport*" cluster was positively enriched in both exposure groups and included up-regulated solute carrier genes, ABC transporters, oxysterol binding proteins, desmogleins, *Cd36* and others. Negatively enriched categories include "*endoplasmic reticulum*" (postnatal exposure group only), "*acute-phase response, HDL, fatty acid binding*," "*metallothionein*," and "*extracellular, glycoprotein.*" The analysis of annotations of genes in the cluster "*endoplasmic reticulum*" showed their functional heterogeneity. Most of these genes grouped in one of three functions: vesicle transport to Golgi (*Ehd4, Golt1b, Lrrc59, Sec23b, Tmed3, Tmed9*), response to ER-stress (*Creb3l2, Creld2, Dnajb9, Hyou1, Manf, Sdf2l1*), and fatty acid metabolism (*Acsl4, Aldh3a2, Elovl3, Elovl7, Fndcb3, Insig2, Mrap, Mrap2*). The

TABLE 3 | Top GSEA enriched gene-sets in livers of 10 months old mice exposed pre- or neonatally to BDE-47.

Gene set	Prenatal exposure			Neonatal exposure		
	NES	**NOM *p*-val**	**FDR *q*-val**	**NES**	**NOM *p*-val**	**FDR *q*-val**
HALLMARK COLLECTION OF GENE-SETS						
Unfolded protein response	**−2.06**	**0.000**	**0.003**	**−1.98**	**0.000**	**0.003**
MYC targets V2	**−2.04**	**0.000**	**0.002**	**−1.81**	**0.006**	**0.017**
MYC targets V1	**−2.01**	**0.000**	**0.002**	**−2.00**	**0.000**	**0.004**
DNA repair	**−1.93**	**0.000**	**0.006**	**−1.62**	**0.011**	**0.054**
Cholesterol homeostasis	**−1.66**	**0.010**	**0.060**	**−1.80**	**0.008**	**0.018**
MTORC1 signaling	**−1.61**	**0.005**	**0.074**	**−1.64**	**0.004**	**0.052**
Interferon gamma response	−1.39	0.050	0.234	**−2.04**	**0.000**	**0.006**
Interferon alpha response	−1.38	0.086	0.205	**−1.84**	**0.001**	**0.016**
Protein secretion	−1.22	0.181	0.365	**−1.65**	**0.007**	**0.052**
Bile acid metabolism	1.62	0.020	0.409	**2.16**	**0.000**	**0.056**
KEGG COLLECTION OF GENE-SETS						
Ribosome	**−2.49**	**0.000**	**0.000**	−1.59	0.019	0.266
Spliceosome	**−1.92**	**0.000**	**0.087**	−1.86	0.000	0.187
RNA polymerase	**−1.90**	**0.007**	**0.097**	−1.48	0.072	0.302
Protein export	−1.85	0.014	0.107	**−2.04**	**0.002**	**0.085**
REACTOME COLLECTION OF GENE-SETS						
Translation	**−2.62**	**0.000**	**0.000**	−1.87	0.000	0.187
SRP dependent cotranslational protein targeting to membrane	**−2.56**	**0.000**	**0.000**	−1.81	0.000	0.196
Influenza viral RNA transcription and replication	**−2.53**	**0.000**	**0.000**	−1.64	0.004	0.247
3 UTR mediated translational regulation	**−2.51**	**0.000**	**0.000**	−1.62	0.009	0.256
Peptide chain elongation	**−2.46**	**0.000**	**0.000**	−1.51	0.031	0.292
Influenza life cycle	**−2.40**	**0.000**	**0.000**	−1.64	0.009	0.247
Nonsense mediated decay enhanced by the exon junction complex	**−2.33**	**0.000**	**0.000**	−1.47	0.034	0.301
Metabolism of proteins	**−2.31**	**0.000**	**0.000**	−1.81	0.000	0.199
Activation of the mRNA upon binding of the cap binding complex and EIFS and subsequent binding to 43S	**−2.29**	**0.000**	**0.001**	−1.52	0.035	0.290
Formation of the ternary complex and subsequently the 43S complex	**−2.25**	**0.000**	**0.001**	−1.54	0.036	0.279
Metabolism of mRNA	**−2.20**	**0.000**	**0.004**	−1.46	0.016	0.307
Metabolism of RNA	**−2.18**	**0.000**	**0.004**	−1.57	0.003	0.271
mRNA splicing minor pathway	**−2.11**	**0.000**	**0.014**	−1.74	0.015	0.224
Protein folding	**−1.95**	**0.000**	**0.072**	−1.77	0.009	0.213
mRNA splicing	**−1.93**	**0.000**	**0.081**	−1.75	0.003	0.219
Activation of chaperone genes by XBP1S	**−1.89**	**0.006**	**0.100**	**−2.03**	**0.000**	**0.094**

NES, normalized enrichment score; NOM p, nominal p-value; FDR q, false discovery q-value. All numbers for gene sets enriched with nominal $p \leq 0.05$ and FDR $q \leq 0.2$ are shown in bold.

"*Acute-phase response, HDL, fatty acid binding*" and the "*extracellular, glycoprotein*" clusters were enriched due mostly to the decreased expression of genes encoding serum lipid-binding proteins. This includes orosomucoid genes (*Orm1, Orm2, and Orm3*), which are carriers of basic and neutrally charged lipophilic compounds, high-density lipoprotein (HDL) associated apolipoproteins (*Saa1, Saa2 and Saa3*), chylomicron associated apolipoprotein A-IV (*Apoa4*) and fatty acid binding proteins (*Fabp4 and Fabp5*). The "*Metallothionein*" cluster was negatively enriched in both exposure groups due to the downregulation of three metallothionein proteins (*Mt1, Mt2, and Mt4*).

We performed an IPA Disease and BioFunctions analysis with default settings. Initially, this analysis was performed for three lists of differentially regulated genes: genes altered in animals exposed to BDE-47 *in utero*, genes altered in animals exposed to BDE-47 neonatally, and a merged list of genes regulated in both groups. The results of this analysis were very similar for all three gene lists, therefore we present here only data for the merged list of genes (see **Supplemental File 3** for details).

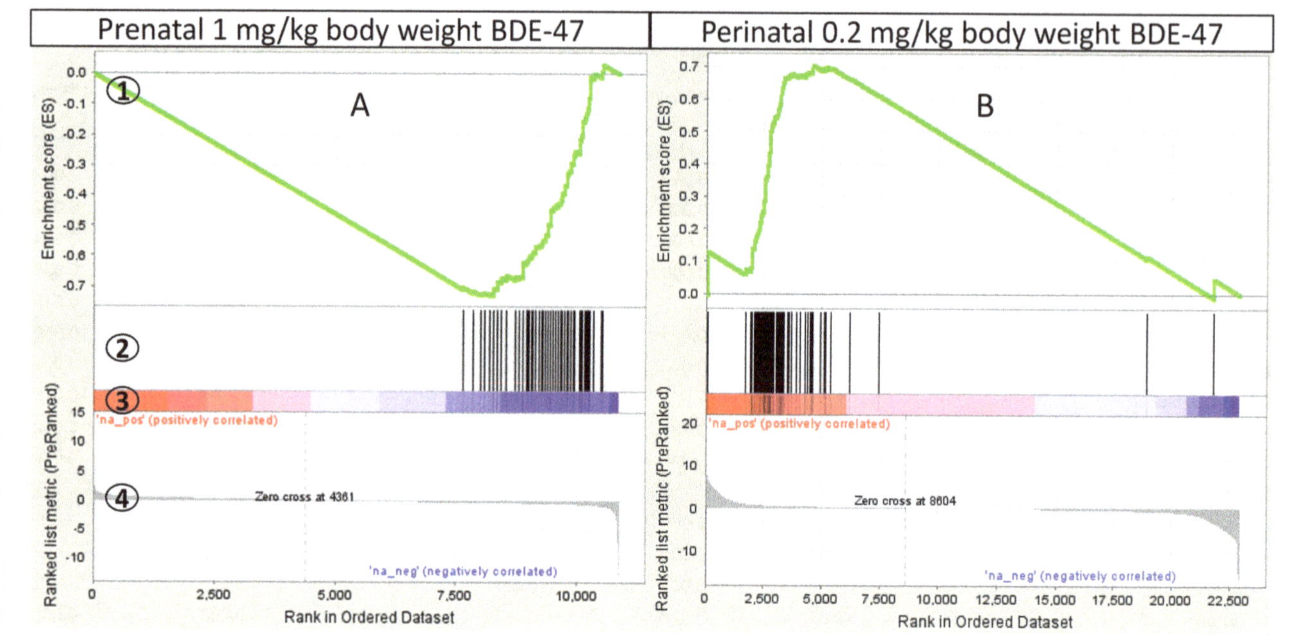

FIGURE 3 | GSEA enrichment of "KEGG Ribosome" gene set in mouse liver: **(A)**–mice were exposed prenatally to 1 mg/kg body weight BDE-47 and gene expression analyzed on PND300; **(B)**–mice were exposed perinatally to 0.2 mg/kg body weight BDE-47 and gene expression analyzed on PND140 (18). GSEA plot legend: 1-running enrichment score for the gene set; 2-vertical lines show where the members of the gene set appear in the ranked list of genes; 3 and 4-ranked list of differentially expressed genes from the most up-regulated (left of each plot) to the most downregulated (right of each plot). Regulation is shown in the heat-bar (3) and in the bar plot (4).

TABLE 4 | Top enriched DAVID clusters in livers of 10 months old mice exposed prenatally or neonatally to BDE-47.

Cluster of enriched terms	Prenatal exposure group		Neonatal exposure group	
	ES*	Benjamini *p*	ES*	Benjamini *p*
POSITIVELY REGULATED FUNCTIONS				
Cytochrome P450	3.13	6.0E-1–2.0E-4	6.14	5.6E-1–1.8E-9
Transmembrane, transmembrane transport			2.22	9.8E-1–5.2E-4
NEGATIVELY REGULATED FUNCTIONS				
Endoplasmic reticulum			4.82	5.8E-3–4.3E-5
Acute-phase response, HDL, fatty acid binding	1.51	9.9E-1–3.2E-1	3.89	9.8E-1–9.9E-5
Metallothionein	3.62	7.5E-1–1.6E-2	3.50	3.1E-1–7.9E-3
Extracellular, glycoprotein	1.86	8.1E-1–1.5E-1	3.43	1.0E0–1.1E-6

ES, enrichment score.

The "*Concentration of lipid*" was the most significantly enriched category ($p = 7.1E\text{-}08$). The "*Hepatic steatosis*" cluster was one of the most significantly enriched categories with high predicted activation ($p = 4.69E\text{-}07$, activation z-score $= 2.89$), while "*Atherosclerosis*" was among the most significant categories with predicted suppression ($p = 5.25E\text{-}06$, activation z-score $= -2.35$; **Figure 4**).

To explore what mechanisms of liver lipid metabolism altered by BDE-47 may be responsible for increased triglycerides in livers of exposed animals we analyzed changes in expression of key enzymes of lipid trafficking, de-novo synthesis and/or disposal (**Supplemental File 1**). *Cd36* is the only gene form this list that was significantly altered in both exposed groups, with 2.3- and 5.6-fold increase in expression in prenatally and postnatally exposed animals, respectively. Higher magnitude of change of *Cd36* in postnatally exposed animals correspond to higher concentrations of triglycerides in their livers. Expression of Cd36 protein was also significantly increased in liver of animals from both exposed groups as confirmed by western blot data (**Figure 5**).

Low and Moderate/High Exposures to PBDE Regulate Expression of Metabolic Genes in Opposite Directions

In both the current study, and our previous study (18), ribosomal genes represented one of the most sensitive groups of genes that underwent coordinated changes in expression following PBDE exposure. However, changes in expression of ribosomal genes had an opposite direction in these studies. Similarly, many other important metabolic genes, including Cd36 were significantly differentially expressed in both studies but the direction of change was different. To test whether variables in the experimental protocol may have contributed to the observed opposite effects in expression of metabolic genes, we analyzed changes in the expression of ribosomal genes in transcriptomic datasets obtained from previously published toxicological experiments with PBDE (18, 43–45) as described

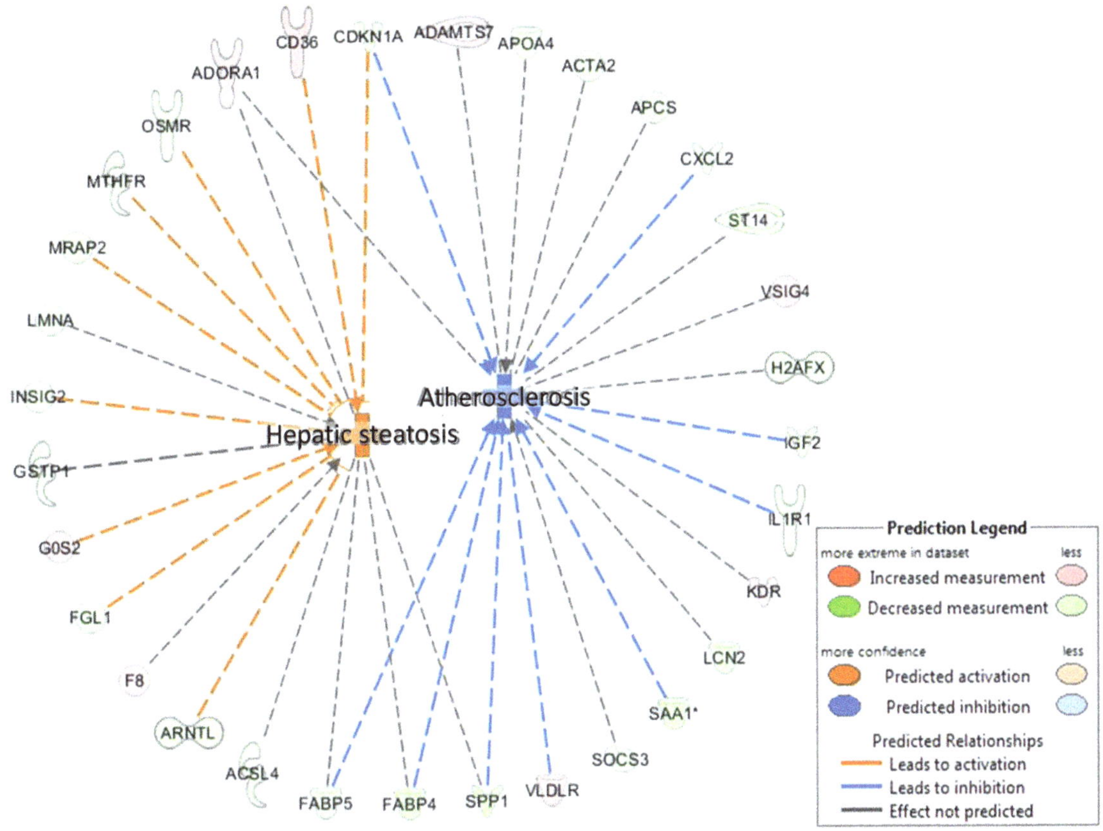

FIGURE 4 | IPA Disease and BioFunctions analysis: hepatic steatosis and atherosclerosis—significantly positively and negatively enriched categories in livers of 10 months old mice developmentally exposed to 1 mg/kg body weight BDE-47.

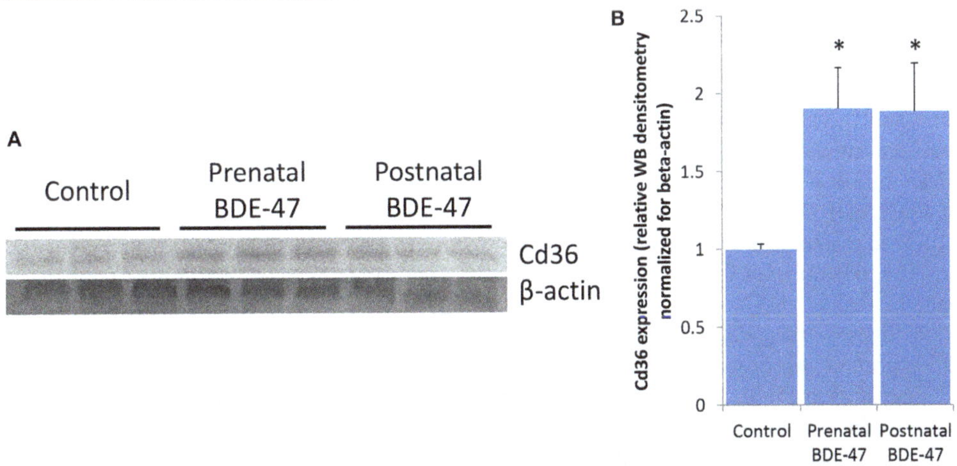

FIGURE 5 | Expression of Cd36 protein is increased in livers of 10 months old mice exposure to BDE-47 during prenatal or neonatal development: **(A)**–expression of Cd36 measured by western blot; **(B)**–quantification of Cd36 protein expression (Mean ± SE, $n = 3$/exposure group, p-value is for T-test).

in Reanalysis of Published Transcriptional Datasets. The results of this analysis are summarized in **Table 2**. In short, (i) the ribosomal gene set was enriched in GSEA analysis with nominal p-value <0.05 in all reanalyzed datasets, supporting our observation that coordinated changes in ribosomal gene expression represent a molecular signature of PBDE exposure. (ii) In the studies that used rats and mice, similar exposures produced similar changes in ribosomal gene expression. For example perinatal exposure to 0.2 mg/kg BW BDE-47 in Wistar rats and in CD-1 mice significantly positively enriched ribosomal dataset in liver tissue (18, 43). (iii) One study focused on gene expression in the brain frontal lobes (44) and it showed similar changes in ribosomal gene expression as studies that used similar exposures to analyze gene expression in liver tissue (43, 44). (iv) Finally, the opposite effects were observed in studies using 0.2 mg/kg BW BDE-47 (18, 43, 44) and studies using 1 mg/kg BW BDE-47 (current study) or 50 mg/kg BW DE-71 (45)—a commercial mix of PBDE, which includes primarily the tetra- through penta- PBDEs and a small component of hexa-BDE.

DISCUSSION

We have found that both prenatal and neonatal exposure to 1 mg/kg body weight of BDE-47 result in similar changes in expression of metabolic genes in 10 months old mouse liver, suggesting permanent reprogramming of the liver metabolism in both exposure groups. This reprogramming includes increased expression of *Cd36* and other lipid transporters and decreased expression of serum lipid-binding proteins which is a likely mechanistic explanation of the observed shift in the balance of triglycerides toward their reduced concentrations in the blood and increased concentrations in the liver. Long-lasting or permanent shift in liver metabolism, leading to excessive accumulation of triglycerides in the liver, may be a risk factor for the development of liver steatohepatitis—the most common form of chronic liver disease among adults and children (46, 47) with 33% to 88% prevalence (48–51). Liver steatohepatitis is a risk factor for type 2 diabetes, dyslipidemia, hypertension, cardiovascular and kidney disease, liver cirrhosis, hepatocellular carcinoma, and mortality (52–57).

Relevance of our Dosing Paradigm

In our previous study (58), exposure of pregnant rats to 0.2 mg/kg body weight of BDE-47 resulted in 234.3 ng BDE-47/g lipid in adipose tissue of dams and 1,054.7 ng BDE-47/g lipid in adipose tissue of pups. These concentrations are comparable with those of the North American human population (mean concentration in adipose tissue of adult subjects = 399 ng/g lipids) (2). Given that the rate of BDE-47 elimination is around 10 times higher in mice than in rats (59, 60) the exposure used in this study may also be relevant to that of the North American human population. To further increase the relevance of our exposure paradigm to human exposures, we dosed animals during pre- or neonatal periods since human PBDE exposure peaks during the perinatal period of life due to the transport of PBDE *via* cord blood and breast milk (19, 20, 22), higher rates of dust ingestion (21), and higher food intake per kilogram of body weight in toddlers (22).

Long Lasting Programming of Liver Metabolism

In our previous studies, we have demonstrated that perinatal exposures to low doses (0.2 mg/kg body weight) of BDE-47 may produce long lasting changes in gene expression in rodent livers. In our rat, study expression of many metabolic genes including genes of cholesterol metabolism and ribosomal proteins, were significantly altered 1 week after the last day of exposure (43). Blood cholesterol was also increased in exposed rats. In a recent study with CD-1 mice similar changes in liver gene expression were observed on postnatal day 140, ~4 months after the last day of exposure (18). Exposed mice had significantly increased blood triglycerides. These findings indicate that metabolic reprogramming of liver by developmental exposure to PBDE is likely permanent. A long-lasting change in liver lipid metabolism by PBDEs is also supported by the current study as it demonstrates altered expression of metabolic genes in liver and increased accumulation of liver triglycerides 10 months after the last day of exposure. A review of extant toxicological evidence linking exposures to different chemicals with hepatic steatosis and steatohepatitis (27) did not list any evidence of liver lipid accumulation in adult organism resulting from developmental exposure. Thus, developmental programming of liver metabolism described in this study is a novel potential risk factor for fatty liver diseases development.

Sensitive Exposure Windows

In previous studies, the perinatal window of exposure, spanning from part of gestation and postnatal development until weaning, was used to study programming effects of PBDE for the liver metabolism (18, 43, 61). In the current study, we aimed to narrow down the sensitive developmental window of liver programming by using prenatal-only and postnatal-only exposures. Surprisingly, both exposed groups developed very similar shift in expression of metabolic genes including upregulation of lipid transporter *Cd36* and suppression of genes encoding ribosomal proteins in the liver. Both exposure groups also had similar shifts in the blood-liver balance of triglycerides, including decreased serum triglycerides and increased liver triglycerides, although triglycerides accumulation in the liver was more pronounced in the neonatal exposure group. Thus, our results demonstrate that the sensitive developmental window of the liver metabolism reprogramming by BDE-47 spans across pre- and neonatal periods of development, i.e., likely corresponds to the period of hepatocyte maturation, which starts at gestation day 18.5 and covers postnatal development at least till postnatal day 45 (62–64). Postnatal exposure used in our experiment covers longer period of hepatocyte maturation than prenatal exposure, which only interferes with the beginning of this process. That fact may explain higher accumulation of triglycerides in the livers of postnatally exposed animals. It should be mentioned that BDE-47 that accumulated in the bodies of fetuses in the prenatal exposure group was not fully eliminated from the organisms by the time of delivery and could affect some molecular mechanisms during the neonatal period, resulting in similar effects in both exposure groups. Given that the half-life of BDE-47 in mice is around 3–4 days (59, 60) we assume that "carry over" of BDE-47 from prenatal life to postnatal life in the prenatal exposure group could have had health consequences only during first few days of neonatal life.

Molecular Mechanisms Underlying Altered Liver/Blood Balance of Triglycerides

It was shown previously that major process that contributes to lipid accumulation in liver is fatty acids uptake by hepatocytes (39, 65, 66), although de novo lipogenesis, triglyceride synthesis, as well as disposal of fatty acids in a form of oxidation and/or VLDL secretion may contribute to triglyceride concentrations in liver. To explore, perturbation of which process may be responsible for the observed accumulation of triglycerides in our study, we analyzed changes in expression of the key enzymes (**Supplemental File 1**) involved in lipid uptake, biosynthesis and disposal. Increased expression of *Cd36* was the only enzyme from this list that was significantly upregulated in both exposed groups at the level of gene expression. Upregulation of *Cd36* was also confirmed at the level of protein expression, suggesting that this change may be the major causative factor responsible for the altered balance of the liver/blood triglycerides. This hypothesis is additionally supported by the concordance in the magnitude of *Cd36* expression and triglycerides concentrations in livers of exposed animals, so that higher upregulation of *Cd36* in postnatally exposed animals (5.7-fold) is concordant with higher increase in concentration of triglycerides (168%) in this group as compared with smaller change in *Cd36* expression (2.3-fold) and triglyceride concentration (125%) in prenatal exposure group. Previous research demonstrates that overexpression of *Cd36* may significantly increase fatty acid uptake in liver. Cd36 upregulation induced by *in vivo* adenoviral delivery of the gene to the livers of mice was sufficient to increased hepatic triglyceride storage and dyslipidemia in mice (67). *Cd36* expression is increased in humans with NAFLD (68–70). Decreased rate of VLDL secretion may also contribute to increased triglycerides in the livers and decreased in blood of exposed mice. Genes of major enzymes involved in VLDL secretion (*Apob, Mttp, Ces1d, Ces1g, Ces3a, Cideb*) were not altered significantly, however many genes responsible for VLDL trafficking between endoplasmic reticulum (ER) and Golgi apparatus (*Ehd4, Golt1b, Lrrc59, Sec23b, Tmed3*, and *Tmed9*) and genes involved in binding of lipids in blood (*Orm1, Orm2, Orm3, Saa1, Saa2, Saa3, Apoa4, Fabp4, and Fabp5*) were significantly downregulated. Triglycerides and other lipid components are synthesized in smooth ER and combine with apolipoprotein B at the junction of smooth and rough ER. The nascent particles are then transferred to the Golgi apparatus for further processing and secretory VLDL vesicles are subsequently released from the Golgi (39, 71, 72). Thus, interruption of ER-Golgi trafficking may slow down VLDL secretion by hepatocytes. Decreased expression of genes encoding serum lipid-binding proteins may also contribute to decreased concentration of triglycerides in blood.

Opposite Effects of Different Dosing Protocols

As previously mentioned our recent study showed that CD-1 mice exposed perinatally to 0.2 mg/kg body weight BDE-47 (**Table 2**) had significantly upregulated genes of ribosomal proteins (**Figure 3B**), significantly downregulated expression of *Cd36*, and almost 2-fold increased concentration of triglycerides in blood (18). Other studies have shown similar effects of genes of ribosomal proteins being upregulated in the livers and brain frontal lobes of rats exposed to the same concentration of BDE-47 perinatally (43, 44). However, experimental data published by Dunnick and others (45) demonstrate opposite effect, genes of ribosomal proteins was the most negatively enriched gene-set. Dunnick and others exposed rats to 50 mg/kg body weight of DE-71, a commercial mix of PBDE, from embryonic day 6 continuously throughout the animals' lifetime until euthanasia (PND22 or PND91). Given that a significant shift (although in different directions) in expression of ribosomal genes was found in all transcriptomic studies of PBDE effects (**Table 2**), we used this "molecular signature" of PBDE to determine whether differences in experimental design were responsible for opposite outcomes. Existing studies used different animal models, timing of exposure, exposure dose, timing of outcome measurement, time interval between exposure and outcome measurement and chemical compound (BDE-47 or DE-71). Interestingly, same dose of BDE-47 produced similar changes in ribosomal gene expression in different tissues (43, 44), in different models (18, 43, 44) and in tissues collected at different time-intervals after exposure (18, 43, 44). However, the same compound used at higher dose produced opposite effect in the current study. This

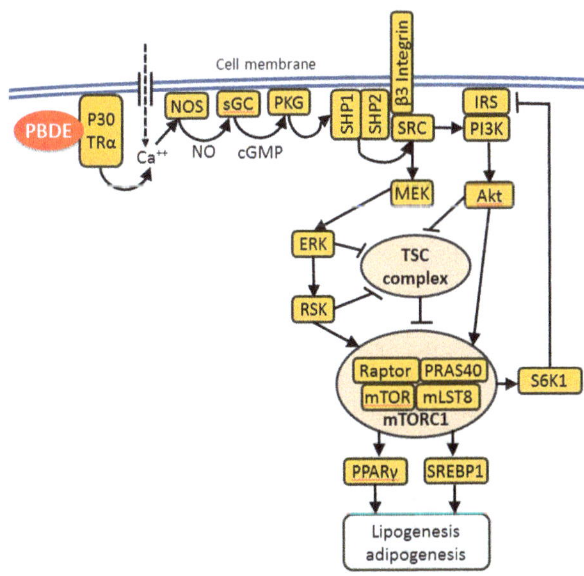

FIGURE 6 | Proposed mechanism of metabolic reprograming by PBDE: PBDEs or their metabolites bind to the plasma membrane associated p30 TRα1 and induce an increase in intracellular Ca^{2+} concentration, which leads to activation of the NO-cGMP-PKGII signaling cascade and the phosphorylation and activation of the SHP1/SHP2 phosphatase complex. This complex activates SRC which in turn activates MEK-ERK and PI3K-AKT signaling. Both cascades merge on and suppress tuberous sclerosis complex (TSC), which is a potent mTORC1 suppressor. Lipogenesis and adipogenesis are regulated by mTORC1 mainly via SREBP1/2 and PPARγ transcription factors that control the expression of genes involved in fatty acid and cholesterol synthesis, lipid uptake and storage. Additionally mTORC1 directly phosphorylates/activates S6K1 which phosphorylates/suppresses IRS1 causing insulin resistance.

effect was similar to the one induced by high dose of PBDE mix (45). Thus, data presented in **Table 2** suggest, that the critical parameter responsible for the direction of change of ribosomal gene expression is likely the dose of the compound. Future research should include targeted dose-response experiments to test this hypothesis.

Concern for Human Health

As discussed in the introduction, approximately one-fifth of the US population (~60 million) experienced their perinatal development when concentrations of PBDE plateaued at their highest environmental levels (17, 18). If the PBDE-induced programming effects described in the current study are seen in humans, we may anticipate long-term adverse consequences of developmental exposures to PBDE. Our study demonstrates that different exposure scenarios in rodents may result in the shift in liver-blood lipid balance in either direction. Our studies indicate, that smaller doses suppress lipid uptake by the liver, resulting in triglyceride accumulation in serum. Higher doses of PBDE induce lipid uptake and accumulation in the liver. Importantly, both smaller and higher doses discussed here are relevant for the general population. Fatty changes in liver were previously shown in juvenile mice exposed for 28 days to 0.45 mg/kg body weight of BDE-47 (73). Liver steatosis associated with increased expression of *Cd36* was recently shown in mice exposed to low doses of BDE-47 perinatally and further kept on high fat diet for 14 weeks (74). Liver fatty degeneration was also demonstrated in adult rats exposed to high dose (2,000 mg/kg body weight) of pentaBDE (75, 76) and in prepubertal rats exposed to high doses (300 and 600 mg/kg body weight) of decaBDE (77). The link between PBDE exposures and lipid imbalance was never tested in human population studies.

Tight regulation of fatty acids (FA) uptake by the liver is the major process that contributes to a healthy balance of lipids between the blood and the liver (65, 66). Abnormal shifts in this balance in either direction may result in increased morbidity and mortality risks. An increase in the uptake of fatty acids and accumulation of triglycerides in lipid droplets results in NAFLD. NAFLD increases the risk of type 2 diabetes, dyslipidemia, hypertension, cardiovascular and kidney disease, liver cirrhosis, hepatocellular carcinoma, and mortality (52–57). Treatment options for NAFLD have very limited efficacy. On the other hand, decreased uptake of fatty acids by the liver may result in hyperlipidemia and atherosclerosis—the primary risk factors for heart attack, which is the most common cause of mortality in the developed world (29, 78–80).

Molecular Mechanisms of Liver Metabolism Programming by PBDE

Molecular mechanisms of metabolic effects of PBDE remain poorly understood. Previously, we demonstrated that BDE-47 activates mTOR (mechanistic target of rapamycin) signaling in mouse livers and in human hepatocellular carcinoma cells (18). mTOR is a serine/threonine protein kinase that emerged over the last decade as a critical signaling node that links nutrient and energy sensing to the coordinated regulation of cellular growth and metabolism (81, 82). Thus, mTOR plays a central role in lipid homeostasis (83, 84). One of the best characterized functions of mTOR pathway consists in the regulation of ribosomal biogenesis (85, 86). In the current study *"mTORC1 signaling"* and *"ribosome"* were among the most negatively enriched categories (**Table 3**) supporting our hypothesis, that mTOR pathway is involved in the long-lasting response to PBDE (18). The mTOR complex one (mTORC1) integrates signals from PI3K-AKT and RAS-ERK pathways upon their activation by receptor tyrosine kinases in response to insulin and insulin-like growth factors (81, 87). A recent study demonstrated the ability of BDE-47 and BDE-85 to activate PI3K-AKT signaling (88) in a thyroid receptor alpha dependent manner. Involvement of TRα and AKT points at recently described non-genomic pathway of thyroid hormone signaling (89) in which binding of T3 to the plasma membrane-associated p30 isoform of TRα1 activates the nitric oxide (NO)/cyclic guanosine monophosphate (cGMP)/protein kinase G II (PKGII) signaling cascade and results in the phosphorylation/activation of the SHP1/SHP2 phosphatase complex. Activation of the tyrosine kinase SRC by this complex results in activation of MEK-ERK and PI3K-Akt signaling. Given that PBDEs are well-characterized thyroid disruptors (90–94), we propose the following hypothesis to link developmental PBDE exposures to long-lasting programming of liver metabolism (**Figure 6**): PBDEs and/or their metabolites interact directly with thyroid receptors and activate downstream PI3K-AKT and MEK-ERK signaling to induce mTORC1 activity; changes in mTORC1 activity during critical windows of liver development change liver metabolic settings and induce long-lasting alterations in lipid and other metabolism. Additional mechanistic research is needed to test this hypothesis.

CONCLUSIONS

We have found that prenatal or neonatal exposures to an environmentally relevant dose (1 mg/kg body weight) of BDE-47 result in permanent reprogramming of the liver metabolism in both exposure groups. The similarity in responses of both exposure groups indicate that the sensitive window of liver metabolism programming spans pre- and postnatal period of development. Observed reprogramming included changes in expression of genes involved in lipid and other metabolism, which resulted in reduced concentrations of triglycerides in the blood and increased concentrations of triglycerides in the liver. Opposite directional changes in expression of many metabolic genes and levels of circulating triglycerides were observed in comparison with previous studies, which used a lower exposure dose (0.2 mg/kg body weight). Both exposure doses are relevant for the general population. If similarity of toxic effects and dose-response relationships between mice and humans will be proven in future research it will indicate that the range of existing and past environmental exposures could produce changes in lipid metabolism in both directions in the general population. The shift in blood-liver balance of lipids may be associated with health conditions, such as NAFLD and atherosclerosis. Based on this study and previously published data, we propose that metabolic effects of developmental exposures to PBDE are mediated by the mTORC1 signaling pathway. Species-specific differences in the involved pathways need to be further investigated to assess the translational relevance of our findings. Additional research is needed to test the mechanistic considerations of this study, establish dose-response relations between developmental exposures and lipid metabolism in adulthood, and elucidate developmental metabolic effects of PBDE in the general population.

AUTHOR CONTRIBUTIONS

AS conceived, designed, and coordinated the study and participated in all steps of laboratory experiments, data analysis and drafting of the manuscript. AK conducted exposure experiment with mice, and protein expression analysis. SC conducted analysis of triglycerides. SH, SK, and MR participated in libraries preparation for RNA-seq and bioinformatic analysis. All authors contributed to the manuscript editing, they read and approved the final manuscript.

FUNDING

This manuscript was produced with funding from a University of Massachusetts start-up fund to AS. RNA-seq experiment was performed as part of laboratory component of the class EHS 667 Environmental & Occupational Toxicology II taught by AS in spring semester, 2016. Cost of all materials and consumables for RNA-seq experiment was covered by the department of Environmental Health Sciences of the University of Massachusetts in Amherst.

ACKNOWLEDGMENTS

We are thankful to Alexandria E. Gillespie, Stephen Paul Hynes and Alehegne W. Yirsaw who participated in library preparation for RNA-seq.

REFERENCES

1. Johnson-Restrepo B, Adams DH, Kannan K. Tetrabromobisphenol A (TBBPA) and hexabromocyclododecanes (HBCDs) in tissues of humans, dolphins, and sharks from the United States. *Chemosphere* (2008) 70:1935–44. doi: 10.1016/j.chemosphere.2007.10.002
2. Johnson-Restrepo B, Kannan K, Rapaport DP, Rodan BD. Polybrominated diphenyl ethers and polychlorinated biphenyls in human adipose tissue from New York. *Environ Sci Technol.* (2005) 39:5177–82. doi: 10.1021/es050399x
3. Geyer HJ, Schramm KW, Darnerud PO, Aune M, Feicht EA, Fried K, et al. (2004). Terminal elimination half-lives of the brominated flame retardants TBBPA, HBCD, and lower brominated PBDEs in humans. Organohalogen Compounds: Vol. 66. (pp. 3867–3872). *Presented at the 24th Int. Symposium on Halogenated Environmental Organic Pollutants and POPs (DIOXIN 2004).* Berlin (2004).
4. Suvorov A, Takser L. Facing the challenge of data transfer from animal models to humans: the case of persistent organohalogens. *Environ Health* (2008) 7:58. doi: 10.1186/1476-069X-7-58
5. Dodson RE, Perovich LJ, Covaci A, Van den Eede N, Ionas AC, Dirtu AC, et al. After the PBDE phase-out: a broad suite of flame retardants in repeat house dust samples from California. *Environ Sci Technol.* (2012) 46:13056–66. doi: 10.1021/es303879n
6. US EPA. *Technical Fact Sheet-Polybrominated Diphenyl Ethers (PBDEs) and Polybrominated Biphenyls (PBBs).* Durham, NC: US Environmental Protection Agency 505-F-14-006:7 (2014).
7. Hites RA. Polybrominated diphenyl ethers in the environment and in people: a meta-analysis of concentrations. *Environ Sci Technol.* (2004) 38:945–56. doi: 10.1021/es035082g
8. Doucet J, Tague B, Arnold DL, Cooke GM, Hayward S, Goodyer CG. Persistent organic pollutant residues in human fetal liver and placenta from Greater Montreal, Quebec: a longitudinal study from 1998 through 2006. *Environ Health Perspect.* (2009) 117:605–10. doi: 10.1289/ehp.0800205
9. Hurley S, Goldberg D, Nelson DO, Guo W, Wang Y, Baek HG, et al. Temporal evaluation of Polybrominated Diphenyl Ether (PBDE) serum levels in middle-aged and older California women, 2011–2015. *Environ Sci Technol.* (2017) 51:4697–704. doi: 10.1021/acs.est.7b00565
10. Bradman A, Castorina R, Gaspar F, Nishioka M, Colon M, Weathers W, et al. Flame retardant exposures in California early childhood education environments. *Chemosphere* (2014) 116:61–6. doi: 10.1016/j.chemosphere.2014.02.072
11. Agarwal V, El Gamal AA, Yamanaka K, Poth D, Kersten RD, Schorn M, et al. Biosynthesis of polybrominated aromatic organic compounds by marine bacteria. *Nat Chem Biol.* (2014) 10:640–7. doi: 10.1038/nchembio.1564
12. Sharma GM, Vig B. Studies on the antimicrobial substances of sponges. VI Structures of two antibacterial substances isolated from the marine sponge *Dysidea* herbacea. *Tetrahedr Lett.* (1972) 13:1715–8. doi: 10.1016/S0040-4039(01)84729-8
13. Carté B, Faulkner DJ. Polybrominated diphenyl ethers from *Dysidea* herbacea, *Dysidea* chlorea and *Phyllospongia foliascens. Tetrahedron* (1981) 37:2335–9. doi: 10.1016/S0040-4020(01)88886-4
14. Calcul L, Chow R, Oliver AG, Tenney K, White KN, Wood AW, et al. NMR strategy for unraveling structures of bioactive sponge-derived oxy-polyhalogenated diphenyl ethers. *J Nat Prod.* (2009) 72:443–9. doi: 10.1021/np800737z
15. Agarwal V, Li J, Rahman I, Borgen M, Aluwihare LI, Biggs JS, et al. Complexity of naturally produced polybrominated diphenyl ethers revealed via mass spectrometry. *Environ Sci Technol.* (2015) 49:1339–46. doi: 10.1021/es505440j
16. Waszak I, Dabrowska H, Gora A. Bioaccumulation of polybrominated diphenyl ethers (PBDEs) in flounder (*Platichthys flesus*) in the southern Baltic Sea. *Mar Environ Res.* (2012) 79:132–41. doi: 10.1016/j.marenvres.2012.06.006
17. Khalil A, Parker M, Brown SE, Cevikae SE, Guo LW, Jensen J, et al. Perinatal exposure to 2,2′,4′4′-tetrabromodiphenyl ether induces testicular toxicity in adult rats. *Toxicology* (2017) 389:21–30. doi: 10.1016/j.tox.2017.07.006
18. Khalil A, Parker M, Mpanga R, Cevik EC, Thorburn C, Suvorov A. Developmental exposure to 2,2′,4,4′-tetrabromodiphenyl ether induces long-lasting changes in liver metabolism in male mice. *J Endocr Soc.* (2017) 1:323–44. doi: 10.1210/js.2016-1011
19. Antignac JP, Cariou R, Maume D, Marchand P, Monteau F, Zalko D, et al. Exposure assessment of fetus and newborn to brominated flame retardants in France: preliminary data. *Mol Nutr Food Res.* (2008) 52:258–65. doi: 10.1002/mnfr.200700077
20. Shi Z, Jiao Y, Hu Y, Sun Z, Zhou X, Feng J, et al. Levels of tetrabromobisphenol A, hexabromocyclododecanes and polybrominated diphenyl ethers in human milk from the general population in Beijing, China. *Sci Total Environ.* (2013) 452–453:10–8. doi: 10.1016/j.scitotenv.2013.02.038

21. Wilford BH, Shoeib M, Harner T, Zhu J, Jones KC. Polybrominated diphenyl ethers in indoor dust in Ottawa, Canada: implications for sources and exposure. *Environ Sci Technol.* (2005) 39:7027–35. doi: 10.1021/es050759g
22. Schecter A, Papke O, Harris TR, Tung KC, Musumba A, Olson J, et al. Polybrominated diphenyl ether (PBDE) levels in an expanded market basket survey of US food and estimated PBDE dietary intake by age and sex. *Environ Health Perspect.* (2006) 114:1515–20. doi: 10.1289/ehp.9121
23. Lotfi L, Puschner B, Elms W, Hertz-Picciottol, Verner M. Plasma levels of polybrominated diphenyl ethers (PBDEs) at 12, 24 and 36 months of age. In: *Society of Toxicology 56th Annual Meeting:Poster #1906* (San Antonio, TX), (2017).
24. Newbold RR, Jefferson WN, Padilla-Banks E, Haseman J. Developmental exposure to diethylstilbestrol (DES) alters uterine response to estrogens in prepubescent mice: low versus high dose effects. *Reprod Toxicol.* (2004) 18:399–406. doi: 10.1016/j.reprotox.2004.01.007
25. NIH. *Funding Opportunity Announcement: Role of Environmental Chemical Exposures in the Development of Obesity, Type 2 Diabetes and Metabolic Syndrome (R21).* Washington, DC (2012).
26. Heindel JJ, vom Saal FS, Blumberg B, Bovolin P, Calamandrei G, Ceresini G, et al. (2015). Parma consensus statement on metabolic disruptors. *Environ Health* 14:54 doi: 10.1186/s12940-015-0042-7
27. Wahlang B, Beier JI, Clair HB, Bellis-Jones HJ, Falkner KC, McClain CJ, et al. Toxicant-associated steatohepatitis. *Toxicol Pathol.* (2013) 41:343–60. doi: 10.1177/0192623312468517
28. Joshi-Barve S, Kirpich I, Cave MC, Marsano LS, McClain CJ. Alcoholic, nonalcoholic, and toxicant-associated steatohepatitis: mechanistic similarities and differences. *Cell Mol Gastroenterol Hepatol.* (2015) 1:356–67. doi: 10.1016/j.jcmgh.2015.05.006
29. Mozaffarian D, Benjamin EJ, Go AS, Arnett DK, Blaha MJ, Cushman M, et al. Heart disease and stroke statistics—2015 update: a report from the American Heart Association. *Circulation* (2015) 131:e29–322. doi: 10.1161/CIR.0000000000000152
30. Vandenberg LN, Welshons WV, Vom Saal FS, Toutain PL, Myers JP. Should oral gavage be abandoned in toxicity testing of endocrine disruptors?. *Environ Health* (2014) 13:46. doi: 10.1186/1476-069X-13-46
31. Suvorov A, Vandenberg LN. To cull or not to cull? Considerations for studies of endocrine disrupting chemicals. *Endocrinology* (2016) 157:2586–94. doi: 10.1210/en.2016-1145
32. Kim D, Pertea G, Trapnell C, Pimentel H, Kelley R, Salzberg SL. TopHat2: accurate alignment of transcriptomes in the presence of insertions, deletions and gene fusions. *Genome Biol.* (2013) 14:R36. doi: 10.1186/gb-2013-14-4-r36
33. Trapnell C, Hendrickson DG, Sauvageau M, Goff L, Rinn JL, Pachter L. Differential analysis of gene regulation at transcript resolution with RNA-seq. *Nat Biotechnol.* (2013) 31:46–53. doi: 10.1038/nbt.2450
34. Boylan JM, Sanders JA, Neretti N, Gruppuso PA. Profiling of the fetal and adult rat liver transcriptome and translatome reveals discordant regulation by the mechanistic target of rapamycin (mTOR). *Am J Physiol Regul Integr Comp Physiol.* (2015) 309:R22–35. doi: 10.1152/ajpregu.00114.2015
35. Subramanian A, Tamayo P, Mootha VK, Mukherjee S, Ebert BL, Gillette MA, et al. Gene set enrichment analysis: a knowledge-based approach for interpreting genome-wide expression profiles. *Proc Natl Acad Sci USA.* (2005) 102:15545–50. doi: 10.1073/pnas.0506580102
36. Mootha VK, Lindgren CM, Eriksson KF, Subramanian A, Sihag S, Lehar J, et al. PGC-1alpha-responsive genes involved in oxidative phosphorylation are coordinately downregulated in human diabetes. *Nat Genet.* (2003) 34:267–73. doi: 10.1038/ng1180
37. Huang da W, Sherman BT, Lempicki RA. Systematic and integrative analysis of large gene lists using DAVID bioinformatics resources. *Nat Protoc.* (2009) 4:44–57. doi: 10.1038/nprot.2008.211
38. Kramer A, Green J, Pollard J Jr, Tugendreich S. Causal analysis approaches in Ingenuity Pathway Analysis. *Bioinformatics* (2014) 30:523–30. doi: 10.1093/bioinformatics/btt703
39. Mashek DG. Hepatic fatty acid trafficking: multiple forks in the road. *Adv Nutr.* (2013) 4:697–710. doi: 10.3945/an.113.004648
40. Nguyen P, Leray V, Diez M, Serisier S, Le Bloc'h J, Siliart B, et al. Liver lipid metabolism. *J Anim Physiol Anim Nutr (Berl).* (2008) 92:272–83. doi: 10.1111/j.1439-0396.2007.00752.x
41. Livak KJ, Schmittgen TD. Analysis of relative gene expression data using real-time quantitative PCR and the 2(-Delta Delta C(T)) method. *Methods* (2001) 25:402–8. doi: 10.1006/meth.2001.1262
42. IHSWorld. *Oil Red O Staining Protocol. Protocols 2017.* (2017). Available online at: http://www.ihcworld.com/_protocols/special_stains/oil_red_o.htm
43. Suvorov A, Takser L. Global gene expression analysis in the livers of rat offspring perinatally exposed to low doses of 2,2′,4,4′-tetrabromodiphenyl ether. *Environ Health Perspect.* (2010) 118:97–102. doi: 10.1289/ehp.0901031
44. Suvorov A, Takser L. Delayed response in the rat frontal lobe transcriptome to perinatal exposure to the flame retardant BDE-47. *J Appl Toxicol.* (2011) 31:477–83. doi: 10.1002/jat.1667
45. Dunnick JK, Brix A, Cunny H, Vallant M, Shockley KR. Characterization of polybrominated diphenyl ether toxicity in Wistar Han rats and use of liver microarray data for predicting disease susceptibilities. *Toxicol Pathol.* (2012) 40:93–106. doi: 10.1177/0192623311429973
46. Kleiner DE, Brunt EM, Van Natta M, Behling C, Contos MJ, Cummings OW, et al. Design and validation of a histological scoring system for nonalcoholic fatty liver disease. *Hepatology* (2005) 41:1313–21. doi: 10.1002/hep.20701
47. Patton HM, Sirlin C, Behling C, Middleton M, Schwimmer JB, Lavine JE. Pediatric nonalcoholic fatty liver disease: a critical appraisal of current data and implications for future research. *J Pediatr Gastroenterol Nutr.* (2006) 43:413–27. doi: 10.1097/01.mpg.0000239995.58388.56
48. Szczepaniak LS, Nurenberg P, Leonard D, Browning JD, Reingold JS, Grundy S, et al. Magnetic resonance spectroscopy to measure hepatic triglyceride content: prevalence of hepatic steatosis in the general population. *Am J Physiol Endocrinol Metab.* (2005) 288:E462–8. doi: 10.1152/ajpendo.00064.2004
49. Browning JD, Szczepaniak LS, Dobbins R, Nuremberg P, Horton JD, Cohen JC, et al. Prevalence of hepatic steatosis in an urban population in the United States: impact of ethnicity. *Hepatology* (2004) 40:1387–95. doi: 10.1002/hep.20466
50. Ryan CK, Johnson LA, Germin BI, Marcos A. One hundred consecutive hepatic biopsies in the workup of living donors for right lobe liver transplantation. *Liver Transpl.* (2002) 8:1114–22. doi: 10.1053/jlts.2002.36740
51. Soejima Y, Shimada M, Suehiro T, Kishikawa K, Yoshizumi T, Hashimoto K, et al. Use of steatotic graft in living-donor liver transplantation. *Transplantation* (2003) 76:344–8. doi: 10.1097/01.TP.0000071205.52835.A4
52. Marchesini G, Bugianesi E, Forlani G, Cerrelli F, Lenzi M, Manini R, et al. Nonalcoholic fatty liver, steatohepatitis, and the metabolic syndrome. *Hepatology* (2003) 37:917–23. doi: 10.1053/jhep.2003.50161
53. Rafiq N, Bai C, Fang Y, Srishord M, McCullough A, Gramlich T, et al. Long-term follow-up of patients with nonalcoholic fatty liver. *Clin Gastroenterol Hepatol.* (2009) 7:234–8. doi: 10.1016/j.cgh.2008.11.005
54. Bonora E, Targher G. Increased risk of cardiovascular disease and chronic kidney disease in NAFLD. *Nat Rev Gastroenterol Hepatol.* (2012) 9:372–81. doi: 10.1038/nrgastro.2012.79
55. Baffy G, Brunt EM, Caldwell SH. Hepatocellular carcinoma in non-alcoholic fatty liver disease: an emerging menace. *J Hepatol.* (2012) 56:1384–91. doi: 10.1016/j.jhep.2011.10.027
56. Otgonsuren M, Stepanova M, Gerber L, Younossi ZM. Anthropometric and clinical factors associated with mortality in subjects with nonalcoholic fatty liver disease. *Dig Dis Sci.* (2013) 58:1132–40. doi: 10.1007/s10620-012-2446-3
57. Anstee QM, Targher G, Day CP. Progression of NAFLD to diabetes mellitus, cardiovascular disease or cirrhosis. *Nat Rev Gastroenterol Hepatol.* (2013) 10:330–44. doi: 10.1038/nrgastro.2013.41
58. Suvorov A, Girard S, Lachapelle S, Abdelouahab N, Sebire G, Takser L. Perinatal exposure to low-dose BDE-47, an emergent environmental contaminant, causes hyperactivity in rat offspring. *Neonatology* (2009) 95:203–9. doi: 10.1159/000155651
59. Sanders JM, Chen LJ, Lebetkin EH, Burka LT. Metabolism and disposition of 2,2′,4,4′-tetrabromodiphenyl ether following administration of single or multiple doses to rats and mice. *Xenobiotica* (2006) 36:103–17. doi: 10.1080/00498250500485107
60. Staskal DF, Diliberto JJ, DeVito MJ, Birnbaum LS. Toxicokinetics of BDE 47 in female mice: effect of dose, route of exposure, and time. *Toxicol Sci.* (2005) 83:215–23. doi: 10.1093/toxsci/kfi018

61. Suvorov A, Battista MC, Takser L. Perinatal exposure to low-dose 2,2′,4,4′-tetrabromodiphenyl ether affects growth in rat offspring: what is the role of IGF-1? *Toxicology* (2009) 260:126–31. doi: 10.1016/j.tox.2009.03.018
62. Gordillo M, Evans T, Gouon-Evans V. Orchestrating liver development. *Development* (2015) 142:2094–108. doi: 10.1242/dev.114215
63. Zhao R, Duncan SA. Embryonic development of the liver. *Hepatology* (2005) 41:956–67. doi: 10.1002/hep.20691
64. Moscovitz JE, Aleksunes LM. Establishment of metabolism and transport pathways in the rodent and human fetal liver. *Int J Mol Sci.* (2013) 14:23801–27. doi: 10.3390/ijms141223801
65. Barrows BR, Parks EJ. Contributions of different fatty acid sources to very low-density lipoprotein-triacylglycerol in the fasted and fed states. *J Clin Endocrinol Metab.* (2006) 91:1446–52. doi: 10.1210/jc.2005-1709
66. Donnelly KL, Smith CI, Schwarzenberg SJ, Jessurun J, Boldt MD, Parks EJ. Sources of fatty acids stored in liver and secreted via lipoproteins in patients with nonalcoholic fatty liver disease. *J Clin Invest.* (2005) 115:1343–51. doi: 10.1172/JCI23621
67. Koonen DP, Jacobs RL, Febbraio M, Young ME, Soltys CL, Ong H, et al. Increased hepatic CD36 expression contributes to dyslipidemia associated with diet-induced obesity. *Diabetes* (2007) 56:2863–71. doi: 10.2337/db07-0907
68. Sheedfar F, Sung MM, Aparicio-Vergara M, Kloosterhuis NJ, Miquilena-Colina ME, Vargas-Castrillon J, et al. Increased hepatic CD36 expression with age is associated with enhanced susceptibility to nonalcoholic fatty liver disease. *Aging (Albany NY)* (2014) 6:281–95. doi: 10.18632/aging.100652
69. Greco D, Kotronen A, Westerbacka J, Puig O, Arkkila P, Kiviluoto T, et al. Gene expression in human NAFLD. *Am J Physiol Gastrointest Liver Physiol.* (2008) 294:G1281–G1287. doi: 10.1152/ajpgi.00074.2008
70. Mitsuyoshi H, Yasui K, Harano Y, Endo M, Tsuji K, Minami M, et al. Analysis of hepatic genes involved in the metabolism of fatty acids and iron in nonalcoholic fatty liver disease. *Hepatol Res.* (2009) 39:366–73. doi: 10.1111/j.1872-034X.2008.00464.x
71. Vance JE, Vance DE. The assembly of lipids into lipoproteins during secretion. *Experientia* (1990) 46:560–9. doi: 10.1007/BF01939694
72. Janero DR, Siuta-Mangano P, Miller KW, Lane MD. Synthesis, processing, and secretion of hepatic very low density lipoprotein. *J Cell Biochem.* (1984) 24:131–52. doi: 10.1002/jcb.240240205
73. Maranghi F, Tassinari R, Moracci G, Altieri I, Rasinger JD, Carroll TS, et al. Dietary exposure of juvenile female mice to polyhalogenated seafood contaminants (HBCD, BDE-47, PCB-153, TCDD): comparative assessment of effects in potential target tissues. *Food Chem Toxicol.* (2013) 56:443–9. doi: 10.1016/j.fct.2013.02.056
74. Wang D, Yan J, Teng M, Yan S, Zhou Z, Zhu W. *In utero* and lactational exposure to BDE-47 promotes obesity development in mouse offspring fed a high-fat diet: impaired lipid metabolism and intestinal dysbiosis. *Arch Toxicol.* (2018) 92:1847–60. doi: 10.1007/s00204-018-2177-0
75. Bruchajzer E, Frydrych B, Sporny S, Szymanska JA. The effect of short-term intoxication of rats with pentabromodiphenyl ether (in mixture mimic commercial products). *Hum Exp Toxicol.* (2011) 30:363–78. doi: 10.1177/0960327110371261
76. Bruchajzer E, Frydrych B, Sporny S, Szymanska JA. Toxicity of penta- and decabromodiphenyl ethers after repeated administration to rats: a comparative study. *Arch Toxicol.* (2010) 84:287–99. doi: 10.1007/s00204-009-0495-y
77. Lee E, Kim TH, Choi JS, Nabanata P, Kim NY, Ahn MY, et al. Evaluation of liver and thyroid toxicity in Sprague-Dawley rats after exposure to polybrominated diphenyl ether BDE-209. *J Toxicol Sci.* (2010) 35:535–45. doi: 10.2131/jts.35.535
78. Zhou SN, Buchar A, Siddique S, Takser L, Abdelouahab N, Zhu J. Measurements of selected brominated flame retardants in nursing women: implications for human exposure. *Environ Sci Technol.* (2014) 48:8873–80. doi: 10.1021/es5016839
79. Zhou SN, Siddique S, Lavoie L, Takser L, Abdelouahab N, Zhu J. Hexachloronorbornene-based flame retardants in humans: levels in maternal serum and milk. *Environ Int.* (2014) 66:11–7. doi: 10.1016/j.envint.2014.01.010
80. Siddique S, Xian Q, Abdelouahab N, Takser L, Phillips SP, Feng YL, et al. Levels of dechlorane plus and polybrominated diphenylethers in human milk in two Canadian cities. *Environ Int.* (2012) 39:50–5. doi: 10.1016/j.envint.2011.09.010
81. Laplante M, Sabatini DM. mTOR signaling in growth control and disease. *Cell* (2012) 149:274–93. doi: 10.1016/j.cell.2012.03.017
82. Dibble CC, Manning BD. Signal integration by mTORC1 coordinates nutrient input with biosynthetic output. *Nat Cell Biol.* (2013) 15:555–64. doi: 10.1038/ncb2763
83. Lamming DW, Sabatini DM. A central role for mTOR in lipid homeostasis. *Cell Metab.* (2013) 18:465–9. doi: 10.1016/j.cmet.2013.08.002
84. Laplante M, Sabatini DM. An emerging role of mTOR in lipid biosynthesis. *Curr Biol.* (2009) 19:R1046–52. doi: 10.1016/j.cub.2009.09.058
85. Conn CS, Qian SB. mTOR signaling in protein homeostasis: less is more? *Cell Cycle* (2011) 10:1940–7. doi: 10.4161/cc.10.12.15858
86. Laplante M, Sabatini DM. Regulation of mTORC1 and its impact on gene expression at a glance. *J Cell Sci.* (2013) 126:1713–9. doi: 10.1242/jcs.125773
87. Duvel K, Yecies JL, Menon S, Raman P, Lipovsky AI, Souza AL, et al. Activation of a metabolic gene regulatory network downstream of mTOR complex 1. *Mol Cell* (2010) 39:171–83. doi: 10.1016/j.molcel.2010.06.022
88. Karandrea S, Yin H, Liang X, Heart EA. BDE-47 and BDE-85 stimulate insulin secretion in INS-1 832/13 pancreatic beta-cells through the thyroid receptor and Akt. *Environ Toxicol Pharmacol.* (2017) 56:29–34. doi: 10.1016/j.etap.2017.08.030
89. Kalyanaraman H, Schwappacher R, Joshua J, Zhuang S, Scott BT, Klos M, et al. Nongenomic thyroid hormone signaling occurs through a plasma membrane-localized receptor. *Sci Signal.* (2014) 7:ra48. doi: 10.1126/scisignal.2004911
90. Hoffman K, Sosa JA, Stapleton HM. Do flame retardant chemicals increase the risk for thyroid dysregulation and cancer? *Curr Opin Oncol.* (2017) 29:7–13. doi: 10.1097/CCO.0000000000000335
91. Miranda ML, Anthopolos R, Wolkin A, Stapleton HM. Associations of birth outcomes with maternal polybrominated diphenyl ethers and thyroid hormones during pregnancy. *Environ Int.* (2015) 85:244–53. doi: 10.1016/j.envint.2015.09.015
92. Chevrier J, Gunier RB, Bradman A, Holland NT, Calafat AM, Eskenazi B, et al. Maternal urinary bisphenol a during pregnancy and maternal and neonatal thyroid function in the CHAMACOS study. *Environ Health Perspect.* (2013) 121:138–44. doi: 10.1289/ehp.1205092
93. Andra SS, Makris KC. Thyroid disrupting chemicals in plastic additives and thyroid health. *J Environ Sci Health C Environ Carcinog Ecotoxicol Rev.* (2012) 30:107–51. doi: 10.1080/10590501.2012.681487
94. Suvorov A, Bissonnette C, Takser L, Langlois MF. (2011). Does 2,2′,4,4′-tetrabromodiphenyl ether interact directly with thyroid receptor? *J Appl Toxicol.* 31:179–84. doi: 10.1002/jat.1580

9

Role of Endocrine-Disrupting Engineered Nanomaterials in the Pathogenesis of Type 2 Diabetes Mellitus

Ayushi Priyam, Pushplata Prasad Singh* and Shweta Gehlout

TERI Deakin Nanobiotechnology Centre, The Energy and Resources Institute, New Delhi, India

***Correspondence:**
Pushplata Prasad Singh
pushplata.singh@teri.res.in

Nanotechnology has enabled the development of innovative technologies and products for several industrial sectors. Their unique physicochemical and size-dependent properties make the engineered nanomaterials (ENMs) superior for devising solutions for various research and development sectors, which are otherwise unachievable by their bulk forms. However, the remarkable advantages mediated by ENMs and their applications have also raised concerns regarding their possible toxicological impacts on human health. The actual issue stems from the absence of systematic data on ENM exposure-mediated health hazards. In this direction, a comprehensive exploration on the health-related consequences, especially with respect to endocrine disruption-related metabolic disorders, is largely lacking. The reasons for the rapid increase in diabetes and obesity in the modern world remain largely unclear, and epidemiological studies indicate that the increased presence of endocrine disrupting chemicals (EDCs) in the environment may influence the incidence of metabolic diseases. Functional similarities, such as mimicking natural hormonal actions, have been observed between the endocrine-disrupting chemicals (EDCs) and ENMs, which supports the view that different types of NMs may be capable of altering the physiological activity of the endocrine system. Disruption of the endocrine system leads to hormonal imbalance, which may influence the development and pathogenesis of metabolic disorders, particularly type 2 diabetes mellitus (T2DM). Evidence from many *in vitro*, *in vivo* and epidemiological studies, suggests that ENMs generally exert deleterious effects on the molecular/hormonal pathways and the organ systems involved in the pathogenesis of T2DM. However, the available data from several such studies are not congruent, especially because of discrepancies in study design, and therefore need to be carefully examined before drawing meaningful inferences. In this review, we discuss the outcomes of ENM exposure in correlation with the development of T2DM. In particular, the review focuses on the following sub-topics: (1) an overview of the sources of human exposure to NMs, (2) systems involved in the uptake of ENMs into human body, (3) endocrine disrupting engineered nanomaterials (EDENMs) and mechanisms underlying the pathogenesis of

T2DM, (4) evidence of the role of EDENMs in the pathogenesis of T2DM from *in vitro*, *in vivo* and epidemiological studies, and (5) conclusions and perspectives.

Keywords: engineered nanomaterial (ENM), type 2 diabetes mellitus (T2DM), endocrine disruptor, insulin resistance, reduced insulin sensitivity, oxidative stress, *in vitro* and *in vivo* studies, epidemiological evidences

BACKGROUND

Materials acquire unique characteristics when the size of the particle is reduced to nanoscale. Nanomaterials (NMs) are a universal set of nanoscale materials having at least one of the dimensions in the nano-range. With having at least one dimension in nanoscale as a common feature, nanoparticles, nanowires, nanosheets, nanotubes, and nanoplates can be stated as the key subsets of NMs (1). The various properties of a nanomaterial (NM), including its melting point, electrical conductivity, magnetic permeability, chemical reactivity and fluorescence, are determined by the particle size (2). Size-reduction of a material to nanoscale enhances its functional aspects and associated technological benefits. Therefore, the use of engineered nanomaterials (ENMs) in the development of advanced technologies for medicine, engineering and natural sciences has significantly increased since the start of the twenty-first century (3). ENMs are being incorporated into our everyday routine as a part of clothing, food, cosmetics, medicines, electronic goods, etc. However, in parallel to the technological advancements, the biosafety issues related to ENMs have also become a matter of apprehension. Whereas, for applications in medicine, ENMs are optimized to enhance their cellular uptake and/or targeting to the desired tissue, an inadvertent exposure to workers may raise health concerns (4, 5). Multiple studies have suggested that unlike their bulk counterparts, the ENMs are highly toxic and may lead to serious human and ecological health risks (6–8). The toxic outcomes of ENM exposure are largely accredited to their small size and increased chemical reactivity, which enhances their permeability to the target tissues which are otherwise not penetrated by larger but chemically identical materials (9). Noticeably, evidence from several research studies indicates functional similarities between the endocrine-disrupting chemicals (EDCs) and ENMs, which supports the view that different types of NMs may be capable of altering the physiological activity of the endocrine system (10–14).

The WHO (World Health Organization) International Programme on Chemical Safety (IPCS) conducts research to understand the basis for the management of chemicals and related risks. According to the IPCS, "a potential endocrine disruptor is an exogenous substance or a mixture, possessing properties that can lead to endocrine disruption in an intact organism, or its progeny, or (sub) populations" (15). Further to add, the EDCs are elements present in our environment, food, and several consumer products that can interfere with synthesis, secretion, transport, metabolism, binding actions and elimination, and mimic the natural hormones. Consequently, this may lead to a deviation from the normal physiological function of the endocrine system to endocrine disruption. The EDCs and endocrine disrupting ENMs (EDENMs) are prevalent in various consumer goods such as agricultural chemicals, notably fertilizers and pesticides (16, 17), therapeutics (18), cosmetics (19, 20), and paints (19). There is accumulating evidence suggesting an increased presence of EDCs and ENMs in the environment, which putatively affects the functioning of the endocrine system, metabolic system and reproductive system (**Figure 1**). Hence, though the ENMs promise remarkable benefits, their successful application requires investigation of their impact on human health.

Both EDCs and NMs are regularly investigated for adverse impacts on health. Studies conducted to evaluate the effects of EDCs on health have generally reported deleterious outcomes like altered reproductive function in males and females (21–25), increased incidence of breast cancer (26–30), abnormal growth patterns (31–33), neurodevelopmental delays in children (34–36), and changes in immune functions (37–39). Similarly, exposure to NMs is found to be associated with

---

Abbreviations: AgNPs, Silver Nanoparticles; Ahr, Aryl Hydrocarbon Receptor; AKT, Alpha Serine/Threonine Kinase; ALS, Alloxan Sensitive; AMPK, AMP Activated Protein Kinase; AR, Androgenic Receptor; AuNPs, Gold Nanoparticles; B7/CD28, Immunoglobulin Superfamily Members; BrdU, Bromodeoxyuridine; CARDIA, Coronary Artery Risk Development In Young Adults; CdTe Qds, Cadmium Telluride Quantum Dots; CeO_2-NPs, Cerium Oxide Nanoparticles; CHOP, CCAAT-Enhancer-Binding Protein Homologous Protein; Cpg-Odns, Cpg Oligodeoxynucleotides; CrNano, Chromium Nanoparticles; CRP, C-Reactive Protein; EDCs, Endocrine-Disrupting Chemicals; EDENM, Endocrine-Disrupting ENM; ENM, Engineered Nanomaterial; ER, Estrogen Receptors; G6PDH, Glucose-6-Phosphate Dehydrogenase; GI, Gastrointestinal tract; GK, Goto-Kakizaki; GLUT, Glucose Transporter; GNPs, Gold Nanoparticles; GPR30, G-Protein-Coupled Receptor For Estrogen; GPX, Glutathione Peroxidase; GR, Glutathione Reductase; GSH, Glutathione; GSK, Glycogen Synthase Kinase; H_2O_2, Hydrogen Peroxide; HIP, Human Amyloid Polypeptide; IFG, Impaired Fasting Glucose; IFN, Interferon; IL, Interleukin; INS-GNPs, Insulin-Coated Gold Nanoparticles; IONPs, Iron Oxide (Fe_2O_3) Nanoparticles; IPCS, International Programme On Chemical Safety; IR, Insulin Receptor; IRE-1, Inositol-Requiring Enzyme 1; IRS, Insulin Receptor Substrate; JNK, C-Jun N-Terminal Kinases; LDL, Low Density Lipoproteins; MCP1, Monocyte Chemoattractant Protein 1; MDA, Malondialdehyde; MIMIC, Modular Immune *in vitro* Construct, An Artificial System Imitating The Human Immune System; MSNs, Mesoporous Silica Nanoparticles; Mtor, Mammalian Target of Rapamycin; NMs, Nanomaterials; NPs, Nanoparticles; PEG-B-PLGA, Biodegradable Polyethylene Glycol And Poly (Lactic-Co-Glycolic Acid) Copolymer; PI3K, Phosphatidylinositol 3-Kinase; PPAR, Peroxisome Proliferator Activated Receptor; PR, Progesterone Receptor; PTP, Phosphotyrosine Phosphotase; rHEGF, Recombinant Human Epidermal Growth Factor; ROS, Reactive Oxygen Species; SD, Sprague–Dawley; SeNPs, Selenium Nanoparticles; SNP, Single Nucleotide Polymorphisms; SOD, Superoxide Dismutase; T2DM, Type 2 Diabetes Mellitus; TiO_2-NPs, Titanium Oxide Nanoparticles; TNF-α, Tumor Necrosis Factor –A; UFPs, Ultrafine Particles; WHO, World Health Organization; ZON, Zinc Oxide Nanoparticles; β-Cells, Beta Cells.

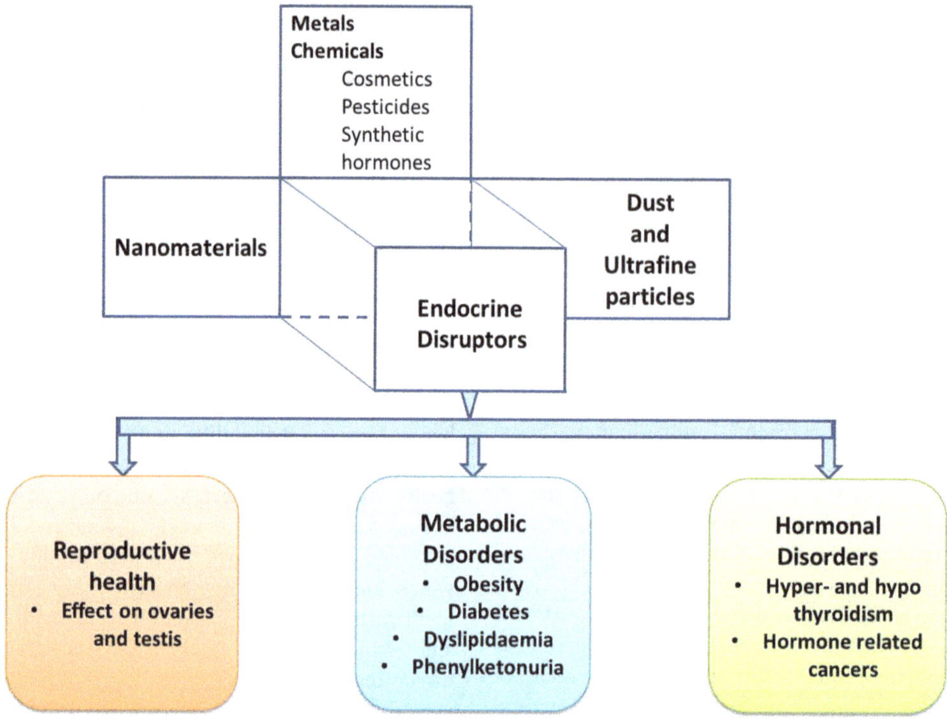

FIGURE 1 | A schematic describing different types of endocrine disruptors and the associated endocrine disorders.

several adverse outcomes such as impaired immune response, inflammation, fibrosis, emphysema, and tumor formation (40–45).

Additionally, EDCs have been reviewed to act as causative agents of metabolic disorders like type 2 diabetes mellitus (T2DM) (46, 47). The prevalence of T2DM has seen a tremendous global upsurge during the last few decades. A report from the International Diabetes Federation (IDF) estimated ~425 million adults (aged between 20 and 79 years) all over the world were living with diabetes in 2017 and predicted that by 2045 this will rise to 629 million. A large number of investigations to define the genetic and environmental bases of T2DM has been done to date but the definite reasons for a rapid increase in diabetes and obesity in the modern world largely remain unclear. Research in the arena increasingly indicates a major role played by environmental chemicals in diabetes and obesity, advocating that the environmental led metabolism disruption could form the "paradox of progress" (48). At present, only a few studies have examined the role of ENMs in the pathogenesis of T2DM. Chevalier and Fénichel reviewed both *in vivo* and *in vitro* experimental data along with epidemiological evidence to support an association of EDC exposure to the induction of insulin resistance and/or disruption of pancreatic β-cell function that leads to glucose homoeostasis related metabolic disorders (49). The evidence of ENM mediated alterations in glucose metabolism, insulin resistance and sensitivity, and homeostasis pathways are mostly indirect. The influence of EDENMs on the candidate genes of T2DM and their further impact on various molecular pathways are scarcely defined at present. Herein, we reviewed the recent literature that presented the effects of ENMs on molecular pathways involved in the development of T2DM. We also identified the knowledge gaps and challenges in the research area, which may provide directions for future research.

AN OVERVIEW OF THE SOURCES OF HUMAN EXPOSURE TO NANOMATERIALS (NMs)

The probability of exposure to NMs in humans (50, 51) increases not only during production and application of ENMs, but also due to their emergence through several natural processes.

Natural Sources of NMs

We generally correlate exposure to NMs with human activities like the automobile industry, building construction and charcoal burning. However, 90% of the nano-particulate matter present in the environment is produced through natural phenomena such as dust storms, forest fires and volcanic eruptions, which significantly pollute natural resources, and affect human health. Dust storms are the main source of environmental NMs which can lead to respiratory issues, especially in subjects suffering from asthma and emphysema. Furthermore, dust rich in metal particles can lead to the generation of reactive oxygen species (ROS) (52), which may lead to an inflammatory response and influence pathogenesis of life style disorders such as T2DM and heart disorders.

Anthropogenic Sources of NMs

ENMs comprise the main category of anthropogenic release of NMs in the environment. These are produced and released into the environment by either intentional or unintentional human activities. The unintentional release of NMs occurs from the burning of natural fuels, wood, and wax (53–56). The intentional release occurs through the discharge of ENMs to rivers, landfills, soils and wastewater-treatment plants as well as from engineered products with embedded NMs. Intentional activities include the commercial synthesis of NMs, combustion of fossil fuel, manufacturing of NM embedded products, etc. Such products have found applications in biomedical, pharmaceutical, and agricultural domains. ENMs are rapidly being used in pharmaceuticals as carriers (57, 58) and as nano-formulations of drugs (59–61) and for electro-analysis of pharmaceuticals (62, 63). ENMs also find diverse applications in agriculture (64) to increase the productivity by providing nano-scaled solutions primarily as pesticides (65), fertilizers (65), and biosensors (66). A fraction of these ENMs may also make their way into soil and water ecosystems, and therefore into drinking water and food products (67–69). Such observations have raised concerns regarding the presence of ENMs in consumer products and plausible association with human health and environmental degradation.

SYSTEMS INVOLVED IN UPTAKE OF ENMs INTO THE HUMAN BODY

Both natural and anthropogenic NMs enter the human body primarily through the respiratory system, skin and gastrointestinal (GI) tract, with further translocation to different tissues and organs as depicted in **Figure 2** (71, 72). Considering the plethora of anthropogenic NMs, many ENMs may not be effectively removed and therefore can accumulate in different organ-systems over a period. Various cell types by which the ENMs are internalized include macrophages (73–75) endothelial cells (76), pulmonary epithelial cells (77–79), the gastrointestinal epithelium (80), blood cells (81), and neurons (82). Depending on their cellular concentration, the nanoscale particulate matter can mediate mutagenesis, damage to cell organelles, and eventually cell death.

Respiratory System

The ENMs most prominently reach the body by inhalation and deposit throughout the entire respiratory tract (41, 70, 83). The soluble kinds of ENMs such as branched polyethylenimine and arginylglycylaspartic acid (RGD) based hydrophilic ENMs can be dissolved in the aqueous fluid lining the epithelium and can escape into the circulatory and lymphatic systems. However, the insoluble ENMs like nano-formulations of Au, Ag, Ti, Si, carbon etc., may accumulate in the lungs upon continued exposure, resulting in injury to the lung tissue (84). Recent research has demonstrated that inhalation of ENMs can deregulate the immune system and diminish the ability to fight infections (85). Also, as depicted in **Figure 2**, ENM exposure through the respiratory tract has been found to be associated with respiratory disorders, namely asthma (86), bronchitis (87, 88), and emphysema (89, 90); neuro-degenerative disorders, namely Alzheimer's (91), and Parkinson's (92, 93); and heart diseases (84).

Skin

The extent of the uptake of ENMs by human skin is still debatable. The outer layer (stratum corneum) of the skin consists of a layer of dead cells and is generally impervious to materials having a pore diameter greater than micron size (94). However, many research studies show that NPs can penetrate the stratum corneum (95–97), especially when the skin is flexed. Dermal exposure of ENM has been reported to be associated with dermatitis (eczema) (98–100).

Gastrointestinal System

ENMs present in food and cosmetics may enter the human body through ingestion by the gastrointestinal (GI) system. Nano-enabled applications, especially those for the food industry, dental care products and cosmetics, may lead to ENM exposure related toxicity (101–103) in humans. Major ENMs that are reported to cause cytotoxicity when ingested include nano-forms of gold, silver, and metal oxides of zinc, silica, and titanium (104–108). As also depicted in **Figure 2**, exposures to these NMs through the GI can lead to Crohn's disease, Colon disease and Gastroenteritis (109).

ENDOCRINE DISRUPTING ENGINEERED NANOMATERIALS (EDENMS) AND MECHANISMS UNDERLYING THE PATHOGENESIS OF TYPE 2 DIABETES MELLITUS (T2DM)

A global spike in the production of ENM has been observed in the twenty-first century, which has enhanced the exposure rate among workers and users. At present no occupational exposure level (OEL) for ENM has been defined and the assessment of exposure to ENM is challenging. Several research groups through various experimental models have demonstrated that ENM can elicit toxic responses that may be inferred from abnormalities in various organ-systems (110–113). The extent of toxicity conferred by ENM has been reported to depend upon their physicochemical properties including size, shape, chemical nature, and surface functionalization. The cytotoxic nature of ENM could eventually lead to cell death in a dose-and time-dependent manner (114). On the other hand, some other research studies that conducted short-term experiments on cultured cells and model organisms in order to evaluate the biocompatibility of ENM (115) suggested a low level of cytotoxicity of ENM. These studies advocated a huge potential for *in vivo* applications of ENM in the form of therapeutic and diagnostic reagents, although the effects related to a long-term exposure remain an unexplored domain at present. The studies on the long-term effects of ENM *in vivo* hold significant importance in

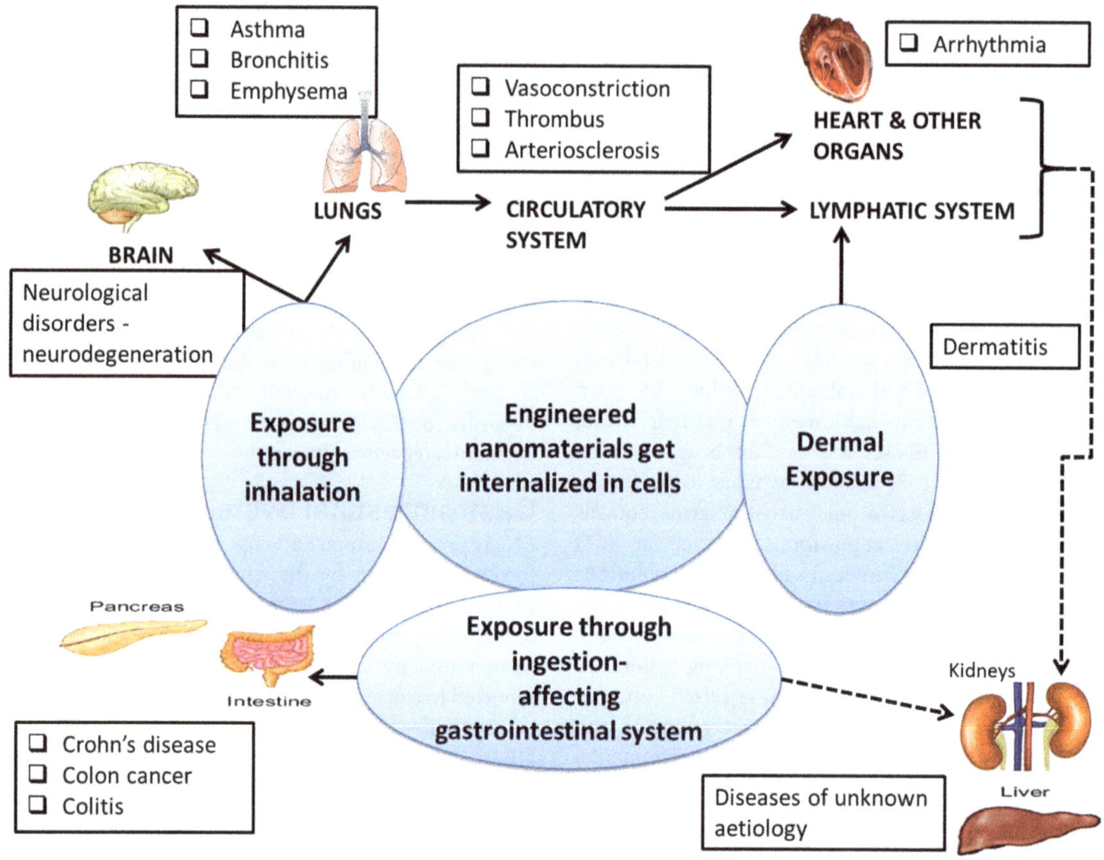

FIGURE 2 | A concise overview of affected organs resulting in various pathological states due to the exposure to ENMs as described in the literature (42, 70). The directly and indirectly affected systems are shown by solid and dashed lines respectively.

designing and development of next-generation materials, but the mechanisms underlying ENM mediated toxicity in humans are less understood (116), Particularly, whether ENM exposure leads to endocrine-disruption and influences development of T2DM among the exposed subjects remains a topic of investigation.

Contemporary *in vitro*, *in vivo* and epidemiological studies link human EDC exposure with obesity, T2DM and metabolic syndrome (47). Endocrine disruptors have a tendency to interact with the cellular receptors either by mimicking the natural hormones (**Figure 3A**) or by blocking the action of hormones (**Figure 3B**) (117).

Some studies have revealed the harmful effects of ENMs on endocrine functions, which suggests that ENMs may behave as potential endocrine disruptors, EDENMs (118–121). It is well acknowledged that endocrine disruption can often lead to the onset of metabolic disorders such as T2DM (122). Therefore, it is suggested that the ENM, which reportedly affects endocrine function, may induce T2DM. The EDENMs can behave in a similar fashion as the EDCs (13, 123, 124). The additional aspects of EDENMs over the traditional EDCs are small size, increased surface area and better uptake capability. Such properties of EDENMs enhance their chances of uptake and bioavailability, which further amplifies the deteriorating effect of the material on metabolic homeostasis (125–129) when compared to the other EDCs.

Working on similar ground as that of endocrine disruptors, ENMs may alter the normal metabolic state by affecting glucose homeostasis, leading to T2DM via the two chief mechanisms (**Figure 4**)—(i) decreasing insulin sensitivity and (ii) impairment of beta (β)-cells, resulting in a deleterious effect on insulin production (130–132).

Reduced Insulin Sensitivity

Several factors lead to a reduction in cellular insulin sensitivity. Using the available *in vitro*, *in vivo* and epidemiological data, here we reviewed and illustrated the prominent mechanisms leading to decreased insulin sensitivity. The major focus in this review has been laid out—impairment of cellular insulin action, interaction with hormonal receptors, inflammation, and variations in homeostatic pathways. Each of these factors is explained in the following sections with evidence to show the deleterious effect of ENM on the pathogenesis of T2DM.

Impairment of Cellular Insulin Action

Cellular metabolic reactions are often mediated by insulin via its action on the plasma membrane, intracellular enzymes and the

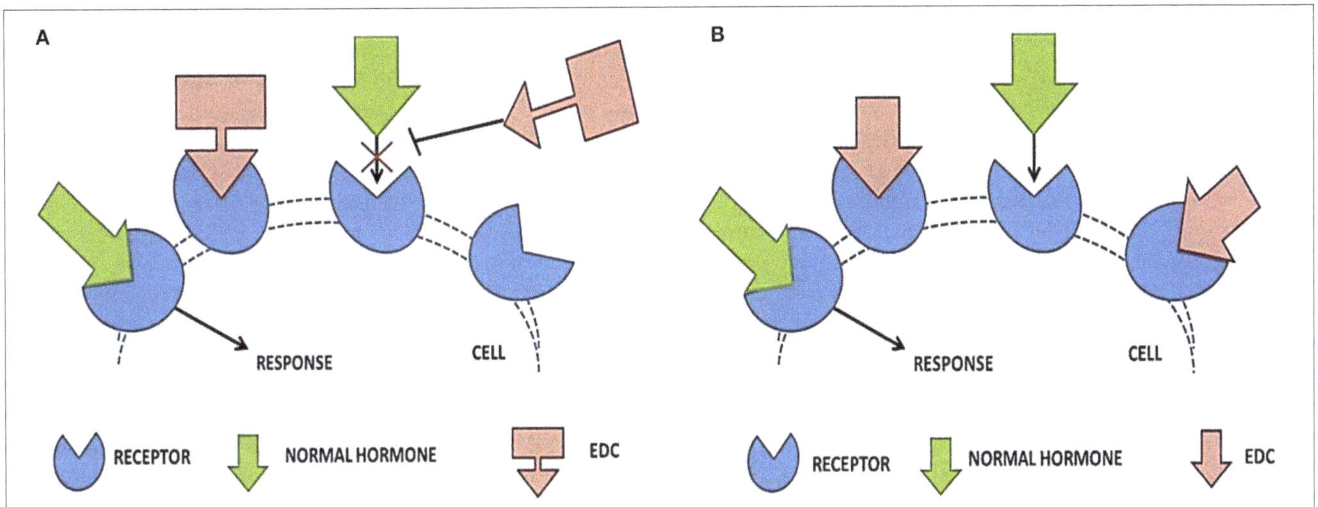

FIGURE 3 | Effect of endocrine disrupting chemicals on receptor—hormone interaction. **(A)** Shows the blocking action of EDCs, where it binds to the receptor within the cell and blocks the endogenous hormone from binding. The normal signaling is blocked and the associated organ system (liver and pancreas) fails to respond properly. In **(B)**, the mimicking action of EDCs is depicted. EDCs completely or partially mimic the naturally occurring hormones, thereby interfering with the obvious physiological responses.

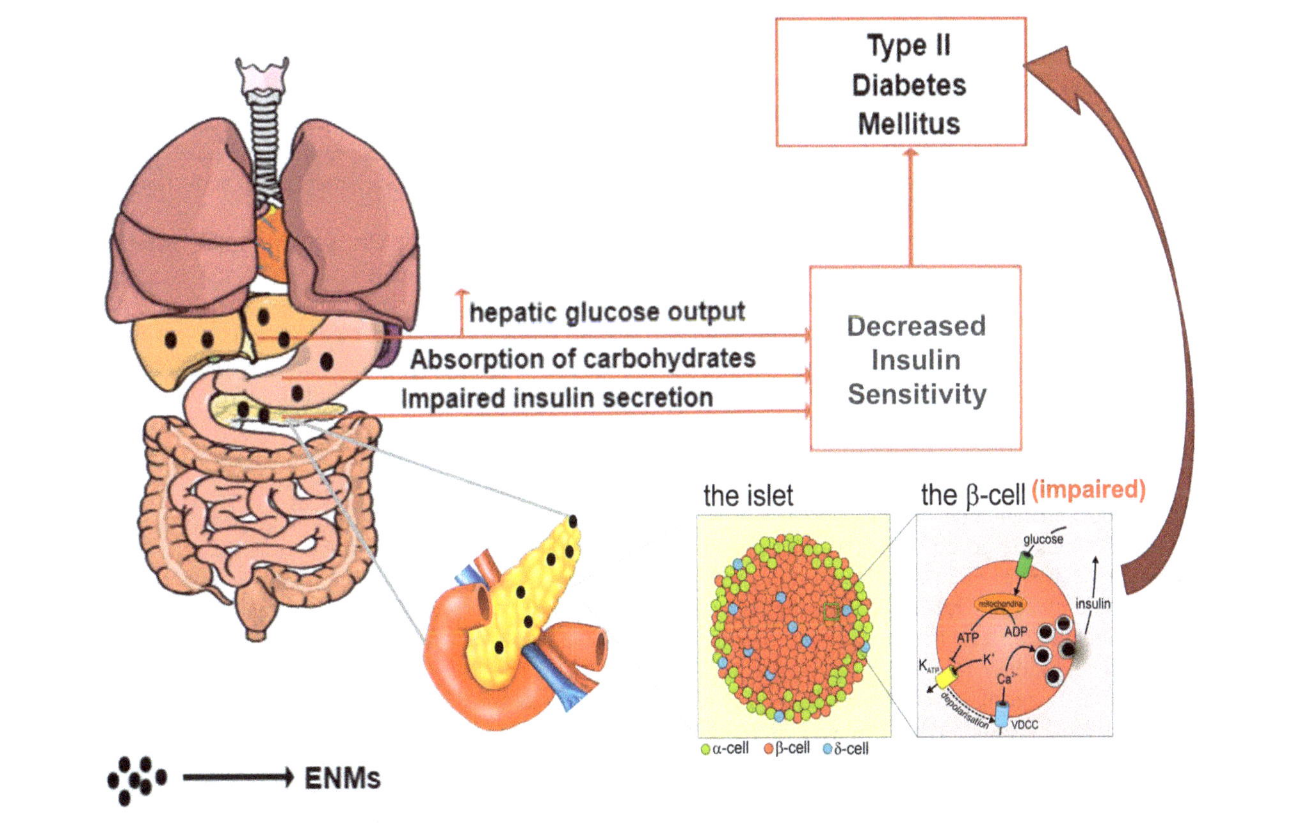

FIGURE 4 | Effects of ENM on the gastrointestinal system, leading to the development of T2DM.

nucleus. The cellular metabolism is regulated by various proteins (e.g., protein kinase C), receptors (e.g., receptor tyrosine kinase) or expression of secondary messengers (e.g., cyclic AMP, calcium, and diacylglycerol). These components control the translocation and activation of glucose transporter proteins (primary effects of insulin) (133). ENMs can influence the signaling mechanism by interfering with the normal actions of cellular messengers (130, 134–137).

The effect of titanium oxide nanoparticles (TiO_2-NPs) on insulin resistance in liver-derived cells was evaluated in a research study (138). Briefly, the dose-dependent action of TiO_2-NPs on Fao cells (rat hepatoma) was investigated. The cells were exposed to various concentrations (10, 50, 100, and 200 μg/mL) of TiO_2-NPs. It was observed that treatment with 50–200 μg/mL of TiO_2-NPs actuated insulin resistance by two mechanisms—directly affecting the hepatic cells to induce hepatic insulin resistance (**Figure 2**) and indirectly eliciting an inflammation response on macrophages (**Figure 6**) and hence releasing inflammatory cytokines such as Tumor Necrosis Factor -α (TNF-α) and Interleukins—1α/β (IL-1α/β). Administration of conditioned media form TiO_2-NP-treated macrophages confirmed the activation of TNF-α, IL-6, IL-8, IL-1α, and IL-1β. These inflammatory cytokines caused insulin resistance in Fao cells. In addition, it was observed that direct exposure of TiO_2–NPs to hepatic cells triggered the activation of stress kinases—c-Jun N-terminal Kinases (JNK) and p38, which attenuated the phosphorylation of Insulin Receptor Substrate (IRS) −1/2, and Glycogen Synthase Kinase (GSK) 3β, and led to abnormal insulin signaling (**Figure 5**).

An 8-week study was conducted to evaluate the effects of chromium nanoparticles (CrNano) on the hormone and immune responses of rats under heat stress conditions (118). Four groups (with 20 individuals per group) of Sprague–Dawley (SD) rats were randomly assigned to different dietary treatments. The first group was offered a basal diet as a control. The second, third, and fourth groups received a basal diet supplemented with 150, 300, and 450 μg/kg of CrNano, respectively. The treatment groups were then studied for various parameters governing overall metabolism. Measurement of sera concentrations of hormones and immunoglobulins with respect to the control group showed a decreased concentration of insulin and an increased concentration of insulin-like growth factor I and immunoglobulin G in the serum.

The same research group conducted another 6-week study to evaluate the effects of seven different levels of dietary CrNano (0, 75, 150, 300, 450, 600, and 1200 ppb Cr) in SD rats (139). Seven groups with 10 individuals per group of SD rats were randomly assigned to different dietary treatments. The results indicated that an addition of 300 and 450 ppb CrNano significantly decreased ($p < 0.05$) the serum insulin level. It was observed that the Cr contents in the liver and kidney were significantly increased ($p < 0.05$) by incremental dosage of CrNano from 150 to 1,200 ppb. The probable mechanism of reduction in peripheral insulin levels was ascribed to the activity of chromium in promoting hormone internalization into cells by increasing the membrane fluidity as explained by Evans and Bowman (140). This possibly led to altered insulin actions including binding of insulin to insulin receptors and the undesired interaction of insulin with various tissues such as adipose tissues and muscle tissues.

Interaction With Estrogenic Receptors

Estrogen receptors (ERs) expressed in adipose tissue, skeletal muscle, liver and pancreatic cells interact with estrogens and regulate metabolism. ER-α and ER-β play an important role in the regulation of glucose homeostasis by modulation of insulin sensitivity (141) and pancreatic insulin secretion (142). Additionally, in order to alter insulin secretion, the estrogen receptors facilitate the action of estrogen via G-protein coupled membrane receptors (137). The available reports suggest an antagonistic action of EDENMs toward the estrogenic receptors (127, 143, 144), which may lead to a decrease in insulin sensitivity and thereby alter glucose homeostasis.

The role of EDENMs in influencing estrogenic activity was demonstrated in a study where time-dependent (1, 3, or 5 h) treatment with 10 nm gold NPs to ovarian granulosa cells resulted in increased levels of estrogen (127). ERs have pathway modulation action via genomic and non-genomic approaches. While the genomic activity involves action of classical nuclear receptors to directly modulate the genes vital to homeostasis, the non-genomic route follows the use of kinases that activate signaling pathways resulting in the activation of ER pathway modulators. The increase in estrogen levels was suggested as indicative of the modulation of processes undergoing nuclear translocation, which might manipulate the normal gene expression for normal insulin signaling.

More evidence to support the endocrine-disrupting action of NMs was generated through illustrating the action of Cadmium Telluride Quantum Dots (CdTe QDs) (143). A dose-dependent study was carried out in uterine cells from female mice. The endocrine disrupting results were confirmed by a BrdU (BromodeoxyUridine) cell proliferation assay and a human ER 1 reporter assay for an assessment of ER activation.

Inflammation as the Cause of Insulin Resistance

In line with the ongoing research on the effect of ENMs on the immune system, research observations have established that the secretion of inflammatory cytokines by various cell types (**Figure 6**) has an impact on insulin resistance (126, 128, 145–147). With their local and global action on different tissues, inflammatory cytokines have contributed to the development of insulin resistance and T2DM (146). The immune system recognizes ENMs as antigens and thus elicits an acute response. Under such circumstances, the adipose tissue upregulates the production of cytokines, which consequently leads to abrupt molecular signaling and the development of T2DM (148). Additionally, a substantial role of various ENMs in causing inflammation mediated toxicity has been previously reported (138, 149, 150).

Evidence from *in silico* experiments has provided insights into the putative mechanistic underlying the toxic response of carbon-based ENMs that causes T2DM. The effects of introducing C60 fullerenes and carbon nanotubes in a living system were modeled in a computational analysis (151). Results demonstrated that carbon NMs could be recognized as pathogens by the Toll-like receptors that may elicit innate immune response. Such a theory was well supported by expression of inflammatory secretory proteins like interleukin IL-8 and chemokine monocyte chemoattractant protein (MCP1). In another study, direct exposure of ENMs, including nano-diamonds and nano-platinum liquid, to human dendritic cells resulted in an enhanced

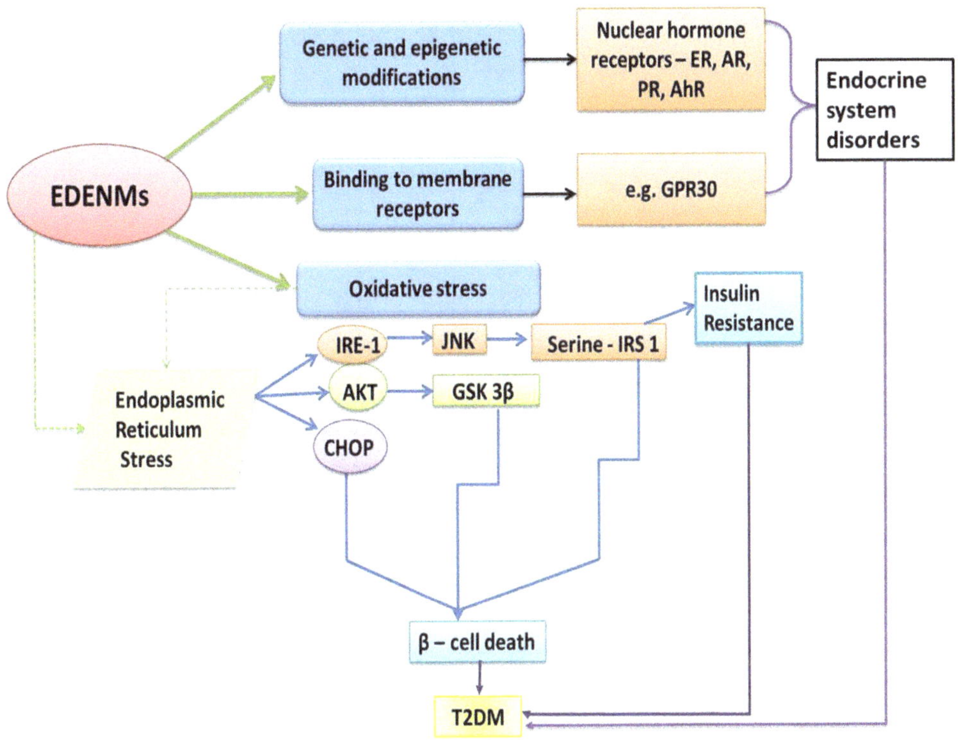

FIGURE 5 | Molecular pathways influenced by EDENM, leading to the development of T2DM. (EDENM, endocrine disrupting engineered nanomaterials; T2 DM, Type 2 Diabetes Mellitus; ER, estrogenic receptor; AR, androgenic receptor; PR, progesterone receptor; AhR, aryl hydrocarbon receptor; GPR30, G-protein-coupled receptor for estrogen; IRE-1, inositol-requiring enzyme 1; AKT, alpha serine/threonine kinase; CHOP, CCAAT-enhancer-binding *protein* homologous *protein; JNK,* c-Jun N-terminal kinase; GSK 3β, Glycogen synthase kinase *3 beta; IRS-1,* Insulin receptor substrate 1). (The green solid arrows show the direct effect of EDENM. The green dashed arrow shows one of the major consequent events later resulting in T2DM, as further described by the blue solid arrows. Black solid arrows point toward the involvement of various receptors resulting in endocrine system disorders. Purple solid arrows infer the T2DM occurrence via various pathways).

expression of IL-1β, IL-6, and TNF-α. These cytokines are known mediators for an inflammatory response (152).

Metallic ENMs were also studied to assess any associated immune response by exploring a variety of mechanisms. Many research groups have conducted various experiments to understand the mechanistic for the inflammatory action of gold nanoparticles (GNPs) (125–127, 153). In one study, two different sized GNPs, 10 and 50nm, were chosen to look for the enhancement of gene expression for cytokines IL-1β, IL-6, and TNF-α by exposure to rat liver (146). The study also included experiments to understand the possibility of oxidative stress mediated damage to hepatic cells. The observations confirmed the generation of ROS in the presence of GNPs. These results clearly suggest that both the inflammation and oxidative stress related molecular pathways induced by ENMs play a significant role in the etiology of T2DM.

Another group investigated the combined effect of ZnO nanoparticle-mediated oxidative stress and immunogenic responses on immune cells. Immune cells, lymphocytes (activated memory and naïve) and monocytes, were assayed for the expression of (Interferon) IFN- γ, TNF- α, and IL-12 upon treatment with ZnO nanoparticles of varying sizes (4, 8, 13 and 20 nm). It was observed that activated memory lymphocytes were the most robust against ZnO exposure, followed by naïve lymphocytes. Monocytes were the most susceptible of the three choices. The effect on immune cells was size-dependent, with the smallest ZnO particles contributing most to the generation of ROS and toxicity (154). Such findings are in line with the previously discussed roles of inflammation and oxidative stress in the etiology of T2DM.

Evidence to support the involvement of metallic ENMs in eliciting immune response was put forward by creating a novel platform, MIMIC (Modular Immune *in vitro* Construct, an artificial system imitating the human immune system). This provides a digitalized platform where the response of the immune system to an antigen can be modeled computationally. Also, it is more flexible and faster as compared to traditional cell or animal models. The study was modeled in a predictive immunological construct for assessment of the effect of nano-TiO_2 on the increase in the expression of IL-1β, IL-6, and TNF-α. The results demonstrated an enhancement in the secretion of pro-inflammatory cytokines on TiO_2 exposure. Additionally, the expression of co-stimulatory B7/CD28 on dendritic cells was observed, which suggested a putative action of T-cells against TiO_2 nanoparticles (145).

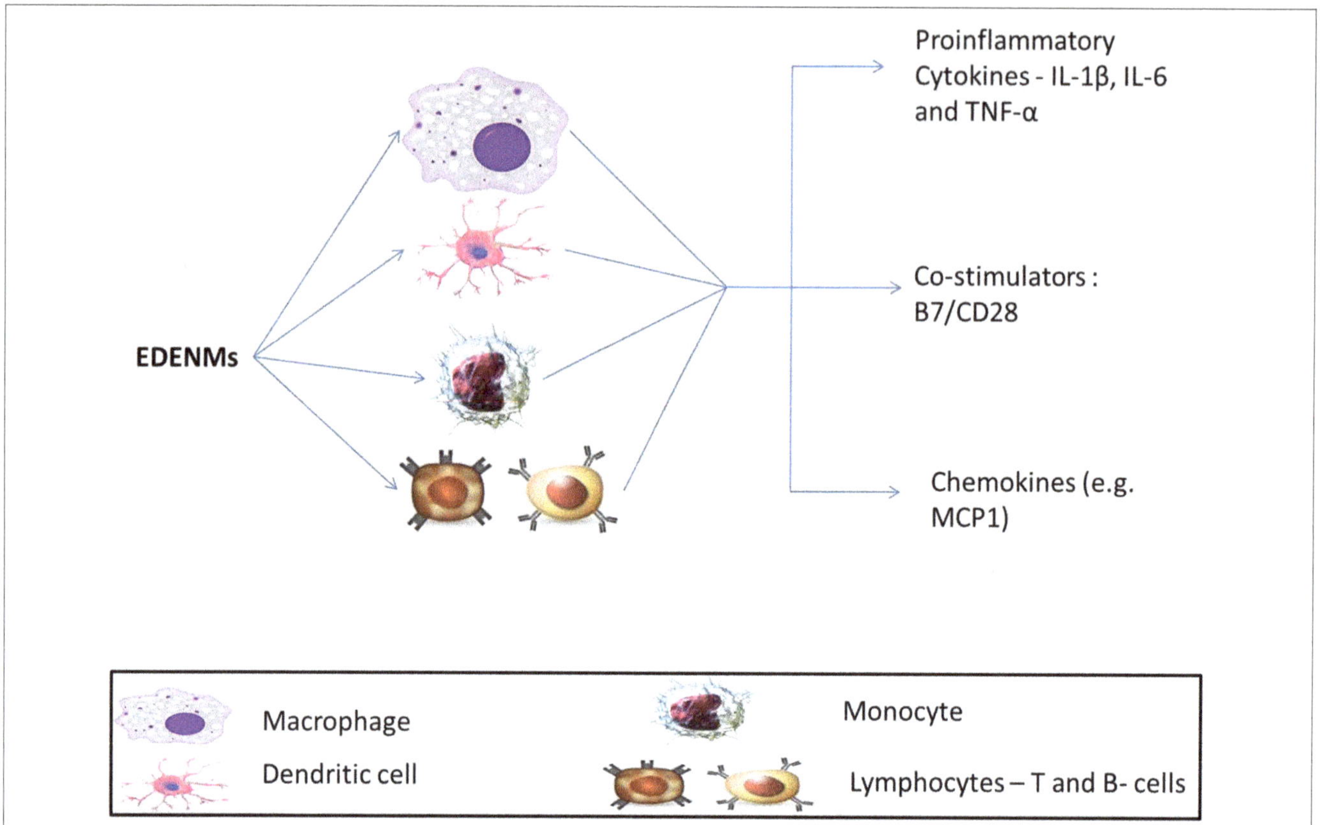

FIGURE 6 | Effect of EDENM on various immune cells resulting in enhancement of expression of various pro-inflammatory cytokines (Interleukins, IL-1β, IL-6; TNF-α, Tumor Necrosis Factor-α), immunoglobulin superfamily members—B7/CD28 and chemokines (MCP-1, Monocyte chemoattractant protein-1).

The available clinical-epidemiological research studies have clearly illustrated the involvement of abrupt immune action and ROS in the occurrence of T2DM. This evidence points toward a predictable association of EDENM-dependent disruption of immune activities and ROS generation that consequently leads to T2DM (155, 156).

Much evidence can be found in literature that establishes a link between the involvement of the immune system and diabetes bridged via inflammation. As substantial evidence, an epidemiological study was conducted to correlate inflammation (as monitored by variations in CRP level) and the development of diabetes (155). Another study evaluated the association between the release of inflammatory cytokines and blood glucose levels. A many-fold increase in cytokine concentration occurred during the low-grade systemic inflammation (157). It was suggested that the accelerated concentrations of interleukins and TNF-α may enable the migration of pro-inflammatory cytokines toward the insulin-signaling pathway. This may interfere with insulin signaling through phosphorylation of serine residues in insulin-receptor- substrate 1 (IRS 1) (158). Insulin-signaling may be blocked and insulin receptor (IR) stays dormant (159). In another epidemiological research, a diabetic Mexican-American population was studied for the effect of inflammation on the occurrence and prevalence of diabetes by testing for cytokines (IL-6, TNF-α, IL-1β, IL-8) and adipokine (adiponectin, resistin and leptin) levels in blood plasma. Increased plasma levels of these chemokines were found to be associated with increased blood glucose levels and T2DM (160). Several genetic association studies have suggested a role of polymorphism in the cytokine genes TNF-α and IL-6 in the development of diabetes and its associated comorbidities, retinopathy (161) and nephropathy (162, 163). Researchers have conducted a meta-analysis to probe into associations between −308 G>A (rs1800629) single nucleotide polymorphisms (SNP) in the TNF-*α* gene and T2DM (156). Another study reported significant association of genetic polymorphism in TNF-*α*, with an increased risk of T2DM in the Han Chinese population (138).

It is evident from the discussion that EDENMs may influence the onset of T2DM by triggering inflammatory pathways. Additionally, the formerly discussed arguments with epidemiological evidence presents a direct link between inflammation and T2DM. Such proof can be used to probe more into inflammation-dependent pathogenesis of T2DM due the exposure to ENMs.

Variations in Homeostatic Pathways

The homeostatic pathways involved in energy metabolism influences the overall development of an organism (136). In the case of metabolic disorders, the normal flow of homeostatic pathway is affected and the regulation is breached

(136, 164). The EDENMs intervene with the factors related to insulin signaling. These factors include various kinases, including phosphatidylinositol 3-kinase (PI3K), protein kinase B, mammalian target of rapamycin (mTOR) and AMPK (AMP-activated protein kinase) which that tightly regulate sugar, lipid and amino acid homeostasis (164). This hampers the transduction of insulin signaling and results in diminished insulin action (165), which is followed by glucose metabolism malfunctions and development of T2DM.

In vitro studies have elucidated the action of metallic ENMs on homeostatic pathways. Findings from one study have established that heavy-metal NPs can elicit hyperglycemia (166). In another study, the influence of iron oxide (Fe_2O_3) NPs exposure on the signaling mechanisms was studied in murine hepatocytes (50). In this dose-dependent study, Fe_2O_3 NPs decreased the cell viability via the PI3K/Akt pathway. The exposure also resulted in a decrement of the intra-cellular antioxidant ability of hepatocytes. The study emphasized the role of exposure to Fe_2O_3 NPs (250 g/ml) in oxidative stress and apoptosis in the hepatic cells (167).

in vivo experiments have been carried out to explore the combined effect of ENM exposure and consequent abrupt functioning of oxidative stress and the homeostatic pathway on the endocrine system. Several *in vivo* studies have shown that the uptake of NMs has induced production of ROS (168). Physiological levels of ROS affected glucose metabolism pathways and insulin sensitivity (169). Moderate but long-standing oxidative stress has been found to be one of the major contributors in the onset of insulin resistance, and consequently T2DM (170). Oral introduction of TiO_2 (anatase) nanoparticles to mice in a dose-dependent manner led to the accumulation of titanium in the liver, spleen, small intestine, kidney, and pancreas. Increased levels of titanium in these organs leads to insulin resistance, which was associated with increased phosphorylation of IRS1 (Ser307), JNK1, and p38 Mitogen activated protein kinase (MAPK), reduced phosphorylation of Akt (Ser473), and increased serum levels of TNF-α and IL-6 in the liver. An increase in the generation of ROS observed in the study also suggests a role for ENM in the induction of oxidative stress (171).

Impairment of β Cells and Influence on Insulin Production

The low doses of endocrine disruptors can alter the functioning of the pancreas by affecting the physiology of both insulin- and glucagon-secretory cells, which can further disrupt the regulation of glucose and lipid metabolism. As depicted in **Figure 5**, loss in β-cell mass is predominantly governed by the pathways involved in oxidative stress and endoplasmic reticulum stress. It is reported that oxidative stress is accounted by the generation of excess ROS and contributes to T2DM through β-cell death (172). It has also been extensively reviewed that endoplasmic reticulum-stress plays a prominent role in causing apoptosis in pancreatic islets, resulting in β-cell death (173, 174).

A few metallic NMs have been shown to affect β-cells indirectly via influencing the kinases involved in transcriptional activation, followed by increased oxidative stress in the cells and finally apoptosis. In a research study carried out in macrophages, AuNPs of various sizes (4, 11, 19, 35, and 45 nm) suppressed NFκβ and JNK pathway activation. The process was observed due to de-methylation of CpG oligodeoxynucleotides (CpG-ODNs) motifs, making them act as immuno-stimulants (150). This effect was size dependent, with 4 nm AuNPs being the strongest suppressor. AuNPs potentially elicited an inflammatory response and induced oxidative stress as reviewed previously (128). Another study demonstrated the ROS generating capacity of Iron oxide (Fe_3O_4) nanoparticles when H_2O_2 was used as the substrate (175). The hydroxyl free-radical generation reaction was biochemically similar to catalase and peroxidase action. It was inferred that the ROS may affect the pancreatic islet by JNK and NFκβ activation (176). Such observations supported the role of oxidative stress mediated inflammatory responses in β-cell damage, which may underlie the pathogenesis to T2DM.

Besides the above-discussed principle mechanisms, several unknown mechanisms underlying the development or pathogenesis of T2DM due to exposure to endocrine disrupters are also discussed in the available literature. The involvement of ultrafine particulate matter (key element of pollution) in the pathogenesis of T2DM is widely argued (52–56). Ultrafine particulate matter constitutes the ultrafine particles (UFPs), which are airborne particles with a thermodynamic/aerodynamic size of <100 nm. Diesel engines as well as automobiles, along with sand dust, fires, hot volcanic lava, and ocean spray along with combustion activities such as the burning of biomass or wood, generate and then release UFPs into the air. The mechanisms underlying the development of T2DM due to exposure to air pollutants have not been completely deciphered to date, however, an epidemiological study has been done to see the effect of ambient UFPs and nitrogen dioxide in a cohort of Canadian-born residents (177). The results clearly indicated that exposure to UFPs led to increased risk of incident hypertension (hazard ratio = 1.03; 95% CI = 1.02, 1.04) and diabetes (hazard ratio = 1.06; 95% CI = 1.05, 1.08).

CONCLUSIONS AND PERSPECTIVES

Evidence suggesting a role of EDENM exposure in the pathogenesis of T2DM is gradually emerging, but a comprehensive understanding of a wide range of nanomaterials and their effect on candidate gene pathways and other causal factors involved in T2DM remain to be completely deciphered. The fact that ENM can disrupt the endocrine system, which may eventually lead to T2DM, has gathered support from several *in vitro*, *in vivo*, and epidemiological studies. Altered glucose metabolism through various molecular mechanisms including insulin resistance, decreased insulin sensitivity, induction of oxidative stress pathways, and altered homeostasis have been reported by numerous laboratory studies that examined the effect of EDENM exposures. On the other hand, a few studies also report a contrasting effect of the same EDENM on T2DM related molecules. Many research groups have come up with a safer application of ENMs by illustrating their ability to work as

TABLE 1 | Different categories of ENM used in therapeutics against T2DM.

Type	Application	Study system	References
NON-METALLIC ENM			
PEG-b-PLGA–biodegradable Polyethylene glycol and Poly (lactic-co-glycolic acid) copolymer (PEG-b-PLGA) Based cationic lipid-assisted nanoparticles (clans)	Anti-inflammatory action	Diet—induced type 2 diabetes mice	(183)
Chitosan	Gene delivery for Glucagon like peptide 1 (GLP-1), dipeptydil peptidase IV (DPP-IV resistant GLP-1 analogs) and siRNA targeting against DPP-IV	HT-29, HepG2, and Caco-2 cell lines	(184)
Insulin-loaded nano-carriers	Transdermal delivery of insulin	Streptozotocin-diabetic male Wistar rats	(185)
Alginic acid nanoparticles containing insulin	Sublingual delivery of insulin	Streptozotocin-induced diabetic male Wistar rats	(186)
Insulin-containing Polyethylene imine-based nanoparticles	Insulin–delivery	Sprague Dawley rats	(187)
PLGA as the carrier to prepare recombinant human epidermal growth factor (rhEGF) nanoparticles	Diabetic wound healing	Diabetic rats	(188)
Insulin encapsulated in polyalkylcyanoacrylate nanocapsules	Hypoglycemia effect	Diabetic rats	(189)
Nanoparticles from dextran, poly (α-1,6 glucose), physically cross-linked with the tetra functional glucose-binding protein, Con A	Controlled delivery of insulin	*In vitro* studies	(190)
Injectable insulin nano-particles	Insulin delivery	Subcutaneous administration in diabetic mice	(191)
BIOSYNTHESIZED ENM			
Eysenhardtia polystachya-loaded silver nanoparticles (EP/AgNPs)	Antidiabetic activity	Pancreatic β cells, INS-1 cells, and *Danio rerio*	(180)
Gold nanoparticles (AuNPs) synthesized using *Gymnema sylvestre R. Br* Plant extract	Antidiabetic activity	Wistar albino rats	(182)
Gold nanoparticles (AuNPs) synthesized using *Cassia auriculata* plant extract	Increasing plasma insulin activity	Alloxan induced albino rats	(181)
METALLIC ENM			
Insulin-coated gold nanoparticles (INS-GNPs)	For controlled and prolonged glucose regulation was reported	Intravenous and subcutaneous administration to diabetic mouse model	(192)
Gold NPs and aspartic acid-capped gold nanoparticles	Insulin delivery	Diabetic Wistar rats	(193)
Gold nanoparticles and Dextran–insulin conjugates	Insulin delivery	Mouse 3T3-L1 cell line	(194)
Mesoporous silica nanoparticles (MSNs)	Gluconic acid-modified insulin (G-Ins) proteins labeled with fluorescein isothiocyanate (FITC-G-Ins) were immobilized on the exterior surface of MSN which served as caps to encapsulate cAMP molecules inside the mesopores of MSN	RIN-5F	(194, 195)
Selenium nanoparticles (SeNPs)	Oral delivery of insulin to enhance the antidiabetic effect	Normal (Sprague-Dawley, SD) and type II DM (Goto-Kakizaki, GK) rats	(196)

therapeutics. Particularly, some of the biologically synthesized ENMs (178, 179) were found to possess therapeutic potential against T2DM (180–182). Other non-metallic and metallic NMs for similar applications are also reported (**Table 1**).

In an interesting study, an increase in cell viability, ATP/ADP ratio and secretion of insulin in response to glucose stimuli in the isolated pancreatic islets when treated with metallic nanoparticles prepared from cerium oxide (CeO_2-NPs) at a concentration of 100 nmol/L, either alone or in combination with 30 nmol/L sodium selenite, was reported (197). These findings could possibly be ascribed to the anti-oxidant potential of CeO_2-NPs, which may exert a different effect on the insulin release. In a similar study, the effect of zinc oxide nanoparticles (ZON) on oxidative stress-mediated pancreatic β-cell death was investigated in rats (RIN5f). The cellular levels of antioxidant factors and the rate of apoptosis were assessed in correlation with ZON uptake. RIN5f cell treatment with ZON (30 and 100 μg/ml) resulted in cytotoxicity, oxidative stress and apoptosis. In contrast, the sub-cytotoxic concentrations (1, 3, 10 μg/ml) protected RIN5f cells from hydrogen peroxide (H_2O_2)-induced oxidative stress by the reducing the cellular levels of ROS, increased SOD activity and GSH, and reduced cell death (198). The findings reported in the above-mentioned studies indicated that nanomaterial-type and size dependencies on the associated cellular toxicity are not precisely explored. An incomplete characterization of ENM may underlie discrepancies observed in available scientific reports. Confusion created from such incomplete explorations demands for the development of a common understanding in the area of ENM characteristics (shape, size, surface area, mass concentration, or a combination of these), which should be a prerequisite to toxic effect determination. This broadens the scope of research to particularly define physicochemical properties of ENM for their sustainable bio-medical applications. Considering this, ENMs for vital bio-medical, pharmaceutical, agricultural, and environmental applications are required to be well characterized for their uptake to various cell/ tissue types, interaction with cellular organelles and cell mechanistic aspects within the intracellular environment (199).

Since *in vitro* systems do not necessarily mimic the human system, results obtained from such experiments need to be replicated through *in vivo* studies conducted in different model animals. Additionally, *in vivo* studies that address potential effects of EDENM on the development of T2DM at a large scale such as a population, a community, or an ecosystem with sufficient power are necessarily required. Further, most of the *in vivo* studies have been conducted on small rodents, specifically rats, mice and hamsters, which may not be optimum for studying the long-term toxic effects of nanomaterial and makes it difficult to extrapolate the observed results to humans. Experiments by including other model systems, which are more closely related to human systems, like *Danio rerio*, *Daphnia magna*, and *Caenorhabditis elegans* need to be conducted in more numbers. Furthermore, pre-clinical *in vitro* studies, such as those using blood samples from a control population, can also be conducted for impact-assessment of EDENMs (200). Additional support to the candidate mechanisms underlying EDENM mediated T2DM and identification of novel pathways can be achieved through the application of the "-omics" approach, which at present is virtually lacking. Also, developing high-throughput pre-screening (HTPS) and quantitative structure-activity relationship (QSAR) methods for *in silico* screening and prediction would be extremely important to comprehend the effect of EDENM (201).

We emphasize the importance of research on safety aspect of ENMs, which would minimize the uncertainties regarding the health and environmental issues surrounding these advance-materials and help in the development of safe applications of nanotechnologies.

AUTHOR CONTRIBUTIONS

PS was the Principal Scientist, involved in conceptualization of the review, study design, data analyses, data compilation, manuscript writing, critical inputs, and finalization of the manuscript. AP contributed toward data analyses, data compilation, manuscript writing, critical inputs, and finalization of the manuscript. SG was involved in data compilation and manuscript writing. All authors have read and approved the final manuscript.

ACKNOWLEDGMENTS

The research activities of the authors are supported by the TERI-Deakin Nanobiotechnology Centre, Gurugram, India.

REFERENCES

1. Chennupati Jagadish AB. Nanoscience: thinking big, working small. In: Chennupati Jagadish AB, editor. *Technology and the Future*. Acton: Australian Academy of Science (2015). Available online at: https://www.science.org.au/curious/nanoscience
2. Schmid G, Fenske D. *Metal Clusters and Nanoparticles*. London: The Royal Society (2010).
3. Pietroiusti A, Stockmann-Juvala H, Lucaroni F, Savolainen K. Nanomaterial exposure, toxicity, and impact on human health. *Wiley Interdiscip Rev Nanomed Nanobiotechnol.* (2018) 10:e1513. doi: 10.1002/wnan.1513
4. Iavicoli I, Fontana L, Pingue P, Todea AM, Asbach C. Assessment of occupational exposure to engineered nanomaterials in research laboratories using personal monitors. *Sci Total Env.* (2018) 627:689–702. doi: 10.1016/j.scitotenv.2018.01.260
5. Guttenberg M, Bezerra L, Neu-Baker NM, del Pilar Sosa Idelchik M, Elder A, Oberdörster G, et al. Biodistribution of inhaled metal oxide nanoparticles mimicking occupational exposure: a preliminary investigation using enhanced darkfield microscopy. *J Biophot.* (2016) 9:987–93. doi: 10.1002/jbio.201600125
6. Catalán J, Ilves M, Järventaus H, Hannukainen KS, Kontturi E, Vanhala E, et al. Genotoxic and immunotoxic effects of cellulose nanocrystals *in vitro*. *Environ Mol Mutagen.* (2015) 56:171–82. doi: 10.1002/em.21913
7. Palomäki J, Välimäki E, Sund J, Vippola M, Clausen PA, Jensen KA, et al. Long, needle-like carbon nanotubes and asbestos activate the NLRP3 inflammasome through a similar mechanism. *ACS Nano* (2011) 5:6861–70. doi: 10.1021/nn200595c
8. Rossi EM, Pylkkänen L, Koivisto AJ, Nykäsenoja H, Wolff H, Savolainen K, et al. Inhalation exposure to nanosized and fine TiO 2 particles inhibits features of allergic asthma in a murine model. *Part Fibre Toxicol.* (2010) 7:35. doi: 10.1186/1743-8977-7-35
9. Kreyling WG, Semmler-Behnke M, Seitz J, Scymczak W, Wenk A, Mayer P, et al. Size dependence of the translocation of inhaled iridium and carbon nanoparticle aggregates from the lung of rats to the blood and secondary target organs. *Inhalat Toxicol.* (2009) 21:55–60. doi: 10.1080/08958370902942517
10. Nel A, Xia T, Mädler L, Li N. Toxic potential of materials at the nanolevel. *Science* (2006) 311:622–7. doi: 10.1126/science.1114397
11. Zhao F, Zhao Y, Liu Y, Chang X, Chen C, Zhao Y. Cellular uptake, intracellular trafficking, and cytotoxicity of nanomaterials. *Small* (2011) 7:1322–37. doi: 10.1002/smll.201100001
12. Rosenkranz P, Fernández-Cruz M, Conde E, Ramírez-Fernández M, Flores J, Fernández M, et al. Effects of cerium oxide nanoparticles to fish and mammalian cell lines: an assessment of cytotoxicity and methodology. *Toxicol Vitro* (2012) 26:888–96. doi: 10.1016/j.tiv.2012.04.019
13. Komatsu T, Tabata M, Kubo-Irie M, Shimizu T, Suzuki KI, Nihei Y, et al. The effects of nanoparticles on mouse testis Leydig cells *in vitro*. *Toxicol Vitro* (2008) 22:1825–31. doi: 10.1016/j.tiv.2008.08.009
14. Bai Y, Zhang Y, Zhang J, Mu Q, Zhang W, Butch ER, et al. Repeated administrations of carbon nanotubes in male mice cause reversible testis damage without affecting fertility. *Nat Nanotechnol.* (2010) 5:683. doi: 10.1038/nnano.2010.153

15. Damstra BST, Bergman A, Kavlock RJ, van der Kraak G. *Global Assessment of the State-of-the-Science of Endocrine Disruptors*. Geneva: World Health Organization (2002).
16. Mnif W, Hassine IHA, Bouaziz A, Bartegi A, Thomas O, Roig B. Effect of endocrine disruptor pesticides: a review. *Int J Env Res Public Health* (2011) 8:2265–303. doi: 10.3390/ijerph8062265
17. Combarnous Y, Endocrine Disruptor Compounds (EDCs) and agriculture: the case of pesticides. *Comp Rendus Biol.* (2017) 340:406–9. doi: 10.1016/j.crvi.2017.07.009
18. Diamanti-Kandarakis E, Bourguignon JP, Giudice LC, Hauser R, Prins GS, Soto AM, et al. Endocrine-disrupting chemicals: an endocrine society scientific statement. *Endocr Rev.* (2009) 30:293–342. doi: 10.1210/er.2009-0002
19. Rudel RA, Perovich LJ. Endocrine disrupting chemicals in indoor and outdoor air. *Atmosph Environ.* (2009) 43:170–81. doi: 10.1016/j.atmosenv.2008.09.025
20. Nicolopoulou-Stamati P, Hens L, Sasco AJ. Cosmetics as endocrine disruptors: are they a health risk? *Rev Endocr Metab Dis.* (2015) 16:373–83. doi: 10.1007/s11154-016-9329-4
21. Knez J. Endocrine-disrupting chemicals and male reproductive health. *Reprod Bio Med Online* (2013) 26:440–8. doi: 10.1016/j.rbmo.2013.02.005
22. Zlatnik G. Endocrine-disrupting chemicals and reproductive health. *J Midwifery Wom Health* (2016) 61:442–55. doi: 10.1111/jmwh.12500
23. Zama AM, Bhurke A, Uzumcu M. Effects of endocrine-disrupting chemicals on female reproductive health. *Open Biotechnol. J.* (2016) 10:54–75. doi: 10.2174/1874070701610010054
24. Jeng HA. Exposure to endocrine disrupting chemicals and male reproductive health. *Front Public Health* (2014) 2:55. doi: 10.3389/fpubh.2014.00055
25. Marques-Pinto A, Carvalho D. Human infertility: are endocrine disruptors to blame? *Endocr Connec.* (2013) 2:R15–29. doi: 10.1530/EC-13-0036
26. Teitelbaum SL, Belpoggi F, Reinlib L. Advancing research on endocrine disrupting chemicals in breast cancer: expert panel recommendations. *Reproduc Toxicol.* (2015) 54:141–7. doi: 10.1016/j.reprotox.2014.12.015
27. Soto AM, Sonnenschein C. Environmental causes of cancer: endocrine disruptors as carcinogens. *Nat Rev Endocrinol.* (2010) 6:363–70. doi: 10.1038/nrendo.2010.87
28. Morgan M, Deoraj A, Felty Q, Roy D. Environmental estrogen-like endocrine disrupting chemicals and breast cancer. *Mol Cell Endocrinol.* (2017) 457:89–102. doi: 10.1016/j.mce.2016.10.003
29. Abdel-Rahman W, Moustafa Y, O Ahmed B, Mostafa R. Endocrine disruptors and breast cancer risk - time to consider the environment. *Asian Pacific J Cancer* (2012) 13:5937. doi: 10.7314/APJCP.2012.13.12.5937
30. Rachon D. Endocrine disrupting chemicals (EDCs) and female cancer: informing the patients. *Rev Endocr Metab Dis.* (2015) 16:359–64. doi: 10.1007/s11154-016-9332-9
31. Greet S, Elly DH, Willem D, Nik VL, Marike L. Endocrine disruptors and abnormalities of pubertal development. *Basic Clin Pharmac Toxicol.* (2008) 102:168–75. doi: 10.1111/j.1742-7843.2007.00180.x
32. Lee HR, Jeung EB, Cho MH, Kim TH, Leung PCK, Choi KC. Molecular mechanism(s) of endocrine-disrupting chemicals and their potent oestrogenicity in diverse cells and tissues that express oestrogen receptors. *J Cell Mol Med.* (2013) 17:1–11. doi: 10.1111/j.1582-4934.2012.01649.x
33. Shahidehnia M. Epigenetic effects of endocrine disrupting chemicals. *J Environ Anal Toxicol.* (2016) 6:381. doi: 10.4172/2161-0525.1000381
34. Colborn T. Neurodevelopment and endocrine disruption. *Environ Health Perspect.* (2004) 112:944–9. doi: 10.1289/ehp.6601
35. Meeker JD. Exposure to environmental endocrine disruptors and child development. *Arch Pediatr Adolesc Med.* (2012) 166:E1–7. doi: 10.1001/archpediatrics.2012.241
36. Pinson A, Bourguignon JP, Parent AS. Exposure to endocrine disrupting chemicals and neurodevelopmental alterations. *Andrology* (2016) 4:706–22. doi: 10.1111/andr.12211
37. Xu H, Yang M, Qiu W, Pan C, Wu M. The impact of endocrine-disrupting chemicals on oxidative stress and innate immune response in zebrafish embryos. *Environ Toxicol Chem.* (2013) 32:1793–9. doi: 10.1002/etc.2245
38. Rogers JA, Metz L, Yong VW. Review: endocrine disrupting chemicals and immune responses: a focus on bisphenol-A and its potential mechanisms. *Mol Immunol.* (2013) 53:421–30. doi: 10.1016/j.molimm.2012.09.013
39. Kuo CH, Yang SN, Kuo PL, Hung CH. Immunomodulatory effects of environmental endocrine disrupting chemicals. *Kaohsiung J Med Sci.* (2012) 28:S37–42. doi: 10.1016/j.kjms.2012.05.008
40. Ferin J. Pulmonary retention and clearance of particles. *Toxicol Lett.* (1994) 72:121–5. doi: 10.1016/0378-4274(94)90018-3
41. Borm PJ, Schins RP, Albrecht C. Inhaled particles and lung cancer, part B: paradigms and risk assessment. *Int J Cancer* (2004) 110:3–14. doi: 10.1002/ijc.20064
42. Oberdörster G, Ferin J, Lehnert BE. Correlation between particle size, *in vivo* particle persistence, and lung injury. *Environ Health Perspect.* (1994) 102:173–9.
43. Dasenbrock C, Peters L, Creutzenberg O, Heinrich U. The carcinogenic potency of carbon particles with and without PAH after repeated intratracheal administration in the rat. *Toxicol Lett.* (1996) 88:15–21. doi: 10.1016/0378-4274(96)03712-5
44. Driscoll KE, Carter JM, Howard BW, Hassenbein DG, Pepelko W, Baggs RB, et al. Pulmonary inflammatory, chemokine, and mutagenic responses in rats after subchronic inhalation of carbon black. *Toxicol Appl Pharmacol.* (1996) 136:372–80. doi: 10.1006/taap.1996.0045
45. Nikula K, Snipes M, Barr E, Griffith W, Henderson R, Mauderly J. Comparative pulmonary toxicities and carcinogenicities of chronically inhaled diesel exhaust and carbon black in F344 rats. *Fundam Appl Toxicol.* (1995) 25:80–94. doi: 10.1006/faat.1995.1042
46. Casals-Casas C, Desvergne B. Endocrine disruptors: from endocrine to metabolic disruption. *Annu Rev Physiol.* (2011) 73:135–62. doi: 10.1146/annurev-physiol-012110-142200
47. Purdel C, Ilie M, Margina D. The involvement of environmental endocrine-disrupting chemicals in type 2 Diabetes Mellitus Development. In: Croniger C. editor. *Treatment of Type 2 Diabetes.* London: IntechOpen (2015) 219–50. doi: 10.5772/59110
48. Piemonte L. *About Diabetes.* International Diabetes Federation (2018).
49. Chevalier N, Fenichel P. Endocrine disruptors: new players in the pathophysiology of type 2 diabetes? *Diabetes Metab.* (2015) 41:107–15. doi: 10.1016/j.diabet.2014.09.005
50. Savolainen K, Alenius H, Norppa H, Pylkkänen L, Tuomi T, Kasper G. Risk assessment of engineered nanomaterials and nanotechnologies—a review. *Toxicology* (2010) 269:92–104. doi: 10.1016/j.tox.2010.01.013
51. Valsami-Jones E, Lynch I. How safe are nanomaterials? *Science* (2015) 350:388–9. doi: 10.1126/science.aad0768
52. Taylor DA. Dust in the wind. *Environ Health Perspect.* (2002) 110:A80–7. doi: 10.1289/ehp.110-a80
53. Dikio D, Bixa N. Carbon nanotubes synthesis by catalytic decomposition of ethyne using Fe/Ni catalyst on aluminium oxide support. *Int J Appl Chem.* (2011) 7:35–42.
54. Shooto DN, Dikio ED. Morphological characterization of soot from the combustion of candle wax. *Int. J. Electrochem. Sci.* (2011) 6:1269–76.
55. Srilatha K, Bhagawan D, Shiva Kumar S, Himabindu V. Sustainable fuel production by thermocatalytic decomposition of methane - A review. *South Afr J Chem Eng.* (2017) 24:156–67. doi: 10.1016/j.sajce.2017.10.002
56. Kumar R, Bharagava RN, Kumar M, Singh S, Kumar G. Enhanced biodegradation of mobil oil hydrocarbons by biosurfactant producing bacterial consortium in wheat and mustard rhizosphere. *J Petrol Environ Biotechnol.* (2013) 4:158. doi: 10.4172/2157-7463.1000158
57. Hu Q, Li H, Wang L, Gu H, Fan C. DNA nanotechnology-enabled drug delivery systems. *Chem Rev.* (2018). doi: 10.1021/acs.chemrev.7b00663. [Epub ahead of print].
58. Sahoo SK, Misra R, Parveen S. Nanoparticles: a boon to drug delivery, therapeutics, diagnostics and imaging. *Nanomed Cancer* (2017) 73–124. doi: 10.1016/j.nano.2011.05.016
59. Xu R, Ferrari M, Shen H. A pro-nanodrug with intratumoral reconstitution and intracellular delivery beyond therapy-resistance molecular pumps. In: *Proceeding of AACR Annual Meeting.* Washington, DC (2017).
60. Xu S, Zhu X, Huang W, Zhou Y, Yan D. Supramolecular cisplatin-vorinostat nanodrug for overcoming drug resistance in cancer synergistic

therapy. *J Contr Release* (2017) 266:36–46. doi: 10.1016/j.jconrel.2017.09.007

61. Ji C, Gao Q, Dong X, Yin W, Gu Z, Gan Z, et al. A size-reducible nanodrug with an aggregation-enhanced photodynamic effect for deep chemo-photodynamic therapy. *Angew Chem Int Ed Engl.* (2018) 57:11384–88. doi: 10.1002/anie.201807602
62. Rahi A, Karimian K, Heli H. Nanostructured materials in electroanalysis of pharmaceuticals. *Analy Biochem.* (2016) 497:39–47. doi: 10.1016/j.ab.2015.12.018
63. Sridhar R, Ramakrishna S. Electrosprayed nanoparticles for drug delivery and pharmaceutical applications. *Biomatter* (2013) 3:e24281. doi: 10.4161/biom.24281
64. Yin J, Wang Y, Gilbertson LM. Opportunities to advance sustainable design of nano-enabled agriculture identified through a literature review. *Environ Sci. Nano* (2018) 5:11–26. doi: 10.1039/C7EN00766C
65. Kah M, Kookana RS, Gogos A, Bucheli TD. A critical evaluation of nanopesticides and nanofertilizers against their conventional analogues. *Nat Nanotechnol.* (2018) 13:677–684. doi: 10.1038/s41565-018-0131-1
66. Srivastava AK, Dev A, Karmakar S. Nanosensors and nanobiosensors in food and agriculture. *Environ Chem Lett.* (2018) 1:161–82. doi: 10.1007/s10311-017-0674-7
67. Mueller NC, Nowack B. Exposure modeling of engineered nanoparticles in the environment. *Environ Sci Technol.* (2008) 42:4447–53. doi: 10.1021/es7029637
68. Gottschalk F, Nowack B. The release of engineered nanomaterials to the environment. *J Environ Monit.* (2011) 13:1145–55. doi: 10.1039/c0em00547a
69. Gottschalk F, Sonderer T, Scholz RW, Nowack B. Possibilities and limitations of modeling environmental exposure to engineered nanomaterials by probabilistic material flow analysis. *Environ Toxicol Chem.* (2010) 29:1036–48. doi: 10.1002/etc.135
70. Oberdorster G. Pulmonary effects of inhaled ultrafine particles. *Int Arch Occupat Environ Health* (2001) 74:1–8. doi: 10.1007/s004200000185
71. Roduner E. Size matters: why nanomaterials are different. *Chem Soc Rev.* (2006) 35:583–92. doi: 10.1039/b502142c
72. Kouwenhoven LP, Austing D, Tarucha S. Few-electron quantum dots. *Rep Prog Phys.* (2001) 64:701. doi: 10.1088/0034-4885/64/6/201
73. Hoet PH, Brüske-Hohlfeld I, Salata OV. Nanoparticles–known and unknown health risks. *J Nanobiotechnol.* (2004) 2:12. doi: 10.1186/1477-3155-2-12
74. Takenaka S, Karg E, Roth C, Schulz H, Ziesenis A, Heinzmann U, et al. Pulmonary and systemic distribution of inhaled ultrafine silver particles in rats. *Environ Health Perspect.* (2001) 109:547–51. doi: 10.1289/ehp.01109s4547
75. Xia T, Kovochich M, Brant J, Hotze M, Sempf J, Oberley T, et al. Comparison of the abilities of ambient and manufactured nanoparticles to induce cellular toxicity according to an oxidative stress paradigm. *Nano Lett.* (2006) 6:1794–807. doi: 10.1021/nl061025k
76. Garcia-Garcia E, Andrieux K, Gil S, Kim HR, Le Doan T, Desmaële D, et al. A methodology to study intracellular distribution of nanoparticles in brain endothelial cells. *Int J Pharmac.* (2005) 298:310–4. doi: 10.1016/j.ijpharm.2005.03.030
77. Gurr JR, Wang AS, Chen CH, Jan KY. Ultrafine titanium dioxide particles in the absence of photoactivation can induce oxidative damage to human bronchial epithelial cells. *Toxicology* (2005) 213:66–73. doi: 10.1016/j.tox.2005.05.007
78. Singal M, Finkelstein JN. Amorphous silica particles promote inflammatory gene expression through the redox sensitive transcription factor, AP-1, in alveolar epithelial cells. *Exp Lung Res.* (2005) 31:581–97. doi: 10.1080/019021490951504
79. Kato T, Yashiro T, Murata Y, Herbert DC, Oshikawa K, Bando M, et al. Evidence that exogenous substances can be phagocytized by alveolar epithelial cells and transported into blood capillaries. *Cell Tissue Res.* (2003) 311:47–51. doi: 10.1007/s00441-002-0647-3
80. Hopwood D, Spiers E, Ross P, Anderson J, McCullough J, Murray F. Endocytosis of fluorescent microspheres by human oesophageal epithelial cells: comparison between normal and inflamed tissue. *Gut* (1995) 37:598–602. doi: 10.1136/gut.37.5.598
81. Rothen-Rutishauser BM, Schürch S, Haenni B, Kapp N, Gehr P. Interaction of fine particles and nanoparticles with red blood cells visualized with advanced microscopic techniques. *Environ Sci Technol.* (2006) 40:4353–9. doi: 10.1021/es0522635
82. Peters A, Veronesi B, Calderón-Garcidueñas L, Gehr P, Chen LC, Geiser M, et al. Translocation and potential neurological effects of fine and ultrafine particles a critical update. *Part Fibre Toxicol.* (2006) 3:13. doi: 10.1186/1743-8977-3-13
83. Elder A, Gelein R, Silva V, Feikert T, Opanashuk L, Carter J, et al. Translocation of inhaled ultrafine manganese oxide particles to the central nervous system. *Environ Health Perspect.* (2006) 114:1172–8. doi: 10.1289/ehp.9030
84. Miller MR, Raftis JB, Langrish JP, McLean SG, Samutrtai P, Connell SP, et al. Inhaled nanoparticles accumulate at sites of vascular disease. *ACS Nano* (2017) 11:4542–52. doi: 10.1021/acsnano.6b08551
85. Lucarelli M, Gatti AM, Savarino G, Quattroni P, Martinelli L, Monari E, et al. Innate defence functions of macrophages can be biased by nano-sized ceramic and metallic particles. *Eur Cytokine Netw.* (2004) 15:339–46. Available online at: http://www.jle.com/fr/revues/ecn/e-docs/innate_defence_functions_of_macrophages_can_be_biased_by_nano_sized_ceramic_and_metallic_particles_264246/
86. Bonner JC. Nanoparticles as a potential cause of pleural and interstitial lung disease. *Proc Am Thor Soc.* (2010) 7:138–41. doi: 10.1513/pats.200907-061RM
87. Byrne JD, Baugh JA. The significance of nanoparticles in particle-induced pulmonary fibrosis. *McGill J Med.* (2008) 11:43–50.
88. Lkhasuren O, Takahashi K, Dash-Onolt L. Occupational lung diseases and the mining industry in Mongolia. *Int J Occup Env Health* (2007) 13:195–201. doi: 10.1179/oeh.2007.13.2.195
89. Chen HW, Su SF, Chien CT, Lin WH, Yu SL, Chou CC, et al. Titanium dioxide nanoparticles induce emphysema-like lung injury in mice. *FASEB J.* (2006) 20:2393–5. doi: 10.1096/fj.06-6485fje
90. You R, Lu W, Shan M, Berlin JM, Samuel ELG, Marcano DC, et al. Nanoparticulate carbon black in cigarette smoke induces DNA cleavage and Th17-mediated emphysema. *eLife* (2015) 4:e09623. doi: 10.7554/eLife.09623
91. Pankhurst Q, Hautot D, Khan N, Dobson J. Increased levels of magnetic iron compounds in Alzheimer's disease. *J Alzheimers Dis.* (2008) 13:49–52. doi: 10.3233/JAD-2008-13105
92. Hawkins SJ, Crompton LA, Sood A, Saunders M, Boyle NT, Buckley A, et al. Nanoparticle-induced neuronal toxicity across placental barriers is mediated by autophagy and dependent on astrocytes. *Nat Nanotechnol.* (2018) 13:427–33. doi: 10.1038/s41565-018-0085-3
93. Li X, Liu B, Li XL, Li YX, Sun MZ, Chen DY, et al. SiO(2) nanoparticles change colour preference and cause Parkinson's-like behaviour in zebrafish. *Sci Rep.* (2014) 4:3810. doi: 10.1038/srep03810
94. Itoh Y, Shimazu A, Sadzuka Y, Sonobe T, Itai S. Novel method for stratum corneum pore size determination using positron annihilation lifetime spectroscopy. *Int J Pharm.* (2008) 358:91–5. doi: 10.1016/j.ijpharm.2008.02.016
95. Borm PJ, Robbins D, Haubold S, Kuhlbusch T, Fissan H, Donaldson K, et al. The potential risks of nanomaterials: a review carried out for ECETOC. *Toxicology* (2006) 3:11. doi: 10.1186/1743-8977-3-11
96. Toll R, Jacobi U, Richter H, Lademann J, Schaefer H, Blume-Peytavi U. Penetration profile of microspheres in follicular targeting of terminal hair follicles. *J Investig Dermatol.* (2004) 123:168–76. doi: 10.1111/j.0022-202X.2004.22717.x
97. Tinkle SS, Antonini JM, Rich BA, Roberts JR, Salmen R, DePree K, et al. Skin as a route of exposure and sensitization in chronic beryllium disease. *Environ Health Perspect.* (2003) 111:1202–8. doi: 10.1289/ehp.5999
98. Mocan T, Matea CT, Iancu C, Agoston-Coldea L, Mocan L, Orasan R. Hypersensitivity and nanoparticles: update and research trends. *Clujul Med.* (2016) 89:216–9. doi: 10.15386/cjmed-574
99. Hirai T, Yoshikawa T, Nabeshi H, Yoshida T, Tochigi S, Ichihashi KI, et al. Amorphous silica nanoparticles size-dependently aggravate atopic dermatitis-like skin lesions following an intradermal injection. *Part Fibre Toxicol.* (2012) 9:3–3. doi: 10.1186/1743-8977-9-3

100. Yanagisawa R, Takano H, Inoue KI, Koike E, Kamachi T, Sadakane K, et al. Titanium dioxide nanoparticles aggravate atopic dermatitis-like skin lesions in NC/Nga mice. *Exp Biol Med.* (2009) 234:314–22. doi: 10.3181/0810-RM-304
101. Martirosyan A, Schneider YJ. Engineered nanomaterials in food: implications for food safety and consumer health. *Int J Environ Res Public Health* (2014) 11:5720–50. doi: 10.3390/ijerph110605720
102. Priyadarsini S, Mukherjee S, Mishra M. Nanoparticles used in dentistry: a review. *J Oral Biol Craniof Res.* (2018) 8:58–67. doi: 10.1016/j.jobcr.2017.12.004
103. Raj S, Jose S, Sumod US, Sabitha M. Nanotechnology in cosmetics: Opportunities and challenges. *J Pharm Bioall Sci.* (2012) 4:186–93. doi: 10.4103/0975-7406.99016
104. Bettini S, Houdeau E. [Oral exposure to titanium dioxide (TiO(2)) nanoparticles: from translocation through oral and intestinal epithelia to fate and effects in the organism]. *Biol Aujourd'hui* (2014) 208:167–75. doi: 10.1051/jbio/20140022
105. Lafuente D, Garcia T, Blanco J, Sánchez DJ, Sirvent JJ, Domingo JL, et al. Effects of oral exposure to silver nanoparticles on the sperm of rats. *Reprod Toxicol.* (2016) 60:133–9. doi: 10.1016/j.reprotox.2016.02.007
106. Balasubramanyam A, Sailaja N, Mahboob M, Rahman MF, Misra S, Hussain SM, et al. Evaluation of genotoxic effects of oral exposure to Aluminum oxide nanomaterials in rat bone marrow. *Mutat Res Gen Toxicol Environ Mutag.* (2009) 676:41–7. doi: 10.1016/j.mrgentox.2009.03.004
107. Susana C, Lucía G, María Pilar V, Dolores V, Gorka S, Yurena L, et al. Safety assessment of chronic oral exposure to iron oxide nanoparticles. *Nanotechnology* (2015) 26:205101. doi: 10.1088/0957-4484/26/20/205101
108. Jia J, Li F, Zhou H, Bai Y, Liu S, Jiang Y, et al. Oral exposure to silver nanoparticles or silver ions may aggravate fatty liver disease in overweight mice. *Environ Sci Technol.* (2017) 51:9334–43. doi: 10.1021/acs.est.7b02752
109. Rabia Riasat NGZR, Imran A. Effects of nanoparticles on gastrointestinal disorders and therapy. *J Clin Toxicol.* (2016) 6:313. doi: 10.4172/2161-0495.1000313
110. Philbert MA. The new toxicology of sophisticated material: Nanotoxicology and beyond. *Toxicol Lett.* (2012) 211:S3. doi: 10.1016/j.toxlet.2012.03.019
111. Sharifi S, Behzadi S, Laurent S, Forrest ML, Stroeve P, Mahmoudi M. Toxicity of nanomaterials. *Chem Soc Rev.* (2012) 41:2323–43. doi: 10.1039/C1CS15188F
112. Stebounova LV, Morgan H, Grassian VH, Brenner S. Health and safety implications of occupational exposure to engineered nanomaterials. *Wiley Interdiscip Rev Nanomed Nanobiotechnol.* (2012) 4:310–21. doi: 10.1002/wnan.174
113. Campagnolo L, Massimiani M, Magrini A, Camaioni A, Pietroiusti A. Physico-chemical properties mediating reproductive and developmental toxicity of engineered nanomaterials. *Curr Med Chem.* (2012) 19:4488–94. doi: 10.2174/092986712803251566
114. Yu P, Sabine N, Annika L, Monika F, Fei W, Ulrich S, et al. Size-dependent cytotoxicity of gold nanoparticles. *Small* (2007) 3:1941–9. doi: 10.1002/smll.200700378
115. Malvindi MA, Brunetti V, Vecchio G, Galeone A, Cingolani R, Pompa PP. SiO2 nanoparticles biocompatibility and their potential for gene delivery and silencing. *Nanoscale* (2012) 4:486–95. doi: 10.1039/C1NR11269D
116. Armstrong N, Ramamoorthy M, Lyon D, Jones K, Duttaroy A. Mechanism of silver nanoparticles action on insect pigmentation reveals intervention of copper homeostasis. *PLoS ONE* (2013) 8 e53186. doi: 10.1371/journal.pone.0053186
117. *Endocrine Disruptors.* U.S. Department of Health and Human Services, National Institutes of Health (2010).
118. Zha L, Zeng J, Sun S, Deng H, Luo H, Li W. Chromium(III) nanoparticles affect hormone and immune responses in heat-stressed rats. *Biol Trace Elem Res.* (2009) 129:157–69. doi: 10.1007/s12011-008-8282-9
119. Wang M, Xu Z, Li W, Jiang Z. Effect of chromium nanocomposite supplementation on growth hormone pulsatile secretion and mRNA expression in finishing pigs. *J Anim Physiol Anim Nutr.* (2009) 93:520–5. doi: 10.1111/j.1439-0396.2008.00836.x
120. Chen Z, Wang Y, Wang X, Zhuo L, Chen S, Tang S, et al. Effect of titanium dioxide nanoparticles on glucose homeostasis after oral administration. *J Appl Toxicol.* (2018) 38:810–23. doi: 10.1002/jat.3589
121. Wang MQ, Xu ZR, Zha LY, Lindemann MD. Effects of chromium nanocomposite supplementation on blood metabolites, endocrine parameters and immune traits in finishing pigs. *Anim Feed Sci Technol.* (2007) 139:69–80. doi: 10.1016/j.anifeedsci.2006.12.004
122. Darbre PD. Endocrine disruption and disorders of energy metabolism. In: Darbre PD. editor. *Endocrine Disruption and Human Health.* Cambridge, MA: Academic Press (2015) p. 273–85.
123. Iavicoli I, Fontana L, Leso V, Bergamaschi A. The effects of nanomaterials as endocrine disruptors. *Int J Mol Sci.* (2013) 14:16732–801. doi: 10.3390/ijms140816732
124. Birnbaum LS, Jung P. From endocrine disruptors to nanomaterials: advancing our understanding of environmental health to protect public health. *Health Aff.* (2011) 30:814–22. doi: 10.1377/hlthaff.2010.1225
125. Abdelhalim MAK, Jarrar BM. Gold nanoparticles administration induced prominent inflammatory, central vein intima disruption, fatty change and Kupffer cells hyperplasia. *Lipids Health Dis.* (2011) 10:133. doi: 10.1186/1476-511X-10-133
126. Sumbayev VV, Yasinska IM, Garcia CP, Gilliland D, Lall GS, Gibbs BF, et al. Gold nanoparticles downregulate interleukin-1β-induced pro-inflammatory responses. *Small* (2013) 9:472–77. doi: 10.1002/smll.201201528
127. Stelzer R, Hutz RJ. Gold nanoparticles enter rat ovarian granulosa cells and subcellular organelles, and alter *in-vitro* estrogen accumulation. *J Reprod Dev.* (2009) 55:685–90. doi: 10.1262/jrd.20241
128. Sharma M, Salisbury RL, Maurer EI, Hussain SM, Sulentic EWC. Gold nanoparticles induce transcriptional activity of NF-[small kappa]B in a B-lymphocyte cell line. *Nanoscale* (2013) 5:3747–56. doi: 10.1039/c3nr30071d
129. Tinkov AA, Gritsenko VA, Skalnaya MG, Cherkasov SV, Aaseth J, Skalny AV. Gut as a target for cadmium toxicity. *Environ Pollut.* (2018) 235:429–34. doi: 10.1016/j.envpol.2017.12.114
130. Shafrir E, Ziv E, Mosthaf L. Nutritionally induced insulin resistance and receptor defect leading to β-cell failure in animal models. *Ann N Y Acad Sci.* (1999) 892:223–46. doi: 10.1111/j.1749-6632.1999.tb07798.x
131. Hasnain SZ, Prins JB, McGuckin MA. Oxidative and endoplasmic reticulum stress in beta-cell dysfunction in diabetes. *J Mol Endocrinol.* (2016) 56:R33–54. doi: 10.1530/JME-15-0232
132. Pilkington EH, Gurzov EN, Kakinen A, Litwak SA, Stanley WJ, Davis TP, et al. Pancreatic beta-cell membrane fluidity and toxicity induced by human islet amyloid polypeptide species. *Sci Rep.* (2016) 6:21274. doi: 10.1038/srep21274
133. Fu Z, Gilbert ER, Liu D. Regulation of insulin synthesis and secretion and pancreatic beta-cell dysfunction in diabetes. *Curr Diabetes Rev.* (2013) 9:25–53. doi: 10.2174/157339913804143225
134. Yun C, Katchko KM, Schallmo MS, Jeong S, Yun J, Chen CH, et al. Aryl hydrocarbon receptor antagonists mitigate the effects of dioxin on critical cellular functions in differentiating human osteoblast-like cells. *Int J Mol Sci.* (2018) 19:E225. doi: 10.3390/ijms19010225
135. Le Marchand-Brustel Y, Jeanrenaud B, Freychet P. Insulin binding and effects in isolated soleus muscle of lean and obese mice. *Am J Physiol Endocrinol Metab.* (1978) 234:E348. doi: 10.1152/ajpendo.1978.234.4.E348
136. Saltiel AR, Kahn CR. Insulin signalling and the regulation of glucose and lipid metabolism. *Nature* (2001) 414799–806. doi: 10.1038/414799a
137. Nadal A, Jm R, Laribi O, Leon-quinto T, Andreu E, Ripoll C, Soria B. Rapid insulinotropic effect of 17 beta-estradiol via a plasma membrane receptor. *FASEB J.* (2012) 12:1341–8. doi: 10.1096/fasebj.12.13.1341
138. Gurevitch D, Shuster-Meiseles T, Nov O, Zick Y, Rudich A, Rudich Y. TiO2 nanoparticles induce insulin resistance in liver-derived cells both directly and via macrophage activation. *Nanotoxicology* (2012) 6:804–12. doi: 10.3109/17435390.2011.625128
139. Zha LY, Xu ZR, Wang MQ, Gu LY. Effects of chromium nanoparticle dosage on growth, body composition, serum hormones and tissue chromium in Sprague-Dawley rats. *J Zhejiang Univ Sci B* (2007) 8:323–30. doi: 10.1631/jzus.2007.B0323
140. Evans GW, Bowman TD. Chromium picolinate increases membrane fluidity and rate of insulin internalization. *J Inorg Biochem.* (1992) 46:243–50. doi: 10.1016/0162-0134(92)80034-S

141. Ropero AB, Alonso-Magdalena P, Quesada I, Nadal A. The role of estrogen receptors in the control of energy and glucose homeostasis. *Steroids* (2008) 73:874–79. doi: 10.1016/j.steroids.2007.12.018
142. Alonso-Magdalena P, Ropero AB, Carrera MP, Cederroth CR, Baquié M, Gauthier BR, et al. Pancreatic insulin content regulation by the estrogen receptor ERα. *PLoS ONE* (2008) 3:e2069. doi: 10.1371/journal.pone.0002069
143. Jain MP, Vaisheva F, Maysinger D. Metalloestrogenic effects of quantum dots. *Nanomedicine* (2012) 7:23–37. doi: 10.2217/nnm.11.102
144. Larson JK, Carvan MJ III, Hutz RJ. Engineered nanomaterials: an emerging class of novel endocrine disruptors. *Biol Reprod* (2014) 91:20. doi: 10.1095/biolreprod.113.116244
145. Schanen BC, Karakoti AS, Seal S, Drake Iii DR, Warren WL, Self WT. Exposure to titanium dioxide nanomaterials provokes inflammation of an *in vitro* human immune construct. *ACS Nano* (2009) 3:2523–32. doi: 10.1021/nn900403h
146. Khan H, Abdelhalim M, Alhomida A, Al Ayed M. Transient increase in IL-1β, IL-6 and TNF-α gene expression in rat liver exposed to gold nanoparticles. *Genet Mol Res.* (2013) 12:5851–7. doi: 10.4238/2013.November.22.12
147. Piret JP, Jacques D, Audinot JN, Mejia J, Boilan E, Noel F, et al. Copper(II) oxide nanoparticles penetrate into HepG2 cells, exert cytotoxicity via oxidative stress and induce pro-inflammatory response. *Nanoscale* (2012) 4:7168–84. doi: 10.1039/c2nr31785k
148. Bruun JM, Lihn AS, Verdich C, Pedersen SB, Toubro S, Astrup A, et al. Regulation of adiponectin by adipose tissue-derived cytokines: *in vivo* and *in vitro* investigations in humans. *Am J Physiol Endocrinol Metab.* (2003) 285:E527–33. doi: 10.1152/ajpendo.00110.2003
149. Han SG, Newsome B, Hennig B. Titanium dioxide nanoparticles increase inflammatory responses in vascular endothelial cells. *Toxicology* (2013) 306:1–8. doi: 10.1016/j.tox.2013.01.014
150. Tsai CY, Lu SL, Hu CW, Yeh CS, Lee GB, Lei HY. Size-dependent attenuation of TLR9 signaling by gold nanoparticles in macrophages. *J Immunol.* (2012) 188:68–76. doi: 10.4049/jimmunol.1100344
151. Turabekova M, Rasulev B, Theodore M, Jackman J, Leszczynska D, Leszczynski J. Immunotoxicity of nanoparticles: a computational study suggests that CNTs and C60 fullerenes might be recognized as pathogens by Toll-like receptors. *Nanoscale* (2014) 6:3488–95. doi: 10.1039/C3NR05772K
152. Ghoneum M, Ghoneum A, Gimzewski J. Nanodiamond and nanoplatinum liquid, DPV576, activates human monocyte-derived dendritic cells *in vitro*. *Anticancer Res.* (2010) 30:4075–9. Available online at: http://ar.iiarjournals.org/content/30/10/4075.short
153. Lasagna-Reeves C, Gonzalez-Romero D, Barria M, Olmedo I, Clos A, Ramanujam VS, et al. Bioaccumulation and toxicity of gold nanoparticles after repeated administration in mice. *Biochem Biophys Res Commun.* (2010) 393:649–55. doi: 10.1016/j.bbrc.2010.02.046
154. Hanley C, Thurber A, Hanna C, Punnoose A, Zhang J, Wingett DG. The influences of cell type and zno nanoparticle size on immune cell cytotoxicity and cytokine induction. *Nanosc Res Lett.* (2009) 4:1409–20. doi: 10.1007/s11671-009-9413-8
155. Freeman DJ, Norrie J, Caslake MJ, Gaw A, Ford I, Lowe GD, et al. West of scotland coronary prevention, C-reactive protein is an independent predictor of risk for the development of diabetes in the West of Scotland Coronary Prevention Study. *Diabetes* (2002) 51:1596–600. doi: 10.2337/diabetes.51.5.1596
156. Liu ZH, Ding Yl, Xiu LC, Pan HY, Liang Y, Zhong SQ, et al. A meta-analysis of the association between TNF-α −308G>A polymorphism and type 2 diabetes mellitus in han chinese population. *PLoS ONE* (2013) 8:e59421. doi: 10.1371/journal.pone.0059421
157. Petersen AM, Pedersen BK. The anti-inflammatory effect of exercise. *J Appl Physiol.* (1985) 98:1154–62. doi: 10.1152/japplphysiol.00164.2004
158. Bastard JP, Jardel C, Bruckert E, Vidal H, Hainque B. Variations in plasma soluble tumour necrosis factor receptors after diet-induced weight loss in obesity. *Diabetes Obes Metab.* (2000) 2:323–5. doi: 10.1046/j.1463-1326.2000.00090.x
159. Fasshauer M, Paschke R. Regulation of adipocytokines and insulin resistance. *Diabetologia* (2003) 46:1594–603. doi: 10.1007/s00125-003-1228-z
160. Mirza S, Hossain M, Mathews C, Martinez P, Pino P, Gay JL, et al. Type (2012) 2-diabetes is associated with elevated levels of TNF-alpha, IL-6 and adiponectin and low levels of leptin in a population of Mexican Americans: a cross-sectional study. *Cytokine* (2012) 57:136–42. doi: 10.1016/j.cyto.2011.09.029
161. Prasad P, Tiwari A, Kumar P, Ammini A, Gupta A, Gupta R, et al. Association of TGFbetal, TNFalpha, CCR2 and CCR5 gene polymorphisms in type-2 diabetes and renal insufficiency among Asian Indians. *BMC Med Genet.* (2007) 8:20. doi: 10.1186/1471-2350-8-20
162. Prasad P, Kumar P, Ammini A, Gupta A, Gupta R, Thelma KB. Association of dopaminergic pathway gene polymorphisms with chronic renal insufficiency among Asian Indians with type-2 diabetes. BMC Genet. (2008) 9:26. doi: 10.1186/1471-2156-9-26
163. Prasad P, Tiwari A, Kumar P, Ammini A, Gupta A, Gupta R, et al. Chronic renal insufficiency among Asian Indians with type 2 diabetes: I. Role of RAAS gene polymorphisms. *BMC Med Genet.* (2006) 7:42. doi: 10.1186/1471-2350-7-42
164. Cantley LC. The phosphoinositide 3-kinase pathway. *Science* (2002) 296:1655–7. doi: 10.1126/science.296.5573.1655
165. Brown EJ, Albers MW, Bum Shin T, Ichikawa K, Keith CT, Lane WS, et al. A mammalian protein targeted by G1-arresting rapamycin–receptor complex. *Nature* (1994) 369:756–8. doi: 10.1038/369756a0
166. Gandhi S, Srinivasan BP, Akarte AS. An experimental assessment of toxic potential of nanoparticle preparation of heavy metals in streptozotocin induced diabetes. *Exp Toxicol Pathol.* (2013) 65:1127–35. doi: 10.1016/j.etp.2013.05.004
167. Sarkar A, Sil PC. Iron oxide nanoparticles mediated cytotoxicity via PI3K/AKT pathway: role of quercetin. *Food Chem Toxicol.* (2014) 71:106–115. doi: 10.1016/j.fct.2014.06.003
168. Jomova K, Valko M. Advances in metal-induced oxidative stress and human disease. *Toxicology* (2011) 283:65–87. doi: 10.1016/j.tox.2011.03.001
169. Loh K, Deng H, Fukushima A, Cai X, Boivin B, Galic S, et al. Reactive oxygen species enhance insulin sensitivity. *Cell Metab.* (2009) 10:260–72. doi: 10.1016/j.cmet.2009.08.009
170. Houstis N, Rosen ED, Lander ES. Reactive oxygen species have a causal role in multiple forms of insulin resistance. *Nature* (2006) 440:944–8. doi: 10.1038/nature04634
171. Hailong H, Qian G, Changlin W, Xiao M, Hongjuan H, Yuri O, et al. Titanium dioxide nanoparticles increase plasma glucose via reactive oxygen species-induced insulin resistance in mice. *J Appl Toxicol.* (2015) 35:1122–32. doi: 10.1002/jat.3150
172. Maiese K. New insights for oxidative stress and diabetes mellitus. *Oxid Med Cell Longev.* (2015) 2015:875961. doi: 10.1155/2015/875961
173. Ashcroft FM, Rorsman P. Diabetes mellitus and the beta cell: the last ten years. *Cell* (2012) 148:1160–71. doi: 10.1016/j.cell.2012.02.010
174. Fonseca SG, Burcin M, Gromada J, Urano F. Endoplasmic reticulum stress in beta-cells and development of diabetes. *Curr Opin Pharmacol.* (2009) 9:763–70. doi: 10.1016/j.coph.2009.07.003
175. Könczöl M, Ebeling S, Goldenberg E, Treude F, Gminski R, Gieré R, et al. Cytotoxicity and genotoxicity of size-fractionated iron oxide (Magnetite) in A549 human lung epithelial cells: role of ROS, JNK, and NF-κB. *Chem Res Toxicol.* (2011) 24:1460–75. doi: 10.1021/tx200051s
176. Nan C, Hui W, Qing H, Jiang L, Juan Y, Dannong H, et al. Long-term effects of nanoparticles on nutrition and metabolism. *Small* (2014) 10:3603–11. doi: 10.1002/smll.201303635
177. Bai L, Chen H, Hatzopoulou M, Jerrett M, Kwong JC, Burnett RT, et al. Exposure to ambient ultrafine particles and nitrogen dioxide and incident hypertension and diabetes. *Epidemiology* (2018) 29:323–32. doi: 10.1097/EDE.0000000000000798
178. Singh P, Kim YJ, Zhang D, Yang DC. Biological synthesis of nanoparticles from plants and microorganisms. *Trends Biotechnol.* (2016) 34:588–99. doi: 10.1016/j.tibtech.2016.02.006
179. Ingale AG, Chaudhari AN. Biogenic synthesis of nanoparticles and potential applications: an eco- friendly approach. *J Nanomed Nanotechnol.* (2013) 4:165. doi: 10.4172/2157-7439.1000165
180. Campoy AHG, Gutierrez RMP, Manriquez-Alvirde G, Ramirez AM. Protection of silver nanoparticles using Eysenhardtia polystachya in peroxide-induced pancreatic β-cell damage and their antidiabetic properties in zebrafish. *Int J Nanomed.* (2018) 13:2601. doi: 10.2147/IJN.S163714

181. Venkatachalam M, Govindaraju K, Mohamed Sadiq A, Tamilselvan S, Ganesh Kumar V, Singaravelu G. Functionalization of gold nanoparticles as antidiabetic nanomaterial. *Spectroch Acta Part A* (2013) 116:331–8. doi: 10.1016/j.saa.2013.07.038
182. Karthick V, Kumar VG, Dhas TS, Singaravelu G, Sadiq AM, Govindaraju K. Effect of biologically synthesized gold nanoparticles on alloxan-induced diabetic rats—An *in vivo* approach. *Coll Surf B Biointerfaces* (2014) 122:505–11. doi: 10.1016/j.colsurfb.2014.07.022
183. Liu Y, Cao ZT, Xu CF, Lu ZD, Luo YL, Wang J. Optimization of lipid-assisted nanoparticle for disturbing neutrophils-related inflammation. Biomaterials (2018) 172:92–104. doi: 10.1016/j.biomaterials.2018.04.052
184. Jean M, Alameh M, De Jesus D, Thibault M, Lavertu M, Darras V, et al. Chitosan-based therapeutic nanoparticles for combination gene therapy and gene silencing of *in vitro* cell lines relevant to type 2 diabetes. *Eur J Pharmac Sci.* (2012) 45:138–49. doi: 10.1016/j.ejps.2011.10.029
185. Rastogi R, Anand S, Koul V. Electroporation of polymeric nanoparticles: an alternative technique for transdermal delivery of insulin. *Drug Dev Industrial Pharma.* (2010) 36:1303–11. doi: 10.3109/03639041003786193
186. Patil NH, Devarajan PV. Insulin-loaded alginic acid nanoparticles for sublingual delivery. *Drug Deliv.* (2016) 23:429–36. doi: 10.3109/10717544.2014.916769
187. Salvioni L, Fiandra L, Del Curto MD, Mazzucchelli S, Allevi R, Truffi M, et al. Oral delivery of insulin via polyethylene imine-based nanoparticles for colonic release allows glycemic control in diabetic rats. *Pharmacol Res.* (2016) 110:122–30. doi: 10.1016/j.phrs.2016.05.016
188. Yuejie C, Demin Y, Penghua W, Jun X, Daiqing L, Min D. Nanotechnology promotes the full-thickness diabetic wound healing effect of recombinant human epidermal growth factor in diabetic rats. *Wound Repair Regener.* (2010) 18:499–505. doi: 10.1111/j.1524-475X.2010.00612.x
189. Damge C, Michel C, Aprahamian M, Couvreur P. New approach for oral administration of insulin with polyalkylcyanoacrylate nanocapsules as drug carrier. *Diabetes* (1988) 37:246–51. doi: 10.2337/diab.37.2.246
190. Zion TC, Tsang HH, Ying JY. Glucose-sensitive nanoparticles for controlled insulin delivery. *Int J Nanomed.* (2003) 12:4037–57. Available online at: http://hdl.handle.net/1721.1/3783
191. Gu Z, Aimetti AA, Wang Q, Dang TT, Zhang Y, Veiseh O, et al. Injectable nano-network for glucose-mediated insulin delivery. *ACS Nano* (2013) 7:4194–201. doi: 10.1021/nn400630x
192. Shilo M, Berenstein P, Dreifuss T, Nash Y, Goldsmith G, Kazimirsky G, et al. Insulin-coated gold nanoparticles as a new concept for personalized and adjustable glucose regulation. *Nanoscale* (2015) 7:20489–96. doi: 10.1039/C5NR04881H
193. Joshi HM, Bhumkar DR, Joshi K, Pokharkar V, Sastry M. Gold nanoparticles as carriers for efficient transmucosal insulin delivery. *Langmuir* (2006) 22:300–5. doi: 10.1021/la051982u
194. Lee KC, Chen WJ, Chen YC. Using dextran-encapsulated gold nanoparticles as insulin carriers to prolong insulin activity. *Nanomedicine* (2017) 12:1823–34. doi: 10.2217/nnm-2017-0019
195. Zhao Y, Trewyn BG, Slowing, II, Lin VS. Mesoporous silica nanoparticle-based double drug delivery system for glucose-responsive controlled release of insulin and cyclic AMP. *J Am Chem Soc.* (2009) 131:8398–400. doi: 10.1021/ja901831u
196. Deng W, Xie Q, Wang H, Ma Z, Wu B, Zhang X. Selenium nanoparticles as versatile carriers for oral delivery of insulin: insight into the synergic antidiabetic effect and mechanism. *Nanomed Nanotechnol Biol Med.* (2017) 13:1965–74. doi: 10.1016/j.nano.2017.05.002
197. Pourkhalili N, Hosseini A, Nili-Ahmadabadi A, Rahimifard M, Navaei-Nigjeh M, Hassani S, et al. Improvement of isolated rat pancreatic islets function by combination of cerium oxide nanoparticles/sodium selenite through reduction of oxidative stress. *Toxicol Mech Methods.* (2012) 22:476–82. doi: 10.3109/15376516.2012.673093
198. Asani SC, Umrani RD, Paknikar KM. Differential dose-dependent effects of zinc oxide nanoparticles on oxidative stress-mediated pancreatic β-cell death. *Nanomedicine* (2017) 12:745–59. doi: 10.2217/nnm-2016-0426
199. Septiadi D, Crippa F, Moore TL, Rothen-Rutishauser B, Petri-Fink A. Nanoparticle–cell interaction: a cell mechanics perspective. *Adv Mater.* (2018) 30:1704463. doi: 10.1002/adma.201704463
200. Wan HT, Leung PY, Zhao YG, Wei X, Wong MH, Wong CK. Blood plasma concentrations of endocrine disrupting chemicals in Hong Kong populations. *J Hazard Mater* (2013) 261:763–9. doi: 10.1016/j.jhazmat.2013.01.034
201. Lai RWS, Yeung KWY, Yung MMN, Djurisic AB, Giesy JP, Leung KMY. Regulation of engineered nanomaterials: current challenges, insights and future directions. *Environ Sci Pollut Res Int.* (2018) 25:3060–77. doi: 10.1007/s11356-017-9489-0

10

Environmental Pollutants and Metabolic Disorders: The Multi-Exposure Scenario of Life

Brigitte Le Magueresse-Battistoni, Hubert Vidal and Danielle Naville*

Univ Lyon, CarMeN Laboratory, INSERM U1060, INRA U1397, INSA Lyon, Université Claude Bernard Lyon1, Oullins, France

***Correspondence:**
Brigitte Le Magueresse-Battistoni
brigitte.lemagueresse@inserm.fr

Obesity and diabetes have reached epidemic proportions the past few decades and continue to progress worldwide with no clear sign of decline of the epidemic. Obesity is of high concern because it is the main risk factor for a number of non-communicable diseases such as cardiovascular diseases and type 2 diabetes. Metabolic diseases constitute a major challenge as they are associated with an overall reduced quality of life and impose a heavy economic burden on countries. These are multifactorial diseases and it is now recognized that environmental exposure to man-made chemical pollutants is part of the equation. Yet, risk assessment procedures are based on a one-by-one chemical evaluation which does not meet the specificities of the multi-exposure scenario of life, e.g., a combined and long-term exposure to even the smallest amounts of chemicals. Indeed, it is assumed that environmental exposure to chemicals will be negligible based on the low potency of each chemical and that they do not interact. Within this mini-review, strong evidences are brought that exposure to low levels of multiple chemicals especially those shown to interfere with hormonal action, the so-called endocrine disrupting compounds do trigger metabolic disturbances in conditions in which no effect was expected if considering the concentration of each individual chemical in the mixture. This is known as the cocktail effect. It means that risk assessment procedures are not protective enough and thus that it should be revisited for the sake of Public Health.

Keywords: cocktail effect, mixture, endocrine disrupting compounds (EDCs), pollutants, sex-dimorphism

INTRODUCTION

Obesity and diabetes have reached epidemic proportions the past few decades and continue to progress worldwide with no clear sign of decline of the epidemic in any country. An estimate of 1.9 billion adults were overweight in 2016 of these over 650 million were obese. Children and teenagers are also of high concern with 380 million overweight or obese in 2016. Latest projections by WHO (World Health Organization) indicate that proportion of overweight and obese males and females will continue to increase and reach 3.3 billion by 2030 (1). Obesity is of high concern because it is the main risk factor for a number of non-communicable diseases such as cardiovascular diseases, certain cancers and type 2 diabetes. Indeed, almost 90% of persons suffering from type 2 diabetes are obese and more than 400 million persons will suffer from diabetes by 2030. Metabolic diseases constitute a major challenge as they are associated with an overall reduced quality of life, psychological problems and several physical disabilities (1, 2). Metabolic diseases also impose a heavy economic burden on countries. It is a major cause of death and it costs an average of $ 2000 billion to the global economy, almost 3 points of GDP (gross domestic product) (3, 4).

Metabolic diseases are multifactorial diseases. Apart from genetic susceptibility, life-style risk factors associating over-nutrition and sedentary behavior are major contributors. Yet these causative factors do not explain the magnitude of metabolic diseases or the kinetics of the epidemic. Among other etiologic factors, it is acknowledged that environmental exposure to man-made chemical pollutants is part of the equation, especially those shown to interfere with hormonal action, the so-called endocrine disrupting compounds (EDCs) (5–12).

Today's non-occupational exposure to chemicals is characterized by exposure to tens of thousands of man-made chemicals at low levels. Occupational exposure will not be considered in this mini-review. Another characteristic of non-occupational exposure is its chronicity, from conception onwards thus encompassing gestation and lactation which are periods highly vulnerable to chemicals. It is indeed recognized that threat during the maternal period (e.g., food restriction, chemical stressors) could trigger diseases later in life including metabolic diseases and some cancers, known as the Developmental Origin of Human adult Diseases (DOHaD) concept (13, 14). In addition, the nature of chemicals and doses to which individuals are exposed may vary across their lifespan. It is also of concern that the number of chemicals to which humans are exposed has continued to grow for more than 100 years as is their spatial distribution while the identification of their possible hazardous effects lags behind. Furthermore, exposure is non-deliberate and the exposed population is seldom aware of the nature of the chemicals, the levels to which it is exposed as well as the health consequences. Hence, it appears that risk assessment procedures need to be revisited because the one-by-one evaluation of chemicals does not meet the specificities of the multi-exposure scenario of life.

Within this mini-review we aim in presenting basic characteristics on environmental pollutants including EDCs and risk assessment principles operating nowadays. We will next summarize evidences gathered using either natural or artificial mixtures in experimental models, that exposures to low levels of multiple chemicals trigger metabolic disorders in conditions in which no effect was expected if considering the concentration of each individual chemical in the mixture. This is defined as the cocktail effect of pollutants which certainly constitutes one of the biggest health challenges in our modern societies.

RISK ASSESSMENT EVALUATION PRINCIPLES AND LIMITS

If industrialization has promoted societal progress improving life expectancy, it also led to the presence of tens of thousands of anthropogenic chemicals transported in the atmosphere and globalizing pollution. Man-made sources of pollution are related to industrial and agricultural activities but also to domestic activities. Pollutants are found in foods, beverages and packaging, clothes, cosmetics and cleaning products, furniture, paints, electronic equipment, plastics, and the list is long. Routes of exposure are mostly through diet but also dermal and by inhalation not to mention transfer via placenta, suckling and mouthing behavior placing babies and small infants at particularly high risk for they lack a mature defensive xenobiotic detoxification system. Pollutants differ according to their natural disposal in degradable and low-degradable or persistent pollutants including the lipophilic persistent organic pollutants (POPs) which bio-accumulate through the food chain in fatty tissues with half-lives of several years in humans (15). Although severely regulated because of environmental toxicity (e.g., the ban of polychlorobiphenyls, PCBs, in the 1970's), POPs still contaminate air, soil and water compartments. Other pollutants may be more quickly degradable, particularly those produced by the plastic industry (phthalates and bisphenols) but because they are produced at very high volumes and massively found in daily consumables they are consistently detected in human body fluids such as plasma or urine, thus reflecting substantial and continuous exposure (16, 17). However regulatory bodies, e.g., the U.S. Environmental Protection agency (EPA) or the European Food Safety Agency (EFSA), do not consider combined exposures in risk assessment procedures or long-term exposure to even the smallest amount of chemicals. Exposure limits are setup for each individual chemical with the definition of reference doses such as the Tolerable Daily Intake (TDI). TDIs are extrapolated from the no or low observed adverse effect level (NoAEL/LoAEL) in experimental studies assuming linearity of the effects and therefore a threshold under which effects will be negligible. With this assumption (which does not apply to genotoxicant carcinogens for which there is no threshold), it can be deduced that risks arising from environmental exposure to chemicals in a real life exposure scenario will be negligible based on the low potency of each chemical of the mixture. But this assumption excludes several aspects linked to environmental exposure and related to the concept of threshold and the supposed linearity of the adverse effects not to mention the effects at low doses. By low doses it is meant environmental doses or concentrations found in biological fluids or doses approaching toxicological reference values (18). This indicates that risk assessment procedures may not be protective enough when it comes to environmental exposure to chemicals and more specifically to EDCs.

EDCS AND SOME OF THEIR CHARACTERISTICS

EDCs are exogenous substances or mixture of chemicals that interfere with any aspect of hormone action, i.e., EDCs can mimic or antagonize hormonal action and interfere with the mechanism of hormonal production, transport or metabolism (12). Energy homeostasis is one of the multiple physiological functions controlled by the endocrine system and as such a target of EDCs. It depends on the integrated action of various hormones including insulin, leptin, growth hormone, thyroid hormones, glucocorticoids but also sex hormones. Importantly, the hormonal interplay intricacies and the nature of the hormones at stake vary with age and sex and the state of maturity of the endocrine function of concern. For example, regulation of metabolism is highly age- and sex- dependent e.g., feeding behavior, distribution of fat masses and insulin

TABLE 1 | Metabolic effects of pollutants in mixture and sex-dimorphism.

Mixture of pollutants	Composition	Animal model	Metabolic effects of the mixture	References
Natural mixture: crude or refined salmon oil in high-fat (HF) diet	mixture of Persistent Organic Pollutants (POPs): organochloride pesticide, Dichlorodiphenyltrichloroéthane (DDTs), dioxins, Polychlorobiphenyls (PCBs)	Adult male Sprague-Dawley rat (28 days of exposure)	HF+ crude oil vs HF: insulin resistance, abdominal obesity, liver steatosis, down-regulation of genes involved in lipid homeostasis (Insig-1 and Lipin 1) in liver	Ruzzin et al. (32)
Very high fat diet (VHF) or Western diet (WD) containing farmed salmon filet (VHF/S and WD/S)	mixture of Persistent Organic Pollutants (POPs): organochloride pesticides, dioxins, furans and Polychlorobiphenyls (PCBs)	8-weeks old male C57BL/6J mice (8 weeks exposure for VHF; 6 weeks for WD)	VHF/S *vs* VHF: aggravation of insulin resistance, visceral obesity and glucose intolerance, adipose tissue inflammation. Increased blood glucose and plasma insulin. WD/S *vs* WD: enhanced body weight, overgrowth of adipose tissue, increased glucose intolerance and insulin resistance with increased plasma insulin	Ibrahim et al. (33)
Combination of four Endocrine Disrupting Chemicals (EDCs) in high fat-high sucrose (HFHS) diet	2,3,7,8-Tetrachlorodibenzo-p-dioxin (TCDD), Polychlorobiphenyls (PCB) 153, Bisphenol A (BPA), di (2-ethylhexyl) phthalate (DEHP) each at reference doses (Tolerable Daily Intake, TDI for Human)	Male and female C57Bl/6J mouse (exposure from pre-conception, gestation to 12 weeks of life)	Sex-dependent metabolic disorders in the absence of weight gain. In males, increased hepatic expression of genes encoding proteins related to cholesterol biosynthesis associated with a decrease in hepatic total cholesterol levels. In females, marked deterioration of glucose tolerance associated with decreased expression of gene encoding ERα as well as estrogen target genes and increased expression of gene encoding the estrogen sulfotransferase SULT1E1.	Naville et al. (34)
Combination of Endocrine Disrupting Chemicals (EDCs) administered intragastrically to the exposed group.	Combination of di (2-ethylhexyl) phthalate, DEHP (15 mg/kg bw) with a mixture of Polychlorobiphenyls, PCBs (Aroclor 1254 at 7.5 mg/Kg bw/day)	female and male mice (12 days of exposure)	Increased liver weight but no difference in body weight; in liver, increased expression of gene encoding Peroxisome Proliferator-Activated Receptor (PPAR)$^{\gamma}$ (males and females), decreased expression of genes encoding Estrogen Receptor (ER)α and phospholipase A (PLA) only in males	Lin et al. (35)
Different combinations of 3 pollutants (2 by 2 or all 3)	Nonylphenol (NP), tert-octylphenol (t-OP), Bisphenol A (BPA) (5 mg/kg bw/day of each)	Juvenile seabream (21 days)	Hepatic steatosis, modulation of the expression of genes involved in lipid metabolism (ppars, lpl, fasn, hsl) mostly using NP+t-OP or BPA+NP. Effects milder than those obtained with one chemical (hypothesis of possible interactions among compounds).	Carnevali et al. (36)
Combination of four Endocrine Disrupting Chemicals (EDCs) in low fat diet	2,3,7,8-Tetrachlorodibenzo-p-dioxin (TCDD), Polychlorobiphenyls (PCB) 153, Bisphenol A (BPA), di (2-ethylhexyl) phthalate (DEHP) each at reference doses (Tolerable Daily Intake, TDI for Human)	female C57Bl6/J mouse (exposure from pre-conception, gestation to 12 weeks of life)	Alteration of lipid homeostasis (increase of hepatic triglycerides) with no difference in body weight or glucose tolerance. Transcriptome analysis in liver highlights dysregulation of genes involved in fatty acid/lipid and circadian clock metabolic pathway. Most of these effects were observed in females and not in males.	Labaronne et al. (37)
Mixture of five prevalent organochlorine pesticides or their metabolites and five Polychlorobiphenyls (PCBs) present in contaminated salmon (32)	Dichlorodiphenyldichloroethylene (p,p'DDE); Dichlorodiphényldichloroéthane (p,p'DDD); hexachlorobenzene, dieldrin, trans-nonachlor, PCB-153, PCB-138, PCB-118, PCB-77, PCB-126 (oral gavage twice weekly during 7 weeks)	5 week-old male wild type C57Bl/6J and male ob/ob mice	Alteration of systemic lipid metabolism in ob/ob mice: increased hepatic triglycerides (TG) with decrease of serum TG levels (no difference either in plasma glucose or insulin levels or in inflammation in liver or adipose tissue). Induction of the expression of *Cyp3a11* in WT mice not in ob/ob mice	Mulligan et al. (38)
Mixture of 13 chemicals	Carbaryl, dimethoate, glyphosate, methomyl, methyl parathion, triadimefon, aspartame, sodium benzoate, Ethylenediaminetetraacetic acid (EDTA), ethylparaben, butylparaben, BPA, acacia gum (6-month exposure in drinking water at three different doses: low, medium and high).	8-week old Female and Male Sprague-Dawley rats	Increased body weight and alteration of hepatotoxic parameters (increased level of total bilirubin, alanine aminotransferase and alkaline phosphatase) even at low dose and only in males. Increased catalase activity with the low doses both in males and females. Also evidence for sex differences in some markers of the redox status (catalase levels, protein carbonyls).	Docea et al. (39)

(Continued)

TABLE 1 | Continued

Mixture of pollutants	Composition	Animal model	Metabolic effects of the mixture	References
Mixture of 4 fungicides and 2 insecticides in standard diet	Ziram; Chlorpyrifos; Thiacloprid; Boscalid; Thiofanate; Captan (52 weeks of exposure; at Tolerable Daily Intake, TDI for Humans)	16-week-old female and male C57BL/6J (WT) and Constitutive Androstane Receptor (CAR)-invalidated mice	In Wild Type (WT) males: increased body weight (not seen in male CAR-/-) and adiposity, hepatic steatosis, fasting hyperglycemia and strong glucose intolerance. In WT females: fasting hyperglycemia and slight glucose intolerance. Pesticide-exposed CAR-/- females exhibited pesticide toxicity with increased body weight and mortality rate. Sexually dimorphic alterations of various metabolic pathways	Lukowicz et al. (40)
Pesticide mixture containing six chemicals at 3 different doses (noted 5–16–37.5%)	Cyromazine, MCPB (4-(4-chloro-2-methylphenoxy) butanoic acid), Pirimicarb, Quinoclamine, Thiram, Ziram (daily oral gavage of pregnant rats from gestation day 7 to pup day 16)	Wistar rats - Male and Female offspring studied until 15 weeks of life	Decreased body weight at birth for both sexes with the highest dose. No difference in body weight after 15 weeks. Differences observed between males and females for several regulatory factors (such as leptin).	Svingen et al. (41)

sensitivity (19). Thus, considering the intrinsic properties of the endocrine system and the definition of the EDCs based on their mode of action and not their chemical structure, the important parameters that should be considered in risk assessment evaluation are: (1) the dose and the non-linearity of the induced effects, (2) the timing and the length of exposure and (3) the simultaneous presence of several chemicals in mixture (18, 20, 21). Additionally, it is emphasized that the less an endocrine function is mature at the time of chemical exposure, the more dramatic health adverse effects will happen defining highly vulnerable periods such as gestation and lactation. For example, ancestral exposure of mice to obesogen chemicals such as organotin tributyltin (TBT) was found to predispose unexposed descendants to obesity (22).

About a thousand of chemicals could display EDC activities (23) and a subset was identified as metabolic disruptors because they favor/aggravate obesity and/or insulin resistance leading to diabetes. Metabolic disruptors may include Bisphenol A (BPA)and dichlorodiphenyltrichloroethane (DDT) but also certain pesticides, perfluorinated compounds and phthalates in addition to TBT. They can target the signaling pathways of different nuclear receptors including the steroid receptors, but also xenobiotic receptors or receptors activated by peroxisome proliferators, PPAR (peroxisome proliferator-activated receptor) and its heterodimeric partner retinoid X receptor (RXR), not to mention non-genomic signaling pathways and cross-talk with the various nuclear receptors (24–27).

EVIDENCES FOR A COCKTAIL EFFECT FROM NATURAL OR ARTIFICIAL MIXTURES ON METABOLIC DISRUPTION AND ITS SEX-DIMORPHISM

First evidences of a cocktail effect resulting from exposure to environmental mixtures were brought by scientists invested in Biology of Reproduction with the demonstration of additive effects in mixtures containing chemicals sharing a similar mechanism of action and combined in mixtures at concentrations that individually do not result in observable adverse effects. This was called the something from "nothing" phenomenon demonstrated originally with a mixture of 8 weak estrogenic chemicals (28) but also using combinations of anti-androgens (29) or more complex mixtures of anti-androgenic pesticides, antioxidants, industrial pollutants and chemicals present in personal care products (30). The concept of additivity was also the basis of the Toxic Equivalent Factor (TEF) set up by the WHO (31) to facilitate risk assessment of "natural" mixtures of dioxins, furans and dioxin-like PCBs, using the dioxin of Seveso (named after the industrial explosion in the village of Seveso, Italy), the most potent in activating the aryl hydrocarbon receptor (AhR), as reference.

First demonstrations of mixture effects in the metabolic disruption field area emerged less than 10 years ago (**Table 1**) when it was observed that rats fed refined salmon oil for 28 days exhibited better metabolic outcomes than rats fed crude salmon oil (32). These experiments suggested that exposure to POPs commonly present in food chains could trigger enhanced body weight and visceral fat, liver steatosis, glucose intolerance and insulin resistance (32) as well as chronic low-grade inflammation in adipose tissue (33). A few years later, we brought (34) the proof-of-concept study that a mixture of low-dosed pollutants not sharing similar mechanisms of action, could trigger metabolic disturbances in mice. Our original model was designed to take into consideration several parameters of the real life including chronic exposure at low doses covering all developmental stages from the fetal period to adult onwards. It even started when dams were immature females of 5 weeks of age. Both male and female mice (and not only adult males as classically studied) were evaluated to explore the sex-biased mechanisms linked to endocrine disruption. The pollutant cocktail was incorporated in either a high-fat high-sucrose (HFHS) diet (34) or a standard diet (37) to reflect different nutritional situations also considering that food is a primary route of exposure. Thus, we selected pollutants known to contaminate food and not sharing similar mechanisms of action to better reflect a "real" scenario of exposure. The mixture was made of two persistent pollutants including the most powerful dioxin (2,3,7,8-Tetrachlorodibenzo-*p*-dioxin, TCDD) and the most abundant of the non-dioxin like PCBs (PCB153). The other two were short-lived pollutants including BPA, one of the substances most investigated for its endocrine disrupting activities (18, 42, 43) and the di-[2-ethylhexyl] phthalate (DEHP) largely used to soften plastics. Each chemical in the mixture was used at a dose in the range of its tolerable daily intake (TDI). With regards to their modes of action, these well-recognized EDCs display mostly estrogeno-mimetic and anti-androgenic activities for BPA and DEHP, respectively, while dioxins interact with AhR and non-dioxin like PCBs may interact with other xenobiotic receptors such as constitutive androstane receptor (CAR) and pregnane X receptor (PXR) (18, 24, 44, 45). Moreover, interaction of pollutants of the mixture may also occur with other receptors like thyroid receptors or glucocorticoid receptors not to mention extensive cross-talks which may occur via direct or indirect interaction with metabolic pathways regulating energy homeostasis as reviewed elsewhere (8, 24). With such a model, we originally demonstrated that the metabolic adverse impact in mice exposed to the mixture lifelong occurs in the absence of any weight gain but was strongly sex-dependent (34, 46), and also related to the age of the animals (47) and their nutritional environment (37). The female offspring exposed to the mixture incorporated in a HFHS diet exhibited aggravated glucose intolerance, impaired estrogen signaling in liver and enhanced expression of inflammatory markers in the adipose tissue at adulthood as compared to non-exposed females. This suggested that pollutants could lessen the protection of estrogens against the development of metabolic diseases. Importantly, these effects were not observed in younger females or in males which are characterized by different hormonal milieu in line with endocrine disrupting effects. Males had impaired cholesterol metabolism resulting from enhancement of genes encoding proteins related to cholesterol synthesis and degradation in bile salts when fed a HFHS diet containing the mixture of pollutants (34, 47). The observed metabolic impact in females was dependent on the nutritional context as female mice fed a standard diet and exposed similarly to the mixture showed alteration of lipid homeostasis with no difference in body weight or glucose tolerance (37). Importantly, pollutants elicited distinct and common features as compared to a HFHS diet as revealed by a comparative hepatic transcriptomic study. Among features resulting from pollutant exposure in the liver was the finding of several dysregulated genes belonging to the circadian clock metabolic pathway including major canonical genes of the core clock (*Period circadian regulators 1-3*, *Arntl1* encoding BMAL1 and *Clock*) and clock regulators thus highlighting circadian disruption (37). None of the described effects observed in females were described in males pointing to the sex-dimorphic impact of pollutants consistent with the sex-dimorphic regulation of energy homeostasis (48) (**Table 1**).

Other combinations of low-dosed pollutants in mixture have later been tested in mouse (35, 38, 40) or rat (41) models as well as in juvenile seabream (36). These studies also reported significant alterations of the hepatic gene signature consistent with the liver being the primary site for detoxification (**Table 1**). Interestingly, whenever males and females have been studied, sex-differences have also been observed (35, 40, 41) as compiled (**Table 1**) which highlights the necessity, as mandated by the National Institutes of Health (NIH), to consider sex as a biological variable (49). Also consistent with our data (34, 37), it was shown that the nutritional component was as well a variable to consider. Indeed, exposure to a mixture of POPs (38), to dioxins (50) or to a pharmaceutical drug cocktail (51) resulted in differential metabolic responses between lean and obese mice. Outcomes surveyed included hepatic steatosis and systemic lipid metabolism (38), hyperglycaemia and hepatic mitochondrial function (51) and hepatic fibrosis (50). Whether this is linked to substantial alterations of the expression of hepatic xenobiotic processed genes (37, 52), resulting in differential ability of the liver to detoxify chemicals, warrants further studies.

CONCLUSIONS

The current legislation on chemical risk assessment is definitely obsolete and needs to be updated to take into account the cocktail effect of mixtures. This is certainly a major challenge for the near future as environmental pollutants are risk factors for numerous pathologies also including cancers and hormono-dependent cancers among them, for which obesity is a risk factor (7). Importantly, it was assumed that the carcinogenic potential of chemical mixtures may be more important than that of individual carcinogens in the real world (53). It will also be critical to enhance our knowledge on chemical toxicity as according to the US EPA, it is available for less than 20% of substances produced at significant amounts, worldwide (54). While additivity was demonstrated for mixture of low-dosed chemicals affecting similar outcomes (55), when it comes to mixtures with molecules acting differently, which better fits the real life scenario, the problem becomes more complex because chemical actions may (41, 56) or may not be independent. For example, in an *in vitro* model of mesenchymal cells, BPA, DEHP and TBT could not be deduced from single compound experiments (57). As well synergistic activation of human PXR was observed in an *in vitro* model of hepatocytes (HepG2) by binary cocktails of pharmaceutical and environmental compounds (58). Another limitation to the additivity concept of cocktail effect lies in the fact that a pollutant can alter the metabolism of another pollutant present in the mixture and potentially its bioavailability (59). Moreover, some products may, by modifying the epigenome, leave an imprint on unexposed generations as recently demonstrated with TBT on RXR activation (60).

The problem posed by the cocktail effect is a virtually insurmountable challenge but it will have to be overcome for the sake of public health. Political authorities should work to reduce the exponential production of industrial chemicals. In addition, integrative approaches combining knowledge gathered in epidemiologic and biomonitoring studies, but also experimental, *in vitro* and *in silico* studies, together with computational approaches to construct predictive models, will certainly help at moving a path forward.

AUTHOR CONTRIBUTIONS

The manuscript was written by BLM. DN created the Table and participated in the editing of the manuscript. HV participated in the editing of the manuscript. All authors approved the final version of the manuscript.

FUNDING

This work was supported by INSERM and University of Lyon1 to INSERM U1060.

REFERENCES

1. WHO. *World Health Organization, Obesity and Overweight, Fact Sheet 311.* (2014). Available online at: http://www.who.int/mediacentre/factsheets/fs311/en/
2. WHO. *World Health Organization, Diabetes, Fact Sheet 312.* (2016). Available online at: http://www.who.int/mediacentre/factsheets/fs312/en/
3. Dobbs R, Sawers C, Thompson F, Manyika J, Woetzel J, Child P, et al. *Overcoming Obesity: An Initial Economic Analysis.* Jakarta: McKinsey Global Institute. (2014). Available online at: https://www.mckinsey.com/~/media/McKinsey/Business%20Functions/Economic%20Studies%20TEMP/Our%20Insights/How%20the%20world%20could%20better%20fight%20obesity/MGI_Overcoming_obesity_Full_report.ashx
4. Tremmel M, Gerdtham UG, Nilsson PM, Saha S. Economic burden of obesity: a systematic literature review. *Int J Environ Res Public Health* (2017) 14:435. doi: 10.3390/ijerph14040435
5. Alonso-Magdalena P, Quesada I, Nadal A. Endocrine disruptors in the etiology of type 2 diabetes mellitus. *Nat Rev Endocrinol.* (2011) 7:346–53. doi: 10.1038/nrendo.2011.56
6. Baillie-Hamilton PF. Chemical toxins: a hypothesis to explain the global obesity epidemic. *J Altern Complement Med.* (2002) 8:185–92. doi: 10.1089/107555302317371479
7. Gore AC, Chappell VA, Fenton SE, Flaws JA, Nadal A, Prins GS, et al. EDC-2: The endocrine society's second scientific statement on endocrine-disrupting chemicals. *Endocr Rev.* (2015) 36:E1–E150. doi: 10.1210/er.2015-1010
8. Le Magueresse-Battistoni B, Labaronne E, Vidal H, Naville D. Endocrine disrupting chemicals in mixture and obesity, diabetes and related metabolic disorders. *World J Biol Chem.* (2017) 8:108–19. doi: 10.4331/wjbc.v8.i2.108
9. Le Magueresse-Battistoni B, Vidal H, Naville D. Lifelong consumption of low-dosed food pollutants and metabolic health. *J Epidemiol Community Health* (2015) 69:512–5. doi: 10.1136/jech-2014-203913
10. Lind PM, and Lind L. Endocrine-disrupting chemicals and risk of diabetes: an evidence-based review. *Diabetologia* (2018) 61:1495–502. doi: 10.1007/s00125-018-4621-3
11. Thayer KA, Heindel JJ, Bucher JR, and Gallo MA. Role of environmental chemicals in diabetes and obesity: a National Toxicology Program workshop review. *Environ Health Perspect.* (2012) 120:779–89. doi: 10.1289/ehp.1104597
12. Zoeller RT, Bergman A, Becher G, Bjerregaard P, Bornman R, Brandt I, et al. A path forward in the debate over health impacts of endocrine disrupting chemicals. *Environ Health* (2014) 13:118. doi: 10.1186/1476-069X-13-118
13. Barouki R, Gluckman PD, Grandjean P, Hanson M, Heindel JJ. Developmental origins of non-communicable disease: implications for research and public health. *Environ Health* (2012) 11:42. doi: 10.1186/1476-069X-11-42
14. Gluckman PD, Hanson MA, Cooper C, Thornburg KL. Effect of in utero and early-life conditions on adult health and disease. *N Engl J Med.* (2008) 359:61–73. doi: 10.1056/NEJMra0708473
15. Milbrath MO, Wenger Y, Chang CW, Emond C, Garabrant D, Gillespie BW, et al. Apparent half-lives of dioxins, furans, and polychlorinated biphenyls as a function of age, body fat, smoking status, and breast-feeding. *Environ Health Perspect.* (2009) 117:417–25. doi: 10.1289/ehp.11781
16. Koch HM, Calafat AM. Human body burdens of chemicals used in plastic manufacture. *Philos Trans R Soc Lond B Biol Sci.* (2009) 364:2063–78. doi: 10.1098/rstb.2008.0208
17. Vandenberg LN, Hauser R, Marcus M, Olea N, Welshons WV. Human exposure to bisphenol A (BPA). *Reprod Toxicol.* (2007) 24:139–77. doi: 10.1016/j.reprotox.2007.07.010
18. Vandenberg LN, Colborn T, Hayes TB, Heindel JJ, Jacobs DR Jr, Lee DH, et al. Hormones and endocrine-disrupting chemicals: low-dose effects and nonmonotonic dose responses. *Endocr Rev.* (2012) 33:378–455. doi: 10.1210/er.2011-1050
19. Mauvais-Jarvis F, Clegg DJ, Hevener AL. The role of estrogens in control of energy balance and glucose homeostasis. *Endocr Rev.* (2013) 34:309–38. doi: 10.1210/er.2012-1055
20. Vandenberg LN, Colborn T, Hayes TB, Heindel JJ, Jacobs DR Jr, Lee DH, et al. Regulatory decisions on endocrine disrupting chemicals should be based on the principles of endocrinology. *Reprod Toxicol.* (2013) 38:1–15. doi: 10.1016/j.reprotox.2013.02.002
21. Barouki R. Endocrine disruptors: Revisiting concepts and dogma in toxicology. *C R Biol.* (2017) 340:410–3. doi: 10.1016/j.crvi.2017.07.005
22. Heindel JJ, Blumberg B. Environmental obesogens: mechanisms and controversies. *Annu Rev Pharmacol Toxicol.* (2018) doi: 10.1146/annurev-pharmtox-010818-021304. [Epub ahead of print].
23. WHO/UNEP. State of the science of endocrine disrupting chemicals—2012. In: Bergman Å, Heindel JJ, Jobling S, Kidd KA, Zoeller RT, editors. *An Assessment of the State of the Science of Endocrine Disruptors Prepared by a Group of Experts for the United Nations Environment Programme (UNEP) and WHO.* (2013). Available online at: http://www.who.int/ceh/publications/endocrine/en/
24. Casals-Casas C, Desvergne B. Endocrine disruptors: from endocrine to metabolic disruption. *Annu Rev Physiol.* (2011) 73:135–62. doi: 10.1146/annurev-physiol-012110-142200
25. Chamorro-Garcia R, Shoucri BM, Willner S, Kach H, Janesick A, Blumberg B. Effects of perinatal exposure to dibutyltin chloride on fat and glucose metabolism in mice, and molecular mechanisms, *in vitro. Environ Health Perspect.* (2018) 126:057006. doi: 10.1289/EHP3030
26. Heindel JJ, Blumberg B, Cave M, Machtinger R, Mantovani A, Mendez MA, et al. Metabolism disrupting chemicals and metabolic disorders. *Reprod Toxicol.* (2017) 68:3–33. doi: 10.1016/j.reprotox.2016.10.001
27. Nadal A, Quesada I, Tuduri E, Nogueiras R, Alonso-Magdalena P. Endocrine-disrupting chemicals and the regulation of energy balance. *Nat Rev Endocrinol.* (2017) 13:536–546. doi: 10.1038/nrendo.2017.51
28. Silva E, Rajapakse N, Kortenkamp A. Something from "nothing"–eight weak estrogenic chemicals combined at concentrations below NOECs produce significant mixture effects. *Environ Sci Technol.* (2002) 36:1751–6. doi: 10.1021/es0101227
29. Hass U, Scholze M, Christiansen S, Dalgaard M, Vinggaard AM, Axelstad M, et al. Combined exposure to anti-androgens exacerbates disruption of sexual differentiation in the rat. *Environ Health Perspect.* (2007) 115(Suppl. 1):122–8. doi: 10.1289/ehp.9360
30. Orton F, Ermler S, Kugathas S, Rosivatz E, Scholze M, Kortenkamp A. Mixture effects at very low doses with combinations of anti-androgenic pesticides, antioxidants, industrial pollutant and chemicals used in personal care products. *Toxicol Appl Pharmacol.* (2014) 278:201–8. doi: 10.1016/j.taap.2013.09.008
31. Van den Berg M, Birnbaum L, Bosveld AT, Brunstrom B, Cook P, Feeley M, et al. Toxic equivalency factors (TEFs) for PCBs, PCDDs, PCDFs for humans and wildlife. *Environ Health Perspect.* (1998) 106:775–92. doi: 10.1289/ehp.98106775
32. Ruzzin J, Petersen R, Meugnier E, Madsen L, Lock EJ, Lillefosse H, et al. Persistent organic pollutant exposure leads to insulin resistance syndrome. *Environ Health Perspect.* (2010) 118:465–71. doi: 10.1289/ehp.0901321

33. Ibrahim MM, Fjaere E, Lock EJ, Naville D, Amlund H, Meugnier E, et al. Chronic consumption of farmed salmon containing persistent organic pollutants causes insulin resistance and obesity in mice. *PLoS ONE* (2011) 6:e25170. doi: 10.1371/journal.pone.0025170
34. Naville D, Pinteur C, Vega N, Menade Y, Vigier M, Le Bourdais A, et al. Low-dose food contaminants trigger sex-specific, hepatic metabolic changes in the progeny of obese mice. *FASEB J.* (2013) 27:3860–70. doi: 10.1096/fj.13-231670
35. Lin Y, Min L, Huang Q, Chen Y, Fang C, Sun X, et al. The combined effects of DEHP and PCBs on phospholipase in the livers of mice. *Environ Toxicol.* (2015) 30:197–204. doi: 10.1002/tox.21885
36. Carnevali O, Notarstefano V, Olivotto I, Graziano M, Gallo P, I. Di Marco Pisciottano, et al. Dietary administration of EDC mixtures: a focus on fish lipid metabolism. *Aquat Toxicol.* (2017) 185:95–104. doi: 10.1016/j.aquatox.2017.02.007
37. Labaronne E, Pinteur C, Vega N, Pesenti S, Julien B, Meugnier-Fouilloux E, et al. Low-dose pollutant mixture triggers metabolic disturbances in female mice leading to common and specific features as compared to a high-fat diet. *J Nutr Biochem.* (2017) 45:83–93. doi: 10.1016/j.jnutbio.2017.04.001
38. Mulligan C, Kondakala S, Yang EJ, Stokes JV, Stewart JA, Kaplan BL, et al. Exposure to an environmentally relevant mixture of organochlorine compounds and polychlorinated biphenyls Promotes hepatic steatosis in male Ob/Ob mice. *Environ Toxicol.* (2017) 32:1399–411. doi: 10.1002/tox.22334
39. Docea AO, Gofita E, Goumenou M, Calina D, Rogoveanu O, Varut M, et al. Six months exposure to a real life mixture of 13 chemicals' below individual NOAELs induced non monotonic sex-dependent biochemical and redox status changes in rats. *Food Chem Toxicol.* (2018) 115:470–81. doi: 10.1016/j.fct.2018.03.052
40. Lukowicz C, Ellero-Simatos C, Régnier M, Polizzi A, Lasserre F, Montagner A, et al. Metabolic effects of achronic dietary exposure to a low-dose pesticide cocktail in mice: sexual dimorphism and role of the constitutive androstane receptor. *Environ Health Perspect.* (2018) 126:067007. doi: 10.1289/EHP2877
41. Svingen T, Ramhoj L, Mandrup K, Christiansen S, Axelstad M, Vinggaard AM, et al. Effects on metabolic parameters in young rats born with low birth weight after exposure to a mixture of pesticides. *Sci Rep.* (2018) 8:305. doi: 10.1038/s41598-017-18626-x
42. Le Magueresse-Battistoni B, Multigner L, Beausoleil C, and Rousselle C. Effects of bisphenol A on metabolism and evidences of a mode of action mediated through endocrine disruption. *Mol Cell Endocrinol.* (2018) 475:74–91. doi: 10.1016/j.mce.2018.02.009
43. Beausoleil C, Emond C, Cravedi JP, Antignac JP, Applanat M, Appenzeller MR, et al. Regulatory identification of BPA as an endocrine disruptor: context and methodology. *Mol Cell Endocrinol.* (2018) 475:4-9. doi: 10.1016/j.mce.2018.02.001.
44. Mimoto MS, Nadal A, and Sargis RM. Polluted pathways: mechanisms of metabolic disruption by endocrine disrupting chemicals. *Curr Environ Health Rep.* (2017) 4:208–22. doi: 10.1007/s40572-017-0137-0
45. Nadal A, Fuentes E, Ripoll C, Villar-Pazos S, Castellano-Munoz M, Soriano S, et al. Extranuclear-initiated estrogenic actions of endocrine disrupting chemicals: Is there toxicology beyond paracelsus? *J Steroid Biochem Mol Biol.* (2018) 176:16–22. doi: 10.1016/j.jsbmb.2017.01.014
46. Le Magueresse-Battistoni B, Vidal H, and Naville D. Sex-specific metabolic alterations induced by environmental pollutants. *Curr Opin Toxicol.* (2018) 8:1–7. doi: 10.1016/j.cotox.2017.11.007
47. Naville D, Labaronne E, Vega N, Pinteur C, Canet-Soulas E, Vidal H, et al. Metabolic outcome of female mice exposed to a mixture of low-dose pollutants in a diet-induced obesity model. *PLoS ONE* (2015) 10:e0124015. doi: 10.1371/journal.pone.0124015
48. Mauvais-Jarvis F. Sex differences in metabolic homeostasis, diabetes, and obesity. *Biol Sex Differ.* (2015) 6:14. doi: 10.1186/s13293-015-0033-y
49. Mauvais-Jarvis F, Arnold AP, Reue K. A Guide for the design of pre-clinical studies on sex differences in metabolism. *Cell Metab.* (2017) 25:1216–30. doi: 10.1016/j.cmet.2017.04.033
50. Duval C, Teixeira-Clerc F, Leblanc AF, Touch S, Emond C, Guerre-Millo M, et al. Chronic exposure to low doses of dioxin promotes liver fibrosis development in the C57BL/6J diet-induced obesity mouse model. *Environ Health Perspect.* (2017) 125:428–36. doi: 10.1289/EHP316
51. Buron N, Porceddu M, Roussel C, Begriche K, Trak-Smayra V, Gicquel T, et al. Chronic and low exposure to a pharmaceutical cocktail induces mitochondrial dysfunction in liver and hyperglycemia: Differential responses between lean and obese mice. *Environ Toxicol.* (2017) 32:1375–89. doi: 10.1002/tox.22331
52. Oshida K, Waxman DJ, Corton JC. Chemical and hormonal effects on STAT5b-dependent sexual dimorphism of the liver transcriptome. *PLoS ONE* (2016) 11:e0150284. doi: 10.1371/journal.pone.0150284
53. Lee DH, Jacobs DR Jr, Park HY, Carpenter DO. A role of low dose chemical mixtures in adipose tissue in carcinogenesis. *Environ Int.* (2017) 108:170–5. doi: 10.1016/j.envint.2017.08.015
54. Sarigiannis DA, Hansen U. Considering the cumulative risk of mixtures of chemicals - a challenge for policy makers. *Environ Health* (2012) 11(Suppl. 1):S18. doi: 10.1186/1476-069X-11-S1-S18
55. Kortenkamp A. Low dose mixture effects of endocrine disrupters and their implications for regulatory thresholds in chemical risk assessment. *Curr Opin Pharmacol.* (2014) 19:105–11. doi: 10.1016/j.coph.2014.08.006
56. Kortenkamp A. Ten years of mixing cocktails: a review of combination effects of endocrine-disrupting chemicals. *Environ Health Perspect.* (2007) 115(Suppl. 1):98–105. doi: 10.1289/ehp.9357
57. Biemann R, Fischer B, Navarrete Santos A. Adipogenic effects of a combination of the endocrine-disrupting compounds bisphenol A, diethylhexylphthalate, and tributyltin. *Obes Facts* (2014) 7:48–56. doi: 10.1159/000358913
58. Delfosse V, Dendele B, Huet T, Grimaldi M, Boulahtouf A, Gerbal-Chaloin S, et al. Synergistic activation of human pregnane X receptor by binary cocktails of pharmaceutical and environmental compounds. *Nat Commun.* (2015) 6:8089. doi: 10.1038/ncomms9089
59. Pollock T, Weaver RE, Ghasemi R, deCatanzaro D. A mixture of five endocrine-disrupting chemicals modulates concentrations of bisphenol A and estradiol in mice. *Chemosphere* (2018) 193:321–8. doi: 10.1016/j.chemosphere.2017.11.030.
60. Shoucri BM, Hung VT, Chamorro-Garcia R, Shioda T, Blumberg B. Retinoid X receptor activation during adipogenesis of female mesenchymal stem cells programs a dysfunctional adipocyte. *Endocrinology* (2018) 159:2863–83. doi: 10.1210/en.2018-00056

11

Persistent Organic Pollutants and Type 2 Diabetes

Yu-Mi Lee [1], *David R. Jacobs Jr.* [2] *and Duk-Hee Lee* [1,3*]

[1] *Department of Preventive Medicine, School of Medicine, Kyungpook National University, Daegu, South Korea,* [2] *Division of Epidemiology and Community Health, School of Public Health, University of Minnesota, Minneapolis, MN, United States,* [3] *BK21 Plus KNU Biomedical Convergence Program, Department of Biomedical Science, Kyungpook National University, Daegu, South Korea*

Correspondence:
Duk-Hee Lee
lee_dh@knu.ac.kr

Low dose persistent organic pollutants (POPs) have emerged as a new risk for type 2 diabetes (T2D). Despite substantial evidence from human and experimental studies, there are several critical issues which have not been properly addressed by POPs researchers. First, as POPs exist as mixtures, findings about POPs from human studies should be interpreted from the viewpoint of lipophilic chemical mixtures which include both measured and unmeasured POPs. Second, as POPs can directly reduce insulin secretion of beta cells, the role of POPs may be more prominent in the development of beta-cell dysfunction-dominant T2D rather than insulin resistance-dominant T2D. Third, there are multidimensional interrelationships between POPs and adipose tissue. Even though POPs are now considered as a new risk factor for T2D, independent of obesity, POPs and obesity are mechanistically linked to each other. POPs are involved in key mechanisms linking obesity and T2D, such as chronic inflammation of adipose tissue and lipotoxicity with ectopic fat accumulation. Also, POPs can explain puzzling human findings which suggest benefits of obesity because healthy adipose tissue can be protective by reducing the amount of POPs reaching other organs. Fourth, non-linear dose-response relationships between POPs and T2D are biologically possible. Although POPs are well-known endocrine disrupting chemicals (EDCs), mitochondrial dysfunction may be a more plausible mechanism due to unpredictability of EDC mixtures. As adipose tissue plays a role as an internal exposure source of POPs, how to manage POPs inside us may be essential to protect against harms of POPs.

Keywords: chemical mixtures, diabetes, insulin resistance, obesity, organochlorine pesticides, persistent organic pollutants, polychlorinated biphenyls

INTRODUCTION

Persistent organic pollutants (POPs) include a wide range of organic compounds which are resistant to degradation by chemical or biological processes. As a result, they are highly persistent in the environment and bio-accumulate in living organisms. Typical examples are chlorinated POPs such as organochlorine pesticides (OCPs), polychlorinated biphenyls (PCBs), or dioxins, brominated POPs such as polybrominated diphenyl ethers, or fluorinated POPs such as perfluoroalkyl and polyfluoroalkyl substances.

Although toxicity of high dose POPs is well-known, the recent concern is the possibility of adverse effects of low dose POPs, similar to the current environmental exposure levels. Among many diseases suspected to be linked to low dose POPs, type 2 diabetes (T2D) is the most convincing, given substantial evidence from both epidemiological and experimental studies.

Since 2010, we identified nine published review articles about human studies on POPs and T2D (1–9). Therefore, rather than adding one more ordinary review article on the same topic, this narrative review was written to bring up several provocative issues which are commonly missed by epidemiologists on POPs and T2D.

First, we briefly summarize the nine published review articles on POPs and T2D based on their own conclusions, rather than presenting our own quantitative analyses. Then we discuss (1) the importance of POPs as mixtures, (2) the role of POPs in inducing beta-cell dysfunction, (3) multi-dimensional interrelationships between POPs and adipose tissue, and (4) non-linear dose response relationships. Consideration of these aspects leads us to debate why currently prevailing actions (including regulations and suggestions for avoidance of POPs) focused on individual chemicals are not effective in protecting the public from POPs-related risk.

In this review, the focus is low dose environmental exposure, not occupational or accidental high dose exposure. Also, among various POP compounds, we deal with chlorinated POPs because they are ones which have shown the most consistent results in human studies. The evidence from brominated or fluorinated POPs is weak and inconsistent (9). Thus, unless we specify brominated or fluorinated, POPs means chlorinated POPs in this review.

TABLE 1 | Summary of review articles about epidemiological studies of persistent organic pollutants (POPs) and type 2 diabetes (T2D).

Authors	Publication year	Verbatim conclusion from each review
Taylor et al. (1)	2013	The overall evidence is sufficient for a positive association of some organochlorine POPs with type 2 diabetes.
Wu et al. (2)	2013	These findings support an association between POP exposure and the risk of T2D.
Lee et al. (3)	2014	The evidence as a whole suggests that, rather than a few individual POPs, background exposure to POP mixtures-including organochlorine pesticides and polychlorinated biphenyls-can increase T2D risk in humans.
Magliano et al. (4)	2014	In summary, while the overall evidence is strongly suggestive of an independent relationship between POPs and diabetes, some inconsistencies exist.
Ngwa et al. (5)	2015	Despite different levels of risk in prospective studies and inconsistent results, the causal effect of POPs on diabetes is supported by *in-vitro* and *in-vivo* experimental studies.
Jaacks et al. (6)	2015	The literature suggests a positive association between select POPs and diabetes.
Song et al. (7)	2016	Serum concentrations of persistent EDCs* were significantly associated with T2D risk.
Evangelou et al. (8)	2016	Data suggest an association between organochlorine exposure and type 2 diabetes
Lind et al. (9)	2018	Evidence is accumulating that EDCs* might be involved in diabetes development. Best evidence exists for p,p'-DDE.

EDCs (endocrine disrupting chemicals), POPs are classified as EDCs.

A BRIEF SUMMARY OF REVIEW ARTICLES ON HUMAN STUDIES ON POPs AND T2D

Table 1 summarizes conclusions from review articles about POPs and T2D which were published since 2010 (1–9). Sentences in the "Conclusion" column were extracted from abstract, highlights, and main findings without any modification. Some reviews focused on POPs while others covered a wide range of endocrine disrupting chemicals (EDCs; POPs were considered to be EDCs).

Although they include systemic reviews, meta-analyses, and narrative reviews, all reviews concluded that there is potentially a role of POPs in the development of T2D despite some inconsistencies and research gaps. However, there are several critical issues which have not been properly considered in most original articles and reviews about POPs and T2D. As they can substantially influence the establishment of causality, the discussion of these issues can be helpful to understand the findings from published articles and plan future epidemiological studies.

CRITICAL ISSUES FOR HUMAN STUDIES OF POPs AND T2D

POPS as a Surrogate Marker of Lipophilic Chemical Mixtures

Most human studies about POPs and T2D have adopted individual chemical-based analyses. Namely, they measured serum concentrations of several or dozens of compounds belonging to POPs, evaluated individual associations between specific compounds and T2D, and interpreted their results focusing on those specific compounds which showed statistical significance. As a result, most reviews also followed the same strategy. In some reviews, only specific compounds such as hexachlorobenzene, p,p'-DDE, and PCBs, but not others, were considered to be linked to the risk of T2D (2, 9).

However, this approach should be reconsidered because recent human studies about POPs and T2D have been performed among general populations. It is well-known that there are substantial positive correlations among serum concentrations of various POP compounds (10, 11). Therefore, the epidemiologic findings on POPs should not be interpreted from the viewpoint of individual compounds which were directly measured and demonstrated statistical significance. The key feature of environmental exposure to POPs is the chronic exposure to the mixture of a variety of lipophilic chemicals at low dose even though absolute concentrations of individual compounds are variable. Focusing only on several compounds can largely distort the whole picture.

In most epidemiological studies, serum concentrations of POPs have been used as an exposure marker of POPs. Although concentrations of most synthetic chemicals measured in blood or urine are indicators of the current or recent exposure levels from the environment, serum concentrations of POPs are different. Humans are exposed to POPs through external exposure sources such as POPs-contaminated food. However, once POPs enter the body, they are primarily stored in adipose tissue and slowly released into the circulation to be eliminated over several years (12). Therefore, ultimately serum concentrations of POPs are largely determined by (1) the amount of POPs released from adipose tissue to circulation and (2) the amount of POPs eliminated from circulation.

In this situation, the findings about POPs in human studies should be interpreted beyond the compounds which are directly measured in each study. Measured POPs should be considered as surrogate markers of lipophilic chemical mixtures which include measured POPs, but also include unmeasured ones. This point has an important implication regarding how to approach the issue of POPs to protect the public. For example, even if we succeeded in completely eliminating specific POPs, this may not lead to the decrease of POPs-related disease because we have done nothing with other lipophilic chemicals which coexist with the eliminated POPs in the mixture. This aspect of POPs suggests that the most effective public health action to reduce harms from POPs should target lipophilic chemical mixtures.

Role of POPs in Inducing Beta-Cell Dysfunction

T2D is increasingly recognized as a heterogeneous condition, ranging from predominantly insulin resistance with relative insulin deficiency to predominantly an insulin secretory defect with insulin resistance (13). Although most epidemiological studies about POPs have evaluated T2D as a whole, the role of POPs may differ depending on subtypes of T2D.

Obesity is the most important risk factor for insulin resistance-dominant T2D, however the role of adiposity is weak in T2D preceded predominantly by beta-cell dysfunction (14). Genetic predisposition has been considered a key determinant of beta-cell function (15), but the role of genes is still largely unknown despite many genome-wide association studies(16).

Environmental chemicals such as POPs can play a role in the development of beta-cell dysfunction (17). Although animal experimental studies have reported that the exposure to POPs can induce insulin resistance (18, 19), human studies evaluating both insulin resistance and insulin secretion have reported that serum concentrations of POPs were more strongly associated with decreased insulin secretion than with increased insulin resistance (20–23). An *in-vitro* cell study demonstrated that POPs can directly reduce insulin secretion at very low dose such as 1 pmol/L (23).

As decreased insulin secretion is a necessary step in developing both types of T2D, POPs can explain both types of T2D. However, the role of POPs may be more salient in beta-cell dysfunction-dominant T2D than insulin resistance-dominant T2D because the overproduction of insulin by pancreatic beta-cells during insulin resistance can mask the direct effect of POPs on beta-cell function (23). Also, POPs can explain why beta-cell dysfunction-dominant T2D is common in Asian and elderly people (24–26) who tend to have high serum concentrations of OCPs (27, 28).

Multi-Dimensional Aspects of Interrelationships Between POPs and Adipose Tissue

POPs have been evaluated as a new risk factor for T2D, independent of traditional risk factors for T2D such as obesity or lack of physical activity. As a result, in epidemiological studies of POPs and T2D, obesity has been considered as a confounder. However, obesity cannot be a simple confounder in the relationship between POPs and T2D. The role of POPs should be comprehensively evaluated and interpreted, considering possibly interactive roles with obesity, due to their innate interrelationship.

Under the current paradigm, obesity is a key risk factor for many insulin resistance-related diseases such as T2D. Several mechanisms explain how obesity can increase these diseases. First, obesity can induce chronic inflammation of adipose tissue and release pro-inflammatory cytokines (29). Second, obesity increases the release of free fatty acid to circulation and promotes fat deposits in ectopic sites such as liver, muscle, and pancreas (30).

However, POPs may participate in all these mechanisms, explained in detail below. Also, POPs can explain some puzzling findings on obesity which cannot be explained by the current paradigm of obesity. We present five different possible dimensions linking POPs and adipose tissue (**Figure 1**). Among them, dimensions 1 and 2 show that POPs can explain traditional obesity-related harmful effects while dimensions 3 and 4 show that POPs can explain puzzling findings on obesity. Dimension 5 casts a question on the current prevailing viewpoint which directly links obesogen-inducing chemicals to diabetes-inducing chemicals. All these issues are critical to understand the role of POPs in humans in a more comprehensive way and also to contrive effective ways to protect the public from POPs.

Dimension 1: POPs in Adipose Tissue Can Induce Inflammation in Adipose Tissue

Adipose tissue is not only a reservoir of chronic internal POPs exposure, but also a possible tissue pathologic target of POPs (31). *In-vivo* and *in-vitro* experimental studies reported that low dose POPs can induce pro-inflammatory change in adipose tissue (18, 19, 31–34). Importantly, POPs-induced inflammation is possible regardless of obesity (19).

A topic for future studies is the interesting speculation that obesity can exacerbate the inflammatory effects of POPs. For example, if POPs are released from lipid droplets of adipocytes to interstitial spaces through necrosis of the hypertrophic adipocytes which are common among obese persons (35), the existence of poorly degradable foreign bodies such as POPs can trigger an adipose tissue immune response.

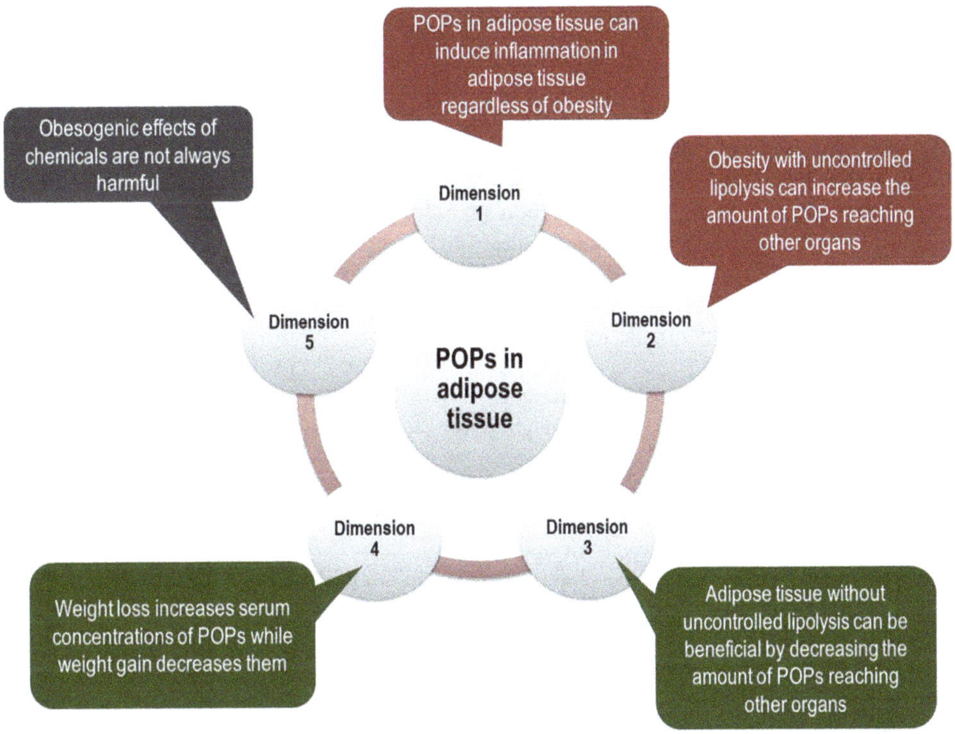

FIGURE 1 | Multi-dimensional aspects of interrelationships between persistent organic pollutants (POPs) and adipose tissue. Even though POPs have been evaluated as a new risk factor for type 2 diabetes (T2D), independent of obesity, the role of POPs should be evaluated together with obesity due to their innate interrelationship. POPs are involved in key mechanisms linking obesity and T2D such as pro-inflammatory adipose tissue and ectopic fat accumulation (Dimensions 1 and 2). In addition, POPs can explain puzzling findings about obesity, which suggest beneficial effects of adipose tissue (Dimensions 3 and 4). Finally, obesogenic effects of chemicals may not always be harmful (Dimension 5). All these issues are critical to understand the role of POPs in the development of T2D.

Dimension 2: Obesity With Uncontrolled Lipolysis Can Increase the Amount of POPs Reaching Other Organs

At normal physiological conditions, lipolysis rates of adipose tissue are tightly regulated through hormonal signals depending on caloric need (36). However, among obese persons, uncontrolled lipolysis is common and increased lipolysis accelerates the efflux of free fatty acids from adipose tissue to the circulation and ectopic fat accumulation (37). Insulin resistance can further enhance lipolysis in adipocytes (38).

Importantly, POPs are also released from adipocytes to circulation during lipid mobilization (39) and POPs in circulation can easily reach other organs (40). Although on average there is a higher risk of uncontrolled lipolysis among obese persons than lean persons, even in non-obese persons, the release of POPs to circulation can increase if uncontrolled lipolysis exists. Toxicokinetics of POPs during lipolysis should be considered in all mechanisms related to lipolysis of adipose tissue.

Dimension 3: Adipose Tissue Without Uncontrolled Lipolysis Can Be Beneficial by Decreasing the Amount of POPs Reaching Other Organs

In contrast to Dimension 2, as far as adipocyte function is physiologically healthy without uncontrolled lipolysis is concerned, greater adipose tissue can be more advantageous than less adipose tissue. The reason is that the storage of POPs in adipose tissue can reduce the amount of POPs reaching other organs (41) even though the storage of POPs in adipose tissue can have a negative side effect such as increasing half-lives of POPs in the long-term.

This aspect of adipose tissue may be helpful in explaining the obesity paradox (42): a better survival among overweight or obese patients or elderly despite a role of obesity as an important risk factor for many chronic diseases. The obesity paradox is also observed among patients with T2D, the exemplary obesity-related disease (43). Although several mechanisms such as body composition, cardiorespiratory fitness, or nutritional status have been suggested as possible explanations for the obesity paradox (42), POPs can provide a better explanation because the beneficial role of adipose tissue may be more important in patients or elderly than in healthy young persons. General features of patients with chronic diseases or elderly are the disturbance of homeostasis. In these conditions, the safe storage of pollutants in adipose tissue can be crucial. Supporting this speculation, there is a human study which showed that the beneficial role of adipose tissue may be increasing as serum concentration of POPs increases (44).

Dimension 4: Weight Loss Increases Serum Concentrations of POPs While Weight Gain Decreases Them

In Dimension 2, we discussed that obesity can increase the release of POPs from adipose tissue to circulation through uncontrolled lipolysis. Ironically, weight loss also increases serum POPs concentrations (45, 46). On the other hand, weight gain can decrease them by sequestering POPs from the circulation into adipose tissue (40, 47). Therefore, possible effects due to dynamics of POPs during weight change are contrary to conventional expected effects of weight change from the viewpoint of fat mass. In that viewpoint, intentional weight loss is beneficial while weight gain is harmful.

Even though the improvement of metabolic risks with weight loss is well-known, the toxicokinetics of POPs during weight loss can negatively affect resting metabolic rate, thyroid hormone levels, and the oxidative potential of skeletal muscle (45, 48, 49). Also, it can be helpful to explain why the intensive lifestyle intervention focusing on weight loss among overweight or obese patients with T2D failed to show a decrease of the development of cardiovascular diseases, compared to the usual management group (50). Repeated experience of weight loss and gain would be the most serious concern due to tissue redistribution of POPs between adipose tissue and other organs (40).

However, the different release pattern of POPs between Dimension 2 and Dimension 4 warrants further discussion. The release of POPs among obese persons through uncontrolled lipolysis is chronic and subtle while the release of POPs during intentional weight loss is temporary and large. Compared to the release of a large amount of POPs for a short period time, the release of a small amount of POPs for a long period can be more harmful because POPs-related health effects do not seem to increase linearly with increasing dose of POPs, as discussed below. In addition, exercise and changes in diet habit which are commonly accompanied with intentional weight loss can increase the elimination of POPs (51) and mitigate possible harms of POPs (52).

Importantly, even though it is intentional, weight loss among the elderly can be problematic. Elderly people can release more POPs into circulation than younger people because of more contamination of adipose tissue with POPs (27), but the capability of metabolizing and excreting xenobiotics is decreasing with aging (53). Therefore, POPs in circulation in the elderly can more easily reach other lipid-rich organs such as the brain. Recently, the dynamics of POPs has been suggested as a key factor to explain a high risk of dementia among patients with T2D as well as puzzling findings on obesity and dementia (54).

Dimension 5: Obesogenic Effects of Chemicals May Not Always Be Harmful

Recently, obesity-inducing effects of environmental chemicals including POPs have gained attention from researchers (55). Obesogens typically act at environmentally relevant doses during critical windows of prenatal or postnatal development to promote obesity later in life and these effects can be transmitted to their descendants (56). Possible mechanisms include increasing number of fat cells, increasing size of fat cells, and modulating hormones affecting appetite, satiety, and energy metabolism (57).

The current prevailing viewpoint on obesogens is that they can also act as diabetogens because they contribute to the development of obesity (58). However, the role of adipose tissue to protect other organs from POPs (Dimension 3) should be incorporated in interpreting the implication of obesogens. Among two mechanisms of the adipose tissue expansion, hypertrophy-dominant obesity (increase in cell size) is harmful due to pro-inflammatory cytokine release and impaired insulin sensitivity, but hyperplasia-dominant obesity (increase in cell number) is known to be beneficial (59). One of the key mechanisms by which obesogens promote adiposity is by increasing adipogenesis (56). Therefore, as far as they can provide healthy adipose tissue, their adipogenesis-promoting effect is not in itself necessarily harmful.

Although the obesogenic effect of DDT and their metabolites have been reported in human, *in-vivo*, and *in-vitro* studies (60), some POPs can suppress adipogenesis (33, 61). From the viewpoint of Dimension 3, these chemicals can be more harmful than obesogens if they diminish the safe storage site for lipophilic chemicals. The reality is much more complicated. For example, the same chemicals can increase adipogenesis at low dose while they can inhibit adipocyte differentiation at high dose (32). Also, there are synergic or antagonistic effects on adipogenesis based on studies of only two chemicals (33). Therefore, it would be almost impossible to predict what will be the net effect of chemical mixtures on the development of obesity.

As we discussed in Dimension 1, adipocytes were observed to be in a pro-inflammatory state regardless of whether POPs induced adipogenesis or reduced adipogenesis (32, 33). Therefore, rather than linking POPs to obesogens, investigation of direct harmful effects of POPs on adipose tissue and other organs would be more worthwhile in future research.

Non-linearity

Body burden of OCPs and PCBs in current general populations are much lower than they were in the era when these chemicals were actively used. Then, why do current low dose POPs reveal significant associations in human studies?

Interestingly, risks of many common environmental chemicals do not increase linearly within the range of environmental low dose exposure (62–64). POPs have also demonstrated the possibility of non-linearity with T2D (3). Within the low dose range, the risk of disease increases linearly within the relatively low dose range, but it does not further increase as dose increases. It can slow down, flatten, or even decrease with increasing doses. This feature is different from the linear dose-response relationship which is commonly observed in the range of high dose toxicity.

This non-linearity has been considered to be biologically implausible and was criticized as artifactual, arising from confounding or bias (65, 66). However, the non-linearity is plausible through several mechanisms. First, if chemicals are harmful through endocrine disruption, they can show non-linearity (67). Second, the activation of stress responses with certain levels of chemicals, called hormesis, can be another mechanism to explain non-linearity (68). The traditional concept of hormesis does not consider possible harmful effects at sub-hormetic very low dose, but only contrasts "beneficial low dose zone" vs. "toxic high dose zone" (69). Within the environmental exposure range, the non-linearity can be the result of the combination of a "sub-hormetic harmful zone" and a "hormetic beneficial zone."

Epidemiologists should understand how non-linearity can affect human studies. Historically, populations with high dose exposure to chemicals have been considered as optimal for investigation of the association between chemical exposure and outcomes. Under non-linearity, however, the association between any exposure and disease should be studied among populations with low dose exposure because the exposure range would correspond to the low dose, linear part of the dose-response relationship. In populations with relatively high dose exposure, the observed result may well be a null association because the exposure range would be in the flattened, higher dose part of the dose-response relationship. This kind of non-linearity can be one reason why current general populations with low body burden of OCPs and PCBs show clear results.

Under non-linearity, conventional quantitative methods of reviews such as meta-analyses or pooled-analyses can be problematic because they assume linearity when summarizing results such as relative risks or odds ratios from individual studies which have been performed in various populations with different levels of POPs.

POPs AS MITOCHONDRIAL TOXIN, NOT CONVENTIONAL EDCs, CAN BETTER EXPLAIN HUMAN FINDINGS ON POPs AND T2D

POPs are well-known EDCs and T2D is an endocrine disease. Therefore, it is common to consider that POPs would be linked to T2D as EDCs, as seen in the titles of some review articles (7, 9). However, it may be difficult to explain human findings about POPs and T2D by the endocrine disrupting properties of POPs.

Several EDCs acting on the same pathway, such as estrogenic chemicals, have gained a lot of attention from researchers due to strong synergic effects (70). However, the unpredictable antagonistic effects of EDCs acting on different pathways are largely ignored (71–74). For example, the mixture of even two different EDCs (estrogenic and androgenic), did not produce predictable mixture effects. POPs are the mixture of diverse EDCs acting as either agonists or antagonists on different hormone receptors which can engage in crosstalk with each other. Therefore, it would be impossible to reliably evaluate the net effect of POPs acting as EDCs in humans.

Considering the complexity of EDC mixtures, other mechanisms might be more plausible as an explanation for the consistent findings about POPs relating to T2D in human studies. In fact, many environmental chemicals are known as mitochondrial toxins (75). Evidence is accumulating that low dose POPs can induce mitochondrial dysfunction and/or reduce oxidative phosphorylation capacities (18, 76–78). Although high dose POPs are well-known direct mitochondrial toxins (79), recent studies highlight functional impairment of mitochondria by low dose POPs. In fact, endocrine disruption can occur as a result of mitochondrial dysfunction because mitochondria are essential sites for steroid hormones biosynthesis in the steroidogenic cells (80).

Mitochondrial dysfunction is currently linked to many common age-related chronic diseases including T2D (81). However, the functional impairment of mitochondria can be reversed by restoration of their function. In the section "Non-linearity," we discussed hormetic stress responses as a mechanism to explain the flattened part of the dose-response curve in the higher part of the low dose range. The activation of mitochondrial function is a typical example of hormetic stress response (82). Therefore, the non-linearity observed in the association between POPs and T2D can be explained by dynamics of mitochondrial function.

Particularly, it is important to note that there are health behaviors which can improve mitochondrial function (83). They include exercise, calorie restriction, and intake of phytochemicals in plant food (84–86). At present, regardless of POPs, these health behaviors are known as beneficial to decrease the risk of T2D and glycemic control among T2D patients. However, POPs may be a piece of the puzzle which has been missed in the relation between healthy behaviors and T2D.

PERSPECTIVE ON FUTURE STUDIES OF POPs

At present, researchers tend to think that even a small increased risk of T2D among persons due to POPs will have huge public health impact because of the ubiquitous presence of POPs and the high prevalence of T2D. However, as issues related to POPs cannot be separated from obesity issues, as we discussed above, a more comprehensive viewpoint about POPs is needed.

As the majority of published human studies about POPs and T2D are still cross-sectional, more prospective studies on POPs and T2D would be desirable. The role of POPs can be better studied among populations in which beta-cell dysfunction-dominant T2D is common, such as Asians or the elderly. In particular, the relationship between POPs and obesity on the development of T2D should be thoroughly investigated. However, the value of long-term follow-up may not be as good as epidemiologists generally believe for reasons discussed below.

First, as the dynamics of adipose tissue continuously affect serum concentration of POPs, the baseline POP value may become less representative of POPs exposure as the follow-up period gets longer. In modern society, many persons repeatedly experience weight gain and weight loss. This experience would be more frequent among obese persons, a high risk group for T2D. Therefore, although POPs are an example of synthetic chemicals with reliable exposure assessment due to their long half-lives (87), the value of baseline serum concentrations of POP decreases as follow-up period gets longer.

Second, in the case of exposure variables such as POPs which are expensive to measure, a nested case control study is generally regarded as the best design for human studies. However, as the value of measurement of POPs at baseline is decreased when the follow-up period increases for the reason we discussed above, the value of a nested case control study is also limited. Additionally, serum stored in periods when POPs were actively used would not be advantageous due to their high serum concentrations among study subjects. Under non-linearity, populations with low dose exposure are better to explore the relationship between exposure and disease than are populations with high dose exposure.

Third, the effects of POPs on the development of T2D may be dynamic. Unlike high dose toxicity with irreversible damage, functional impairment due to low dose exposure can be reversible. For example, as we discussed above, healthy lifestyles can reverse harmful effects of POPs through the improvement of mitochondrial function. Therefore, the interaction between healthy behaviors and POPs can dynamically influence the development of T2D.

All these issues suggest that a prospective study or a nested case control study with only baseline information may fail to uncover a role of POPs in the development of T2D. This problem becomes more serious as the follow-up period gets longer. Considering the necessity of repeated measurements of POPs, obesity, and other relevant variables, epidemiologists need to plan a reasonable follow-up period. The development of cheap and quick bioassay methods to assess POPs in bio-specimens would be useful for large-scale human studies with repeated measurements.

Considering the difficulties in human studies, laboratory studies mimicking human exposure would be crucial. For this purpose, animal models using lipolysis of adipose tissue such as hypertrophic adipocytes with uncontrolled lipolysis or repeated weight cycling can be useful. Mitochondrial dysfunction by the environmentally-relevant doses of POPs and the possibility of their restoration by the activation of mitohormesis would be another important study topic in the field of laboratory research.

CONCLUSION

If POPs are a new risk factor for T2D, what can we do? POPs are different from traditional risk factors such as cigarette smoking which can be avoided through education, policy, etc. In modern society, complete avoidance of exposure to POPs is not possible due to the wide contamination of the food chain. Also, a large amount of POPs is already stored in our adipose tissue and they are continuously released to circulation. Furthermore, most problematic POPs such as OCPs or PCBs were already banned in most countries several decades ago.

Therefore, how to manage POPs in adipose tissue and circulation is the foremost issue in humans. Routine application of health behaviors such as exercise, calorie restriction, and high intake of phytochemicals have been suggested as practical ways to increase the continuous elimination of POPs from human bodies or mitigate harmful effects of POPs at the cellular level based on physiology of metabolism of xenobiotics and mitochondrial function (51, 52). Even though their effects need to be evaluated in randomized controlled trials, short-term clinical trials may fail to discover solid evidence due to the dynamic nature of serum concentrations of POPs. However, as these behaviors are currently well-accepted as healthy even without any consideration on POPs, they can be safely recommended to the public. Besides health behaviors, future research focusing on the development of more effective methods of eliminating POPs is needed.

AUTHOR CONTRIBUTIONS

Y-ML wrote the first draft of the manuscript. DJ contributed to the revision of draft. D-HL devised the main concept of manuscript and contributed to the revision of draft. All read and approved the submitted version.

FUNDING

This study was supported by the Kyungpook National University Research Fund, 2015 (No. 201514690000).

REFERENCES

1. Taylor KW, Novak RF, Anderson HA, Birnbaum LS, Blystone C, Devito M, et al. Evaluation of the association between persistent organic pollutants (POPs) and diabetes in epidemiological studies: a national toxicology program workshop review. *Environ Health Perspect.* (2013) 121:774–83. doi: 10.1289/ehp.1205502
2. Wu H, Bertrand KA, Choi AL, Hu FB, Laden F, Grandjean P, et al. Persistent organic pollutants and type 2 diabetes: a prospective analysis in the nurses' health study and meta-analysis. *Environ Health Perspect.* (2013) 121:153–61. doi: 10.1289/ehp.1205248
3. Lee DH, Porta M, Jacobs DR Jr, Vandenberg LN. Chlorinated persistent organic pollutants, obesity, and type 2 diabetes. *Endocr Rev.* (2014) 35:557–601. doi: 10.1210/er.2013-1084
4. Magliano DJ, Loh VH, Harding JL, Botton J, Shaw JE. Persistent organic pollutants and diabetes: a review of the epidemiological evidence. *Diabetes Metab.* (2014) 40:1–14. doi: 10.1016/j.diabet.2013.09.006
5. Ngwa EN, Kengne AP, Tiedeu-Atogho B, Mofo-Mato EP, Sobngwi E. Persistent organic pollutants as risk factors for type 2 diabetes. *Diabetol Metab Syndr.* (2015) 7:41. doi: 10.1186/s13098-015-0031-6
6. Jaacks LM, Staimez LR. Association of persistent organic pollutants and non-persistent pesticides with diabetes and diabetes-related health outcomes in Asia: a systematic review. *Environ Int.* (2015) 76:57–70. doi: 10.1016/j.envint.2014.12.001
7. Song Y, Chou EL, Baecker A, You NC, Song Y, Sun Q, et al. Endocrine-disrupting chemicals, risk of type 2 diabetes, and diabetes-related metabolic traits: a systematic review and meta-analysis. *J Diabetes* (2016) 8:516–32. doi: 10.1111/1753-0407.12325
8. Evangelou E, Ntritsos G, Chondrogiorgi M, Kavvoura FK, Hernandez AF, Ntzani EE, et al. Exposure to pesticides and diabetes: a systematic review and meta-analysis. *Environ Int.* (2016) 91:60–8. doi: 10.1016/j.envint.2016.02.013
9. Lind PM, Lind L. Endocrine-disrupting chemicals and risk of diabetes: an evidence-based review. *Diabetologia* (2018) 61:1495–502. doi: 10.1007/s00125-018-4621-3
10. Lee DH, Lee IK, Song K, Steffes M, Toscano W, Baker BA, et al. A strong dose-response relation between serum concentrations of persistent organic

pollutants and diabetes: results from the National Health and Examination Survey 1999–2002. *Diabetes Care* (2006) 29:1638–44. doi: 10.2337/dc06-0543
11. Porta M, Gasull M, Puigdomenech E, Gari M, Bosch de Basea M, Guillen M, et al. Distribution of blood concentrations of persistent organic pollutants in a representative sample of the population of Catalonia. *Environ Int.* (2010) 36:655–64. doi: 10.1016/j.envint.2010.04.013
12. Birnbaum LS. The role of structure in the disposition of halogenated aromatic xenobiotics. *Environ Health Perspect.* (1985) 61:11–20.
13. American Diabetes Association. Diagnosis and classification of diabetes mellitus. *Diabetes Care* (2014) 37 (Suppl. 1):S81–90. doi: 10.2337/dc14-S081
14. Imamura F, Mukamal KJ, Meigs JB, Luchsinger JA, Ix JH, Siscovick DS, et al. Risk factors for type 2 diabetes mellitus preceded by beta-cell dysfunction, insulin resistance, or both in older adults: the cardiovascular health study. *Am J Epidemiol.* (2013) 177:1418–29. doi: 10.1093/aje/kws440
15. McCarthy MI. Genomics, type 2 diabetes, and obesity. *N Engl J Med.* (2010) 363:2339–50. doi: 10.1056/NEJMra0906948
16. Ma RC, Chan JC. Type 2 diabetes in East Asians: similarities and differences with populations in Europe and the United States. *Ann N Y Acad Sci.* (2013) 1281:64–91. doi: 10.1111/nyas.12098
17. Fabricio G, Malta A, Chango A, De Freitas Mathias PC. Environmental contaminants and pancreatic beta-cells. *J Clin Res Pediatr Endocrinol.* (2016) 8:257–63. doi: 10.4274/jcrpe.2812
18. Ruzzin J, Petersen R, Meugnier E, Madsen L, Lock EJ, Lillefosse H, et al. Persistent organic pollutant exposure leads to insulin resistance syndrome. *Environ Health Perspect.* (2010) 118:465–71. doi: 10.1289/ehp.0901321
19. Ibrahim MM, Fjaere E, Lock EJ, Naville D, Amlund H, Meugnier E, et al. Chronic consumption of farmed salmon containing persistent organic pollutants causes insulin resistance and obesity in mice. *PLoS ONE* (2011) 6:e25170. doi: 10.1371/journal.pone.0025170
20. Jensen TK, Timmermann AG, Rossing LI, Ried-Larsen M, Grontved A, Andersen LB, et al. Polychlorinated biphenyl exposure and glucose metabolism in 9-year-old Danish children. *J Clin Endocrinol Metab.* (2014) 99:E2643–51. doi: 10.1210/jc.2014-1683
21. Jorgensen ME, Borch-Johnsen K, Bjerregaard P. A cross-sectional study of the association between persistent organic pollutants and glucose intolerance among Greenland Inuit. *Diabetologia* (2008) 51:1416–22. doi: 10.1007/s00125-008-1066-0
22. Park SH, Ha E, Hong YS, Park H. Serum Levels of Persistent organic pollutants and Insulin secretion among children Age 7–9 Years: A Prospective Cohort Study. *Environ Health Perspect.* (2016) 124:1924–30. doi: 10.1289/EHP147
23. Lee YM, Ha CM, Kim SA, Thoudam T, Yoon YR, Kim DJ, et al. Low-dose persistent organic pollutants impair insulin secretory function of pancreatic beta-cells: human and in vitro evidence. *Diabetes* (2017) 66:2669–80. doi: 10.2337/db17-0188
24. Morimoto A, Tatsumi Y, Deura K, Mizuno S, Ohno Y, Miyamatsu N, et al. Impact of impaired insulin secretion and insulin resistance on the incidence of type 2 diabetes mellitus in a Japanese population: the Saku study. *Diabetologia* (2013) 56:1671–9. doi: 10.1007/s00125-013-2932-y
25. Yoon KH, Lee JH, Kim JW, Cho JH, Choi YH, Ko SH, et al. Epidemic obesity and type 2 diabetes in Asia. *Lancet* (2006) 368:1681–8. doi: 10.1016/S0140-6736(06)69703-1
26. Chang AM, Halter JB. Aging and insulin secretion. *Am J Physiol Endocrinol Metab.* (2003) 284:E7–12. doi: 10.1152/ajpendo.00366.2002
27. Hue O, Marcotte J, Berrigan F, Simoneau M, Dore J, Marceau P, et al. Plasma concentration of organochlorine compounds is associated with age and not obesity. *Chemosphere* (2007) 67:1463–7. doi: 10.1016/j.chemosphere.2006.10.033
28. Tanabe S, Minh TB. Dioxins and organohalogen contaminants in the Asia-Pacific region. *Ecotoxicology* (2010) 19:463–78. doi: 10.1007/s10646-009-0445-8
29. Tilg H, Moschen AR. Adipocytokines: mediators linking adipose tissue, inflammation and immunity. *Nat Rev Immunol.* (2006) 6:772–83. doi: 10.1038/nri1937
30. Shulman GI. Ectopic fat in insulin resistance, dyslipidemia, and cardiometabolic disease. *N Engl J Med.* (2014) 371:2237–8. doi: 10.1056/NEJMc1412427
31. La Merrill M, Emond C, Kim MJ, Antignac JP, Le Bizec B, Clement K, et al. Toxicological function of adipose tissue: focus on persistent organic pollutants. *Environ Health Perspect.* (2013) 121:162–9. doi: 10.1289/ehp.1205485
32. Arsenescu V, Arsenescu RI, King V, Swanson H, Cassis LA. Polychlorinated biphenyl-77 induces adipocyte differentiation and proinflammatory adipokines and promotes obesity and atherosclerosis. *Environ Health Perspect.* (2008) 116:761–8. doi: 10.1289/ehp.10554
33. May P, Bremond P, Sauzet C, Piccerelle P, Grimaldi F, Champion S, et al. *In vitro* cocktail effects of PCB-DL (PCB118) and Bulky PCB (PCB153) with BaP on Adipogenesis and on expression of genes involved in the establishment of a pro-inflammatory state. *Int J Mol Sci.* (2018) 19:E841. doi: 10.3390/ijms19030841
34. Pestana D, Teixeira D, Meireles M, Marques C, Norberto S, Sa C, et al. Adipose tissue dysfunction as a central mechanism leading to dysmetabolic obesity triggered by chronic exposure to p,p'-DDE. *Sci Rep.* (2017) 7:2738. doi: 10.1038/s41598-017-02885-9
35. Cinti S, Mitchell G, Barbatelli G, Murano I, Ceresi E, Faloia E, et al. Adipocyte death defines macrophage localization and function in adipose tissue of obese mice and humans. *J Lipid Res.* (2005) 46:2347–55. doi: 10.1194/jlr.M500294-JLR200
36. Rosen ED, Spiegelman BM. Adipocytes as regulators of energy balance and glucose homeostasis. *Nature* (2006) 444:847–53. doi: 10.1038/nature 05483
37. de Ferranti S, Mozaffarian D. The perfect storm: obesity, adipocyte dysfunction, and metabolic consequences. *Clin Chem.* (2008) 54:945–55. doi: 10.1373/clinchem.2007.100156
38. Morigny P, Houssier M, Mouisel E, Langin D. Adipocyte lipolysis and insulin resistance. *Biochimie* (2016) 125:259–66. doi: 10.1016/j.biochi.2015.10.024
39. Louis C, Tinant G, Mignolet E, Thome JP, Debier C. PCB-153 shows different dynamics of mobilisation from differentiated rat adipocytes during lipolysis in comparison with PCB-28 and PCB-118. *PLoS ONE* (2014) 9:e106495. doi: 10.1371/journal.pone.0106495
40. Jandacek RJ, Anderson N, Liu M, Zheng S, Yang Q, Tso P. Effects of yo-yo diet, caloric restriction, and olestra on tissue distribution of hexachlorobenzene. *Am J Physiol Gastrointest Liver Physiol.* (2005) 288:G292–9. doi: 10.1152/ajpgi.00285.2004
41. Ahotupa M, Mantyla E. Adipose tissue content as a modifier of the tissue distribution, biological effects, and excretion of a hexachlorobiphenyl in C57BL/6J and DBA/JBOMf mice. *Mol Pharmacol.* (1983) 24:464–70.
42. Antonopoulos AS, Oikonomou EK, Antoniades C, Tousoulis D. From the BMI paradox to the obesity paradox: the obesity-mortality association in coronary heart disease. *Obes Rev.* (2016) 17:989–1000. doi: 10.1111/obr.12440
43. Hainer V, Aldhoon-Hainerova I. Obesity paradox does exist. *Diabetes Care* (2013) 36 (Suppl. 2):S276–81. doi: 10.2337/dcS13-2023
44. Hong NS, Kim KS, Lee IK, Lind PM, Lind L, Jacobs DR, et al. The association between obesity and mortality in the elderly differs by serum concentrations of persistent organic pollutants: a possible explanation for the obesity paradox. *Int J Obes.* (2012) 36:1170–5. doi: 10.1038/ijo.2011.187
45. Imbeault P, Tremblay A, Simoneau JA, Joanisse DR. Weight loss-induced rise in plasma pollutant is associated with reduced skeletal muscle oxidative capacity. *Am J Physiol Endocrinol Metab.* (2002) 282:E574–9. doi: 10.1152/ajpendo.00394.2001
46. Jansen A, Lyche JL, Polder A, Aaseth J, Skaug MA. Increased blood levels of persistent organic pollutants (POP) in obese individuals after weight loss-A review. *J Toxicol Environ Health B Crit Rev.* (2017) 20:22–37. doi: 10.1080/10937404.2016.1246391
47. Lim JS, Son HK, Park SK, Jacobs DR Jr, Lee DH. Inverse associations between long-term weight change and serum concentrations of persistent organic pollutants. *Int J Obes.* (2011) 35:744–7. doi: 10.1038/ijo.2010.188
48. Pelletier C, Doucet E, Imbeault P, Tremblay A. Associations between weight loss-induced changes in plasma organochlorine concentrations, serum T_3 concentration, and resting metabolic rate. *Toxicol Sci.* (2002) 67:46–51. doi: 10.1093/toxsci/67.1.46
49. Tremblay A, Pelletier C, Doucet E, Imbeault P. Thermogenesis and weight loss in obese individuals: a primary association with organochlorine pollution. *Int J Obes Relat Metab Disord.* (2004) 28:936–9. doi: 10.1038/sj.ijo.0802527
50. Look ARG, Wing RR, Bolin P, Brancati FL, Bray GA, Clark JM, et al. Cardiovascular effects of intensive lifestyle intervention in type 2 diabetes. *N Engl J Med.* (2013) 369:145–54. doi: 10.1056/NEJMoa1212914

51. Lee YM, Kim KS, Jacobs DR Jr, Lee DH. Persistent organic pollutants in adipose tissue should be considered in obesity research. *Obes Rev.* (2017) 18:129–39. doi: 10.1111/obr.12481
52. Kim SA, Lee YM, Choi JY, Jacobs DR Jr, Lee DH. Evolutionarily adapted hormesis-inducing stressors can be a practical solution to mitigate harmful effects of chronic exposure to low dose chemical mixtures. *Environ Pollut.* (2017) 233:725–34. doi: 10.1016/j.envpol.2017.10.124
53. McLachlan AJ, Pont LG. Drug metabolism in older people–a key consideration in achieving optimal outcomes with medicines. *J Gerontol A Biol Sci Med Sci.* (2012) 67:175–80. doi: 10.1093/gerona/glr118
54. Lee DH, Porta M, Lind L, Lind PM, Jacobs DR Jr. Neurotoxic chemicals in adipose tissue: A role in puzzling findings on obesity and dementia. *Neurology* (2018) 90:176–82. doi: 10.1212/WNL.0000000000004851
55. Chamorro-Garcia R, Blumberg B. Transgenerational effects of obesogens and the obesity epidemic. *Curr Opin Pharmacol.* (2014) 19:153–8. doi: 10.1016/j.coph.2014.10.010
56. Janesick AS, Shioda T, Blumberg B. Transgenerational inheritance of prenatal obesogen exposure. *Mol Cell Endocrinol.* (2014) 398:31–5. doi: 10.1016/j.mce.2014.09.002
57. Heindel JJ, Newbold R, Schug TT. Endocrine disruptors and obesity. *Nat Rev Endocrinol.* (2015) 11:653–61. doi: 10.1038/nrendo.2015.163
58. Thayer KA, Heindel JJ, Bucher JR, Gallo MA. Role of environmental chemicals in diabetes and obesity: a National Toxicology Program workshop review. *Environ Health Perspect.* (2012) 120:779–89. doi: 10.1289/ehp.1104597
59. Kloting N, Fasshauer M, Dietrich A, Kovacs P, Schon MR, Kern M, et al. Insulin-sensitive obesity. *Am J Physiol Endocrinol Metab.* (2010) 299:E506–15. doi: 10.1152/ajpendo.00586.2009
60. Cano-Sancho G, Salmon AG, La Merrill MA. Association between Exposure to p,p'-DDT and Its Metabolite p,p'-DDE with Obesity: integrated systematic review and meta-analysis. *Environ Health Perspect.* (2017) 125:096002. doi: 10.1289/EHP527
61. Alexander DL, Ganem LG, Fernandez-Salguero P, Gonzalez F, Jefcoate CR. Aryl-hydrocarbon receptor is an inhibitory regulator of lipid synthesis and of commitment to adipogenesis. *J Cell Sci.* (1998) 111 (Pt 22):3311–22.
62. Bowe B, Xie Y, Li T, Yan Y, Xian H, Al-Aly Z. The 2016 global and national burden of diabetes mellitus attributable to $PM_{2.5}$ air pollution. *Lancet Planet Health* (2018) 2:e301–12. doi: 10.1016/S2542-5196(18)30140-2
63. Lanphear BP. Low-level toxicity of chemicals: no acceptable levels? *PLoS Biol.* (2017) 15:e2003066. doi: 10.1371/journal.pbio.2003066
64. Lanphear BP, Rauch S, Auinger P, Allen RW, Hornung RW. Low-level lead exposure and mortality in US adults: a population-based cohort study. *Lancet Public Health* (2018) 3:e177-e84. doi: 10.1016/S2468-2667(18)30025-2
65. Banner W, Kahn CM. Low blood lead level effects on intelligence: can a dose-response curve be determined from the epidemiological data? *Clin Toxicol.* (2014) 52:113–7. doi: 10.3109/15563650.2013.876544
66. Bowers TS, Beck BD. What is the meaning of non-linear dose-response relationships between blood lead concentrations and IQ? *Neurotoxicology* (2006) 27:520–4. doi: 10.1016/j.neuro.2006.02.001
67. Vandenberg LN, Colborn T, Hayes TB, Heindel JJ, Jacobs DR Jr, Lee DH, et al. Hormones and endocrine-disrupting chemicals: low-dose effects and nonmonotonic dose responses. *Endocr Rev.* (2012) 33:378–455. doi: 10.1210/er.2011-1050
68. Calabrese EJ, Mattson MP. How does hormesis impact biology, toxicology, and medicine? *NPJ Aging Mech Dis.* (2017) 3:13. doi: 10.1038/s41514-017-0013-z
69. Lee DH, Jacobs DR Jr. Hormesis and public health: can glutathione depletion and mitochondrial dysfunction due to very low-dose chronic exposure to persistent organic pollutants be mitigated? *J Epidemiol Community Health* (2015) 69:294–300. doi: 10.1136/jech-2014-203861
70. Kortenkamp A. Low dose mixture effects of endocrine disrupters and their implications for regulatory thresholds in chemical risk assessment. *Curr Opin Pharmacol.* (2014) 19:105–11. doi: 10.1016/j.coph.2014.08.006
71. Carnevali O, Notarstefano V, Olivotto I, Graziano M, Gallo P, Di Marco Pisciottano I, et al. Dietary administration of EDC mixtures: a focus on fish lipid metabolism. *Aquat Toxicol.* (2017) 185:95–104. doi: 10.1016/j.aquatox.2017.02.007
72. Hu Y, Wang R, Xiang Z, Qian W, Han X, Li D. Antagonistic effects of a mixture of low-dose nonylphenol and di-n-butyl phthalate (monobutyl phthalate) on the Sertoli cells and serum reproductive hormones in prepubertal male rats *in vitro* and *in vivo*. *PLoS ONE* (2014) 9:e93425. doi: 10.1371/journal.pone.0093425
73. Ribeiro E, Ladeira C, Viegas S. EDCs mixtures: a stealthy hazard for human health? *Toxics* (2017) 5:5. doi: 10.3390/toxics5010005
74. Sarria MP, Santos MM, Reis-Henriques MA, Vieira NM, Monteiro NM. The unpredictable effects of mixtures of androgenic and estrogenic chemicals on fish early life. *Environ Int.* (2011) 37:418–24. doi: 10.1016/j.envint.2010.11.004
75. Meyer JN, Leung MC, Rooney JP, Sendoel A, Hengartner MO, Kisby GE, et al. Mitochondria as a target of environmental toxicants. *Toxicol Sci.* (2013) 134:1–17. doi: 10.1093/toxsci/kft102
76. Lim S, Ahn SY, Song IC, Chung MH, Jang HC, Park KS, et al. Chronic exposure to the herbicide, atrazine, causes mitochondrial dysfunction and insulin resistance. *PLoS ONE* (2009) 4:e5186. doi: 10.1371/journal.pone.0005186
77. Liu Q, Wang Q, Xu C, Shao W, Zhang C, Liu H, et al. Organochloride pesticides impaired mitochondrial function in hepatocytes and aggravated disorders of fatty acid metabolism. *Sci Rep.* (2017) 7:46339. doi: 10.1038/srep46339
78. Mailloux RJ, Florian M, Chen Q, Yan J, Petrov I, Coughlan MC, et al. Exposure to a northern contaminant mixture (NCM) alters hepatic energy and lipid metabolism exacerbating hepatic steatosis in obese JCR rats. *PLoS ONE* (2014) 9:e106832. doi: 10.1371/journal.pone.0106832
79. Byczkowski JZ. The mode of action of p,p'=DDT on mammalian mitochondria. *Toxicology* (1976) 6:309–14.
80. Miller WL. Steroid hormone synthesis in mitochondria. *Mol Cell Endocrinol.* (2013) 379:62–73. doi: 10.1016/j.mce.2013.04.014
81. Chan DC. Mitochondria: dynamic organelles in disease, aging, and development. *Cell* (2006) 125:1241–52. doi: 10.1016/j.cell.2006.06.010
82. Sano M, Fukuda K. Activation of mitochondrial biogenesis by hormesis. *Circ Res.* (2008) 103:1191–3. doi: 10.1161/CIRCRESAHA.108.189092
83. Yun J, Finkel T. Mitohormesis. *Cell Metab.* (2014) 19:757–66. doi: 10.1016/j.cmet.2014.01.011
84. Merry TL, Ristow M. Mitohormesis in exercise training. *Free Radic Biol Med.* (2016) 98:123–30. doi: 10.1016/j.freeradbiomed.2015.11.032
85. Ristow M, Zarse K. How increased oxidative stress promotes longevity and metabolic health: the concept of mitochondrial hormesis (mitohormesis). *Exp Gerontol.* (2010) 45:410–8. doi: 10.1016/j.exger.2010.03.014
86. Grabacka MM, Gawin M, Pierzchalska M. Phytochemical modulators of mitochondria: the search for chemopreventive agents and supportive therapeutics. *Pharmaceuticals* (2014) 7:913–42. doi: 10.3390/ph7090913
87. Lee DH, Jacobs DR Jr. Methodological issues in human studies of endocrine disrupting chemicals. *Rev Endocr Metab Disord.* (2015) 16:289–97. doi: 10.1007/s11154-016-9340-9

12

Preconceptional, Gestational and Lactational Exposure to an Unconventional Oil and Gas Chemical Mixture Alters Energy Expenditure in Adult Female Mice

*Victoria D. Balise[1,2], Jennifer N. Cornelius-Green[1], Christopher D. Kassotis[3], R. Scott Rector[4,5,6], John P. Thyfault[7,8] and Susan C. Nagel[1,2]**

[1] Department of Obstetrics, Gynecology and Women's Health, University of Missouri, Columbia, MO, United States, [2] Department of Biological Sciences, University of Missouri, Columbia, MO, United States, [3] Nicholas School of the Environment, Duke University, Durham, NC, United States, [4] Department of Nutrition and Health Exercise Physiology, University of Missouri, Columbia, MO, United States, [5] Medicine-Division of Gastroenterology and Hepatology, University of Missouri, Columbia, MO, United States, [6] Research Service, Harry S Truman Memorial Veterans Medical Center, Columbia, MO, United States, [7] Department of Molecular and Integrative Physiology, University of Kansas Medical Center, Kansas City, KS, United States, [8] Kansas City VA Medical Center, Research Service, Kansas City, MO, United States

***Correspondence:**
Susan C. Nagel
nagels@health.missouri.edu

Previous studies conducted in our laboratory have found altered adult health outcomes in animals with prenatal exposure to environmentally relevant levels of unconventional oil and gas (UOG) chemicals with endocrine-disrupting activity. This study aimed to examine potential metabolic health outcomes following a preconception, prenatal and postnatal exposure to a mixture of 23 UOG chemicals. Prior to mating and from gestation day 1 to postnatal day 21, C57BL/6J mice were developmentally exposed to a laboratory-created mixture of 23 UOG chemicals in maternal drinking water. Body composition, spontaneous activity, energy expenditure, and glucose tolerance were evaluated in 7-month-old female offspring. Neither body weight nor body composition differed in 7-month female mice. However, females exposed to 1.5 and 150 μg/kg/day UOG mix had lower total and resting energy expenditure within the dark cycle. In the light cycle, the 1,500 μg//kg/day group had lower total energy expenditure and the 1.5 μg/kg/day group had lower resting energy expenditure. Females exposed to the 150 μg/kg/day group had lower spontaneous activity in the dark cycle, and females exposed to the 1,500 μg/kg/day group had lower activity in the light cycle. This study reports for the first time that developmental exposure to a mixture of 23 UOG chemicals alters energy expenditure and spontaneous activity in adult female mice.

Keywords: unconventional oil and gas, energy expenditure, endocrine disrupting chemicals, developmental origins of health and disease, hydraulic fracturing, metabolism, metabolic disruptors

INTRODUCTION

Unconventional oil and gas (UOG) extraction combines directional drilling and hydraulic fracturing to liberate oil and gas that was previously inaccessible by traditional drilling methods, including sources of shale gas, coal bed methane, and tight gas. Across the industry, over 1,000 chemicals have been reportedly used in the hydraulic fracturing process. Varying mixtures of these chemicals are combined with millions of gallons of water to fracture underground rock. UOG extraction has been identified as a potential source of EDCs, developmental and reproductive toxicants. We have previously reported that out of 24 UOG chemicals tested, 23 exhibited antagonist activity for one or more of the estrogen, androgen, progesterone, thyroid, and glucocorticoid receptors; and a mixture of 23 of these UOG chemicals exhibited antagonistic activity for all five receptors (1).

UOG activities, including drilling, hydraulic fracturing, and wastewater removal and storage, can contaminate surface and ground water with endocrine-disrupting chemicals (EDCs), defined as exogenous chemicals that can interfere with normal hormone action [(2–6) and reviewed in (7–9)]. We have previously observed an association between endocrine-disrupting activity in surface water and UOG activities. For example, we measured greater antagonistic activities for the estrogen, androgen, progesterone, thyroid, and glucocorticoid receptors immediately downstream of a UOG wastewater disposal facility relative to upstream (4). Our laboratory has reported that prenatal exposure to a laboratory-created mixture of 23 UOG chemicals was associated with altered organ weights, reproductive endpoints, and body weight in adult offspring of gestationally-exposed C57BL/6 mice, suggestive of developmental programming (1, 10, 11). Previous studies on hydraulic fracturing flowback and produced water also support the hypothesis that UOG chemical mixtures can alter fetal development, as developmentally-exposed zebrafish exhibited reduced reproduction, developmental malformations, and developmental toxicity (12, 13). Additionally, a systematic review by Elliot et al. found that 40% of 240 UOG chemicals with publicly-available reproductive and/or developmental toxicity information had been shown to exhibit developmental toxicity (14).

Developmental exposure to EDCs has also been associated with metabolic disease later in life (15), and these chemicals have been termed "metabolic disruptors" (16, 17). Exposure to multiple EDCs, e.g., bisphenol A (BPA), phthalates, dichlorodiphenyltrichloroethane (DDT), and nicotine, among others, has been associated with one or more altered metabolic endpoints, such as obesity, insulin sensitivity, adipose tissue regulation, and lipid disorders [reviewed in (18) and (19)]. UOG chemicals also have the potential to be metabolic disruptors. We have shown that both a 23-UOG mixture and UOG-impacted surface water samples had adipogenic activity *in vitro* (20). Studies in zebrafish have shown that exposure to UOG wastewater resulted in decreased metabolic rates (12, 21). Two studies reported an association between maternal residential proximity to UOG sites and low birth weight infants, while another found an association between maternal residential proximity to UOG sites and increased birth weights (22–24). Both high and low birth weights are associated with later-life development of obesity (25). We have previously demonstrated that female mice prenatally exposed to a mixture of 23 UOG chemicals from gestation day 11 through birth had increased body weights at postnatal days 7, 13, and 21. Body weight and composition can be indicative of energy imbalance.

Taken together, there is limited but suggestive data linking UOG chemicals and altered metabolism. However, no studies have examined the direct of effects of developmental exposure to UOG chemicals and energy expenditure and activity in adulthood. We hypothesized that preconceptional, gestational and lactational exposure to a laboratory-created mixture of UOG chemicals would alter energy balance in adult mice through modulation of energy expenditure. To test this hypothesis, we exposed female C57BL/6 mice to a mixture of 23 UOG chemicals 5 weeks prior to mating, and from gestation day (GD) 1 to postnatal day (PND) 21, and evaluated body composition, energy expenditure, activity, and glucose tolerance in adult offspring.

MATERIALS AND METHODS

Animals

This study was carried out in accordance with the recommendations of the National Research Council's Guide for the Care and Use of Laboratory Animals. The protocol was approved by the University of Missouri Animal Care and Use Committee. C57BL/6J mice (purchased from Jackson Laboratories) were housed in polysulfone cages, in a barrier facility with a 12 h light/dark cycle. Feed (LabDiet 5053: 13% kcal fat, 3.25% kcal sucrose) and acidified water (in glass bottles) were sterilized and provided *ad libitum*.

Chemical Mixture and Treatment

C57BL/6 dams used in this study were 8 months old at initiation of treatment, and 9 months of age when mated. These dams were used in a previous study. Offspring outcomes from the first experiment were reported in Kassotis et al. (1, 11). Each female received the same concentration of chemical mixture that was randomly assigned in the previous study (1). Dams (n = 14, 9, 11, 8, and 10) were exposed to the chemical mixture (at concentrations of 0, 0.01, 0.10, 1.0, or 10 μg/mL, respectively) for 5 weeks prior to mating (**Figure 1**). Chemical exposure was paused while females were mated in order to bypass the window of fertilization, and to avoid consumption of treatment chemicals by the males (**Figure 1**). Treatment was resumed at gestational day 1 (1 day after presence of copulatory plug) and continued through weaning of the F1 generation at PND 21. "Developmental exposure" will be used throughout the manuscript to describe the inclusive exposure to the dam preconception and GD 1 to PND 21 exposure.

The 23 chemicals were mixed equimass in 200 proof ethanol and added to drinking water such that each individual chemical was present at a concentration of 0.01, 0.10, 1.0, and or 10 μg/mL in a 0.2% ethanol vehicle. Water bottles were changed twice per week to ensure consistent chemical concentrations throughout the dosing period. Water consumption was calculated as the difference in the weight of the water bottle before and after use every time the bottle was changed. Dosages based on weight of the dam and the amount of water consumed were calculated as 1.5, 15, 150, and 1,500 μg/kg/day.

To be included in further analysis, litters had to meet minimum inclusion criteria: Each litter had to have $\geq$ 3 pups, $\geq$ 1 male, and $\geq$ 1 female. After application of

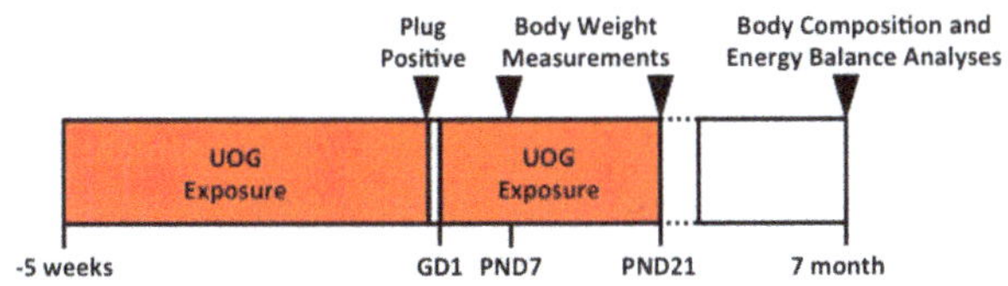

FIGURE 1 | Experimental timeline. Dams ($n = 14, 9, 11, 8$, and 10) that were exposed to the 23 UOG chemical mixture (at concentrations of 0, 0.01, 0.10, 1.0, or 10 μg/mL, respectively) for 5 weeks prior to mating. Chemical exposure was paused while females were mated in order to bypass the window of fertilization, and to avoid consumption of treatment chemicals by the males. Treatment was resumed at gestational day 1 (1 day after presence of copulatory plug) and continued through weaning of the F1 generation at PND 21. Body composition was measured at PND 7, PND 21, and at 7 months of age. Energy balance analyses including energy expenditure, activity, food intake, and glucose tolerance were measured at 7 months of age.

inclusion criteria, $n = 6, 4, 5, 4$, and 4 unique litters; and $n = 9, 11, 9, 10$, and 10 individual animals from vehicle, 1.5, 15, 150, and 1,500 μg/kg/day treatment groups, respectively (**Supplementary Table 1**).

At PND 7, F1 pups were toe clipped and anogenital distance (AGD) was determined by caliper measurement. At PND 21, pups were weaned and rehoused with pups of the same treatment group and sex.

Animal Rehousing

Female offspring at 6 months of age were transferred to an open-top conventional facility for body composition and metabolic assessments. Mice were allowed to acclimate to the new environment for a month prior to initiation of metabolic testing. This facility was temperature controlled and kept on a 12-h light/dark cycle. In this facility, the experimental animals received non-sterilized feed (LabDiet 5053) and non-acidified, non-sterilized water.

Body Composition

Body weight was measured at PND 7, PND 21, and 7 months of age. Fat and lean mass were assessed at 7 months of age, using an EchoMRI-900 (EchoMRI, Houston, TX). Fat and lean percentages were calculated by dividing fat or lean mass by body weight.

Indirect Calorimetry

Energy expenditure via indirect calorimetry, activity, and behavior were measured using the Promethion from Sable Systems Int., (Las Vegas, NV). Oxygen consumption, energy expenditure, and activity were calculated with macros provided by the manufacturer (26).

Total energy expenditure was measured for a 12-h cycle. Resting energy expenditure was extrapolated from the lowest average energy expenditure in a 30-min window within a 12-h cycle and calculated to be representative of the resting energy expenditure for a complete 12-h period. Non-resting energy expenditure was calculated for each 12-h cycle by subtracting 12-h calculated resting energy expenditure from 12-h total energy expenditure (27).

Activity and meters traveled were measured by infrared beams that track movement in horizontal (X and Y plane) and vertical directions (Z plane). Spontaneous activity was defined as activity in the X, Y, and Z directions, ambulatory activity in the X and Y directions, and rearing activity in the Z direction. Meters traveled counted all meters in the X, Y, and Z direction. Food consumption was also measured in this system.

Energy expenditure, activity, and behavior were assessed for a random subset of 7 animals per treatment group on the first day of estrus. Energy expenditure was calculated from measured oxygen consumption using the Kaiyala-Simple equation. Valid data (barring system malfunctions) were collected for $n = 7$, 4, 6, 6, and 6 animals in the vehicle, 1.5, 15, 150, and 1,500 μg/kg/day groups, respectively (**Supplementary Table 1**). Mice were individually housed in the system's cages for 48 h. The first 24 h were used as an acclimation period, and the second 24 h were analyzed separately as the 12-h light cycle or the 12-h dark cycle. Oxygen consumption, energy expenditure, and activity were calculated with macros provided by the manufacturer (26).

Glucose Tolerance Test

Glucose tolerance tests were performed only in females in blocks of mice in estrus ($n = 16$/block). Mice were weighed at 1000 h, and fasted from 1000 to 1600 h. A baseline (0 min) blood sample was collected via tail snip at 1600–1630 h, and blood glucose was determined using a glucose monitor (Accu-Chek Aviva Plus). Immediately after the baseline measurement was taken, 250 mg/mL glucose was injected intraperitoneally at 1 mg/kg body weight. Blood glucose concentrations were measured at 30, 60, and 120 min post injection, as described previously (28).

Statistics

Data were analyzed with a linear mixed model, using SPSS version 32. This model was selected so that litter could be incorporated as a random effect. Treatment and date of measurement (if more than 1 day) were included as fixed effects for body weight, fat mass, lean mass, fat percent, lean percent, food consumption, and activity. For analysis of energy expenditure, body weight and size of litter were also considered as fixed effects. Data were normally distributed or transformed to achieve normality. Results are displayed in all figures as the estimated marginal means, back transformed for presentation if transformation was necessary, except for **Supplemental Figure 1C**. Differences between vehicle and treatment groups were analyzed using Fisher's Least Significant Difference tests, with 95% confidence intervals. The percent dams that delivered (**Supplemental Figure 1C**) was analyzed by Fisher's exact test. All tests were compared to vehicle.

RESULTS

Maternal and Birth Outcomes

The body weights of pregnant dams were measured in order to monitor health and calculate treatment dosage. The body weights of the dams exposed to the UOG chemical mixture did not differ from those of dams exposed to the vehicle at gestation day 0 after 5 weeks of treatment (**Supplementary Figure 1A**). Treatment did not alter dam body weight or water consumption (**Supplementary Figures 1A,B**). The percentage of dams per group that delivered tended to be decreased in the 150 and 1,500 µg/kg/day groups (p<0.20) (**Supplementary Figure 1C**). The number of live pups per litter did not differ relative to vehicle (**Supplementary Figure 1D**).

Offspring Body Composition

Developmental exposure to the UOG chemical mixture altered the body weights of female offspring at PND 7. Body weight at PND 7 in F1 females developmentally exposed to the UOG chemical mixture was 10–26% lower in the 1.5, 15, and 1,500 µg/kg/day treatment groups relative to vehicle (**Figure 2A**). At PND 21 and at 7 months of age, these females no longer displayed differences in body weight relative to vehicle (**Figures 2B,C**). Fat mass, percent fat mass, lean mass, and percent lean mass at 7 months of age also did not differ relative to vehicle (**Supplemental Figure 2**).

Offspring Energy Expenditure

Developmental exposure to the UOG chemical mixture was associated with altered energy expenditure in the dark cycle in females. After 24 h of acclimation, energy expenditure was assessed for the final 24 h. Energy expenditure data were divided into 12-h light and dark cycles for analysis. In the dark cycle, total energy expenditure was 16 and 19% lower and resting energy expenditure was 20 and 18% lower in the 1.5 and 150 µg/kg/day treatment groups respectively (**Figures 3A,B**). Non-resting energy expenditure tended to be 22 and 20% lower in the 15 ($p = 0.054$) and 150 ($p = 0.054$) µg/kg/day treatment groups relative to vehicle (**Figure 3C**).

In the light cycle, total energy expenditure was 20% lower in the 1,500 µg/kg/day treatment group relative to vehicle (**Figure 3A**). Resting energy expenditure was 17% lower in the 1.5 µg/kg/day group relative to vehicle, while non-resting energy expenditure was not altered relative to vehicle in any treatment group (**Figures 3B,C**).

Offspring Activity

Developmental exposure to the UOG chemical mixture was associated with altered spontaneous activity in both the light and dark cycles in females. In the dark cycle, spontaneous activity was 27% lower in the 150 µg/kg/day treatment group relative to vehicle (**Figure 4A**). In the light cycle, spontaneous activity was 34% lower in the 1,500 µg/kg/day treatment group relative to vehicle (**Figure 4B**). No differences were detected in ambulatory, rearing activity, or meters traveled for any treatment group relative to vehicle in the light or the dark cycles (**Supplementary Figure 3**).

Offspring Glucose Homeostasis

Glucose tolerance tests were performed at 7 months of age on the day of estrus. No differences were detected in basal glucose levels, glucose levels at subsequent time points using basal glucose as a baseline, or in area under the curve for any treatment groups in females (**Supplementary Figure 4**).

Offspring Food Consumption

Food consumption during the dark cycle did not differ between vehicle and treatment groups in 7-month-old female offspring. However, food consumption during the light cycle increased by 60% in the 150 µg/kg/day treatment group relative to vehicle (**Figure 5**), but no differences were detected in the other treatment groups when compared to vehicle.

DISCUSSION

We report for the first time that developmental exposure to a mixture of 23 oil and gas chemicals altered adult energy expenditure in 7-month-old female mice, particularly in the dark cycle when mice are more active. Mice in the 15 µg/kg/day group had a lower non-resting energy expenditure. Females in the 1.5 and 150 µg/kg/day groups had lower total and resting energy expenditure within the dark cycle, and the 150 µg/kg/day group had lower spontaneous activity and tended to have lower non-resting energy expenditure in the dark cycle. This decrease in energy expenditure did not result in altered body weight or body composition at 7 months of age. This study supports the hypothesis that developmental exposure to EDCs can contribute to the programming of energy expenditure and activity in adulthood.

Hormones are essential in regulating metabolism throughout development and programming metabolic function in adulthood, and developmental exposure to EDCs has been

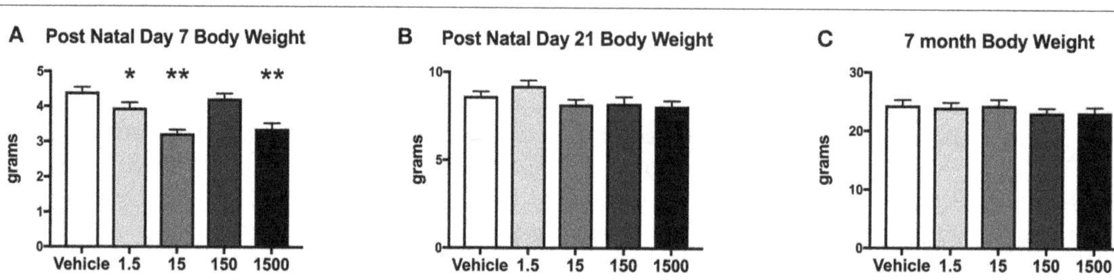

FIGURE 2 | Body weights of offspring. Estimated marginal means (±) SEM of body weight at post-natal day 7 **(A)**, post-natal day 21 **(B)**, and at 7 months of age **(C)**. *$p < 0.05$ relative to vehicle **$p < 0.0125$ relative to vehicle (n = 9, 11, 9, 10, 10 respectively for vehicle, 1.5, 15, 150, and 1,500 µg/kg/day treatment groups). Models included covariates: litter, date body weight was taken and litter size.

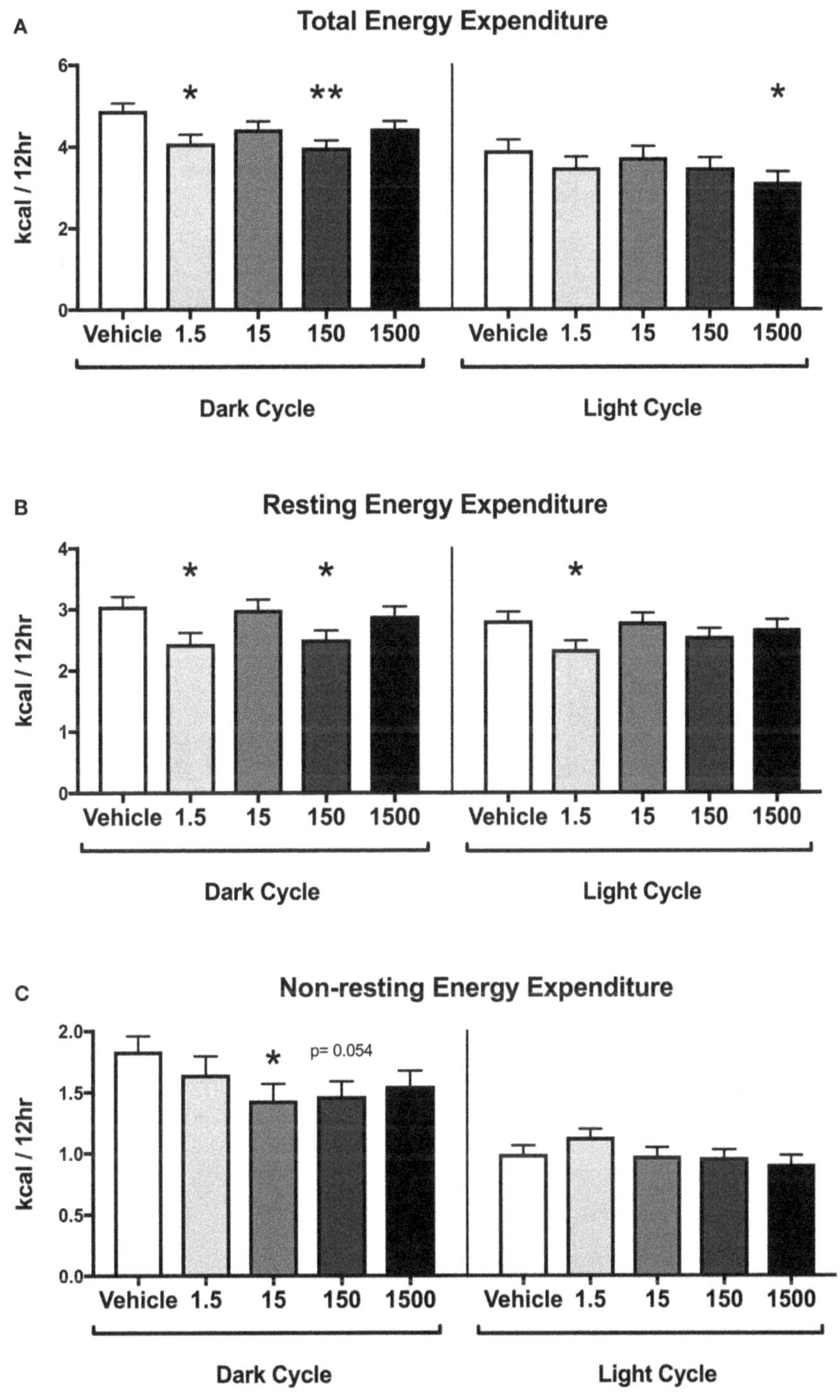

FIGURE 3 | Energy Expenditure in Female Offspring at 7 months of age. Estimated marginal means (±) SEM in 12-h average increments of total energy expenditure **(A)**, resting energy expenditure **(B)**, non-resting expenditure **(C)** ($n = 7, 4, 6, 6, 5$ respectively for vehicle, 1.5, 15, 150, and 1,500 μg/kg/day treatment groups). *$p < 0.05$ relative to vehicle **$p < 0.0125$ relative to vehicle. Models included covariates: litter, date of recording, litter size, and body weight.

reported to alter body composition, energy expenditure, activity, glucose homeostasis and adipogenesis (29–32). Developmental exposure to EDCs, including BPA, lead, arsenic, diethylstilbestrol (DES), and perfluorooctanoic acid (PFOA) has been associated with altered metabolism (19, 29–39). While these EDCs are reported to disrupt one or more hormone receptors, including estrogen, androgen, progesterone, glucocorticoid, thyroid hormone, and others, they have all been reported to agonize the estrogen receptor (33, 35–37, 39–41). Developmental exposure to estrogen receptor agonists from preconception to weaning is

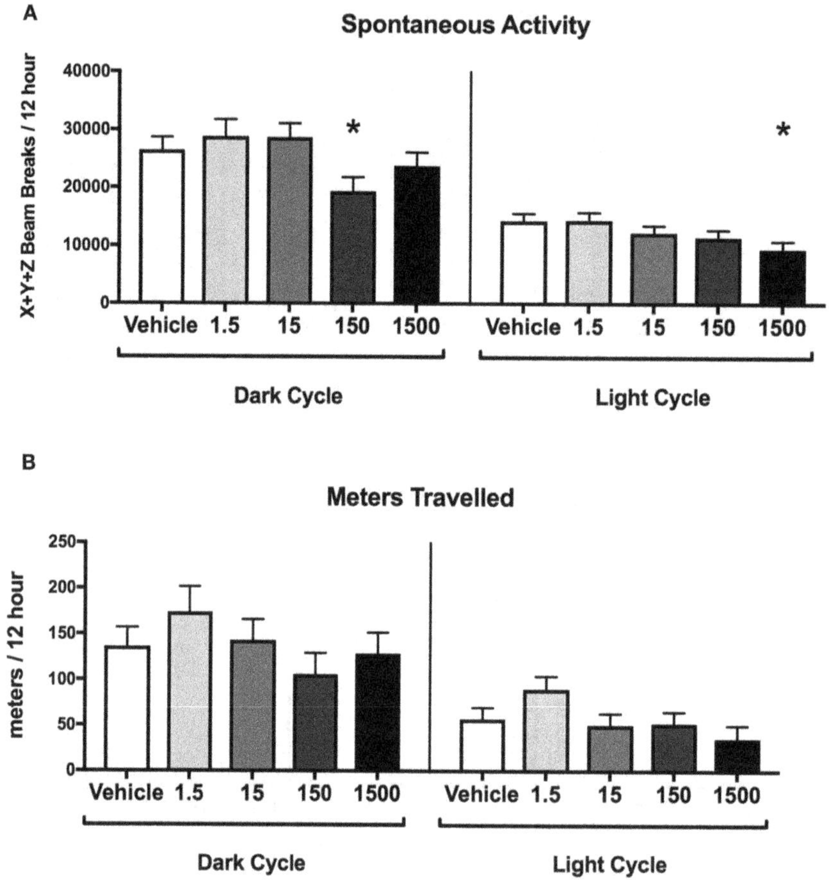

FIGURE 4 | Activity of female offspring at 7 months of age. Estimated marginal means (±) SEM in 12-h average increments of total spontaneous activity **(A)**, and meters travelled **(B)** ($n = 7, 4, 6, 6, 5$ respectively for vehicle, 1.5, 15, 150, and 1,500 μg/kg/day treatment groups). $^*p < 0.05$ relative to vehicle. Models included covariates: litter and date of recording.

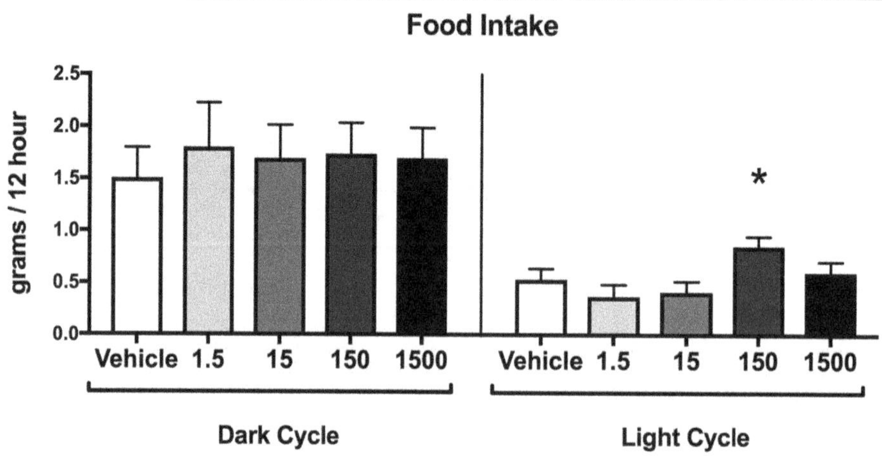

FIGURE 5 | Food consumption in female offspring at 7 months of age. Estimated marginal means (±) SEM of food intake at 7 months of age in 12 h increments of both light and dark cycle ($n = 7, 4, 6, 6, 5$ respectively for vehicle, 1.5, 15, 150, and 1,500 μg/kg/day treatment groups). $^*p < 0.05$ relative to vehicle. Models included date of recording as a covariate.

associated with increased energy expenditure and spontaneous activity in female Agouti (lead and BPA) and C57BL/6JxFVB (BPA) mice (29, 34, 38). These effects may be strain specific as no difference in energy expenditure was seen in CD-1 and California mice (42–46).

The role of androgens in metabolic dysfunction are well-appreciated, though are not likely to play a role in the observed effects herein. Acute androgen exposure is generally considered anti-adipogenic and anti-androgen exposure is adipogenic using *in vitro* or *in vivo* models (47, 48). However, dissimilar effects can be observed in specific cases. Women, such as those with polycystic ovarian syndrome (PCOS), have increased serum androgens and suffer increased visceral white adipose tissue deposition (47), potentially mediated by reduced insulin sensitivity (48, 49). These effects also appear reversed with developmental androgen exposure. For example, prenatal exposure to androgen results in metabolic dysfunction in adult female rodents and monkeys, including increased body weight, adiposity, insulin, serum lipids profiles, and decreased energy expenditure (1, 49–51).

We have previously reported that the UOG mix has antagonist activity for estrogen, androgen, glucocorticoid, progesterone, and thyroid hormone receptors suggesting the UOG mix may antagonize one or more of these receptors during development to alter metabolic endpoints in adulthood (10). In this study, females exposed to the 1.5 and 150 μg/kg/day 23-UOG mix had lower total and resting energy expenditure and 15 μg/kg/day had lower non-resting energy expenditure in the dark cycle. Further, females developmentally exposed to the 15 and 150 μg/kg/day 23-UOG mix had lower spontaneous activity. These effects are the opposite of the increased energy expenditure and spontaneous activity after developmental exposure to estrogen receptor agonists (34, 38); thus, the UOG mixture may have programmed reduced energy expenditure and spontaneous activity at 7 months of age due to estrogen receptor antagonism during development. While there is little information on the developmental effects of estrogen receptor antagonists and adult energy expenditure, depletion of estrogen receptor activity (estrogen receptor-alpha knockout and g-protein coupled estrogen receptor knockout) has been associated with lower total energy expenditure suggesting estrogen receptor activity may modulate development of energy homeostasis in adulthood (50, 51). Androgenic effects during gestation could elicit some of the effects reported herein; however, since the UOG mix contains anti-androgenic activity rather than agonist activity, the effects observed in the current study in 7-month-old female mice, do not appear to be mediated through AR (1, 10). Taken together, while the lower energy expenditure and activity seen in the current study is consistent with antiestrogenic activity in the 23-UOG mixture, future studies are needed to delineate the exact developmental receptor pathways modulated by the 23-UOG mixture during development that alter adult energy expenditure.

In the current study, we expanded the exposure window from our prior work using a prenatal exposure (GD 11–18) to combine pre-conception, prenatal, and lactational exposure to assess impacts of adult maternal exposure prior to fertilization and to bracket fetal development from GD 1 to PND 21. Exposure during GD 1–11 covers development of the placenta, pancreas, and liver, and maternal high fat diet during this period has been shown to cause adverse metabolic outcomes in offspring (52). Also, a prolonged exposure through PND 21 includes development of the brain including expression of neurotransmitters and their receptors (53). The brain is a key modulator of energy balance regulating food intake, energy expenditure, and insulin secretion (54). UOG chemicals are cleared from the body within hours, so the exposure window for this study did not cover the time of mating to avoid male exposure as it has been shown male sperm can effect the epigenetics of offspring leading to obesity (55). Exposure started at GD 1, which is 24–36 h after mating depending on exactly when copulation occurred. This exposure paradigm is largely after the major wave of the zygotic activation phase between ~24 and 36 h, when the embryo is becoming transcriptionally active, which will result in some heterogeneity of exposure depending on when copulation occurred (56, 57). Epigenetic remodeling occurs during this developmental phase and experiments should specifically target this phase for exposure to determine if UOG chemical exposure alters epigenetic reprogramming (56, 58). Future work is needed to systematically assess the impacts of UOG exposure on the epigenetics of offspring and the unique impacts of different exposure windows.

In the current study, we report that a combined pre-conceptional, prenatal, and lactational exposure from GD 1 to PND 21 to a mixture of 23 UOG chemicals was associated with decreased body weights at PND 7 in females. Previously our lab has shown that a prenatal exposure from GD 11 to GD 18 to the same 23-UOG mixture resulted in the opposite–increased body weight at PND 7 and 21 (11). This may be due in part to the different exposure windows as developmental exposure to environmental chemicals can have quantitatively and qualitatively different effects depending on the exposure windows (59–61). Alternatively, decreased body weight at PND 7 in the current study could have been a transient acute effect from lactational exposure to the 23-UOG mixture or a result of altered maternal behavior as EDCs have been shown to disrupt maternal behavior (62–64).

Many factors contribute to energy balance, body composition, and body mass regulation. In this study, pre- and post-natal exposure to the 23-UOG mixture decreased total and resting energy expenditure in some UOG mix groups, but this did not result in altered body weight, lean mass, or fat mass in 7-month-old females. Although one would typically expect higher body mass or fat mass to track with lower energy expenditure, this is not always the case. For example, Wan et al. also found that AKT knockout mice displayed an increase in energy expenditure compared to control mice matched for body mass (65). A limitation of indirect calorimetry is that it is taken at one point in time and does not represent energy metabolism throughout the lifespan of the animal. It is possible that the lower energy expenditure measured in the 23-UOG mixture may have led to greater body mass if mice were aged longer-a question directly assessed in a companion paper in this journal, Balise et al. (submitted). In addition, although efforts were made to reduce any stress caused by the indirect calorimetry cages by providing an acclimation period and using the same bedding as home cages, it is possible that a change to a new environment impacted control mice and 23 UOG exposed mice differently during the defined period of time. Energy homeostasis is maintained with different compensating mechanisms such as differences in digestion, skeletal muscle metabolism, adipose storage, or fecal deposition. In addition, although we carefully measured food intake at defined periods of time, it is possible that small reductions in food intake allowed 23-UOG mixture treated animals to maintain normal body mass despite reduced energy expenditure. Future long-term studies can be conducted to determine if these significant decrements in energy expenditure have long term ramifications for body mass and metabolic health. At this age, an impact on body weight might not be seen unless the system is challenged beyond compensatory mechanisms. For example, a high-fat diet or western style diet challenge has revealed underlying metabolic programming following developmental exposure to other EDCs, such as DEHP, atrazine, and BPA (66–68). Further studies challenging these animals with a high fat high sugar diet might reveal underlying metabolic differences by challenging the homeostatic mechanisms that regulate metabolism (see Balise et al., submitted).

Overall, we have reported that the 23-UOG mixture can alter developmental programming and result in altered energy expenditure and activity of 7-month-old females. The results shown thus far highlight the need for additional research on metabolic health effects in humans and animals in drilling-dense regions. More studies should be aimed at understanding exposure to UOG and other environmental chemicals on metabolic health outcomes (69).

AUTHOR CONTRIBUTIONS

VB and JC-G performed animal experiments. VB analyzed the data. SN secured funding, directed experiments and assisted in data analysis and interpretation. All authors have contributed to the design of experiments, interpretation of the data, and writing the manuscript.

FUNDING

Funding was received from NIH R21ES026395 (SN), R01ES021394-04S1 (SN and VB), and from the department of Obstetrics, Gynecology and Women's Health, University of Missouri (SN and VB), VA-Merit Grant I01BX003271-01 (RR), and NIH DK088940 (JT), VA Merit Award 1I01BX002567-01 (JT), and United States Environmental Protection Agency Science To Achieve Results Fellowship Assistance Agreement FP-91747101 (CK).

ACKNOWLEDGMENTS

We wish to thank members of the Nagel lab for helping with animal husbandry, particularly Sierra Baxter, Brittany Parmenter, Leighton McCabe, Anne Maas, Katelyn Cinnamon, and Kara Klemp.

REFERENCES

1. Kassotis CD, Klemp KC, Vu DC, Lin CH, Meng CX, Besch-Williford CL, et al. Endocrine-disrupting activity of hydraulic fracturing chemicals and adverse health outcomes after prenatal exposure in male mice. *Endocrinology.* (2015) 156:4458–73. doi: 10.1210/en.2015-1375
2. Burton GA Jr., Basu N, Ellis BR, Kapo KE, Entrekin, S, Nadelhoffer K. Hydraulic "fracking": are surface water impacts an ecological concern? *Environ Toxicol Chem.* (2014) 33:1679–89. doi: 10.1002/etc.2619
3. Ingraffea AR, Wells MT, Santoro RL, Shonkoff SB. Assessment and risk analysis of casing and cement impairment in oil and gas wells in Pennsylvania, 2000-2012. *Proc Natl Acad Sci USA.* (2014) 111:10955–60. doi: 10.1073/pnas.1323422111
4. Kassotis CD, Iwanowicz LR, Akob DM, Cozzarelli IM, Mumford AC, Orem WH, et al. Endocrine disrupting activities of surface water associated with a West Virginia oil and gas industry wastewater disposal site. *Sci Total Environ.* (2016) 557–558:901–10. doi: 10.1016/j.scitotenv.2016.03.113
5. Mauter MS, Alvarez PJ, Burton A, Cafaro DC, Chen W, Gregory KB, et al. Regional variation in water-related impacts of shale gas development and implications for emerging international plays. *Environ Sci Technol.* (2014) 48:8298–306. doi: 10.1021/es405432k
6. Rozell DJ, Reaven SJ. Water pollution risk associated with natural gas extraction from the Marcellus Shale. *Risk Anal.* (2012) 32:1382–93. doi: 10.1111/j.1539-6924.2011.01757.x
7. Vengosh A, Jackson RB, Warner N, Darrah TH, Kondash A. A critical review of the risks to water resources from unconventional shale gas development and hydraulic fracturing in the United States. *Environ Sci Technol.* (2014) 48:8334–48. doi: 10.1021/es405118y
8. Zoeller RT, Brown TR, Doan LL, Gore AC, Skakkebaek NE, Soto AM, et al. Endocrine-disrupting chemicals and public health protection: a statement of principles from The Endocrine Society. *Endocrinology.* (2012) 153:4097–110. doi: 10.1210/en.2012-1422
9. Diamanti-Kandarakis E, Bourguignon JP, Giudice LC, Hauser R, Prins GS, Soto AM, et al. Endocrine-disrupting chemicals: an Endocrine Society scientific statement. *Endocr Rev.* (2009) 30:293–342. doi: 10.1210/er.2009-0002
10. Kassotis CD, Tillitt DE, Davis JW, Hormann AM, Nagel SC. Estrogen and androgen receptor activities of hydraulic fracturing chemicals and surface and ground water in a drilling-dense region. *Endocrinology.* (2014) 155:897–907. doi: 10.1210/en.2013-1697
11. Kassotis CD, Bromfield JJ, Klemp KC, Meng CX, Wolfe A, Zoeller RT, et al. Adverse Reproductive and developmental health outcomes following prenatal exposure to a hydraulic fracturing chemical mixture in female C57Bl/6 Mice. *Endocrinology.* (2016) 157:3469–81. doi: 10.1210/en.2016-1242

12. Folkerts EJ, Blewett TA, He Y, Goss GG. Alterations to Juvenile Zebrafish (*Danio rerio*) swim performance after acute embryonic exposure to sub-lethal exposures of hydraulic fracturing flowback and produced water. *Aquat Toxicol.* (2017) 193:50–9. doi: 10.1016/j.aquatox.2017.10.003
13. He Y, Sun C, Zhang Y, Folkerts EJ, Martin JW, Goss GG. Developmental toxicity of the organic fraction from hydraulic fracturing flowback and produced waters to early life stages of Zebrafish (*Danio rerio*). *Environ Sci Technol.* (2018) 52:3820–30. doi: 10.1021/acs.est.7b06557
14. Elliott EG, Ettinger AS, Leaderer BP, Bracken MB, Deziel NC. A systematic evaluation of chemicals in hydraulic-fracturing fluids and wastewater for reproductive and developmental toxicity. *J Expo Sci Environ Epidemiol.* (2017) 27:90–9. doi: 10.1038/jes.2015.81
15. Schug TT, Janesick A, Blumberg B, Heindel JJ. Endocrine disrupting chemicals and disease susceptibility. *J Steroid Biochem Mol Biol.* (2011) 127:204–15. doi: 10.1016/j.jsbmb.2011.08.007
16. Grun, F, Blumberg B. Environmental obesogens: organotins and endocrine disruption via nuclear receptor signaling. *Endocrinology.* (2006) 147:S50–5. doi: 10.1210/en.2005-1129
17. Heindel JJ, Vom Saal FS, Blumberg B, Bovolin P, Calamandrei G, Ceresini G, et al. Parma consensus statement on metabolic disruptors. *Environ Health.* (2015) 14:54. doi: 10.1186/s12940-015-0042-7
18. Darbre PD. Endocrine disruptors and obesity. *Curr Obes Rep.* (2017) 6:18–27. doi: 10.1007/s13679-017-0240-4
19. Heindel JJ, Blumberg B, Cave M, Machtinger R, Mantovani A, Mendez MA, et al. Metabolism disrupting chemicals and metabolic disorders. *Reprod Toxicol.* (2017) 68:3–33. doi: 10.1016/j.reprotox.2016.10.001
20. Kassotis CD, Hoffman, K, Stapleton HM. Characterization of adipogenic activity of house dust extracts and semi-volatile indoor contaminants in 3T3-L1 cells. *Environ Sci Technol.* (2017) 51:8735–45. doi: 10.1021/acs.est.7b01788
21. Folkerts EJ, Blewett TA, He Y, Goss GG. Cardio-respirometry disruption in zebrafish (*Danio rerio*) embryos exposed to hydraulic fracturing flowback and produced water. *Environ Pollut.* (2017) 231:1477–87. doi: 10.1016/j.envpol.2017.09.011
22. Stacy SL, Brink LL, Larkin JC, Sadovsky Y, Goldstein BD, Pitt BR, et al. Perinatal outcomes and unconventional natural gas operations in Southwest Pennsylvania. *PLoS ONE.* (2015) 10:e0126425. doi: 10.1371/journal.pone.0126425
23. McKenzie LM, Guo R, Witter RZ, Savitz DA, Newman LS, Adgate JL. Birth outcomes and maternal residential proximity to natural gas development in rural Colorado. *Environ Health Perspect.* (2014) 122:412–7. doi: 10.1289/ehp.1306722
24. Currie J, Greenstone, M, Meckel K. Hydraulic fracturing and infant health: new evidence from Pennsylvania. *Sci Adv.* (2017) 3:e1603021. doi: 10.1126/sciadv.1603021
25. Johnsson IW, Haglund B, Ahlsson, F, Gustafsson J. A high birth weight is associated with increased risk of type 2 diabetes and obesity. *Pediatr Obes.* (2015) 10:77–83. doi: 10.1111/ijpo.230
26. Park YM, Kanaley JA, Padilla J, Zidon T, Welly RJ, Will MJ, et al. Effects of intrinsic aerobic capacity and ovariectomy on voluntary wheel running and nucleus accumbens dopamine receptor gene expression. *Physiol Behav.* (2016) 164:383–9. doi: 10.1016/j.physbeh.2016.06.006
27. Morris EM, Jackman MR, Johnson GC, Liu TW, Lopez JL, Kearney ML, et al. Intrinsic aerobic capacity impacts susceptibility to acute high-fat diet-induced hepatic steatosis. *Am J Physiol Endocrinol Metab.* (2014) 307:E355–64. doi: 10.1152/ajpendo.00093.2014
28. Angle BM, Do RP, Ponzi D, Stahlhut RW, Drury BE, Nagel SC, et al. Metabolic disruption in male mice due to fetal exposure to low but not high doses of bisphenol A (BPA): evidence for effects on body weight, food intake, adipocytes, leptin, adiponectin, insulin and glucose regulation. *Reprod Toxicol.* (2013) 42:256–68. doi: 10.1016/j.reprotox.2013.07.017
29. Faulk C, Barks A, Sanchez BN, Zhang Z, Anderson OS, Peterson KE, et al. Perinatal lead (Pb) exposure results in sex-specific effects on food intake, fat, weight, and insulin response across the murine life-course. *PLoS ONE.* (2014) 9:e104273. doi: 10.1371/journal.pone.0104273
30. Hatch EE, Troisi R, Palmer JR, Wise LA, Titus L, Strohsnitter WC, et al. Prenatal diethylstilbestrol exposure and risk of obesity in adult women. *J Dev Orig Health Dis.* (2015) 6:201–7. doi: 10.1017/S2040174415000033
31. Jensen ET, Longnecker MP. Pharmacologic sex hormones in pregnancy in relation to offspring obesity. *Obesity (Silver Spring).* (2014) 22:2406–12. doi: 10.1002/oby.20778
32. Rodriguez KF, Ungewitter EK, Crespo-Mejias Y, Liu C, Nicol B, Kissling GE, et al. Effects of *in utero* exposure to arsenic during the second half of gestation on reproductive end points and metabolic parameters in female CD-1 Mice. *Environ Health Perspect.* (2016) 124:336–43. doi: 10.1289/ehp.1509703
33. Abbott BD, Wood CR, Watkins AM, Tatum-Gibbs K, Das KP, Lau C. Effects of perfluorooctanoic acid (PFOA) on expression of peroxisome proliferator-activated receptors (PPAR) and nuclear receptor-regulated genes in fetal and postnatal CD-1 mouse tissues. *Reprod Toxicol.* (2012) 33:491–505. doi: 10.1016/j.reprotox.2011.11.005
34. Anderson OS, Peterson KE, Sanchez BN, Zhang Z, Mancuso P, Dolinoy DC. Perinatal bisphenol A exposure promotes hyperactivity, lean body composition, and hormonal responses across the murine life course. *FASEB J.* (2013) 27:1784–92. doi: 10.1096/fj.12-223545
35. Davey JC, Nomikos AP, Wungjiranirun M, Sherman JR, Ingram L, Batki C, et al. Arsenic as an endocrine disruptor: arsenic disrupts retinoic acid receptor-and thyroid hormone receptor-mediated gene regulation and thyroid hormone-mediated amphibian tail metamorphosis. *Environ Health Perspect.* (2008) 116:165–72. doi: 10.1289/ehp.10131
36. Doumouchtsis KK, Doumouchtsis SK, Doumouchtsis EK, Perrea DN. The effect of lead intoxication on endocrine functions. *J Endocrinol Invest.* (2009) 32:175–83. doi: 10.1007/BF03345710
37. Ronis MJ, Gandy J, Badger T, Endocrine mechanisms underlying reproductive toxicity in the developing rat chronically exposed to dietary lead. *J Toxicol Environ Health A.* (1998) 54:77–99. doi: 10.1080/009841098158935
38. van Esterik JC, Dolle ME, Lamoree MH, van Leeuwen SP, Hamers T, Legler JLT, et al. Programming of metabolic effects in C57BL/6JxFVB mice by exposure to bisphenol A during gestation and lactation. *Toxicology.* (2014) 321:40–52. doi: 10.1016/j.tox.2014.04.001
39. Yin Y, Lin C, Veith GM, Chen H, Dhandha M, Ma L. Neonatal diethylstilbestrol exposure alters the metabolic profile of uterine epithelial cells. *Dis Model Mech.* (2012) 5:870–80. doi: 10.1242/dmm.009076
40. Behr AC, Lichtenstein D, Braeuning A, Lampen A, Buhrke T. Perfluoroalkylated substances (PFAS) affect neither estrogen and androgen receptor activity nor steroidogenesis in human cells *in vitro*. *Toxicol Lett.* (2018) 291:51–60. doi: 10.1016/j.toxlet.2018.03.029
41. Jana K, Jana, S, Samanta PK. Effects of chronic exposure to sodium arsenite on hypothalamo-pituitary-testicular activities in adult rats: possible an estrogenic mode of action. *Reprod Biol Endocrinol.* (2006) 4:9. doi: 10.1186/1477-7827-4-9
42. Johnson SA, Painter MS, Javurek AB, Ellersieck MR, Wiedmeyer CE, Thyfault JP, et al. Sex-dependent effects of developmental exposure to bisphenol A and ethinyl estradiol on metabolic parameters and voluntary physical activity. *J Dev Orig Health Dis.* (2015) 6:539–52. doi: 10.1017/S2040174415001488
43. Ryan KK, Haller AM, Sorrell JE, Woods SC, Jandacek RJ, Seeley RJ. Perinatal exposure to bisphenol-a and the development of metabolic syndrome in CD-1 mice. *Endocrinology.* (2010) 151:2603–12. doi: 10.1210/en.2009-1218
44. Mackay H, Patterson ZR, Khazall R, Patel S, Tsirlin D, Abizaid A. Organizational effects of perinatal exposure to bisphenol-A and diethylstilbestrol on arcuate nucleus circuitry controlling food intake and energy expenditure in male and female CD-1 mice. *Endocrinology.* (2013) 154:1465–75. doi: 10.1210/en.2012-2044
45. Dolinoy DC, Weidman JR, Waterland RA, Jirtle RL. Maternal genistein alters coat color and protects Avy mouse offspring from obesity by modifying the fetal epigenome. *Environ Health Perspect.* (2006) 114:567–72. doi: 10.1289/ehp.8700
46. Mosci P, Pietrella D, Ricci G, Pandey N, Monari C, Pericolini E, et al. Mouse strain-dependent differences in estrogen sensitivity during vaginal candidiasis. *Mycopathologia.* (2013) 175:1–11. doi: 10.1007/s11046-012-9589-9
47. Delitala AP, Capobianco G, Delitala G, Cherchi PL, Dessole S. Polycystic ovary syndrome, adipose tissue and metabolic syndrome. *Arch Gynecol Obstet.* (2017) 296:405–19. doi: 10.1007/s00404-017-4429-2
48. M't Mannetje M, van Houten ELAF, McLuskey A, Kramer P, Themmen APN, Visser JA. The effect of androgens on adipose tissue in PCOS.

Endocrine Abstracts. (2011) 26:P322. Available online at: https://www.endocrine-abstracts.org/ea/0026/ea0026p322

49. Buffington CK, Givens JR, Kitabchi AE. Opposing actions of dehydroepiandrosterone and testosterone on insulin sensitivity. *In vivo* and *in vitro* studies of hyperandrogenic females. *Diabetes.* (1991) 40:693–700. doi: 10.2337/diabetes.40.6.693
50. Ban Z, Maurischat P, Benz V, Brix S, Sonnenburg A, Schuler G, et al. High-fat diet induces unexpected fatal uterine infections in mice with aP2-cre-mediated deletion of estrogen receptor alpha. *Sci Rep.* (2017) 7:43269. doi: 10.1038/srep43269
51. Davis KE, Carstens EJ, Irani BG, Gent LM, Hahner LM, Clegg DJ. Sexually dimorphic role of G protein-coupled estrogen receptor (GPER) in modulating energy homeostasis. *Horm Behav.* (2014) 66:196–207. doi: 10.1016/j.yhbeh.2014.02.004
52. Williams L, Seki Y, Vuguin, PM, Charron MJ. Animal models of *in utero* exposure to a high fat diet: a review. *Biochim Biophys Acta.* (2014) 1842:507–19. doi: 10.1016/j.bbadis.2013.07.006
53. Semple BD, Blomgren K, Gimlin K, Ferriero DM, Noble-Haeusslein LJ. Brain development in rodents and humans: identifying benchmarks of maturation and vulnerability to injury across species. *Prog Neurobiol.* (2013) 106–107:1–16. doi: 10.1016/j.pneurobio.2013.04.001
54. Roh E, Song DK, Kim MS. Emerging role of the brain in the homeostatic regulation of energy and glucose metabolism. *Exp Mol Med.* (2016) 48:e216. doi: 10.1038/emm.2016.4
55. Houfflyn S, Matthys C, Soubry A. Male obesity: epigenetic origin and effects in sperm and offspring. *Curr Mol Biol Rep.* (2017) 3:288–96. doi: 10.1007/s40610-017-0083-5
56. Eckersley-Maslin MA, Alda-Catalinas C, Reik W. Dynamics of the epigenetic landscape during the maternal-to-zygotic transition. *Nat Rev Mol Cell Biol.* (2018) 19:436–50. doi: 10.1038/s41580-018-0008-z
57. Tadros W, Lipshitz HD. The maternal-to-zygotic transition: a play in two acts. *Development.* (2009) 136:3033–42. doi: 10.1242/dev.033183
58. Herrera BM, Keildson, S, Lindgren CM. Genetics and epigenetics of obesity. *Maturitas.* (2011) 69:41–9. doi: 10.1016/j.maturitas.2011.02.018
59. Gioiosa L, Fissore E, Ghirardelli G, Parmigiani, S, Palanza P. Developmental exposure to low-dose estrogenic endocrine disruptors alters sex differences in exploration and emotional responses in mice. *Horm Behav.* (2007) 52:307–16. doi: 10.1016/j.yhbeh.2007.05.006
60. Gioiosa L, Parmigiani S, Vom Saal FS, Palanza P. The effects of bisphenol A on emotional behavior depend upon the timing of exposure, age and gender in mice. *Horm Behav.* (2013) 63:598–605. doi: 10.1016/j.yhbeh.2013.02.016
61. Mendez MA, Torrent M, Ferrer C, Ribas-Fito N, Sunyer J. Maternal smoking very early in pregnancy is related to child overweight at age 5-7 y. *Am J Clin Nutr.* (2008) 87:1906–13. doi: 10.1093/ajcn/87.6.1906
62. Johnson SA, Javurek AB, Painter MS, Peritore MP, Ellersieck MR, Roberts RM, et al. Disruption of parenting behaviors in california mice, a monogamous rodent species, by endocrine disrupting chemicals. *PLoS ONE.* (2015) 10:e0126284. doi: 10.1371/journal.pone.0126284
63. Palanza P, Nagel SC, Parmigiani, S, Vom Saal FS. Perinatal exposure to endocrine disruptors: sex, timing and behavioral endpoints. *Curr Opin Behav Sci.* (2016) 7:69–75. doi: 10.1016/j.cobeha.2015.11.017
64. Palanza PL, Howdeshell KL, Parmigiani, S, vom Saal FS. Exposure to a low dose of bisphenol A during fetal life or in adulthood alters maternal behavior in mice. *Environ Health Perspect.* (2002) 110(Suppl. 3):415–22. doi: 10.1289/ehp.02110s3415
65. Wan M, Easton RM, Gleason CE, Monks BR, Ueki K, Kahn CR, et al. Loss of Akt1 in mice increases energy expenditure and protects against diet-induced obesity. *Mol Cell Biol.* (2012) 32:96–106. doi: 10.1128/MCB.05806-11
66. Strakovsky RS, Lezmi S, Shkoda I, Flaws JA, Helferich WG, Pan YX. *In utero* growth restriction and catch-up adipogenesis after developmental di (2-ethylhexyl) phthalate exposure cause glucose intolerance in adult male rats following a high-fat dietary challenge. *J Nutr Biochem.* (2015) 26:1208–20. doi: 10.1016/j.jnutbio.2015.05.012
67. Lim S, Ahn SY, Song IC, Chung MH, Jang HC, Park KS, et al. Chronic exposure to the herbicide, atrazine, causes mitochondrial dysfunction and insulin resistance. *PLoS ONE.* (2009) 4:e5186. doi: 10.1371/journal.pone.0005186
68. Wei J, Lin Y, Li Y, Ying C, Chen J, Song L, et al. Perinatal exposure to bisphenol A at reference dose predisposes offspring to metabolic syndrome in adult rats on a high-fat diet. *Endocrinology.* (2011) 152:3049–61. doi: 10.1210/en.2011-0045
69. Legler J, Fletcher T, Govarts E, Porta M, Blumberg B, Heindel JJ, et al. Obesity, diabetes, and associated costs of exposure to endocrine-disrupting chemicals in the European Union. *J Clin Endocrinol Metab.* (2015) 100:1278–88. doi: 10.1210/jc.2014-4326

13

Analysis of Lipid Metabolism, Immune Function, and Neurobehavior in Adult C57BL/6JxFVB Mice After Developmental Exposure to Di (2-Ethylhexyl) Phthalate

*Liana Bastos Sales [1], Joantine C. J. van Esterik [2], Hennie M. Hodemaekers [3], Marja H. Lamoree [1], Timo Hamers [1], Leo T. M. van der Ven [3] and Juliette Legler [4,5]**

[1] Department of Environment and Health, Vrije Universiteit Amsterdam, Amsterdam, Netherlands, [2] Department of Pathobiology, Faculty of Veterinary Medicine, Utrecht University, Utrecht, Netherlands, [3] Center for Health Protection, National Institute for Public Health and the Environment (RIVM), Bilthoven, Netherlands, [4] Institute for Risk Assessment Sciences (IRAS), Utrecht University, Utrecht, Netherlands, [5] Utrecht Institute for Pharmaceutical Sciences, Utrecht University, Utrecht, Netherlands

Correspondence:
Juliette Legler
j.legler@uu.nl

Background: Developmental exposure to di (2-ethylhexyl) phthalate (DEHP) has been implicated in the onset of metabolic syndrome later in life. Alterations in neurobehavior and immune functions are also affected by phthalate exposure and may be linked to the metabolic changes caused by developmental exposure to DEHP.

Objectives: Our goal was to study the effects of developmental exposure to DEHP in the context of metabolic syndrome by integrating different parameters to assess metabolic, neurobehavioral, and immune functions in one model.

Methods: Female C57BL/6J mice were exposed to DEHP through the diet during gestation and lactation at doses ranging from 3.3 to 100,000 μg/kg body weight/day (μkd). During a 1-year follow-up period, a wide set of metabolic parameters was assessed in the F1 offspring, including weekly body weight measurements, food consumption, physical activity, glucose homeostasis, serum lipids, and endocrine profile. In addition, neurobehavioral and immune functions were assessed by sweet preference test, object recognition test, acute phase protein, and cytokines production. Animals were challenged with a high fat diet (HFD) in the last 9 weeks of the study.

Results: Increased free fatty acids (FFA) and, high density lipoprotein (HDL-C) were observed in serum, together with a decrease in glycated hemoglobin levels in blood of 1-year old male DEHP-exposed offspring after HFD challenge. For the most sensitive endpoint measured (FFA), a lower bound of the 90%-confidence interval for benchmark dose (BMD) at a critical effect size of 5% (BMDL) of 2,160 μkd was calculated. No persistent changes in body weight or fat mass were observed. At 33,000 μkd altered performance was found in the object recognition test in males and changes in interferon (IFN)γ production were observed in females.

Conclusions: Developmental exposure to DEHP combined with HFD in adulthood led to changes in lipid metabolism and neurobehavior in male offspring and cytokine production in female offspring. Our findings contribute to the evidence that DEHP is a developmental dyslipidemic chemical, however, more research is needed to further characterize adverse health outcomes and the mechanisms of action associated with the observed sex-specific effects.

Keywords: early-life exposure, DEHP, lipid metabolism, neurobehavior, immunofunction, sex-specificity, mouse model, developmental exposure and adult disease

INTRODUCTION

Metabolic syndrome (MetS) is a pathologic condition characterized by abdominal obesity, insulin resistance, hypertension, dyslipidemia, and hyperglycemia (1). The MetS prevalence among adults in the US (24–34%) (2) and in China (24.5%) (3) indicates its epidemic proportions. Many interventions have targeted excessive food intake and sedentary lifestyle without success, indicating the need for a better understanding of the factors involved in the pathogenesis of MetS (4). Increasing attention has been given to the developmental origins of health and disease (DOHaD) hypothesis (5), in which early exposure to stressors during critical periods of life may induce effects that manifest later in life. Exposure to environmental chemicals is one of the stressors which has been linked to the high MetS prevalence rates, and evidence is growing that exposure during periods when adipocytes are differentiating and/or organs as pancreas, liver, and brain are developing can lead to disruption of normal development and alterations in the homeostatic control of adipogenesis and energy balance (6).

Di(2-ethylhexyl) phthalate (DEHP) is an example of an environmental chemical which has been linked to metabolic disorders. It is used to add flexibility to polyvinyl chloride polymers (7). Human exposure occurs mainly orally, by migration of the chemical from the packaging to food such as fatty fish, meat and milk (8). DEHP metabolites have been detected in human samples of blood and urine, confirming the ubiquitous presence of DEHP (8, 9). DEHP is an endocrine disrupting chemical (EDC) and has putative obesogenic properties as reported in epidemiological, animal and *in vitro* studies (10). The first line of evidence that developmental exposure to DEHP may promote metabolic disorders was the increases in serum cholesterol (CHOL), triglycerides (TGs) and glucose reported in multiple studies (11–13). Recently, Wassenaar and Legler (14) conducted a systematic review and meta-analysis of experimental rodent studies with DEHP, and reported a statistically significant positive association between developmental exposure to DEHP and increased fat pad weight. However, further associations with triglycerides, free fatty acids (FFA) and leptin could not be analyzed due to few or no data available. The second line of evidence for a role for DEHP in metabolic disorder is its effects on neurobehavior, given the interaction of the brain with other key metabolic organs via signaling molecules and neuronal connections at the basis of pathways such as regulation of appetite (15). Schmidt et al. (16) reported an alteration in food intake in female C3H/N mice after an 8-week exposure to DEHP, and Barakat et al. (17) reported an impairment in neurobehavior and recognition memory in male CD-1 mice after prenatal exposure to DEHP. In addition, inflammation and activation of the immune system have been observed in abdominal obesity and may have a role in the pathogenesis of obesity-related metabolic disorders (18). Specifically, *in utero* exposure to DEHP increased serum levels of C-reactive protein (CRP) and tumor necrosis factor (TNF), increased TNF levels in adipose tissue homogenates, and promoted a focal macrophage infiltration in whole-adipose tissue, suggesting a systemic and local adipose inflammation in the adult male offspring of Sprague-Dawley rats (19).

Given the previous findings in separate studies and the need to have a global view of the effects of developmental exposure to DEHP, we hypothesized that early exposure to DEHP may affect metabolic, neurobehavioral, and immunological domains in an integrated manner. Our aim was to perform a combined assessment of metabolism disruptive properties, neurobehavior, and immune function following developmental exposure to DEHP. To achieve this, metabolic alterations in adult mouse offspring were studied after maternal dietary exposure during gestation and lactation, using seven doses ranging from doses relevant to human diet exposure (20) to a dose approximating the no observed adverse effect level (NOAEL) for developmental toxicity in CD-1 mice (21). The offspring was followed for one year and parameters related to energy balance (weekly body weight measurements, food consumption, and physical activity) and metabolism (glucose homeostasis, serum lipids, and endocrine profile) were assessed. In the last 9 weeks of the follow-up, offspring was challenged with a high fat diet (HFD) to test potential disturbances in their metabolic homeostatic capacity. A sweet preference test and an object recognition test were

Abbreviations: BMD, Benchmark dose; BMDL/BMDU, lower/upper bound of the 90%-confidence interval for BMD at a critical effect size of 5%; CHOL, cholesterol; conA, concanavalin A; CRP, C-reactive protein; DEHP, di (2-ethylhexyl) phthalate; DOHaD, developmental origins of health and disease; FFA, free fatty acids; GTT, glucose tolerance test; HbA1c, Glycated hemoglobin; HDL-C, high density lipoprotein cholesterol; HFD, high fat diet; IFN-γ, interferon γ; ITT, insulin tolerance test; LOQ, limit of quantification; LPS, lipopolysaccharide; MECPP, mono(2-ethyl-5-carboxypentyl)phthalate; MEHHP, mono(2-ethyl-5-hydroxyhexyl) phthalate; MEHP, mono (2-ethylhexyl) phthalate; MEOHP, mono(2-ethyl-5-oxohexyl)phthalate; MetS, metabolic syndrome; NOAEL, no observed adverse effect level; NO, nitric oxide; PND, postnatal day; ORT, object recognition test; TGs, triglycerides; TNF, tumor necrosis factor; T1, training session; T2, test session; μkd, μg/kg body weight/day.

performed to assess neurobehavior whereas levels of CRP and pro- and anti-inflammatory cytokines were measured to assess immunological function.

MATERIALS AND METHODS

Test Chemical and Test Diets

DEHP (D201154, purity ≥99.5%, Sigma-Aldrich, Zwijndrecht, The Netherlands) was dissolved in soy oil (Research Diet Services, Wijk bij Duurstede, The Netherlands), by gently stirring at room temperature for 2 min. Serial dilutions of this master solution and blank soy oil were mixed with the diet (NIH-07 diet, Research Diet Services, Wijk bij Duurstede, The Netherlands) before pelleting, aiming at concentrations in a range of 0.018–555.6 mg DEHP/kg feed, corresponding to targeted exposures of 0, 3.3, 33, 330, 3,300, 10,000, 33,000, and 100,000 μg/kg body weight/day (μkd) based on an average food consumption of 4.5 g/mouse (average body weight of 25 g)/day(d).

Experimental Conditions

This study was approved by the Animal Experimentation Ethical Committee of National Institute for Public Health and Environment under permit number 201100086 and carried out in accordance with prevailing legislation.

Nulliparous 13–14 weeks old female C57BL/6J mice (Charles River, Sulzfeld, Germany) were mated with 12–16 weeks old male FVB mice (GLP, Bilthoven, The Netherlands) to produce hybrid offspring with a known background information of phenotype and development (22). Mice were housed as previously reported (23). After an acclimatization period of 2 weeks, F0 female mice were fed experimental diets for 9 weeks starting 2 weeks pre-mating. Each dose group had six F0 females, which, to accommodate time and space restrictions, were mated in groups of three with one F0 male. Body weight and feed consumption of F0 females were monitored during pre-mating, gestation, and lactation. Anogenital distance of the offspring was assessed at post-natal day (PND) 4 and PND7 in the control, 3,300 and 100,000 μkd dose groups. Litter size was assessed at PND4 and PND21. At PND 21, after sacrifice by cervical dislocation under ketamine/xylazine anesthesia, serum of the dams was collected for DEHP metabolite determination.

From PND 21, offspring was weaned and housed individually (males M) or in groups of 2–3 animals (females F). Six litters of 5 or less pups (in dose groups 0, 33, 330, 10,000, 33,000 and 100,000 μkd) were discarded to avoid the effect of small litters on postnatal growth (23). After weaning, an average of 9 mice per sex (range 6–11) were included per dose group for follow-up through juvenile and adult stages. The control group consisted of 23 male and 19 female mice. Mice from available litters were randomly allocated to dose group using a computer-generated sequence, obtaining the following total number of individuals and litters, respectively per dose group/sex: 0 (M: 23/10; F:19/8), 3.3 (M:10/5; F:9/3), 33 (M:9/4; F:8/5), 330 (M:8/3; F:10/3), 3,300 (M:9/4; F:10/4), 10,000 (M:10/4; F:11/5), 33,000 (M:10/5;F:9/5) and 100,000 (M: 6/3; F:10/3). DEHP containing diet was discontinued at PND21 and offspring was further fed with the control NIH-07 diet. During the final 9 weeks of the study (starting at 46 weeks of age in males and at 48 weeks in females), all F1 offspring was challenged with a NIH-07 based HFD (D12451) containing 45 kcal% fat (lard) compared to 15 kcal% fat in the NIH-07 diet. Body weight was measured weekly from 5 to 55–57 weeks of age. In some experiments described below, a selection of control, middle (330 μkd) and/or high (33,000 μkd) DEHP dose groups was made to allow better allocation of resources and was based on evaluation of body weight changes such as for glucose homeostasis study or on the importance of observed parameter to middle or high exposures.

In vivo Experiments in Adult F1 Mice

Feed consumption was measured weekly in all F1 offspring at 21–23 weeks of age. Physical activity was measured in control and 33,000 μkd at 27–29 weeks of age. For this purpose, 10 animals per sex and per group were transferred to polysulfone cages mounted on Laboras platforms (Metris BV, Hoofddorp, The Netherlands). After an acclimatization period of at least 6 h, time spent in locomotion was continuously monitored for 36 h (males, individually caged) and 60 h (females, group caged) starting at 6.30 p.m. (begin dark phase) and expressed as kinetic energy indices per cage per 15 min as described in van Esterik et al. (23). At 30 and 31 weeks of age, a glucose tolerance test (GTT) with a 18-h fasting period and insulin tolerance test (ITT) were performed in both control and 33,000 μkd males and females offspring (24). Briefly, for the GTT a baseline glucose blood sample (0 min) in tail vein was taken before D-glucose injection i.p. at a concentration of 1.5 g/kg bw. At 15, 30, 60, and 120 min after injection, glucose was measured with a FreeStyle Lite meter (Abbott, Hoofddorp, The Netherlands). For ITT, glucose was measured before (0 min) and 15, 30, 45, and 60 min after insulin injection i.p. at a concentration of 0.75 IU/kg bw.

At 37–39 weeks of age, control and 33,000 μkd mice (n = 8–10 per sex per group) were subjected to an object recognition test (ORT) (24). Briefly, after habituation in the test cage, a training session (T1) started in which animals were exposed to two identical objects during 5 min. After a retention time of 120 min, test session (T2) took place by which animals were exposed to one familiar object and one novel object during 5 min. During both sessions, the time spent exploring each object was recorded with a stopwatch by the observer situated in front of the cage at 1 meter distance.

At 40 weeks of age, control and 33,000 μkd mice (n = 8–10 per sex per group) were subjected to a sucrose preference test as described previously (24). Briefly, animals were placed in a cage with two bottles filled with tap water and habituated for 4 days. Afterwards, a 4-day-test session was started in which a bottle filled with water and one with 1% w/v sucrose solution were available. Bottles were daily weighed and sucrose preference was calculated as percentage of sucrose water consumption out of total liquid consumption.

Necropsy F1 Mice

At termination of the *in vivo* study, after being fasted for 18 h to induce a general basal metabolic state, mice were sacrificed under ketamine/xylazine anesthesia. Nose-anus length, right femur length, body weight and glucose levels were assessed at dissection time. Liver, pancreas, spleen, brain, *m. quadriceps femoris*, thymus, adrenals, femur, testis, perigonadal fat, interscapular fat, and perirenal fat were weighed and fixed in formalin and/or liquid nitrogen. Formalin-fixed organs were stored at 4°C (except femur at room temperature), and after 24 h transferred to 70% alcohol. Blood samples were collected at the time of dissection by orbital puncture, treated with Pefabloc SC PLUS (Roche, Mannheim, Germany) to neutralize proteases, allowed to clot and centrifuged. Serum samples, snap-frozen organs and adipose tissue were stored at −80°C until further analysis. All F1 animals at this stage were fed a HFD so the measurements performed were under HFD condition.

Ex vivo Experiments

Internal Dose Measurement in F0

To avoid incorrect conclusions on internal exposure to DEHP due to contamination of samples with background levels of DEHP or its primary metabolite mono (2-ethylhexyl) phthalate (MEHP), secondary metabolites are preferred as biomarkers of DEHP exposure (8). Serum samples of 200 μl from dams on PND21 were analyzed for the presence of DEHP secondary metabolites: mono(2-ethyl-5-carboxypentyl)phthalate (MECPP), mono(2-ethyl-5-hydroxyhexyl) phthalate (MEHHP), and mono(2-ethyl-5-oxohexyl)phthalate (MEOHP) (9). Briefly, the analytical method includes an enzymatic deconjugation step, followed by solid phase extraction and quantitative analysis using isotope dilution. The chemical analysis was performed on an on-line trapping column in combination with liquid chromatography with mass spectrometric detection. In doses below 33 μkd, most metabolite concentrations were below the limit of quantification (LOQ), and for those samples, the equation $LOQ/\sqrt{2}$ was used to generate values for mean calculation (25).

Immune Assessments in F1

Single-cell splenocyte suspensions were prepared from adult F1 mice controls, 330 and 33,000 μkd DEHP dose groups after exposure to a HFD by using fresh spleen as described in Tonk et al. (26). Splenocytes were plated 4×10^6 cells/well in 24-well culture plates. Adherent splenocytes were stimulated with 15 μg/ml lipopolysaccharide (LPS) (Sigma) for 24 h and the supernatants were used to measure nitric oxide (NO) production using the Griess reaction, and tumor necrosis factor (TNF)-α production and IL-6 levels using an ELISA kit (eBioscience, San Diego, CA). Protein content was analyzed using the bicinchoninic acid method (Pierce Biochemicals, Rockford, IL) for cell number correction. Furthermore, splenocytes were seeded in a 96- well plate at 4×10^5 cells/well and stimulated with 5 μg/ml concanavalin A (conA) or 15 μg/ml LPS for 48 and 24 h, respectively. Supernatants were used for the determination of interleukins: IL-1β, IL-2, IL-4, IL-10, IL-13 using a Milliplex Map kit (Millipore, Billerica, MA, USA) and interferon (IFN)-γ levels using an ELISA kit (eBioscience) as a measure of activation responsivity of these cells.

Serum Chemistry in F1

Serum total cholesterol (CHOL), triglycerides (TGs), free fatty acids (FFAs), and high-density lipoproteins cholesterol (HDL-C) were analyzed as described (23). Adiponectin, leptin, ghrelin, insulin, glucagon, and C- reactive protein (CRP) were measured in sera by Milliplex Map Kit (Millipore) according to manufacturers' instructions. Glycated hemoglobin (HbA1c) was used as a marker for average glucose levels over the last 3 months (27), and assessed in full blood on a Beckman Coulter LX20 Clinical Chemistry Analyzer using the Direct Enzymatic HbA1c Assay kit (Diazyme Europe GmbH, Dresden, Germany). These measurements were performed after F1 animals switched to HFD.

Uncoupled Protein 1 (*Ucp1*) Gene Expression Analysis in F1

Gene expression of *Ucp1* was measured in the intrascapular fat tissue of controls and 100,000 μkd animals under HFD by qPCR as described previously (23). *Ucp1* is a marker of energy expenditure through thermogenesis, and contributes to regulation of body weight (28). In addition to *Ucp1*, expression levels of *Cidea* were determined as a marker of brown adipose tissue adipocytes (29) and were used to normalize the contents of brown adipose tissue adipocytes in the tissue extracts. Relative quantification was performed by the comparative CT method (ddCt).

Statistical Analyses

Data obtained from the whole range of doses tested, such as body weight measurements, endocrine, and lipid profile, were analyzed for statistically significant dose-response relationships using the benchmark dose (BMD) approach (30) with PROAST software (www.rivm.nl/proast), version 65.5. In this approach, models from exponential and Hill families were fitted to data covering the entire study population, and a BMD with its 5% lower (BMDL) and upper bounds (BMDU) of the 90% confidence interval was derived from the fitted models at a predefined benchmark response (CES = critical effect size) of 5%. The goodness of the fit was determined by Akaike information criterion (AIC). AIC integrates log-likelihood and the number of model parameters in one single value. The model with relatively low AIC gives a good fit without using too many parameters (31). The bootstrap method was used to calculate the 90% confidence interval of BMD so that individuals from the same litter were clustered to account for litter effects. Data which did not produce a statistically significant dose-response with exponential and Hill models as well as data with a wide confidence interval (BMDU/BMDL ratio>100) were considered not suitable for a valid BMD determination. Males and females were analyzed separately.

Measurements that included only a selection of dose groups such as neurobehavioral and immunological assessments were analyzed by a nested (to account for litter size covariance) ANOVA (using a custom R script), followed by Bonferroni *post-hoc* analysis ($p < 0.025$) to account for multiple testing (24). Males and females were analyzed separately.

RESULTS

Internal Exposure Assessment

Analysis of the serum concentrations of MECPP, MEHHP, and MEOHP in dams following a 9-week dietary exposure to DEHP confirmed the presence of DEHP metabolites in the samples and, hence, internal exposure (**Table 1**). A positive correlation in serum concentrations of the secondary metabolites in relation to the nominal external DEHP doses was observed ($R^2 = 0.93$ for MECPP, $R^2 = 0.99$ for MEHHP, and $R^2 = 0.99$ for MEOHP, **Figure S1**). Concentrations of secondary metabolite MEHHP and MEOHP in serum were in the same order of magnitude while the concentration of MECPP was the lowest (**Table 1**).

General Toxicity and Reproductive Parameters

In dams, dietary exposure to DEHP had no effect on survival, behavior or body weight (**Figure S2**) Feed consumption was not affected by DEHP in the gestation weeks (3.9 ± 0.5 g/day) and in the lactation weeks (12.5 ± 5.5 g/day). Average reproduction rate was 87% (67–100% per dose group). The average litter size in the total of 45 litters was 7.0 (range 4–10), and litter sizes were evenly distributed over doses (**Figure S3**). No difference in the anogenital distance in F1 was observed (**Figure S4**). The overall F/M sex ratio in the F1 generation was 1.2 and the overall survival rate was 97%, with no effects of DEHP observed on these parameters.

Energy Balance

A summary of dose-related effects on endpoints measured in F1 offspring exposed to DEHP during development is given in **Table 2**. No persistent changes in body weight were observed in F1 animals in either sex at the end of the follow-up period (55–57 weeks; **Table 2**, **Figures 1A,B**, **Figure S5**). In males, a dose-dependent decrease in body weight was observed until 4 weeks of age, but no effects on body weight were found after this period (**Figures S6A,B**). No effects on feed consumption were observed with the exception of a decrease in males at 23 weeks of age (data not shown), which did not coincide with a change in body weight. From 46 weeks of age until the end of the study (55–57 weeks), all animals were challenged with a HFD. No dose-dependent effects were observed in the body weight response during this period (**Table 2**). No difference in physical activity was observed between controls and 33,000 μkd exposed group in both sexes (**Figure S7**). No significant difference was observed in fat mass by individual analysis of perigonadal and perirenal fat weights in both sexes. In addition, no difference in *Ucp1* gene expression in intrascapular brown fat tissue between controls and exposed group 100,000 μkd was observed (data not shown).

In adult males, among all measured organs after necropsy, only muscle weight (*m.quadriceps femoris*) showed a dose-dependent decrease (**Figure 2A**). This 8% decrease persisted when expressed relative to body weight. However, a wide confidence interval (BMDU/BMDL ratio = 130) was observed and renders this parameter as not informative (**Table 2**). In adult females, a 9% increase in femur weight and a 22% increase in spleen weight were observed (**Table 2**). However, there was no effect in femur weight when analyzed relative to body weight, while the increase in spleen weight remained when expressed relative to body weight (**Figure 2B**), with a BMDL of 8,350 μkd.

In adult male offspring, dose-dependent increases in serum FFA and HDL-C (**Figures 3A,B**), but not TGs and CHOL (**Figure 3C**) were observed with FFA levels at the top dose 115% higher relative to background (**Table 2**). Considering the effect size and the BMDL of 2,160 μkd, the most critical parameter was the increase in FFA (**Table 2**). No effects on adiponectin, leptin, and ghrelin serum levels were observed. In females, no effects on serum lipids nor on endocrine parameters were observed (**Table 2**).

Glucose homeostasis appeared not to be affected by developmental DEHP exposure, as no difference between control and the 33,000 μkd exposed group was found in the GTT and ITT performed before start of HFD challenge. In addition, serum insulin and glucagon levels were not affected by exposure to DEHP when all dose groupswere analyzed. Fasting glucose levels measured during necropsy were also not altered. However, in

TABLE 1 | Concentration of secondary metabolites MEOHP, MEHHP, and MECPP in serum of dams exposed via diet to DEHP.

DEHP dose group (μkd)	N	MEOHP (ng/ml)	LOQ	<LOQ (%)	MEHHP (ng/ml)	LOQ	<LOQ (%)	MECPP (ng/ml)	LOQ	<LOQ (%)
0	10	0.18 ± 0.06	0.17–0.41	100%	0.15 ± 0.04	0.14–0.34	80%	0.06 ± 0.03	0.04–0.10	40%
3.3	5	0.13 ± 0.01	0.18–0.22	100%	0.12 ± 0.02	0.15–0.18	20%	0.07 ± 0.04	0.04–0.05	NA
33	5	0.19 ± 0.10	0.18–0.43	100%	0.22 ± 0.06	0.15–0.35	60%	0.06 ± 0.02	0.04–0.11	60%
330	4	0.48 ± 0.16	0.17–0.30	25%	0.67 ± 0.40	0.13–0.25	25%	0.13 ± 0.05	0.04–0.08	25%
3300	6	3.18 ± 1.75	0.5–0.54	17%	5 ± 3	0.42–0.44	17%	1.05 ± 0.59	0.13	NA
10000	5	17 ± 3.16	0.3–0.53	NA	30.60 ± 10.06	0.25–0.43	NA	5.98 ± 2.38	0.08–0.13	NA
33000	6	27.92 ± 22.07	0.5–0.8	NA	54.04 ± 43.70	0.26–0.83	NA	8.05 ± 7.62	0.08–0.25	NA
100000	4	85.43 ± 56.03	1.7–1.9	NA	198.23 ± 131.83	1.4–1.6	NA	16.67 ± 14.75	0.43–0.48	NA

N, number of samples; SD, standard deviation; LOQ, limit of quantification; <LOQ (%), percentage of the samples under the LOQ; NA, all samples above LOQ. Data shown as average± SD.

TABLE 2 | Overview of dose-response results in the offspring after *in utero* and lactational exposure to DEHP.

	Males				Females			
	Dose response	**BMDL μkd**	**BMDU μkd**	**Max effect size (%)**	**Dose response**	**BMDL μkd**	**BMDU μkd**	**Max effect size (%)**
Body weight (bw)								
Week 46 (m)/48 (f)	–				–			
Week 55 (m), 57(f)	–				–			
Body size								
Body length	–				–			
Femur length	–				–			
Femur length /bw	–				–			
Growth[a]								
Bw week 46/5 (m), 48/5 (f)	–				–			
Bw 55/46 (m), 57/48 (f)	–				–			
Food consumption/bw								
Organ weights								
Adrenal glands	–				–			
Brain	–				–			
Femur	–				↑	34,450	230,400	9
Liver	–				–			
m.quadr.fem.	↓	ni	ni	−8	–			
Pancreas	–				–			
Spleen	–				↑	8,350	24,800	22
Testes	–				–			
Thymus	–				–			
Relative organ weights(/bw[b]***)***	↓	ni	ni	−11				
m.quadr.fem								
pancreas					↑	19,760	135,900	17
spleen								
Fat pad weights								
Interscapular	–				–			
Perigonadal	–				–			
Perirenal	–				–			
Metabolic parameters								
Cholesterol					–			
Free fatty acids	↑	2160	60,600	115	–			
High–density lipoproteins	↑	149	27,400	19	–			
Triglycerides	–				–			
Glucose(HbA1c)	↓	17,400	96,600	−13	–			
Glucose	–				–			
C–reactive protein	–				–			
Leptin	–				–			
Ghrelin	–				–			
Adiponectin	–				–			
Insulin	–				–			
Glucagon	–				–			

↑,↓,- significant increase, decrease dose-responses, or absence of effect. Effects were significant with exponential (E) and Hill (H) modeling. BMDL and BMDU (lower and upper bounds of the 90%-confidence interval for BMD at a critical effect size of 5%); effects with a wide confidence interval of the BMD (ratio BMDU/BMDL> 100) are not considered informative (ni) for risk assessment. A maximum effect size is derived from the c-parameter if present in the dose-response function, otherwise calculated as a relative difference between top dose and control (background); reported value is an average of E and H maximum effect sizes. [a]Growth is determined by the ratio bw in week 46 (males) or week 48 (females) to bw in week 5 and for the period in which animals are fed a HFD by the ratio bw in week 55 (males) or week 57 (females) to bw in week 46/48. [b]Relative weight data are provided when significant dose-response in the parameter is observed.

males, HbA1c was decreased by 13% with a BMDL of 17,400 μkd (**Figure 4**).

Neurobehavioral Assessment

We examined the preference for a sucrose solution in adult F1 mice after developmental exposure to 33,000 μkd DEHP. No effect was observed compared to controls (data not shown).

In the ORT, total exploration time did not differ among control and 33,000 μkd exposed F1 mice within the sessions. During T2, exposed males showed a decrease in time exploring the familiar object (T2fam; **Table 3**) when compared to controls, which is reflected in a just significant ($p = 0.0481$) increase in the ratio between exploration time of the foreign object and the familiar object (ratio = T2for/T2fam), while in females the same trend but non-significant ($p = 0.0589$) was observed (**Figure 5**).

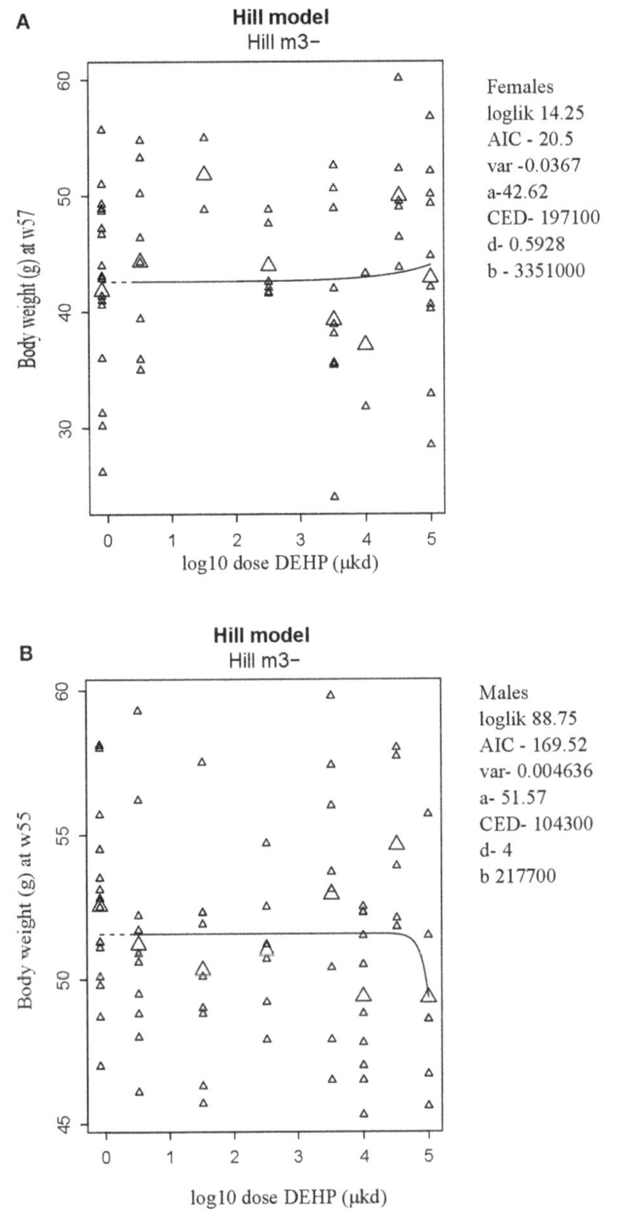

FIGURE 1 | Body weight at 57 weeks of age in female **(A)** and at 55 weeks of age in male **(B)** offspring after developmental exposure to 3.3 to 100,000 DEHP µkd. Explanation of dose-response graphs is in **Figure 2** legend.

Immunological Assessment

Serum levels of CRP were not affected in adult offspring exposed to DEHP during development (**Table 2**). No significant differences were observed in NO, IL-6 (**Figures S8A,B**) and TNFα production in adherent splenocytes after *ex vivo* stimulation with LPS in both sexes after developmental exposure to DEHP at 330 and 33,000 µkd. Concerning cytokine production after ConA stimulation, *post-hoc* analysis showed a non-significant decrease in IL-2 levels in F1 males toward the 33,000 µkd DEHP exposed group ($p < 0.08$, **Figure 6A**). In F1 females, a significant increase in IFNγ ($p < 0.01$) was observed at 33,000 µkd DEHP exposed group (**Figure 6B**). No other cytokine was affected by the exposure to DEHP during development as shown in the examples for IL-2 in females and IFNγ in males (**Figures 6C,D**).

DISCUSSION

In this study we investigated the metabolism disrupting properties of developmental exposure to DEHP in combination with effects on neurobehavior and immunological functions. We mimicked human dietary exposure to DEHP by including low doses to our range of studied concentrations. We observed alterations in lipid metabolism, glucometabolism, and neurobehavior in adult C57BL/6JxFVB hybrid male mice, as well as in immune function in adult female mice.

Initially, we measured the internal concentrations of DEHP secondary metabolites MEOHP, MEHHP, and MECPP in serum from dams. An increased concentration of all metabolites highly correlated with the external dose, confirming internal exposure. We show here that in the serum from DEHP exposed dams, MEHHP, and MEOHP are present in the highest concentrations, followed by MECPP. This is in line with previous studies examining concentrations of DEHP metabolites in mouse urine (32). Limited studies have measured DEHP in human serum samples, in either cord blood (9) or adult plasma (33). Levels of these three metabolites at our external DEHP exposure of 330 µkd were similar to background levels observed in human cord blood [0.29–0.31 ng/ml; (9)]. In contrast to data in rodents, likely due to inter-species metabolic capacity and pathways (32), concentrations of MEOHP, MEHHP, and MECPP in humans are similar in cord blood, whereas in adult blood, higher levels of MECPP are found relative to the other secondary metabolites. In a recent study, Quinnies et al. (34) reported serum levels of MEOHP in dams exposed to 40 and 400 µkd DEHP. MEOHP values of 0.54 ng/ml for the lowest dose and 1.6 ± 0.4 ng/ml for the highest dose were within the range of our exposures of 330 µkd and 3,300 µkd, respectively. They also report similar levels of MEOHP for the dose of 400 µkd in embryos, confirming that secondary metabolites reach the offspring. The primary DEHP metabolite MEHP is considered the active metabolite of DEHP, but Engel et al. (35) reported that the secondary metabolites are PPARα and/or PPARγ agonists *in vitro*, indicating that also the secondary metabolites may be involved in the molecular mechanisms behind the DEHP effects. Although the metabolites all have short half-lives ranging from 5 to 15 h (8), exposure at a developmental stage is likely to be implicated in the persistent effects of DEHP as discussed below.

During the first 26 weeks of life, we mainly focused on exploring changes in body weight and feed consumption in the offspring. We observed transient increases in body weight in females and transient decreases in body weight in males in a few weeks, but taking the entire follow up period into account, no clear impact on body weight was observed. In line with our findings, recent studies report a lack of effects on body weight after developmental exposure to DEHP (34, 36, 37). After 27 weeks of age, we continued with the body weight measurements,

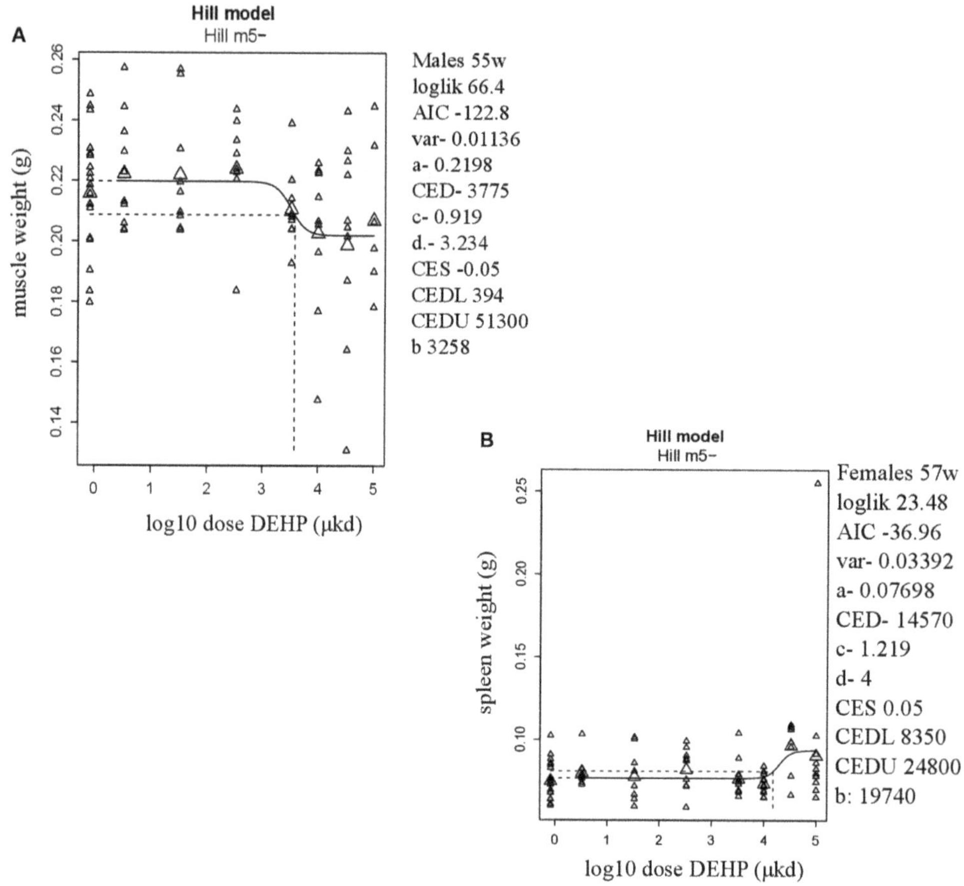

FIGURE 2 | Dose-dependent changes in organ weights after 9 weeks of developmental exposure to DEHP. **(A)** decrease in muscle weight (*m.quadriceps femoris*) in 55 weeks of age male offspring; **(B)** increase in spleen weight in 57 weeks of age female offspring. The function of the curve is shown on the top of the chart. In the right corner version 65.5 of PROAST, parameters of significance of the fit [loglikelihood (loglik), AIC (Akaike information criterion) and variation (var)] together with the function parameters (a = background response, b = potency of chemical, c = maximum fold change in response compared to background response, and d = steepness of curve) that shape the curve are shown. CES, critical effect size. CEDL/CEDU, critical effect dose lower and upper bound of the (2-sided) 90%-confidence interval for the CED. Small triangles represent individuals and large triangles represent the geometric mean per dose.

performed a locomotion test and studied the glucose homeostasis via glucose and insulin tolerance tests. With no further changes in body weight nor fat mass, no alteration in physical activity and normal glucose and insulin levels, we did not detect any changes which could be an indication of metabolic disruption through adipogenesis or endocrine pancreas function by developmental exposure to DEHP. Our findings do not support the results of a recent meta-analysis (14) which showed that early life exposure to DEHP is significantly associated with increased fat weight, but not body weight. It should be noted, however, that the authors judged the quality of evidence for body weight and fat weight to be low due to concerns regarding risk of bias and unexplained inconsistency (i.e., substantial heterogeneity).

We performed a sweet preference test and an object recognition test to check whether early exposure to DEHP could promote changes in neurobehavior between 37 and 40 weeks of life. Using these tests, we report that male offspring had changes affecting their attention span, particularly toward the familiar object. Although these changes were not accompanied by an increased preference for a sweet beverage, it is an indication of impaired neurobehavior in line with Barakat et al. (17). Barakat reported elevated anxiety and impaired memory function in male mice exposed early in life to DEHP as signs of developmental defects in the neural system or neurodegeneration caused by inflammation and/or oxidative damage in the hippocampus. More research is needed to investigate the mechanisms underlying such neurobehavioral changes and the impact of those changes in the context of MetS.

To further study the effects of developmental exposure to DEHP, we measured lipids levels in serum of 55–57 weeks of age mice and report a dose-related increase in free fatty acids and high density lipoprotein cholesterol in our male offspring. In lipid metabolism, triglycerides stored in adipose tissue are hydrolyzed to glycerol and free fatty acids. When lipolysis is stimulated, an increase in free fatty acids is expected. As fatty acids are the precursors of cholesterol, an increase in cholesterol may occur. To cope with cholesterol increase, HDL may be mobilized to transport cholesterol to the liver and facilitate removal (38). Gu

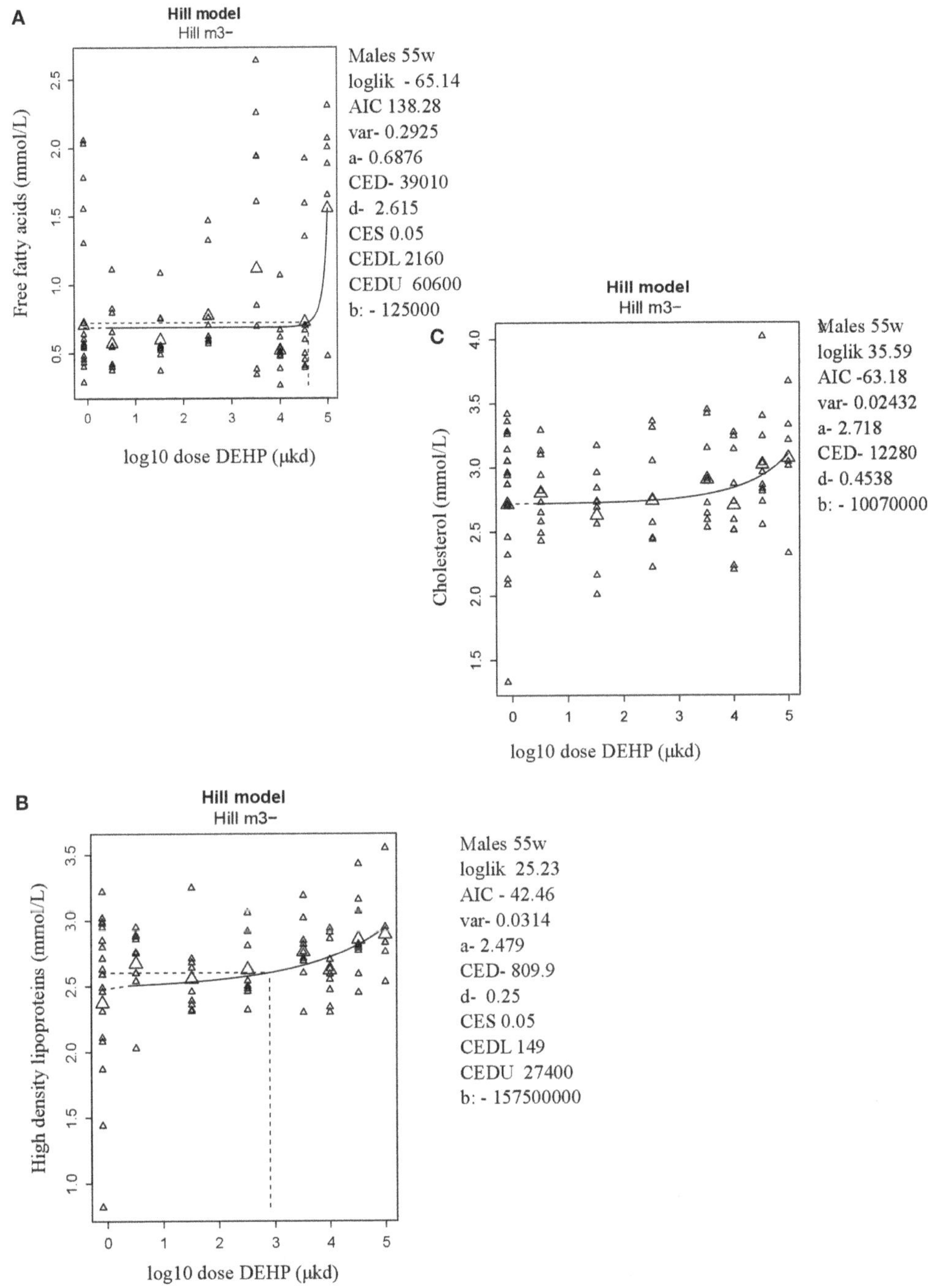

FIGURE 3 | Dose-dependent increases in **(A)** Free fatty acids (FFA) and **(B)** High density lipoprotein (HDL-C) and no alteration in **(C)** Cholesterol in 55 weeks of age male offspring after developmental exposure to DEHP. Explanation of dose-response graphs is in **Figure 2** legend.

et al. (36) reported that after gestational exposure to 50 μkd to DEHP via gavage, 9 weeks old male and females had an increase in visceral fat weights associated with elevated levels of triglycerides and total cholesterol. Hao et al. (11) also showed that maternal exposure from gestational day 12 to PND 7 to 250 μkd DEHP via gavage results in elevated cholesterol and triglycerides at 8 weeks of age while maternal exposure to 30,000 μkd DEHP by gavage from 4 weeks prior to gestation to PND 28 resulted in a significant increase in serum cholesterol, but not triglycerides, in offspring at 8 weeks of age (39). The studies above report alteration in serum lipids under a normal diet. In our experimental setting, we studied for the first time the effect of developmental exposure to DEHP in combination with a HFD challenge as calorie-rich diets are tightly linked to the pandemic

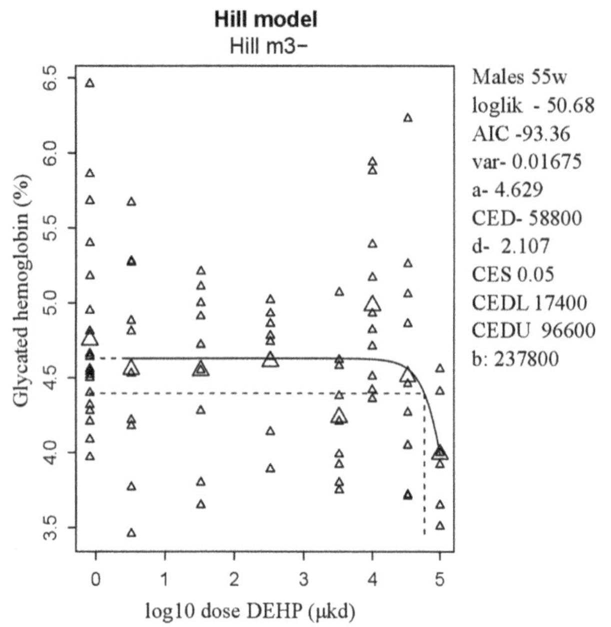

FIGURE 4 | Dose-dependent decrease in glycated hemoglobin (HbA1c) in 55 weeks of age male after developmental exposure to DEHP. Explanation of dose-response graphs is in **Figure 2** legend.

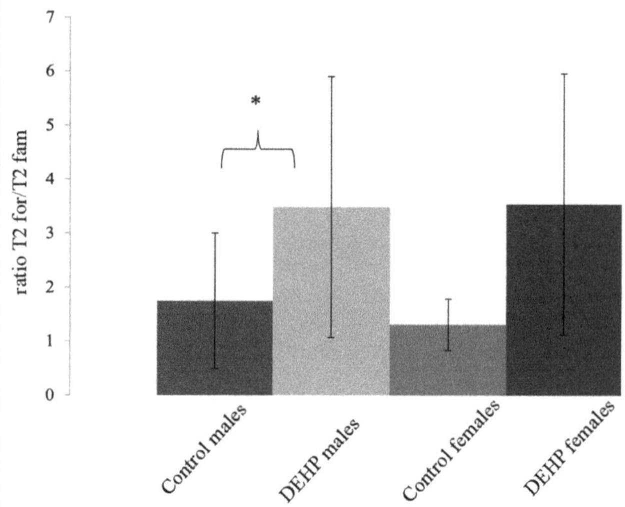

FIGURE 5 | Effect of 33,000 DEHP µkd developmental exposure on the exploration performance during the object recognition test. The index Ratio T2for/T2fam is used and means the time exploring the foreign object (Tfor) divided by the time exploring the familiar object (Tfam) during the test session (T2). Columns represent average of the index calculated in males and females (controls × DEHP exposed with $n = 8$–10 animals/sex) and error bars depict standard deviation. Data was analyzed by a nested ANOVA, comparing exposed to control animals within sexes. *$p = < 0.05$ ($p = 0.0481$, males; $p = 0.0589$, females).

TABLE 3 | Overview of exploration times and ratio during object recognition test (ORT).

ORT	Males		Females	
	Control	DEHP	Control	DEHP
Total T1 (s)	28.8 ± 11.6	27.6 ± 10.5	28.1 ± 13.6	18.8 ± 8.4
T2for (s)	11.5 ± 6.9	10.3 ± 4.1	17.1 ± 12.2	11.1 ± 9.2
T2fam (s)	7.8 ± 3.4	4.4 ± 3.3	13.4 ± 7.7	4.5 ± 3.7
Total T2 (s)	19 ± 7.8	15 ± 6.3	31 ± 19.1	16 ± 12.2
ratio T2for/T2fam	1.7 ± 1.3	3.5 ± 2.4[a]	1.3 ± 0.5	3.5 ± 2.4[a]

Total T1: total exploration time during training session in seconds (sec); T2for: exploration time of foreign object during test session; T2fam: exploration time of familiar object during test session. Total T2: total exploration time during test session. Data shown as average ± SD. N (control males) = 10; N (DEHP males) = 10; N (control females) =10; N (DEHP females) = 8. [a]significance compared to controls within the same sex (p = 0.0481, males; p = 0.0589, females).

of metabolic disorders (37). We pinpoint here increases in 2 parameters out of 4 related to lipid metabolism studied (TG's, FFA, CHOL, HDL-C). Although these should be interpreted with caution in view of limited effect sizes, our findings strengthen the body of evidence that developmental exposure to DEHP disrupts lipid metabolism.

Experimental studies indicate that DEHP targets lipid and cholesterol metabolism. *In vitro* and *in vivo* studies suggest that cholesterol transport into mitochondria needed for steroid biosynthesis is inhibited by DEHP, leading to accumulation of lipid droplets, while *de novo* synthesis of cholesterol is stimulated by DEHP (40). Although our offspring was indirectly exposed to DEHP via maternal diet, it is likely that direct effects of DEHP on somatic cells of the developing embryo/fetus may affect proliferation, differentiation and organ development. Recent data suggest that the adrenals are specific target organs of developmental DEHP exposure that may play an important role in the metabolic effects of DEHP, as global gene expression study has revealed changes in lipid metabolism and PPAR pathways affected in adult adrenal glands after *in utero* exposure in a rat model (41). In addition, another developmental *in vivo* study in mice related increased serum cholesterol levels in the offspring to decreased hepatic clearance of cholesterol, as suggested by decreased protein expression of cholesterol clearance-related regulators (39). These reports point to adrenals and liver as target organs and give insight into the long term effects of DEHP exposure on lipid metabolism, but the mechanism is still not fully understood. In the case of adrenals as a target organ of DEHP, involvement of epigenetic regulation remains to be elucidated as the differential DNA methylation identified did not affect directly gene expression (42).

In addition to effects on lipid metabolism, our study indicated that glucose homeostasis may be affected by developmental DEHP exposure. Serum levels of glycated hemoglobin, a marker of long term glucose levels, were decreased in adult male offspring. In previous studies, it has been shown that developmental exposure of rodents to DEHP alone or in combination with a high-fat dietary challenge disrupts glucose homeostasis in offspring (13, 43, 44). In these studies, disruption of glucose homeostasis was accompanied by effects on glucose and insulin tolerance. In our study, we performed GTT and ITT in one treatment group only

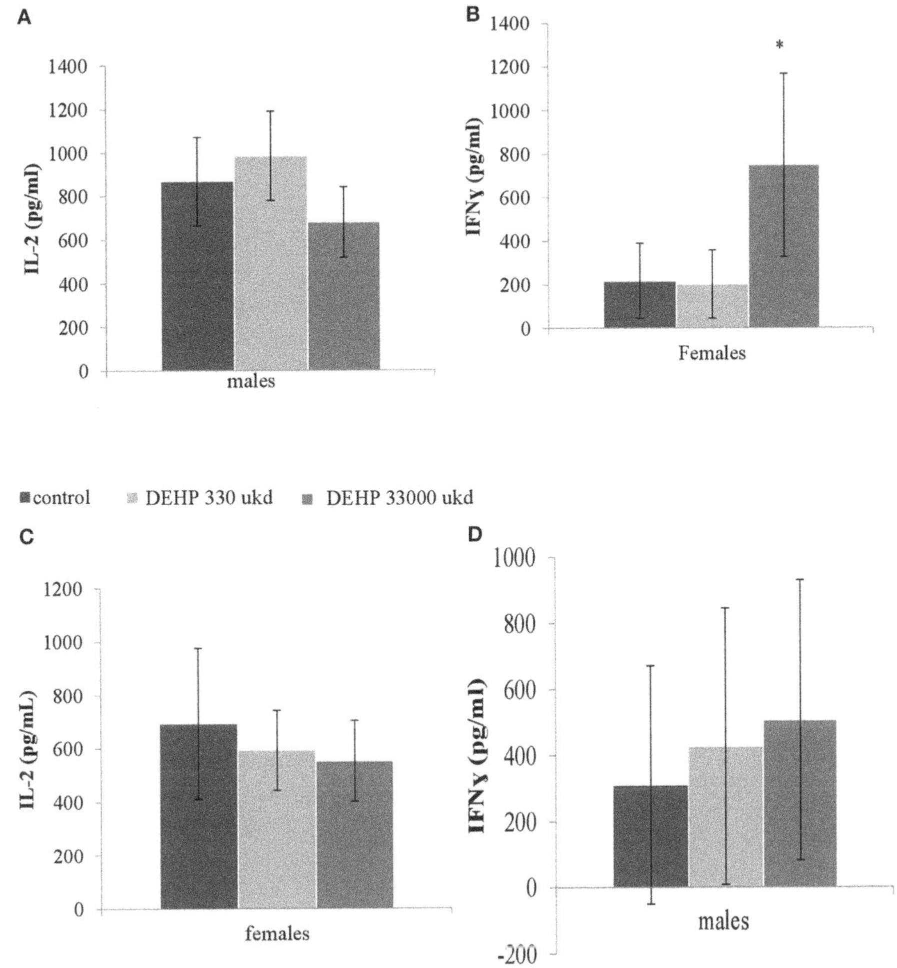

FIGURE 6 | Sex-specific effects of developmental exposure to DEHP on immunological parameters measured *ex vivo* in splenocytes culture after ConA stimulation. No effect on IL-2 in males **(A)** and a significant effect on IFNγ in females (* means $p = 0.01$) **(B)**. No effects on IL-2 in females **(C)** nor on IFNγ in males **(D)**. Columns represent average of concentrations measured in males and females (controls × DEHP exposed with $n = 8$–10 animals/sex) and error bars depict standard deviation. Data was analyzed by a nested ANOVA followed by a *post-hoc* analysis ($p < 0.025$).

(33,000 µkd) and observed no effects. Non-monotonic dose-response relationships have been reported for several EDCs, making it difficult to predict effects at lower doses by using higher doses (45). However, as all other endpoints measured in this study to investigate glucose regulation at 55–57 weeks of age (i.e., serum levels of fasting glucose, insulin and glucagon levels and glycated hemoglobin) did not show non-monotonic dose-responses, lower dose effects on GTT ad ITT are not expected. Overall, as our finding of decreased glycated hemoglobin is limited to alteration in one single parameter and is in opposite direction of the effects mostly associated with insulin resistance, it should be interpreted with caution.

We also measured a range of immune parameters in the cell population present in spleen after stimulation and observed sex-specific effects on cytokines, but not on CRP, a marker of chronic low grade systemic inflammation. Following developmental exposure to 33,000 µkd, splenocytes isolated from adult females produced an increase in IFNγ after stimulation with Con A, which is a T-cell response. Female offspring also showed a dose-related decrease in spleen weight, with a BMDL of 9,189 µkd, suggesting that developmental exposure to DEHP may affect immune functions in female offspring. Low grade inflammation plays a role in the development of obesity and metabolic disorders and in a recent report (19), elevated serum levels of CRP and TNF-α in 300,000 µkd DEHP *in utero* exposed offspring were detected. IFNγ is a pro-inflammatory cytokine and contributes to metabolic dysfunction by the repression of the expression and activity of SIRT1, an energy sensor, resulting in altered expression of genes involved in cellular metabolism and energy expenditure (46). In addition, patients with type 2 diabetes show elevated IFNγ circulating levels (46). However, it cannot be excluded that an elevated IFNγ represents a non-adverse physiological response to DEHP in combination with ConA exposure (47). In contrast to our findings, in another study with younger animals with follow-up until 13 weeks of age, *in utero* exposure of CD female rats from GD 6-12 by gavage to DEHP at doses of 37,500, 75,000, 150,000, or 300,000 μkd DEHP showed no effects on immune organ weights, antibody levels and *ex vivo* cytokine production (48). Taken together, the evidence in animal studies on the effects of developmental exposure to DEHP on the immune system in the context of metabolic disorders is limited and more research is needed.

The strength of our study is the wide range of doses studied, from 3.3 to 100,000 μkd DEHP. The dose regime applied also mimicked the relevant human exposure route, i.e., through the diet, and included the important periods of development encompassing both gestation and lactation. The lower dose ranges applied approximated human external exposure concentrations, which have been estimated to range from 2.5 to 15.7 μkd for an average adult of 60 kg, and about 24 μkd for an infant in the first year of life (20). The highest dose used is slightly above NOAEL levels, i.e., 91,000 μkd reported for a two generation developmental toxicity study in CD-1 mice (21). The results observed in our study are exclusively at the higher external dose range and the most critical BMDL of 2,160 μkd for FFA, if used to calculate a margin of safety (MOS), is >100 times higher than an average human exposure (49), though it should be noted that the internal serum concentrations of DEHP secondary metabolites in dams at this BMDL approximated those reported human cord blood (9). We did not observe developmental toxicity in terms of anogenital distance in offspring or otherwise, but we did observe a transient decrease in the body weight of the dams during the first weeks of gestation. To rule out possible toxic effects of the top dose (100,000 μkd) tested, we excluded this dose group from subsequent analyses of glucose homeostasis, immune function, and neurobehavior. In addition, we had a year follow-up, with parameters measured during the whole study period, so we could investigate the development of adult disease following the initial early exposure to DEHP.

We observed sex-specific effects of DEHP on lipid metabolism, neurobehavior, and immune function, though the mechanisms underlying these effects warrant further study. The sex-specific anti-androgenic effects of DEHP on male sexual development and reproduction are well known (50, 51) and sexual dimorphic expression of genes controlling hepatic lipid metabolism could play a role in the different outcome between sexes as, in an obesity context, transcription factors/nuclear receptors response to pollutants is sex-dependent (52). There is also evidence that sex influences innate and adaptive immune responses. Sex chromosome genes and sex hormones, including estrogens, progesterone, and androgens, contribute to the differential regulation of immune responses between the sexes (53). For instance, half of the activated genes in female T cells have estrogen response elements (ERE) in their promoters, suggesting that sex steroids may directly cause dimorphic immune responses (54). Therefore, it is expected that environmental factors such as DEHP exposure may alter the development and function of the immune system differently in males and females.

Our research suggests that developmental exposure to DEHP is a long term dyslipidemic factor, due to the observed changes in total cholesterol, FFA and HDL-C reported at adulthood. Dyslipidemia is a leading cardiovascular risk factor characterized by high circulating triglycerides, total cholesterol and LDL-C and low HDL-C; it affects 20% of children and adolescents in the U.S. (55) and is associated with future cardiovascular and metabolic disease risk (56). Therefore, developmental exposure to DEHP should be further investigated to understand potential risks to human health. Our most critical parameter was the circulating FFA levels. Although an increase in FFA cannot be claimed as adverse, it is suggested that FFA can mediate adverse metabolic effects such as insulin resistance (57). Developmental exposure to DEHP may either directly activate fatty acid catabolism (58) or indirectly via changes in expression of genes related to beta-oxidation (58), leading to increased levels of FFA at adulthood observed here. FFA are also important signaling molecules and an increase may affect brain and endocrine pancreas functions (15). Therefore, the neurobehavior and lipid metabolism effects detected in our study could be linked with one another by the circulating FFA.

In conclusion, developmental exposure to DEHP *in utero* and during lactation resulted in modest metabolic changes in lipids and glucose in combination with a neurobehavioral change in the area of attention span in adult C57BL/6JxFVB male mice at 55 weeks of age. The most critical and sensitive alteration was on FFA in serum which warrants further investigation on adversity.

AUTHOR CONTRIBUTIONS

JL, LvdV, and TH supervised the project. LvdV, JL, JvE, and LB designed the experiments. JvE and LB carried out the experiments. HH contributed to sample preparation. ML and TH assisted with metabolites analysis. LB wrote the manuscript with input of all authors.

FUNDING

This project received funding from the European Community's Seventh Framework Programme [FP7/2007-2013] under grant agreement OBELIX n° 227391 and the Netherlands Organization for Scientific Research (NWO-VIDI 864.09.005).

ACKNOWLEDGMENTS

The authors acknowledge the support of the biotechnicians from the team of Hans Strootman at the RIVM animal facilities and the technical support provided by Eric Gremmer, Jacco Koekkoek, Piet Beekhof, and Sandra Imholz.

REFERENCES

1. Grundy SM, Brewer HB, Cleeman JI, Smith SC, Lenfant C. Definition of metabolic syndrome:report of national heart, lung and blood Institute/American heart association conference on scientif issues related to definition. *Circulation* (2004) 109:433–8. doi: 10.1161/01.CIR.0000111245.75752.C6
2. Aguilar M, Bhuket T, Torres S, Liu B, Wong RJ. Prevalence of the metabolic syndrome in the United States: 2003-2012. *JAMA* (2015) 313:1973–4. doi: 10.1001/jama.2015.4260
3. Li R, Li W, Lun Z, Zhang H, Sun Z, Kanu JS, et al. Prevalence of metabolic syndrome in mainland china: a meta-analysis of published studies. *BMC Public Health* (2016) 16:296. doi: 10.1186/s12889-016-2870-y
4. Saklayen MG. The global epidemic of the metabolic syndrome. *Curr Hypertension Rep.* (2018) 20:12. doi: 10.1007/s11906-018-0812-z
5. Barker DJ, Clark PM. Fetal undernutrition and disease in later life. *Rev Reproduc.* (1997) 2:105–12. doi: 10.1530/ror.0.0020105
6. Heindel JJ, Blumberg B, Cave M, Machtinger R, Mantovani A, Mendez MA, et al. Metabolism disrupting chemicals and metabolic disorders. *Reprod Toxicol.* (2017) 68:3–33. doi: 10.1016/j.reprotox.2016.10.001
7. Agency for Toxic Substances and Disease Registry (ATSDR). *Toxicological Profile for Di(2-ethylhexyl)phthalate (DEHP).* Atlanta, GA: U.S. Department of Health and Human Services, Public Health Service (2002).
8. Koch HM, Preuss R, Angerer J, Foster P, Sharpe R, Toppari J. Di(2-ethylhexyl)phthalate (DEHP): human metabolism and internal exposure - an update and latest results. *Int J Androl.* (2006) 29:155–65. doi: 10.1111/j.1365-2605.2005.00607.x
9. de Cock M, De Boer M, Lamoree M, Legler J, Van De Bor M. Prenatal exposure to endocrine disrupting chemicals in relation to thyroid hormone levels in infants – a Dutch prospective cohort study. *Environ Health* (2014) 13:106. doi: 10.1186/1476-069X-13-106
10. Gore AC, Chappell VA, Fenton SE, Flaws JA, Nadal A, Prins GS, et al. Executive Summary to EDC-2: the endocrine society's second scientific statement on endocrine-disrupting chemicals. *Endocrine Rev.* (2015) 36:593–602. doi: 10.1210/er.2015-1093
11. Hao C, Cheng X, Guo J, Xia H, Ma X. Perinatal exposure to diethyl-hexyl-phthalate induces obesity in mice. *Front Biosci.* (2013) 5:725–33. doi: 10.2741/E653
12. Hao CJ, Cheng XJ, Xia HF, Ma X. The endocrine disruptor mono-(2-ethylhexyl) phthalate promotes adipocyte differentiation and induces obesity in mice. *Biosci Rep.* (2012) 32:619–29. doi: 10.1042/BSR20120042
13. Rajesh P, Balasubramanian K. Phthalate exposure *in utero* causes epigenetic changes and impairs insulin signalling. *J Endocrinol.* (2014) 223:47–66. doi: 10.1530/JOE-14-0111
14. Wassenaar PNH, Legler J. Systematic review and meta-analysis of early life exposure to di(2-ethylhexyl)phthalate and obesity related outcomes in rodents. *Chemosphere* (2017) 188:174–81. doi: 10.1016/j.chemosphere.2017.08.165
15. Nadal A, Quesada I, Tudurí E, Nogueiras R, Alonso-Magdalena P. Endocrine-disrupting chemicals and the regulation of energy balance. *Nat Rev Endocrinol.* (2017) 13:536–46. doi: 10.1038/nrendo.2017.51
16. Schmidt J, Schaedlich K, Fiandanese N, Pocar P, Fischer B. Effects of di(2-ethylhexyl) phthalate (DEHP) on female fertility and adipogenesis in C3H/N mice. *Environ Health Perspect.* (2012) 180:1123–9. doi: 10.1289/ehp.1104016
17. Barakat R, Lin PC, Park CJ, Best-Popescu C, Bakery HH, Abosalum ME, et al. Prenatal exposure to DEHP induces neuronal degeneration and neurobehavioral abnormalities in adult male mice. *Toxicol Sci.* (2018) 164:439–52. doi: 10.1093/toxsci/kfy103
18. Ouchi N, Parker JL, Lugus JJ, Walsh K. Adipokines in inflammation and metabolic disease. *Nat Rev Immunol.* (2011) 11:85–97. doi: 10.1038/nri2921
19. Campioli E, Martinez-Arguelles DB, Papadopoulos V. *In utero* exposure to the endocrine disruptor di-(2-ethylhexyl) phthalate promotes local adipose and systemic inflammation in adult male offspring. *Nutr Diabetes* (2014) 4:1–10. doi: 10.1038/nutd.2014.13
20. European Food Safety Authority. Opinion of the Scientific Panel on Food Additives, Flavourings, Processing Aids and Materials in Contact with Food (AFC) on a request from the Commission related to Bis(2-ethylhexyl)phthalate (DEHP) for use in food contact materials. *EFSA J.* (2006) 299:243. doi: 10.2903/j.efsa.2005.243
21. Tyl RW, Price CJ, Marr MC, Kimmel CA. Developmental toxicity evaluation of dietary di(2-ethylhexyl)phthalate in Fischer 344 rats and CD-1 mice. *Fundamental Appl Toxicol.* (1988) 10:395–412. doi: 10.1016/0272-0590(88)90286-2
22. Dollé ME, Kuiper RV, Roodbergen M, Robinson J, de Vlugt S, Wijnhoven SW, et al. Broad segmental progeroid changes in short-lived Ercc(-/Delta7) mice. *Pathobiol Aging Age Related Dis.* (2011) 1:7219. doi: 10.3402/pba.v1i0.7219
23. Van Esterik JCJ, Dollé MET, Lamoree MH, van Leeuwen SPJ, Hamers T, Legler J, et al. Programming of metabolic effects in C57BL/6JxFVB mice by exposure to bisphenol A during gestation and lactation. *Toxicology* (2014) 321:40–52. doi: 10.1016/j.tox.2014.04.001
24. van Esterik JCJ, Verharen HW, Hodemaekers HM, Gremmer ER, Nagarajah B, Kamstra JH, et al. Compound- and sex-specific effects on programming of energy and immune homeostasis in adult C57BL/6JxFVB mice after perinatal TCDD and PCB 153. *Toxicol Appl Pharmacol.* (2015) 289:262–75. doi: 10.1016/j.taap.2015.09.017
25. Govarts E, Nieuwenhuijsen M, Schoeters G, Ballester F, Bloemen K, de Boer M, et al. Prenatal Exposure to Polychlorinated Biphenyls (PCB) and Dichlorodiphenyldichloroethylene (DDE) and Birth Weight: a meta-analysis within 12 European birth cohorts. *Environ Health Perspect* (2012) 120:162–70. doi: 10.1289/ehp.1103767
26. Tonk ECM, de Groot DMG, Penninks AH, Waalkens-Berendsen IDH, Wolterbeek APM, Slob W, et al. Developmental immunotoxicity of methylmercury: the relative sensitivity of developmental and immune parameters. *Toxicol Sci.* (2010) 117:325–35. doi: 10.1093/toxsci/kfq223
27. Saudek CD, Brick JC. The clinical use of hemoglobin A1c. *J Diabetes Sci Technol.* (2009) 3:629–34. doi: 10.1177/193229680900300402
28. Kozak LP, Anunciado-Koza R. 2005.UCP1: its involvement and utility in obesity. *Int J Obesity* (2008) 32(Suppl 7):S32–8. doi: 10.1038/ijo.2008.236
29. Zhou Z, Yon Toh S, Guo K, Ng CP, Ponniah S, Lin SC, et al. *Cidea*-deficient mice have lean phenotype and are resistant to obesity. *Nat Genet.* (2003) 35:49–56. doi: 10.1038/ng1225
30. Slob W. Dose-response modeling of continuous endpoints. *Toxicol Sci.* (2002) 66:298–312. doi: 10.1093/toxsci/66.2.298
31. EFSA Scientific Committee, Hardy A, Benford D, Halldorsson T, Jeger MJ, Knutsen KH, et al. Update: guidance on the use of the benchmark dose approach in risk assessment. *EFSA J.* (2017) 15:4658. doi: 10.2903/j.efsa.2017.4658
32. Ito Y, Kamijima M, Hasegawa C, Tagawa M, Kawai T, Miyake M, et al. Species and inter-individual differences in metabolic capacity of di(2-ethylhexyl)phthalate (DEHP) between human and mouse livers. *Environ Health Prevent Med* (2014) 19:117–25. doi: 10.1007/s12199-013-0362-6
33. Frederiksen H, Jørgensen N, Andersson A. Correlations between p phthalate metabolites in urine, serum,and seminal plasma from young Danish men determined by Isotope Dilution Liquid Chromatography TandemMass Spectrometry. *J Anal Toxicol.* (2010) 34:400–10. doi: 10.1093/jat/34.7.400
34. Quinnies KM, Harris EP, Snyder RW, Sumner SS, Rissman EF. Direct and transgenerational effects of low doses of perinatal di-(2-ethylhexyl) phthalate (DEHP) on social behaviors in mice. *PLoS ONE* (2017) 12:e0171977. doi: 10.1371/journal.pone.0171977
35. Engel A, Buhrke T, Imber F, Jessel S, Seidel A, Völkel W, et al. Agonistic and antagonistic effects of phthalates and their urinary metabolites on the steroid hormone receptors ERα, ERβ, and AR. *Toxicol Lett.* (2017) 277:54–63. doi: 10.1016/j.toxlet.2017.05.028
36. Gu H, Liu Y, Wang W, Ding L, Teng W, Liu L. In utero exposure to di-(2-ethylhexyl) phthalate induces metabolic disorder and increases fat accumulation in visceral depots of C57BL/6J mice offspring. *Exp Ther Med.* (2016) 12:3806–12. doi: 10.3892/etm.2016.3820
37. Hunt BG, Wang Y, Chen M, Wang S, Watls SE. Maternal diethylhexyl phthalate exposure affects adiposity and insulin tolerance in offspring in a PCNA-dependent manner. *Environ Res.* (2017) 159:588–94. doi: 10.1016/j.envres.2017.09.004
38. Kingsbury KJ, Bondy G. Understanding the essentials of blood lipid metabolism. *Prog Cardiovasc Nurs Winter* (2003) 18:13–8. doi: 10.1111/j.0889-7204.2003.01176.x

39. Lee KI, Chiang CW, Lin HC, Zhao JF, Li CT, Shyue SK, et al. Maternal exposure to di-(2-ethylhexyl) phthalate exposure deregulates blood pressure, adiposity, cholesterol metabolism and social interaction in mouse offspring. *Arch Toxicol.* (2015) 90:1211–24. doi: 10.1007/s00204-015-1539-0
40. Martinez-Arguelles DB, Papadopoulos V. Mechanisms meadiating environmental chemical-induced endocrine disruption in the adrenal gland. *Front Endocrinol.* (2016) 6:29. doi: 10.3389/fendo.2015.00029
41. Martinez-Arguelles DB, Campioli E, Lienhart C, Fan J, Culty M, Zirkin BR, et al. *In utero* exposure to the endocrine disruptor di-(2-ethylhexyl) phthalate induces long-term changes in gene expression in the adult male adrenal gland. *Endocrinology* (2014) 155:1667–78. doi: 10.1210/en.2013-1921
42. Martinez-Arguelles DB, Papadopoulos V. *Prenatal phthalate exposure: epigenetic changes leading to lifelong impact on steroid* formation. *Andrology* (2016) 1–12. doi: 10.1111/andr.12175
43. Lin Y, Wei J, Li Y, Chen J, Zhou Z, Song L, et al. Developmental exposure to di(2-ethylhexyl) phthalate impairs endocrine pancreas and leads to long-term adverse effects on glucose homeostasis in the rat. *Am J Physiol Endocrinol Metabol.* (2011) 301:E527–38. doi: 10.1152/ajpendo.00233.2011
44. Strakovsky RS, Lezmi S, Shkoda I, Flaws JA, Helferich WG, Pan YX. *In utero* growth restriction and catch-up adipogenesis after developmental di (2-ethylhexyl) phthalate exposure cause glucose intolerance in adult male rats following a high-fat dietary challenge. *J Nutr Biochem.* (2015) 26:1208–20. doi: 10.1016/j.jnutbio.2015.05.012
45. vandenBerg L, Colborn T, Hayes TB, Heindel JJ, Jacobs DR, Lee D, et al. Hormones and endocrine disrupting chemicals: low-dose effects and nonmonotonic dose responses. *Endocr Rev.* (2012) 33:378–455. doi: 10.1210/er.2011-1050
46. Li P, Zhao Y, Wu X, Xia M, Fang M, Iwasaki Y, et al. Interferon gamma (IFN-c) disrupts energy expenditure and metabolic homeostasis by suppressing SIRT1 transcription. *Nucleic Acids Res.* (2012) 40:1609–20. doi: 10.1093/nar/gkr984
47. Hessel EVS, Tonk ECM, Bos PMJ, van Loveren H, Piersma AH. Developmental immunotoxicity of chemicals in rodents and its possible regulatory impact. *Critic Rev Toxicol.* (2015) 45:68–82. doi: 10.3109/10408444.2014.959163
48. Piepenbrink MS, Hussain I, Marsh JA, Dietert RR. Developmental immunotoxicology of Di-(2-Ethylhexyl)phthalate (DEHP): age-based assessment in the female rat. *J Immunotoxicol.* (2005) 2:21–31. doi: 10.1080/15363750490429435
49. EU. Summary Risk Assessment Report for DEHP, Final report, European Commission, 2008, EUR 23384EN, European Union Risk Assessment Report, Volume 80, Luxembourg: Office for Official Publications of the European Communities, *ISSN* (2008) 1018–5593.
50. Howdeshell KL, Rider CV, Wilson VS, Gray LE. Mechanisms of action of phthalate esters, individually and in combination, to induce abnormal reproductive development in male laboratory rats. *Environ Res.* (2008) 108:168–76. doi: 10.1016/j.envres.2008.08.009
51. Martinez-Arguelles DB, Campioli E, Culty M, Zirkin BR, Papadopoulos V. Fetal origin of endocrine dysfunction in the adult: the phthalate model. *J Steroid Biochem Mol Biol.* (2013) 137:5–17. doi: 10.1016/j.jsbmb.2013.01.007
52. Naville D, Pinteur C, Vega N, Menade Y, Vigier M, Bourdais A, et al. Low-dose food contaminants trigger sex-specific hepatic metabolic changes in the progeny of obese mice. *FASEB J.* (2013) 27:3860–69. doi: 10.1096/fj.13-231670
53. Klein SL, Flanagan KL. Sex differences in immune responses. *Nat Rev Immunol.* (2016) 626–38. doi: 10.1038/nri.2016.90
54. Hewagama A, Patel D, Yarlagadda S, Strickland FM, Richardson BC. Stronger inflammatory/cytotoxic T-cell response in women identified by microarray analysis. *Genes Immun.* (2009) 10:509–16. doi: 10.1038/gene.2009.12
55. Kit BK, Kuklina E, Carroll MD. Prevalence of and trends in dyslipidemia and blood pressure among us children and adolescents. *JAMA Pediatr* (2015) 169:272–79. doi: 10.1001/jamapediatrics.2014.3216
56. Juonola M, Viikari JS, Ronnemaa T, Marniemi J. Associations of dyslipidemias from childhood to adulthood with carotid intimedia thickness, elasticty, and brachial flow-mediated dilatation in adulthood: the cardiovascular risk in young finns study.Arterioscer. *Thromb Vasc Biol.* (2008) 28:1012–17. doi: 10.1161/ATVBAHA.108.163329
57. Karpe F, Dickmann JR, Frayn KN. Fatty acids, obesity, and insulin resistance: time for a reevaluation. *Diabetes* (2011) 60:2441–9. doi: 10.2337/db11-0425
58. Feige JN, Gerber A, Casals-Casas C, Yang Q, Winkler C, Bedu E, et al. The pollutant diethylhexyl phthalate regulates hepatic energy metabolism via species-specific PPARα-dependent mechanisms. *Environ Health Perspect* (2010) 118:234–41. doi: 10.1289/ehp.0901217

14

History of the Obesogen Field: Looking Back to Look Forward

*Jerrold J. Heindel**

Program on Endocrine Disruption Strategies, Commonweal, Bolinas, CA, United States

Correspondence:
Jerrold J. Heindel
jerryheindel@gmail.com

The Obesogen field developed from two separate scientific research areas, endocrine disruptors and the Developmental Origins of Health and Disease (DOHaD). Endocrine Disrupting Chemicals (EDCs) are exogenous chemicals or mixtures of chemicals that interfere with the action of hormones. Exposure to EDCs during early development (DOHaD) has been shown to increase susceptibility to a variety of diseases including infertility, asthma, breast and prostate cancer, early puberty, susceptibility to infections, heart disease, autoimmune disease, and attention deficit hyperactivity disorder/learning disability. The effects of EDCs on obesity and fat cell development first gained attention around the turn of the twenty-first century. In 2002 Dr. Paula Baillie-Hamilton wrote the first review article focusing on environmental chemicals and obesity. She suggested that the obesity epidemic correlated with the increased production of chemicals after World War II. Baillie-Hamilton identified studies showing that exposures to a variety of chemicals led to weight gain. Shortly after that a commentary on an article showing that nonylphenol would increase fat cell differentiation *in vitro* noted the Baillie-Hamilton article and made the point that perhaps obesity was due in part to exposure to EDCs. In 2006 the field of DOHaD/EDCs and obesity made a giant leap forward when Dr. Bruce Blumberg published a paper showing that tributyltin could lead to weight gain in mice and coined the term obesogen for a chemical that caused weight gain and lead to obesity. In 2011, the NIEHS developed the first funding initiative focused on obesogens. In the following years there have been several workshops focused on obesogens. This paper describes these early days that lead to the obesogen hypotheses and the growth of the field for a decade, leading to its prominence today, and provides some insight into where the field is moving.

Keywords: endocrine disruptor, obesogen, metabolism disruptor, developmental origins of disease, obesity

INTRODUCTION

It is never easy to determine when a scientific paradigm shift has occurred that will lead to the development of a new scientific field, including the development of the obesogen field. Before moving into the history of obesogens *per se*, it is important to note that data supported the concept before anyone thought that unintentional chemical exposures could make people fat. These data came from the pharmaceutical arena, where certain drugs developed for a specific disease had a side effect of causing weight gain. For instance, many individuals on selective serotonin uptake inhibitors, atypical anti-psychotics, tricyclic antidepressants, and thiazolidines antidiabetics experienced weight gains of 5–10 kg (1). The data are particularly strong for rosiglitazone, used to treat type 2 diabetes, which acts as a selective PPAR gamma receptor agonist; a pathway that is known to stimulate fat cell development (2). Monosodium glutamate, a widely used food additive, has a side effect of being a known activator of brain pathways that cause weight gain in animal models (3). Thus, these studies provided proof of principle that chemicals could interfere with metabolism, resulting in weight gain.

ENDOCRINE DISRUPTORS

In the case of environmental chemicals and obesity, this field emerged from research on endocrine disruptors and the concept of developmental origins of adult disease, now called developmental origins of health and disease (DOHaD). Endocrine disrupting chemicals (EDCs), for the most part, are chemicals designed for a specific purpose, for example, a pesticide or plasticizer, but they also mimic natural hormone actions in the body leading to increased susceptibility to a variety of diseases. The endocrine disruption field began at a Wingspread Conference in 1991 where the term endocrine disruptor was first coined [reviewed in (4)]. There are now around 1,000 chemicals designated as EDCs (https://endocrinedisruption.org/). EDCs are found in a wide variety of products including pesticides/herbicides/fungicides, flame retardants, surfactants, plastics, sunscreens, cosmetics, and personal care products, etc. [reviewed in (5)]. Exposure to EDCs is ubiquitous, such that exposure occurs from air, dust, water and food via ingestion, inhalation, the skin, and the placenta. Some EDCs have short half-lives in minutes or hours while others are highly persistent with half-lives in years (6). Originally, EDCs were shown to interfere with estrogen, androgen and thyroid hormone signaling (7, 8) resulting in diseases and dysfunctions in reproduction, learning, memory, and behavior.

DEVELOPMENTAL ORIGINS OF HEALTH AND DISEASE

The DOHaD field posits that development, when tissues are forming, is a highly orchestrated and coordinated process controlled by altering gene expression to make specific tissues with specific genes and functions (9, 10). Hormones and growth factors control this process. Poor nutrition, stress or EDCs can interfere with this developmental trajectory, leading to functional changes in tissues (altered gene expression, altered cell numbers or locations) leading to increased sensitivity/susceptibility to disease and dysfunction over the lifespan (11).

As scientists studied the role of exposure to EDCs in reproductive diseases (e.g., the DOHaD hypothesis), they discovered that these same EDCs could cause weight gain which led to the development of a new scientific field.

SERENDIPITY AND THE BIRTH OF A NEW FIELD: INTEGRATION OF EDC AND DOHaD FIELDS

Serendipity, sometimes called unexpected good luck, involves finding something unexpected, realizing its importance and acting on it. Thus, while the initial discovery might be due to luck, the realization of its importance and acting on it is a key component of science. Serendipity played a key role in the birth of the obesogen field.

The first serendipitous discovery came in 1997 when Paula Baillie-Hamilton, a physician, noted that "After the birth of my second son, I gained a significant amount of weight. And I happened to read an article in a national newspaper on how chemical toxins at today's levels of environmental exposure are damaging animals' health by meddling with their hormones. My academic background and previous experience as a doctor had given me the ability to see the connection between these toxins and that perhaps there was a connection to our growing weight problem." (12). She serendipitously put two scientific fields together for the first time.

In 2002, she published the first paper that focused on a new hypothesis, that chemical toxins could explain the global obesity epidemic (12). In the article she noted, "Therefore it can be posited that the relatively recent presence of synthetic chemicals in the environment may be a significant causative factor in the current worldwide obesity epidemic. These chemicals may be causing weight gain via toxic effects on the body's natural weight-control mechanisms."

A figure in this publication showed that the increase in obesity followed by several decades the increase in production of chemicals, thus suggesting a link between the two. It further showed that since the early 1970s there had been numerous publications that showed that environmental chemical exposures to rodents could lead to weight gain. However, these were toxicity studies, and the authors did not consider weight gain as a toxic endpoint. The chemicals that she noted as having the ability to cause weight gain include organochlorine pesticides, carbamates, polychlorinated biphenols, plastics such as phthalates and bisphenol A (BPA), heavy metals and solvents. It should be noted that recent studies have indeed confirmed that exposures to these chemicals during development can lead to weight gain in offspring (13). She also noted, "Researchers have reportedly found a positive association between levels of certain toxic chemicals in the children's and adults body tissues and increased weight in these subjects." Thus, the Baillie-Hamilton review of the literature led her to develop a hypothesis for a new field, which did not exist: an amazing scientific deduction. Unfortunately, the article was published in the Journal of Alternative and Comparative Medicine and therefore was not initially widely noted and cited.

SERENDIPITY: THE FIRST PUBLICATIONS

Two of the articles noted in the Baillie-Hamilton literature review were published by reproductive biologists who were studying the effects of BPA. The authors serendipitously discovered that developmental exposure to BPA would not only result in reproductive effects but would also lead to weight gain (14, 15). While both publications were focused on the reproductive effects of BPA and noted effects on body weight, the Rubin et al. (15) paper mentioned—in the title—that BPA affected body weight. In 2002, several articles showed that childhood obesity is associated with maternal smoking during pregnancy (16, 17), another unexpected result as smoking led initially to lower birth weight. These data led to a review of the fetal origins of obesity focusing on *in utero* nutrition and later-life obesity (18, 19).

At the turn of the twenty-first century, two research areas were coming together, the first of which was the fetal origins of adult disease (now called DOHaD). DOHaD started with a focus on nutrition and the field of environmental chemicals and disease, which initially focused on reproduction. The discovery that developmental exposure to BPA would lead to weight gain led to the development of a new field: the developmental origins of obesity and the role of EDCs.

Data showing that BPA and nonylphenol could stimulate differentiated 3T3-L1 cells into adipocytes followed these initial studies (20–22). These articles were the first to show that an environmental chemical can cause differentiation into adipocytes. In 2003 a commentary (23) on the nonylphenol manuscript was published in Toxicological Sciences (22). This commentary noted the prior Baillie-Hamilton (12) publication and the developing new research area (the fetal basis of adult disease), showing that nutrition *in utero* and early life can have profound influences on birth weight and on lifelong health. It also noted, "the authors of this article on adipocyte differentiation by nonylphenol opened the door to a potentially very exciting new area of research on the action of estrogenic endocrine-disrupting chemicals: one that has enormous implications for public health." It asked thought provoking questions: "Will these results extrapolate to the *in vivo* situation in rodents and other animal models? Will humans be sensitive to the *in utero* exposure to environmental estrogens about the development of adipocytes? Will toxicology and environmental health sciences play a key role in addressing the obesity epidemic via a reduction in exposures to environmental chemicals *in utero* and throughout life? Only time will tell, but the door has been opened…" While just a commentary, it alerted toxicologists to the Baillie-Hamilton article and the new area of fetal origins of obesity.

In 2005, Newbold et al. (24) first showed that neonatal exposure to low doses of diethylstilbestrol (DES) would cause obesity as measured both by increased weight and increased fat in females. The picture, published in 2009 (25) on the effect of neonatal DES exposure on weight gain in adults has, in today's vernacular, gone viral as it has been shown as a key example of an estrogenic chemical and obesity many times.

EPIDEMIOLOGY STUDIES ON EDCS AND OBESITY

Smoking during pregnancy is a proof of principle for the ability of chemicals to cause increased risk for overweight in childhood. The first publications showing that smoking during pregnancy would increase weight gain in children were published in 2002 and 2003, predating an obesogen field. In 2008, Oken et al. conducted a meta-analysis of 14 epidemiology studies that showed a strong association between smoking during pregnancy and weight gain in the children (18). Smoking throughout pregnancy has the largest effect on childhood weight, and there was a dose response with more smoking leading to a larger effect on the children's weight. By 2013, there were over 30 separate epidemiology publications that all showed the same effect; increased weight gain in children from the mother's smoking during pregnancy, something unheard of in the epidemiology literature (26). These results were confirmed in human studies that examined nicotine administration to pregnant mothers [reviewed in (18)] and in animal studies showing that nicotine increased body weight and fat disposition, adipocyte size and gene markers of adipogenesis as well as decreases physical activity (27, 28). Even today, smoking during pregnancy represents the strongest data point supporting both the importance of development as a sensitive period for weight gain later in life and for nicotine being an endocrine disruptor. Interestingly, in this instance, epidemiological data was the first to show the association between smoking and weight gain, and the data appeared before anyone thought that chemicals (EDCs) could cause weight gain.

Beth Gladen, who had a history of studying polychlorinated biphenyls (PCBs) and dioxins in breast milk and pregnancy outcomes in humans, appears to have published the first epidemiology study on EDCs and obesity (29). They showed that girls born from mothers with the highest PCB and DDE (metabolite of DDT) exposures during pregnancy were heavier for their heights than other girls. In 2004, this same group showed that prenatal exposure to DDT was not associated with BMI (30). Despite this dubious start in the early 2000s, by 2014, 33 publications examined either overweight, BMI or general growth. Twenty-two publications examined organochlorine pesticides (DDT, hexachlorobenzene), and seven examined PCBs. There were also publications that assessed the effects of polyaromatic hydrocarbons, perfluorooctanoic acid(PFOA)/perfluorooctane sulfonate (PFOS), BPA and dioxins (31). The first comprehensive review of childhood obesity and environmental chemicals appeared in 2011(32).

SERENDIPITY AND THE OBESOGEN HYPOTHESIS

What is in a name? A lot. In 2006, the focus of the Blumberg lab was on orphan receptors, with an emphasis on PPARγ and RXR. They noted that tributyltin which activates PPARγ and RXR in mollusks also increased fat in this model. This serendipitous discovery changed the direction of the lab to a focus on the ability of tributyltin to cause weight gain in mice and differentiation of 3T3-L1 cells into lipid accumulating adipocytes. These data lead Grun and Blumberg to publish their classic paper which introduced the term "environmental obesogen." They defined an obesogen as molecules that inappropriately regulates lipid metabolism and adipogenesis to promote obesity (33). The obesogen hypothesis stimulated the field in general by giving a catchy, easy-to-remember name to a subset of EDCs that can stimulate obesity.

They noted, "the existence of chemical obesogens in and of themselves suggests that the prevailing paradigm, which holds that diet and decreased physical activity alone are the causative triggers for the burgeoning epidemic of obesity, should be reassessed."

As an indication of the growth of this new field, or perhaps to stimulate this new field, several reviews appeared in 2007, 2008, and 2009 (7, 25, 34–39), and this trend continues today (13, 40–44).

WORKSHOPS

The first workshop that focused on the role of developmental exposures to environmental chemicals and obesity was held at Duke University and sponsored by the National Institute of Environmental Health Sciences (NIEHS) and the Duke University Integrated Toxicology Program in 2004 (45). The goal of the workshop was to highlight the available data as a proof-of-concept in animals and to stimulate interest in this research area. The workshop focused on *in utero* nutrition and obesity, basic biology of fat cells and their control and several talks related to the effects of developmental exposure to environmental chemicals and later onset of obesity.

In 2011, the National Toxicology Program at the National Institute of Environmental Health Sciences held a workshop, "Role of Environmental Chemicals in the Development of Diabetes and Obesity." At this workshop, a diverse group of scientists was asked to evaluate the current literature for consistency and biological plausibility (46). The strongest conclusion from the workshop was that nicotine is an obesogen, followed by the animal and *in vitro* data for tributyltin being an obesogen and the human data on some persistent organic pollutants and diabetes. The data on BPA were considered suggestive of effects on glucose homeostasis, insulin release and adipogenesis (26, 46–48). The workshop proceedings identified research gaps including more research on type 1 diabetes, lack of human studies, more studies on the basic biology of adipocytes, and a need for more information on the biology that controls body weight and metabolic set points that change with life stage. There was also a discussion of how high throughput screening could provide valuable information about chemicals, pathways, and endpoints.

The first International workshops on obesity, "Obesity and Environmental Contaminants," were held in Uppsala, Sweden, in 2013 and 2015. A consensus statement was published as a result of the 2nd International Workshop on Obesity and Environmental Contamination, held in 2015 (49). It discussed several actions that could be taken to restrict the use of potentially harmful contaminants on metabolism.

In 2014, a small group of scientists met in Parma, Italy, to address how to help move the obesogen field forward. This was the first meeting to focus not just on obesogens and obesity, but to expand the focus to metabolic disruptors, chemicals that can cause obesity, diabetes, and fatty liver disease including metabolic syndrome. This workshop resulted in two key publications: the Parma Consensus statement (50) and a review of metabolism and the chemicals that have been shown to disrupt metabolism (13).

FUNDING AND SCIENTIFIC SUPPORT

Funding for the research area of environmental chemicals and obesity has come mainly from the NIEHS in the USA. Indeed, from the first publications noted above (14, 15), essentially all the publications related to *in vitro* and *in vivo* obesogen animal models and human studies were supported by NIEHS. Nonetheless, it took until 2011 for the NIEHS to release a specific funding announcement that focused on the role of environmental chemicals and obesity and diabetes. This announcement led to the funding of more than a dozen animal and human birth cohort studies which stimulated research and interest in the field over 3 years. This has been the only major funding focused specifically on understanding the role of EDCs in the obesity epidemic.

There is no EDC Society to specifically support and coordinate EDC, and therefore obesogen, research. However, in 2005 the Endocrine Society committed itself to EDCs as an important issue (http://press.endocrine.org/doi/10.1210/en.2005-1367) (51). In 2009, the Endocrine Society developed a position statement on EDCs followed by a Scientific Statement on EDCS (52), which established EDC research as a policy priority backed by a strong foundation of science. EDC-2. The Endocrine Society's Second Scientific Statement on Endocrine-Disrupting Chemicals was published in 2015 and contained a focus on obesogens (5). Thus, the Endocrine Society can be considered a home for obesogen research.

SUMMARY OF THE FIRST DECADE

The first 10 years of the obesogen hypothesis has led to research which has identified chemicals of concern and developmental windows of sensitivity (*in utero* and neonatal). In addition, publications showed sexually dimorphic differences in the effects of obesogens: developmental exposure to DES or BPA resulted in obesity only in the female offspring (24, 53). There are now numerous chemicals that can be designated as obesogens (13, 40, 54, 55). See **Box 1** and **Figure 1.**

The animal and human data developed in the first decade have led to the following conclusions outlined in Heindel (50):

- Susceptibility to obesity is at least in part "programmed" *in utero* and early postnatal life by exposures to environmental stressors including obesogens. This developmental programming can be considered to alter the "set point" or sensitivity to develop obesity. Indeed, it is likely that obesogens, due to their actions on programming metabolism, alter the amount of food needed to result in weight gain and the amount of exercise needed to lose weight.
- Programming may alter the number, size and function of fat cells, as well as effects on the brain appetite and/or satiety centers, control of the GI tract, muscle, pancreas, and liver, leading to altered sensitivity for gaining weight.
- It is likely that we are underestimating the importance of obesogens because of the focus of current research on a single or small subset of chemicals at a time, during limited windows of sensitivity, in single tissues and focusing on endpoints related to only one metabolic disease.

BOX 1 | Examples of obesogenic chemicals and their sources.

Antimicrobial: Triclosan, Paraben(s).

Biogenic compounds: Isoflavones (genistein, daidzein), Nicotine, Permethrins.

Byproducts/intermediate reactants: Dioxin, Nonylphenol, Acrylamide, Bisphenol A(BPA), Perfluorooctanoic acid (PFOA), Tributyltin, Benzo(a)pyrene.

Flame retardants: Tetrabromobisphenol A (TBBPA), Polybrominated diphenyl ethers (PBDE), Firemaster 550.

Food additives and contact materials: Monosodium glutamate, Tributyltin, High fructose corn syrup, nonmetabolizable sugars.

Household product ingredient: Acrylamide, di(2-ethylhexyl) phthalate (DEHP), Tributyltin, Triclosan, Bisphenol A diglycidyl ether (BADGE), Parabens.

Industrial additive: di (2 ethylhexyl) phthalate (DEHP), dibutyl phthalate (DBP),Tributyltin, Persistent Organic Pollutants (POPs).

Medical/veterinary research: Acrylamide, Bisphenol A diglycidyl ether (BADGE), Butyl benzyl phthalate (BBzP), Neonicotinoid Insecticide -imidacloprid, Permethrins, Tetrabromobisphenol A (TBBPA), Tributyltin, Diethylstilbestrol, Thiazolinedione antidiabetics (rosiglitazone), Tricyclic antidepressants (amitrriiptyline, Miratazapine), Selective serotonin uptake inhibitors.

Metabolite/degradate: Butyl benzl phthalate (metabolite of BBzP), Mono-(2-ethylhexyl) phthalate (metabolite of DEHP), Butyl phthalate (metabolite of DBP), o, p'DDE (metabolite of DDT).

Metal/metalurgy: Lead, Arsenic, Cadmium.

Personal care products/cosmetic ingredients: Perfluorooctanoic acid (PFOA), Perfluroooctane sulfonate (PFOS), butyl paraben, methyl paraben, di(2-ethylhexyl) Phthalate (DEHP), dibutyl phthalate (DBP), triclosan.

Pesticide/fungicide and ingredient: di(2-ethylhexyl)phthalate (DEHP), Dibutyl phthalate (DBP), Methyl paraben, Perfluorooctane sulfonic acid (PFOA), triclosan, Parathion, Organophosphate Pesticides (Diazinon, Chlorpyrifos) Imidacloprid, Triflumizole, Zoxamide, Quinoxyfen, Fludioxonil, Organochlorine Pesticides (Dichlorophenyltrichlorethane (DDT), Hexachlorobenzene (HCB),Lindane), Pyrethroid Pesticides (Permethrin, Deltamethrin), Phenylpyrazole Pesticide (Fipronil), Fungicide (Pyraclostrobin).

Plastic/rubber: Octyl phenol, acrylamide, Bisphenol A(BPA), Bisphenol A diglycidyl ether (BADGE), Bisphenol S, di(2-ethylhexyl) phthalate (DEHP), Perfluorooctanoic acid (PFOA), Tributyl tin, Triclosan.

Solvent: Dibutyl phthalate (DBP).

Air pollutants: Poly Aromatic Hydrocarbons (PAH), PM 2.5.

Note that some chemicals occur in multiple classes indicating several venues for exposure. This list is derived from review articles noted in this review as well as the listing of EDCs found on The Endocrine Disruption Exchange website: https://endocrinedisruption.org/

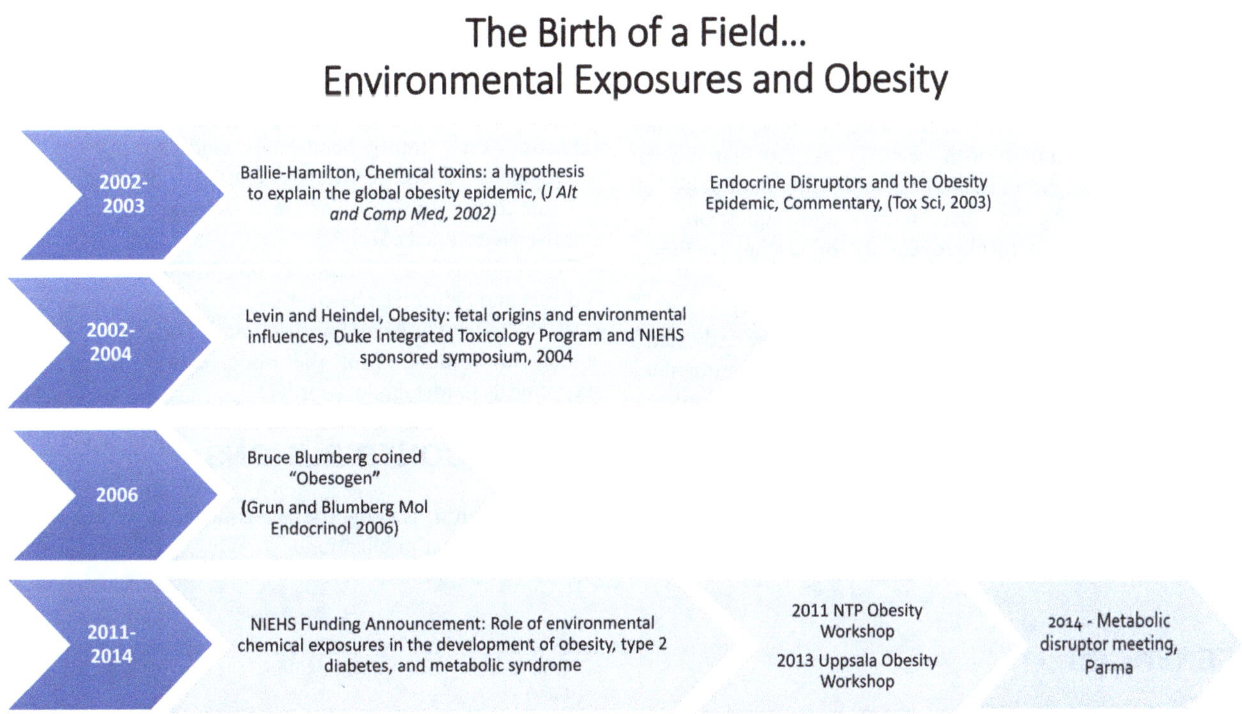

FIGURE 1 | Timeline of obesogen field.

THE OBESOGEN FIELD TODAY

In the last few years there have been two major advances in the field: a focus on transgenerational inheritance by obesogens and a change from a focus on obesogens to metabolism disruptors.

Transgenerational epigenetic inheritance due to exposure to environmental chemicals was first shown in 2005 (56) and it focused on reproductive endpoints. The first report of obesity being inherited transgenerationally by environmental chemicals appeared in 2013 (57). There are currently publications linking ancestral exposure to dichlopdiphenyltrichloroethane (DDT) (57), a combination of BPA, diethyl hexyl phthalate and dibutyl phthalate (58) tributyltin (59, 60) and jet fuel (61) to obesity. These transgenerational inheritance studies are the most disturbing as they show that the effects of obesogen exposure during pregnancy may be apparent in future generations. Perhaps some of the global obesity epidemics noted today are due to exposures to past generations in addition to current exposures.

While the term obesogen is still valid, it soon became apparent that some obesogens had activity at other tissues leading to type 2 diabetes, fatty liver and indeed metabolic syndrome. The first publication that changed the focus from obesogens *per se* to metabolic disruption and metabolic disruptors appeared in 2011 (62). This expansion from obesogen to metabolic disruptors was developed further in 2015 (13, 50) and again in 2017 (13, 55) in reviews that discussed moving to the new term metabolism disrupting chemicals (MDCs) for chemicals that cause not just weight gain but also type 2 diabetes and non-alcoholic fatty liver disease.

FUTURE DIRECTIONS

As the obesogen field moves into its second decade, an iceberg may be a good representation of the state of the science. The current data are just the tip of the iceberg, the part that shows above the water. The part of the iceberg under the water is likely to be larger, indicating that there remain many questions to answer including, how many obesogens are there, what are their molecular targets, what are the critical windows of exposure, how many windows of exposure are there and how do they interact?

Indeed, the field is still quite small, with only a few dedicated researchers focused on understanding the role of environmental chemicals in the epidemics of obesity, diabetes, and liver diseases. Thus, the first and main objective must be to expand the cadre of researchers. Just as the first researchers came from other fields, it is imperative that animal, epidemiology and clinical researchers from other fields use their expertise to help understand the role of environment in these metabolic diseases. The obesogen field, along with the focus on metabolism disruptors, has no society or specific training or coordination. The development of some oversight and coordination would be helpful to the science, outreach to clinicians and public as well as interaction with policy makers. Finally, since it is now clear that developmental exposures to obesogens/MDCs play a role in the obesity epidemic, there needs to be a concerted effort to focus on prevention by reducing exposures during windows of susceptibility and across the lifespan. Making an effort to prevent disease is always the best strategy!

Also, the field would be improved by

- Development of an integrated conceptual approach linking animal studies and endpoints with longitudinal human cohort studies.
- Development of studies that focus on the ability of obesogens/MDCs to not cause obesity or other metabolic diseases *per se*, but to show how altering the "set point" or sensitivity for gaining weight and the ability to lose weight, can alter the amount of food needed to gain or lose weight or the amount of exercise needed to lose weight.
- Assessment of multiple chemicals, mixture studies, and integration of environmental chemical studies with other stressors including stress, drugs nutrition, and infections.
- Identification of windows of sensitivity, how many are there, what mechanisms underly a window of sensitivity, how multiple windows interact across the lifespan and generations.
- Focus on environmentally relevant doses of chemicals when assessing their obesogenic effects.
- Focus on assessment of both males and females as obesogenic effects tend to be sexually dimorphic.
- Assessment of the interaction of diet including high-fat and/or high carbohydrate diets with obesogen exposures, since diet can modulate obesogen activity.
- Focus on transgenerational inheritance. Will all obesogens/MDCs be transgenerational obesogens or just a subset; if a subset, what are the characteristics that allow transgenerational effects?
- Development and validation of *in vivo* and *in vitro* screens to detect and prioritize obesogens/MDCs.
- Work with clinicians and clinical societies to improve their understanding of the importance of environmental chemicals in metabolic disorders.

AUTHOR CONTRIBUTIONS

The author confirms being the sole contributor of this work and has approved it for publication.

REFERENCES

1. Serretti A, Mandelli L. Antidepressants and body weight: a comprehensive review and meta-analysis. *J Clin Psychiatry* (2010) 71:1259–72. doi: 10.4088/JCP.09r05346blu
2. Zhang J, Liu X, Xie XB, Cheng XC, Wang RL. Multitargeted bioactive ligands for PPARs discovered in the last decade. *Chem Biol Drug Des.* (2016) 88:635–63. doi: 10.1111/cbdd.12806
3. Roman-Ramos R, Almanza-Perez JC, Garcia-Macedo R, Blancas-Flores G, Fortis-Barrera A, Alarcon-Aguilar FJ. Monosodium glutamate neonatal intoxication associated with obesity in adult stage is characterized by chronic inflammation and increased mRNA expression of peroxisome proliferator-activated receptors in mice. *Basic Clin*

Pharmacol Toxicol. (2011) 108:406–13. doi: 10.1111/j.1742-7843.2011.00671.x
4. Schug TT, Johnson AF, Birnbaum LS, Colborn T, Guillette LJ, Heindel JJ. Minireview: endocrine disruptors: past lessons and future directions. *Mol Endocrinol.* (2016) 30:833–47. doi: 10.1210/me.2016-1096
5. Gore AC, Chappell VA, Fenton SE, Flaws JA, Nadal A, Zoeller RT. EDC-2: the endocrine society's second scientific statement on endocrine-disrupting chemicals. *Endocr Rev.* (2015) 36:E1–e150. doi: 10.1210/er.2015-1010
6. Lee DH, Porta M, Jacobs DR Jr, Vandenberg LN. Chlorinated persistent organic pollutants, obesity, and type 2 diabetes. *Endocr Rev.* (2014) 35:557–601. doi: 10.1210/er.2013-1084
7. Newbold RR, Padilla-Banks E, Snyder RJ, Jefferson WN. Perinatal exposure to environmental estrogens and the development of obesity. *Mol Nutr Food Res.* (2007) 51:912–7. doi: 10.1002/mnfr.200600259
8. Newbold RR. Developmental exposure to endocrine-disrupting chemicals programs for reproductive tract alterations and obesity later in life. *Am J Clin Nutr.* (2011) 94(Suppl 6):1939S–42. doi: 10.3945/ajcn.110.001057
9. Hanson M, Godfrey KM, Lillycrop KA, Burdge GC, Gluckman PD. Developmental plasticity and developmental origins of non-communicable disease: theoretical considerations and epigenetic mechanisms. *Prog Biophys Mol Biol.* (2011) 106:272–80. doi: 10.1016/j.pbiomolbio.2010.12.008
10. Hanson MA, Gluckman PD. Developmental origins of health and disease– global public health implications. *Best Pract Res Clin Obstet Gynaecol.* (2015) 29:24–31. doi: 10.1016/j.bpobgyn.2014.06.007
11. Grandjean P, Barouki R, Bellinger DC, Casteleyn L, Chadwick LH, Heindel JJ. Life-long implications of developmental exposure to environmental stressors: new perspectives. *Endocrinology* (2015) 156:3408–15. doi: 10.1210/EN.2015-1350
12. Baillie-Hamilton PF. Chemical toxins: a hypothesis to explain the global obesity epidemic. *J Altern Complement Med.* (2002) 8:185–92. doi: 10.1089/107555302317371479
13. Heindel JJ, Blumberg B, Cave M, Machtinger R, Mantovani A, Mendez, M. et al. Metabolism disrupting chemicals and metabolic disorders. *Reprod Toxicol.* (2017) 68:3–33. doi: 10.1016/j.reprotox.2016.10.001
14. Howdeshell KL, Hotchkiss AK, Thayer KA, Vandenbergh JG, vom Saal FS. Exposure to bisphenol A advances puberty. *Nature* (1999) 401:763–4. doi: 10.1038/44517
15. Rubin BS, Murray MK, Damassa DA, King JC, Soto AM. Perinatal exposure to low doses of bisphenol A affects body weight, patterns of estrous cyclicity, and plasma LH levels. *Environ Health Perspect.* (2001) 109:675–80. doi: 10.1289/ehp.01109675
16. Toschke AM, Koletzko B, Slikker W Jr, Hermann M, von Kries R. Childhood obesity is associated with maternal smoking in pregnancy. *Eur J Pediatr.* (2002) 161:445–8. doi: 10.1007/s00431-002-0983-z
17. von Kries R, Toschke AM, Koletzko B, Slikker W Jr. Maternal smoking during pregnancy and childhood obesity. *Am J Epidemiol.* (2002) 156:954–61. doi: 10.1093/aje/kwf128
18. Oken E, Levitan EB, Gillman MW. Maternal smoking during pregnancy and child overweight: systematic review and meta-analysis. *Int J Obes.* (2008) 32:201–10. doi: 10.1038/sj.ijo.0803760
19. Oken E, Gillman MW. Fetal origins of obesity. *Obes Res.* (2003) 11:496–506. doi: 10.1038/oby.2003.69
20. Masuno H, Kidani T, Sekiya K, Sakayama K, Shiosaka T, Yamamoto, H. et al. Bisphenol A in combination with insulin can accelerate the conversion of 3T3-L1 fibroblasts to adipocytes. *J Lipid Res.* (2002) 43:676–84.
21. Masuno H, Iwanami J, Kidani T, Sakayama K, Honda K. Bisphenol a accelerates terminal differentiation of 3T3-L1 cells into adipocytes through the phosphatidylinositol 3-kinase pathway. *Toxicol Sci.* (2005) 84:319–27. doi: 10.1093/toxsci/kfi088
22. Masuno H, Okamoto S, Iwanami J, Honda K, Shiosaka T, Kidani, T. et al. Effect of 4-nonylphenol on cell proliferation and adipocyte formation in cultures of fully differentiated 3T3-L1 cells. *Toxicol Sci.* (2003) 75:314–20. doi: 10.1093/toxsci/kfg203
23. Heindel JJ. Endocrine disruptors and the obesity epidemic. *Toxicol Sci.* (2003) 76:247–9. doi: 10.1093/toxsci/kfg255
24. Newbold RR, Padilla-Banks E, Snyder RJ, Jefferson WN. Developmental exposure to estrogenic compounds and obesity. *Birth Defects Res A Clin Mol Teratol.* (2005) 73:478–80. doi: 10.1002/bdra.20147
25. Newbold RR, Padilla-Banks E, Jefferson WN. Environmental estrogens and obesity. *Mol Cell Endocrinol.* (2009) 304:84–9. doi: 10.1016/j.mce.2009.02.024
26. Behl M, Rao, D. Aagaard K, Davidson TL, Levin ED, Holloway AC. Evaluation of the association between maternal smoking, childhood obesity, and metabolic disorders: a national toxicology program workshop review. *Environ Health Perspect* (2013) 121:170–80. doi: 10.1289/ehp.1205404
27. Gao Q, Horvath TL. Neuronal control of energy homeostasis. *FEBS Lett.* (2008) 582:132–41. doi: 10.1016/j.febslet.2007.11.063
28. Somm E, Schwitzgebel VM, Vauthay DM, Camm EJ, Chen CY, Huppi PS. Prenatal nicotine exposure alters early pancreatic islet and adipose tissue development with consequences on the control of body weight and glucose metabolism later in life. *Endocrinology* (2008) 149:6289–99. doi: 10.1210/en.2008-0361
29. Gladen BC, Ragan NB, Rogan WJ. Pubertal growth and development and prenatal and lactational exposure to polychlorinated biphenyls and dichlorodiphenyl dichloroethene. *J Pediatr.* (2000) 136:490–6. doi: 10.1016/S0022-3476(00)90012-X
30. Gladen BC, Klebanoff MA, Hediger ML, Katz SH, Barr DB, Longnecker MP. Prenatal DDT exposure in relation to anthropometric and pubertal measures in adolescent males. *Environ Health Perspect.* (2004) 112:1761–7. doi: 10.1289/ehp.7287
31. Heindel JJ, Skalla LA, Joubert BR, Dilworth CH, Gray KA. Review of developmental origins of health and disease publications in environmental epidemiology. *Reprod Toxicol.* (2017) 68:34–48. doi: 10.1016/j.reprotox.2016.11.011
32. La Merrill M, Birnbaum LS. Childhood obesity and environmental chemicals. *Mt Sinai J Med.* (2011) 78:22–48. doi: 10.1002/msj.20229
33. Grun F, Blumberg B. Environmental obesogens: organotins and endocrine disruption via nuclear receptor signaling. *Endocrinology* (2006) 147(Suppl. 6):S50–5. doi: 10.1210/en.2005-1129
34. Tuma RS. Environmental chemicals–not just overeating–may cause obesity. *J Natl Cancer Inst.* (2007) 99:835. doi: 10.1093/jnci/djk230
35. Elobeid MA, Allison DB. Putative environmental-endocrine disruptors and obesity: a review. *Curr Opin Endocrinol Diabetes Obes.* (2008) 15:403–8. doi: 10.1097/MED.0b013e32830ce95c
36. Newbold RR, Padilla-Banks E, Jefferson WN, Heindel JJ. Effects of endocrine disruptors on obesity. *Int J Androl* (2008) 31:201–8. doi: 10.1111/j.1365-2605.2007.00858.x
37. Chen JQ, Brown TR, Russo J. Regulation of energy metabolism pathways by estrogens and estrogenic chemicals and potential implications in obesity associated with increased exposure to endocrine disruptors. *Biochim Biophys Acta* (2009) 1793:1128–43. doi: 10.1016/j.bbamcr.2009.03.009
38. Grun F, Blumberg B. Minireview: the case for obesogens. *Mol Endocrinol.* (2009) 23:1127–34. doi: 10.1210/me.2008-0485
39. Heindel JJ, vom Saal FS. Role of nutrition and environmental endocrine disrupting chemicals during the perinatal period on the aetiology of obesity. *Mol Cell Endocrinol..* (2009) 304:90–6. doi: 10.1016/j.mce.2009.02.025
40. Janesick AS, Blumberg B. Obesogens: an emerging threat to public health. *Am J Obstet Gynecol.* (2016). doi: 10.1016/j.ajog.2016.01.182
41. Darbre PD. Endocrine Disruptors and Obesity. *Curr Obes Rep.* (2017) 6:18–27. doi: 10.1007/s13679-017-0240-4
42. Le Magueresse-Battistoni B, Labaronne E, Vidal H, Naville D. Endocrine disrupting chemicals in mixture and obesity, diabetes and related metabolic disorders. *World J Biol Chem.* (2017) 8:108–19. doi: 10.4331/wjbc.v8.i2.108
43. Muscogiuri G, Barrea L, Laudisio D, Savastano S, Colao A. Obesogenic endocrine disruptors and obesity: myths and truths. *Arch Toxicol.* (2017) 91:3469–75. doi: 10.1007/s00204-017-2071-1
44. Stojanoska MM, Milosevic N, Milic N, Abenavoli L. The influence of phthalates and bisphenol A on the obesity development and glucose metabolism disorders. *Endocrine* (2017) 55:666–81. doi: 10.1007/s12020-016-1158-4
45. Heindel JJ. The fetal basis of adult disease: Role of environmental exposures– introduction. *Birth Defects Res A Clin Mol Teratol.* (2005) 73:131–2. doi: 10.1002/bdra.20119
46. Thayer KA, Heindel JJ, Bucher JR, Gallo MA. Role of Environmental chemicals in diabetes and obesity: a National Toxicology Program Workshop Report. *Environ Health Perspect.* (2012). doi: 10.1289/ehp.1104597

47. Maull EA, Ahsan H, Edwards J, Longnecker MP, Navas-Acien A, Loomis D. Evaluation of the association between arsenic and diabetes: a National Toxicology Program workshop review. *Environ Health Perspect.* (2012) 120:1658–70. doi: 10.1289/ehp.1104579
48. Taylor KW, Novak RF, Anderson HA, Birnbaum LS, Blystone C, Lind L. Evaluation of the association between persistent organic pollutants (POPs) and diabetes in epidemiological studies: a national toxicology program workshop review. *Environ Health Perspect.* (2013) 121:774–83. doi: 10.1289/ehp.1205502
49. Lind L, Lind PM, Lejonklou MH, Dunder L, Bergman A, Birnbaum LS. Uppsala Consensus Statement on Environmental Contaminants and the Global Obesity Epidemic. *Environ Health Perspect.* (2016) 124:A81–83. doi: 10.1289/ehp.1511115
50. Heindel JJ, vom Saal FS, Blumberg B, Bovolin P, Calamandrei G, Palanza P. Parma consensus statement on metabolic disruptors. *Environ Health* (2015) 14:54. doi: 10.1186/s12940-015-0042-7
51. Gore AC, Heindel JJ, Zoeller RT. Endocrine disruption for endocrinologists (and others). *Endocrinology* (2006) 147(Suppl. 6):S1–3. doi: 10.1210/en.2005-1367
52. Diamanti-Kandarakis E, Bourguignon JP, Guidice LC, Hauser R, Prins GS, Gore AC. Endocrine-disrupting chemical: an Endocrine Society scientific statement. *Endocr Rev.* (2009) 30:293–342. doi: 10.1210/er.2009-0002
53. Rubin BS, Paranjpe M, DaFonte T, Schaeberle C, Soto AM, Greenberg AS. Perinatal BPA exposure alters body weight and composition in a dose specific and sex specific manner: The addition of peripubertal exposure exacerbates adverse effects in female mice. *Reprod Toxicol.* (2017) 68:130–44. doi: 10.1016/j.reprotox.2016.07.020
54. Kim JT, Lee HK. Childhood obesity and endocrine disrupting chemicals. *Ann Pediatr Endocrinol Metab.* (2017) 22:219–25. doi: 10.6065/apem.2017.22.4.219
55. Mimoto MS, Nadal A, Sargis RM. Polluted pathways: mechanisms of metabolic disruption by endocrine disrupting chemicals. *Curr Environ Health Rep.* (2017) 4:208–22. doi: 10.1007/s40572-017-0137-0
56. Anway MD, Cupp AS, Uzumcu M, Skinner MK. Epigenetic transgenerational actions of endocrine disruptors and male fertility. *Science* (2005) 308:1466–9. doi: 10.1126/science.1108190
57. Skinner MK, Manikkam M, Tracey R, Guerrero-Bosagna C, Haque M, Nilsson EE. Ancestral dichlorodiphenyltrichloroethane (DDT) exposure promotes epigenetic transgenerational inheritance of obesity. *BMC Med.* (2013) 11:228. doi: 10.1186/1741-7015-11-228
58. Manikkam M, Tracey R, Guerrero-Bosagna C, Skinner MK. Plastics derived endocrine disruptors (BPA, DEHP and DBP) induce epigenetic transgenerational inheritance of obesity, reproductive disease and sperm epimutations. *PLoS ONE* (2013) 8:e55387. doi: 10.1371/journal.pone.0055387
59. Janesick AS, Shioda T, Blumberg B. Transgenerational inheritance of prenatal obesogen exposure. *Mol Cell Endocrinol.* (2014) 398:31–5. doi: 10.1016/j.mce.2014.09.002
60. Chamorro-Garcia R, Diaz-Castillo C, Shoucri BM, Kach H, Leavitt R, Blumberg B. Ancestral perinatal obesogen exposure results in a transgenerational thrifty phenotype in mice. *Nat Commun.* (2017) 8:2012. doi: 10.1038/s41467-017-01944-z
61. Tracey R, Manikkam M, Guerrero-Bosagna C, Skinner MK. Hydrocarbons (jet fuel JP-8) induce epigenetic transgenerational inheritance of obesity, reproductive disease and sperm epimutations. *Reprod Toxicol.* (2013) 36:104–16. doi: 10.1016/j.reprotox.2012.11.011
62. Casals-Casas C, Desvergne B. Endocrine disruptors: from endocrine to metabolic disruption. *Annu Rev Physiol.* (2011) 73:135–62. doi: 10.1146/annurev-physiol-012110-142200

15

Prenatal Exposure to Traffic Pollution and Childhood Body Mass Index Trajectory

Abby F. Fleisch[1,2*], *Izzuddin M. Aris*[3,4], *Sheryl L. Rifas-Shiman*[3], *Brent A. Coull*[5], *Heike Luttmann-Gibson*[6], *Petros Koutrakis*[6], *Joel D. Schwartz*[6], *Itai Kloog*[6,7], *Diane R. Gold*[6,8] *and Emily Oken*[3,9]

[1] *Pediatric Endocrinology and Diabetes, Maine Medical Center, Portland, ME, United States,* [2] *Center for Outcomes Research and Evaluation, Maine Medical Center Research Institute, Portland, ME, United States,* [3] *Division of Chronic Disease Research Across the Lifecourse, Department of Population Medicine, Harvard Medical School and Harvard Pilgrim Health Care Institute, Boston, MA, United States,* [4] *Department of Obstetrics and Gynecology, Yong Loo Lin School of Medicine, National University of Singapore, Singapore, Singapore,* [5] *Department of Biostatistics, Harvard School of Public Health, Boston, MA, United States,* [6] *Department of Environmental Health, Harvard School of Public Health, Boston, MA, United States,* [7] *Department of Geography and Environmental Development, Ben-Gurion University of the Negev, Beersheba, Israel,* [8] *Channing Laboratory, Brigham and Women's Hospital, Boston, MA, United States,* [9] *Department of Nutrition, Harvard School of Public Health, Boston, MA, United States*

***Correspondence:**
Abby F. Fleisch
afleisch@mmc.org

Background: Limited evidence suggests an association between prenatal exposure to traffic pollution and greater adiposity in childhood, but the time window during which growth may be most affected is not known.

Methods: We studied 1,649 children in Project Viva, a Boston-area pre-birth cohort. We used spatiotemporal models to estimate prenatal residential air pollution exposures and geographic information systems to estimate neighborhood traffic density and roadway proximity. We used weight and stature measurements at clinical and research visits to estimate a BMI trajectory for each child with mixed-effects natural cubic spline models. In primary analyses, we examined associations of residential $PM_{2.5}$ and black carbon (BC) exposures during the third trimester and neighborhood traffic density and home roadway proximity at birth address with (1) estimated BMI at 6 month intervals through 10 years of age, (2) magnitude and timing of BMI peak and rebound, and (3) overall BMI trajectory. In secondary analyses, we examined associations of residential $PM_{2.5}$ and BC exposures during the first and second trimesters with BMI outcomes.

Results: Median (Interquartile range; IQR) concentration of residential air pollution during the third trimester was 11.4 (1.7) $\mu g/m^3$ for $PM_{2.5}$ and 0.7 (0.3) $\mu g/m^3$ for BC. Participants had a median (IQR) of 13 (7) clinical or research BMI measures from 0 to 10 years of age. None of the traffic pollution exposures were significantly associated with any of the BMI outcomes in covariate-adjusted models, although effect estimates were in the hypothesized direction for neighborhood traffic density and home roadway proximity. For example, greater neighborhood traffic density [median (IQR) 857 (1,452) vehicles/day x km of road within 100 m of residential address at delivery] was associated with a higher BMI throughout childhood, with the strongest associations in early childhood [e.g., per IQR increment natural log-transformed neighborhood traffic density, BMI at 12 months of age was 0.05 (−0.03, 0.13) kg/m^2 higher and infancy peak BMI was 0.05 (−0.03, 0.14) kg/m^2 higher].

Conclusions: We found no evidence for a persistent effect of prenatal exposure to traffic pollution on BMI trajectory from birth through mid-childhood in a population exposed to modest levels of air pollution.

Keywords: air pollution, particulate matter, traffic, growth, childhood

INTRODUCTION

Childhood obesity often tracks into adulthood (1), leading to costly comorbidities and lower life expectancy in affected individuals (2). Obesity is primarily a result of high caloric intake and low physical activity, but eating less and exercising more has proven very difficult to maintain (3). Prenatal and early life exposure to some environmental toxicants may also predispose children to obesity (4). It is a public health imperative to evaluate early life determinants of obesity and identify vulnerable windows of exposure because of the potential for preventive interventions.

In rodents, early life air pollution exposure results in systemic and adipose inflammation and leads to greater visceral adiposity (5). Consistent with this observation, epidemiologic studies have demonstrated an association between air pollution exposure during childhood and increased risk of overweight or obesity (6–10). Greater maternal air pollution exposure during pregnancy also may be associated with greater offspring adiposity and increased risk of overweight or obesity in childhood (11–15). Prenatal air pollution may affect child weight directly by increasing inflammatory potential of fetal adipose tissue or indirectly by restricting fetal growth or disrupting maternal glycemia, which have both been associated with prenatal air pollution exposure in our cohort (11, 12) and others (16, 17) and may prime children for greater weight or adiposity later in life (18, 19). In our cohort, late prenatal traffic pollution exposure was associated with greater weight gain during infancy (12), and infants of mothers living closer to a major roadway at the time of delivery had greater adiposity but no difference in BMI in mid-childhood (11). Despite the fact that obesity is more prevalent as children age (20), there has been no prior evaluation of the extent to which prenatal traffic pollution exposure may differentially impact growth at different time windows during childhood.

In the present analysis, we used a growth trajectory approach to evaluate the impact of traffic pollution exposure on critical windows of growth across childhood. Our primary objective was to evaluate the extent to which late prenatal exposures to fine particulate matter ($PM_{2.5}$) and black carbon (BC) (a traffic-related component of $PM_{2.5}$), as well as residential traffic density and roadway proximity, were associated with trajectory of body mass index (BMI) from birth to mid-childhood. In secondary analyses, we also evaluated the role of early and mid-prenatal exposures to traffic pollution on BMI trajectory. We hypothesized that higher prenatal traffic pollution exposure would be associated with lower BMI at birth and greater gains in BMI throughout childhood.

MATERIALS AND METHODS

Study Population and Design

Participants were recruited during 1999–2002 to Project Viva, a prospective observational cohort study of prenatal exposures and offspring health. We recruited women during their first prenatal visit (median 10 weeks gestation) at Atrius Harvard Vanguard Medical Associates, a multi-specialty group practice in eastern Massachusetts. Children had study visits at the time of birth and in infancy (median: 6.0 months of age), early childhood (median: 3.3 years of age), and mid-childhood (median: 7.7 years of age). We have previously published details of our recruitment procedures and study protocol (21).

Of 2,128 live singleton births, we modeled BMI trajectories in 1,649 (77.5%) offspring who had data for at least 3 measurements of BMI from birth to mid-childhood (our criterion for inclusion in the growth trajectory model) and at least one air pollution exposure metric. Children included vs. excluded in this analysis were more likely to have older and more educated mothers, had a larger gestational age at delivery, and were more likely to be white or other race/ethnicity and less likely to be black, Hispanic, or Asian (**Supplemental Table 1**).

Mothers provided written informed consent at enrollment and for their child at each in-person visit. Project Viva has been reviewed and approved by the Institutional Review Board of Harvard Pilgrim Health Care. The present secondary data analysis was deemed exempt by the Maine Medical Center Institutional Review Board.

Air Pollution Exposures

We used aerosol optical depth data to estimate $PM_{2.5}$ exposure at each participant's residence at a 1 × 1 km spatial grid resolution (mean daily "out-of-sample" ten-fold cross-validation $R^2 = 0.88$) (22). We used a land-use regression model to estimate daily BC exposure at each residence (mean "out-of-sample" 10-fold cross-validation $R^2 = 0.73$) (23). Our $PM_{2.5}$ model encompassed addresses in the New England region, and our BC model encompassed addresses in Eastern Massachusetts.

Because we have previously shown 3rd trimester exposure to traffic pollution to be most closely associated with fetal and infant growth in Project Viva (12), in primary analyses, we used estimates of residential traffic pollution during the 3rd trimester, which we obtained by averaging daily exposures from the 188th day (i.e.—27 weeks gestation) after the last menstrual period (LMP) to the day before birth. For secondary analyses, we used estimated average residential traffic pollution during the 1st trimester [date of LMP to 93rd day after LMP (i.e.—13 weeks gestation)] and 2nd trimester (94th day after LMP to 187th day after LMP). We assigned exposures to addresses where we had data available for at least 90% of days in the trimester. Our estimates of $PM_{2.5}$ and BC exposure accounted for residential moves during pregnancy.

We used the 2002 road inventory from the Massachusetts Executive Office of Transportation to calculate traffic density at each participant's residential address at the time of delivery by multiplying annual average daily traffic (vehicles/day) by length of road (km) within 100 m of participants' residential address. We used 2005 ESRI Street Map™ North America ArcGIS 10 Data and Maps to estimate home roadway proximity at the time of delivery as distance to Census Feature Class Code A1 or A2 roads (i.e.—highways).

Child Anthropometric Measures

We obtained anthropometric measures from study visits and from clinical records. At study visits, research assistants measured participants' weight using an electronic scale [Seca scale in infancy and early childhood (Hanover, MD); Tanita scale in mid-childhood (Arlington Heights, IL)] and length/height in infancy and early childhood using a Shorr measuring board and height in mid-childhood using a stadiometer (Shorr Productions, Olney, MD). We also reviewed data from each participant's pediatrician's office to obtain length/height and weight data from clinical visits during infancy and childhood. We have previously shown clinical measurements of length, obtained by the paper and pencil method, to systematically overestimate research measures by 1.8 cm in children <2 years of age (24), so we included this correction factor for clinical lengths obtained in this age group. Using both research and clinical measures, we calculated BMI as weight in kilograms divided by length or height in meters squared.

Covariates

We collected information on maternal race/ethnicity, education, parity, and smoking habits by questionnaire at study enrollment and on child race/ethnicity by questionnaire in early childhood. We obtained child sex, birth weight, and date of birth from the hospital medical record. We calculated length of gestation by last menstrual period, and we updated it with mid-pregnancy ultrasound if the two estimates differed by >10 days. We abstracted residential census tract median annual household income and percent below poverty at the time of delivery from 2000 US Census data (25).

Statistical Analyses

Modeling BMI Trajectory

We fit individual BMI curves using mixed-effects models with natural cubic spline functions for age, as previously described (26). The fixed effects component of the model was:

$$BMI = \beta_{00} + \beta_{10}(\text{age}) + \sum_{j=1}^{m} \beta j\{(\text{age} - k_j)_+^3 - \lambda j(\text{age} - k_{\min})_+^3 - (1 - \lambda j)(\text{age} - k_{\max})_+^3\} + e_{ij} \quad (1)$$

where k_{min} and k_{max} = boundary knots, k_j = interior knot point j between boundary knots; m = number of interior knots between boundary knots; $j = 1, 2, \ldots$, m; e = residual and $(\text{age-k}_j)_+^3$ is defined as age–k if age $\geq k_j$. We included random effects for the intercept, linear age slopes and spline functions to account for repeated measures in the same child and capture the non-linear trend in BMI. Our final model included interactions of child sex with spline terms as fixed parameters, as BMI trajectories derived were similar using this approach as compared to modeling BMI trajectories separately for boys and girls.

We considered two approaches to select knot locations: at equally spaced percentiles or at the median, minimum and maximum ages of each of three developmental periods: infancy and early and mid-childhood. We used Bayesian information criterion to determine the optimal number (six) and location (0.1, 4.9, 10.6, 37.9, 92.5, and 131.1 months of age) of knots for both fixed and random effects.

We estimated child age at peak and rebound by differentiation of the subject-specific BMI curve; the peak and rebound are located at ages where the derivative of the curve equals zero. We estimated the magnitude (kg/m^2) at peak and rebound as the highest and lowest points, respectively, of the child-specific BMI curve. We defined velocity (kg/m^2/month) to BMI peak as the linear velocity from birth to the BMI peak, and velocity to rebound as the linear velocity from BMI peak to rebound. We also used the modeled trajectory to predict BMI at 6-monthly intervals from birth to 10 years for each child. Among the 1,649 children, 1,578 (74.2%) had estimable BMI peak and rebound, 41 had no BMI peak (i.e., showed no decline in BMI after the rise in infancy) and 30 had no BMI rebound (i.e., showed no rise in BMI after the decline in early childhood).

Examining Associations of Prenatal Air Pollution Exposure With BMI Trajectory

We ran separate linear regression models to examine the associations of exposure to each air pollutant with BMI in childhood. In primary analyses, we examined average $PM_{2.5}$ exposure during the 3rd trimester, average BC exposure during the 3rd trimester, traffic density based on address at delivery, and major roadway proximity based on address at delivery. In secondary analyses, we examined average $PM_{2.5}$ and BC exposures during the 1st and 2nd trimesters. For all analyses, our outcomes included (1) BMI predicted by the cubic spline model at 6 month intervals, and (2) age of child (months), magnitude (kg/m^2), and velocity (kg/m^2/month) at BMI peak and BMI rebound. We also estimated the association of each exposure with overall BMI trajectory by including the exposures as fixed effects in the mixed-effects models. For analyses of BMI peak and rebound, we restricted the analyses to children with estimable BMI peak and rebound (n = 1,396–1,649).

To account for the exponential spatial decay of traffic pollution (27), we *a priori* categorized residential proximity to major roadway as > 200 m, 100 to < 200 m, 50 to < 100 m, and < 50 m, as we have done previously (11, 12). We initially modeled BC, $PM_{2.5}$, and neighborhood traffic density in quartiles. We did not observe non-linearity in exposure–outcome relationships, and so we also modeled these variables as continuous measures, scaled by the interquartile range (IQR) of each exposure. We log-transformed neighborhood traffic density, which was right-skewed, using natural logarithms.

We first fit models adjusted only for child sex, followed by full multivariable models for each exposure–outcome relationship. We included additional covariates potentially associated with air pollution exposure and/or childhood growth: maternal age (continuous), education (with or without college degree), smoking habits (smoked during pregnancy, formerly smoked, never smoked), and parity (nulliparous or multiparous); child race/ethnicity (white, black, Hispanic, Asian or other); and census tract median household income (continuous) and percent below poverty (continuous). To account for trends in traffic pollution and growth by season and over time, we also included season (continuous sine and cosine of date) and date (continuous) of birth in multivariable models. We did not include gestational weight gain, maternal glucose tolerance, or gestational age in our models because these variables may be on the causal pathway, and their inclusion could introduce collider bias (28). We substituted maternal for child race/ethnicity in 10% of participants missing data on child race/ethnicity. Between 98.7 and 99.5% of participants had complete covariate information for the multivariable models. We assessed for effect modification by child sex, based on prior data suggesting the possibility of sex-specific associations in relation to prenatal air pollution exposure (29, 30). We found no effect modification, so we present all results without stratification or inclusion of an interaction term for child sex.

We used Stata 15 (StataCorp LP, Texas, USA) for all analyses.

TABLE 1 | Characteristics of participants overall and by quartile of 3rd trimester $PM_{2.5}$.

$PM_{2.5}$ (μg/m^3), Max-Min	**Overall (7.7–17.3)**	**Quartiles of $PM_{2.5}$**			
		Q1 (7.7-10.5)	**Q2 (10.5–11.4)**	**Q3 (11.4–12.2)**	**Q4 (12.2–17.3)**
MEAN (SD) OR %					
Maternal characteristics					
Age at enrollment (years)	32.0 (5.2)	32.2 (4.6)	31.9 (5.3)	31.7 (5.4)	32.5 (5.3)
College graduate	66	72	67	66	63
Smoking habits					
Never	68	64	65	73	71
Prior to pregnancy	20	23	21	16	17
During pregnancy	12	13	13	10	12
Nulliparous	48	45	46	52	46
Household characteristics					
Census tract median income (US dollars/year)	57,921 (21,310)	64,794 (22,397)	60,855 (20,411)	53,698 (19,171)	52,423 (20,778)
Census tract% below poverty	10 (9)	7 (8)	8 (8)	11 (10)	12 (10)
Child characteristics					
Gestational age at delivery (weeks)	39.5 (1.8)	39.2 (2.0)	39.7 (1.6)	39.5 (1.9)	39.6 (1.5)
Female	49	47	48	50	51
Race/ethnicity					
White	64	73	69	59	57
Black	16	12	15	18	20
Hispanic	5	4	3	7	6
Asian	4	4	4	5	3
Other	10	8	8	10	13
MEDIAN (IQR) OR %					
Traffic pollution					
3rd trimester black carbon (μg/m^3)	0.7 (0.3)	0.5 (0.2)	0.6 (0.3)	0.7 (0.3)	0.8 (0.3)
Neighborhood traffic density at delivery (km*vehicles/day)	857 (1,452)	531 (1,190)	658 (1,420)	1,016 (1,373)	1,223 (1,697)
Home proximity to major roadway at delivery					
<50 m	3	3	3	4	5
50–<100 m	3	1	3	3	4
100–<200 m	6	3	7	9	7
≥200 m	88	93	87	84	84

RESULTS

Population Characteristics

Sixty six percent of mothers were college graduates, 69% were non-smokers, and 52% were nulliparous. 64% of children were white. Third trimester median (IQR, range) $PM_{2.5}$ concentration was 11.4 (1.7, 7.7–17.3) μg/m^3 which is below the Environmental Protection Agency air quality standard for annual $PM_{2.5}$ exposure (15 μg/m^3 at the time of the study and 12 μg/m^3 currently in 2018). Third trimester median (IQR, range) BC concentration was 0.7 (0.3, 0.1–1.6) μg/m^3 which is consistent with the annual US urban average (ranged from 0.2 to 1.9 μg/m^3) during 2005–2007 (31). At the time of delivery, median (IQR, range) neighborhood traffic density was 857 (1,452, 0–30,900) vehicles/day x km of road within 100 m of residential address; most mothers (88%) lived > 200 m from a major roadway, and 3% lived <50 m (**Table 1**). Correlations between exposures were moderate (Spearman correlation coefficients ranged from −0.37 to 0.51) and reported previously in detail in a similar subset of the Project Viva cohort (11).

Each child had a median [interquartile range (IQR)] of 13 (7) BMI measures between birth and mid-childhood. The mean (SD) of age at BMI peak was 8.4 (2.7) months and at BMI rebound was 59.4 (19.4) months. The mean (SD) of the magnitude of the BMI peak was 18.0 (1.4) kg/m^2 and of the BMI rebound was 16.0 (1.2) kg/m^2. The mean (SD) of velocity to BMI peak was 0.5 (0.2) kg/m^2/month and to BMI rebound was −0.04 (0.02) kg/m^2/month. As compared to boys, girls were older at peak BMI (8.9 vs. 8.1 months), younger at BMI rebound (55.5 vs. 63.1 months), had a lower magnitude at BMI peak (17.7 vs. 18.3 kg/m^2) and rebound (15.9 vs. 16.1 kg/m^2), and had a slower velocity to BMI peak (0.5 vs. 0.6 kg/m^2/month).

Traffic Pollution Exposure and Childhood BMI Trajectory

Exposures to $PM_{2.5}$, BC, neighborhood traffic density, and home roadway proximity in late pregnancy were not associated with any of the BMI outcomes at any age in sex-adjusted or covariate-adjusted models, regardless of whether the exposure was represented in quartiles (**Figures 1–3**), per IQR increment (**Supplemental Tables 2–4**), or by category of roadway proximity (**Figure 4; Supplemental Table 5**). Effect estimates were in the hypothesized direction for neighborhood traffic density and home roadway proximity, although confidence intervals crossed

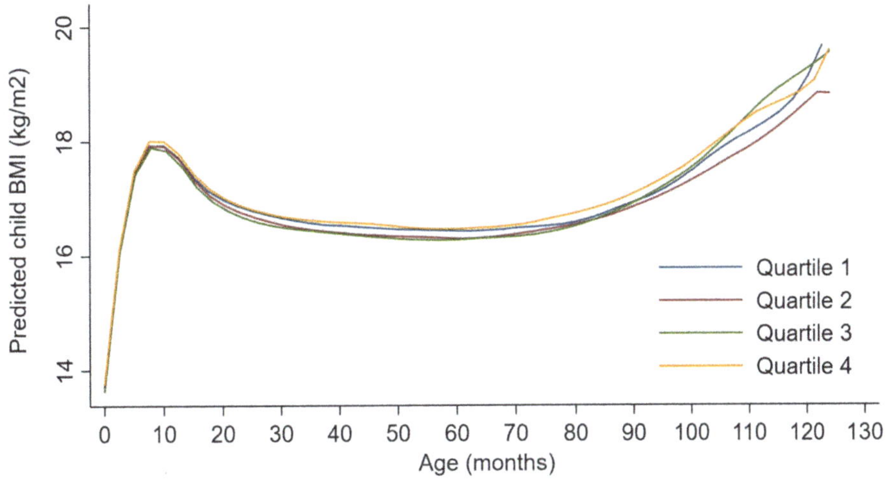

FIGURE 1 | Child BMI trajectories from birth to mid-childhood according to quartiles of 3rd trimester $PM_{2.5}$ exposure. Trajectories were additionally adjusted for date of birth, sine/cosine of the date of birth, maternal age, educational attainment, parity, smoking history, median household income, census tract% below poverty, child sex, and race/ethnicity.

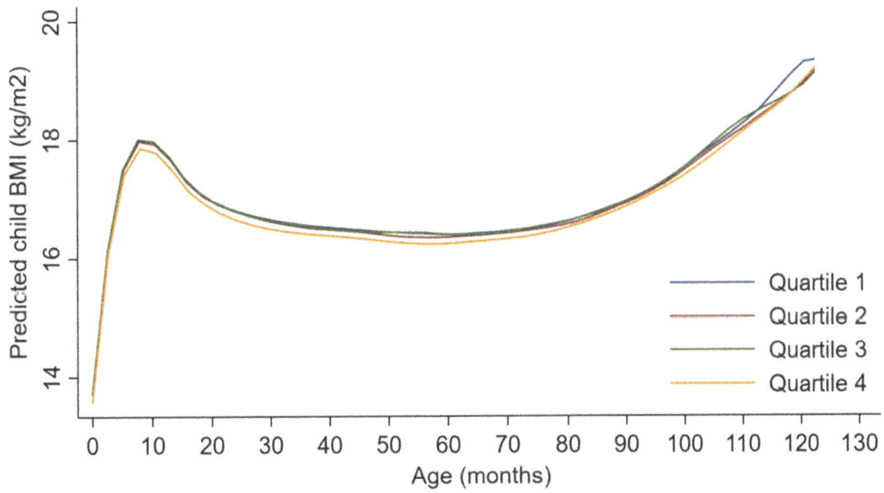

FIGURE 2 | Child BMI trajectories from birth to mid-childhood according to quartiles of 3rd trimester black carbon exposure. Trajectories were additionally adjusted for date of birth, sine/cosine of the date of birth, maternal age, educational attainment, parity, smoking history, median household income, census tract% below poverty, child sex, and race/ethnicity.

the null and estimates were quite small in magnitude. For example, each IQR increment greater natural log-transformed neighborhood traffic density was associated with a 0.01 (95% CI: −0.06, 0.04) kg/m^2 lower BMI at birth, a peak BMI 0.05 (−0.03, 0.14) kg/m^2 higher, and a higher BMI throughout childhood, with the strongest associations with childhood BMI at 12–18 months of age [e.g., 0.05 (-0.03, 0.13) kg/m^2 higher BMI per IQR increment neighborhood traffic density at 12 months of age]. The associations of home roadway proximity and childhood BMI trajectory were also in the hypothesized direction, with stronger associations as children approached 120 months (10 years) of age, although associations were non-monotonic and confidence intervals consistently crossed the null. For example, children of mothers who lived closest (<50 m) vs. farthest (>200 m) from the nearest major roadway had a BMI that was 0.46 (−0.21, 0.59) kg/m^2 higher at 120 months of age.

In secondary analyses, 1st and 2nd trimester residential $PM_{2.5}$ and BC exposures were not associated with BMI trajectory (data not shown), and directionality and magnitude of effect estimates were similar to 3rd trimester exposures.

DISCUSSION

In a large, prospective Massachusetts pre-birth cohort, prenatal exposures to $PM_{2.5}$ and BC were not related to BMI trajectory. Neighborhood traffic density and home roadway proximity were

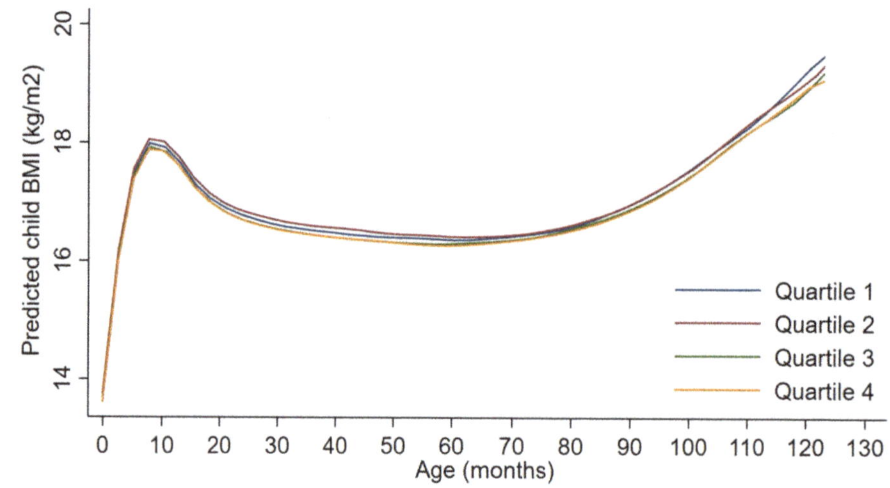

FIGURE 3 | Child BMI trajectories from birth to mid-childhood according to quartiles of ln-transformed neighborhood traffic density. Trajectories were additionally adjusted for date of birth, sine/cosine of the date of birth, maternal age, educational attainment, parity, smoking history, median household income, census tract% below poverty, child sex and, race/ethnicity.

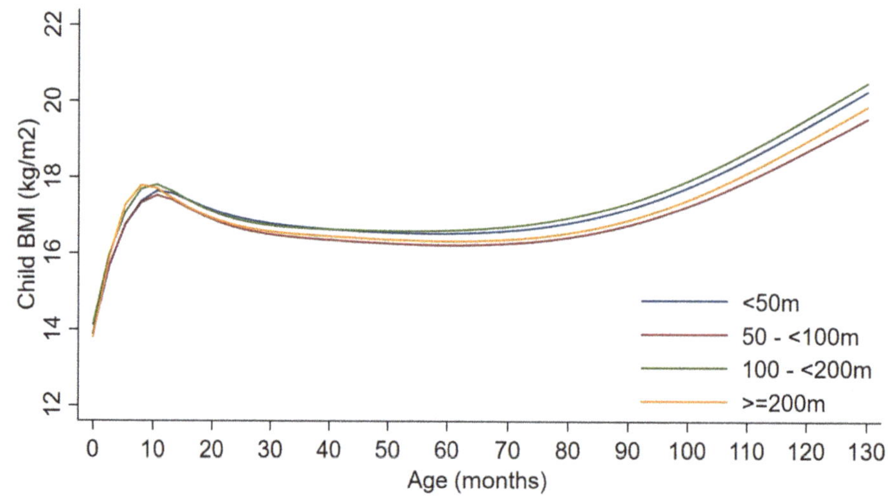

FIGURE 4 | Child BMI trajectories from birth to mid-childhood according to distance to nearest major roadway. Trajectories were additionally adjusted for date of birth, sine/cosine of the date of birth, maternal age, educational attainment, parity, smoking history, median household income, census tract% below poverty, child sex, and race/ethnicity.

associated with lower BMI at birth and greater gains in BMI throughout childhood, but effect sizes were small and confidence intervals consistently crossed the null.

In the present study, we leveraged clinical and research data to estimate BMI trajectories for each participant from birth through mid-childhood. Our findings are partly consistent with previously reported observations in this cohort of prenatal traffic pollution on discrete research measures of growth and adiposity. We previously observed late prenatal exposures to BC, neighborhood traffic density, and home roadway proximity to be associated with lower birth weight-for-gestational age z-score, greater neighborhood traffic density to be associated with more rapid weight-for-length (WFL) gain in infancy (12), and home roadway proximity to be associated with greater BMI z-score in early childhood and higher central and total adiposity in early and mid-childhood (11).

We are aware of only two cohorts besides ours that have examined prenatal air pollution exposure and growth/adiposity in childhood (13, 14). The Boston-based Asthma Coalition on Community, Environment, and Social Stress (ACCESS) cohort ($n = 239$) observed associations of prenatal residential $PM_{2.5}$ exposure with BMI z-score and total fat mass at 4 years of age in boys only (13). The Boston Birth Cohort (BBC) ($n =$

1,446) observed associations between prenatal residential $PM_{2.5}$ exposure and greater odds of overweight or obesity as assessed at each participant's last recorded well-child check from 2 to 9 years of age (14). In both the ACCESS cohort and the BBC, associations with child adiposity were most pronounced for $PM_{2.5}$ exposures during the 2nd trimester. We previously reported associations of prenatal $PM_{2.5}$ exposure with early and mid-childhood BMI to be null regardless of trimester of exposure (11), and in the present study, prenatal residential $PM_{2.5}$ exposure in any trimester was similarly not associated with childhood BMI trajectory. As compared to Project Viva, both the ACCESS cohort and the BBC comprise a greater number of children of lower socioeconomic status with obese mothers, factors which may increase susceptibility to prenatal air pollution exposure. Consistent with this observation, the BBC showed the strongest associations between prenatal air pollution exposure and child overweight/obesity in children of obese mothers (14). Furthermore, rates of breastfeeding in Project Viva (88%) (32) were higher than in the ACCESS cohort (68%) (33) or BBC (64%) (14), and recent studies suggest that breastfeeding may protect against $PM_{2.5}$-induced health effects (34, 35). Thus, while our null findings are in contrast to studies of prenatal air pollution and child adiposity published in two other Boston cohorts, this discrepancy may be a result of differences in study population.

The present study is the first of which we are aware to examine prenatal air pollution exposure in relation to BMI trajectory across childhood. Examining a BMI trajectory outcome is advantageous because it flexibly allows identification of the time window during childhood when growth may be most affected by prenatal exposures. We found no association between prenatal exposure to traffic pollution and BMI estimated at multiple timepoints through 10 years of age, and we also found no association with overall BMI trajectory or with the timing or magnitude of BMI peak or rebound, which are known to predict greater susceptibility to cardio-metabolic disease later in life (36, 37). Additional studies of prenatal air pollution exposure and child growth trajectory, particularly in cohorts of children potentially more susceptible to air pollution exposure based on socioeconomic status or maternal weight, will help to further elucidate this potential association.

Our cohort is the first, so far as we know, to examine prenatal exposure to markers of traffic pollution other than regional $PM_{2.5}$ in relation to growth in later childhood. Although associations did not reach statistical significance, we found neighborhood traffic density and home roadway proximity to be associated with lower BMI at birth, higher peak BMI in infancy, and a higher BMI throughout childhood—the directionalities expected based on our *a priori* hypotheses. As we have noted previously (11), the possible stronger impact of roadway/traffic as compared to $PM_{2.5}$ or BC on child growth and adiposity in our cohort may be explained by independent associations of noise (38), light (39), ultrafine particles (40), or other roadway features distinct from air pollution or from the pollutants we measured, with child growth.

A strength of our study is that it is the largest prospective cohort to date that has analyzed prenatal air pollution exposure and growth in later childhood. In addition, we employ a growth trajectory approach and examine multiple pollutants. Limitations that may have prevented us from observing an association between prenatal air pollution exposure and growth in later childhood are lack of information on maternal time-activity patterns, a relatively high socioeconomic status cohort with a lower incidence of maternal overweight compared to previously published studies, and generally low levels of air pollution. Also, we assessed maternal smoking by questionnaire but did not biochemically validate the exposure. In addition, we did not have data to evaluate repeated measures of body composition, and we predicted BMI trajectories from statistical models rather than directly measuring BMI at each time point, but our models are precise as evidenced by mean residual errors (differences between observed and predicted BMI) close to zero across all ages (26).

In summary, neighborhood traffic density and home roadway proximity were associated with lower BMI at birth and greater gains in BMI throughout childhood, but observed effects were small and confidence intervals consistently crossed the null. We found no association between residential $PM_{2.5}$ or BC exposure and childhood BMI trajectory. Thus, while there may be a role for roadway features distinct from the pollutants we measured, we found no persistent effect of prenatal traffic pollution on childhood BMI trajectory in a population exposed to modest levels of air pollution.

AUTHOR CONTRIBUTIONS

AF, BC, DG, and EO conceived this analysis. JS, PK, IK, HL-G, and DG developed air pollution models and/or applied them to this cohort. IA and SR-S performed the analysis. AF drafted the manuscript. All authors critically reviewed the manuscript.

FUNDING

The authors have received support from the National Institutes of Health (K23ES024803, R01HD034568, P30DK092924, P03ES000002, P01ES009825, R01AI102960, UG3OD023286) and the Environmental Protection Agency (RD83587201). IA is additionally supported by the National University of Singapore Overseas Postdoctoral Fellowship (NUS OPF/2017). This publication's contents are solely the responsibility of the grantee and do not necessarily represent the official views of the US EPA. Further, US EPA does not endorse the purchase of any commercial products or services mentioned in the publication.

ACKNOWLEDGMENTS

We thank Lisa Rokoff for her contributions during the study design and assistance with manuscript formatting. We appreciate the work of past and present Project Viva staff and the ongoing participation of the Project Viva participants.

REFERENCES

1. Singh AS, Mulder C, Twisk JW, van Mechelen W, Chinapaw MJ. Tracking of childhood overweight into adulthood: a systematic review of the literature. *Obes Rev.* (2008) 9:474–88. doi: 10.1111/j.1467-789X.2008.00475.x
2. Finkelstein EA, Brown DS, Wrage LA, Allaire BT, Hoerger TJ. Individual and aggregate years-of-life-lost associated with overweight and obesity. *Obesity* (2010) 18:333–9. doi: 10.1038/oby.2009.253
3. Ebbeling CB, Pawlak DB, Ludwig DS. Childhood obesity: public-health crisis, common sense cure. *Lancet* (2002) 360:473–82. doi: 10.1016/S0140-6736(02)09678-2
4. Heindel JJ, Newbold R, Schug TT. Endocrine disruptors and obesity. *Nat Rev Endocrinol.* (2015) 11:653–61. doi: 10.1038/nrendo.2015.163
5. Xu X, Yavar Z, Verdin M, Ying Z, Mihai G, Kampfrath T, et al. Effect of early particulate air pollution exposure on obesity in mice: role of p47phox. *Arterioscler Thromb Vasc Biol.* (2010) 30:2518–27. doi: 10.1161/ATVBAHA.110.215350
6. Jerrett M, McConnell R, Chang CC, Wolch J, Reynolds K, Lurmann F, et al. Automobile traffic around the home and attained body mass index: a longitudinal cohort study of children aged 10-18 years. *Prev Med.* (2010) 50 (Suppl. 1):S50–8. doi: 10.1016/j.ypmed.2009.09.026
7. Jerrett M, McConnell R, Wolch J, Chang R, Lam C, Dunton G, et al. Traffic-related air pollution and obesity formation in children: a longitudinal, multilevel analysis. *Environ Health* (2014) 13:49. doi: 10.1186/1476-069X-13-49
8. Dong G, Qian Z, Liu M, Wang D, Ren W, Flick L, et al. Ambient air pollution and the prevalence of obesity in chinese children: the seven northeastern cities study. *Obesity* (2014) 22:795–800. doi: 10.1002/oby.20198
9. McConnell R, Shen E, Gilliland FD, Jerrett M, Wolch J, Chang CC, et al. A longitudinal cohort study of body mass index and childhood exposure to secondhand tobacco smoke and air pollution: the Southern California Children's Health Study. *Environ Health Perspect.* (2015) 123:360–6. doi: 10.1289/ehp.1307031
10. Toledo-Corral CM, Alderete TL, Habre R, Berhane K, Lurmann FW, Weigensberg MJ, et al. Effects of air pollution exposure on glucose metabolism in Los Angeles minority children. *Pediatr Obes.* (2018) 13:54–62. doi: 10.1111/ijpo.12188
11. Fleisch AF, Luttmann-Gibson H, Perng W, Rifas-Shiman SL, Coull BA, Kloog I, et al. Prenatal and early life exposure to traffic pollution and cardiometabolic health in childhood. *Pediatr Obes.* (2017) 12:48–57. doi: 10.1111/ijpo.12106
12. Fleisch AF, Rifas-Shiman SL, Koutrakis P, Schwartz JD, Kloog I, Melly S, et al. Prenatal exposure to traffic pollution: associations with reduced fetal growth and rapid infant weight gain. *Epidemiology* (2015) 26:43–50. doi: 10.1097/EDE.0000000000000203
13. Chiu YH, Hsu HH, Wilson A, Coull BA, Pendo MP, Baccarelli A, et al. Prenatal particulate air pollution exposure and body composition in urban preschool children: Examining sensitive windows and sex-specific associations. *Environ Res.* (2017) 158:798–805. doi: 10.1016/j.envres.2017.07.026
14. Mao G, Nachman RM, Sun Q, Zhang X, Koehler K, Chen Z, et al. Individual and joint effects of early-life ambient exposure and maternal prepregnancy obesity on childhood overweight or obesity. *Environ Health Perspect.* (2017) 125:067005. doi: 10.1289/EHP261
15. Rundle A, Hoepner L, Hassoun A, Oberfield S, Freyer G, Holmes D, et al. Association of childhood obesity with maternal exposure to ambient air polycyclic aromatic hydrocarbons during pregnancy. *Am J Epidemiol.* (2012) 175:1163–72. doi: 10.1093/aje/kwr455
16. Stieb DM, Chen L, Eshoul M, Judek S. Ambient air pollution, birth weight and preterm birth: a systematic review and meta-analysis. *Environ Res.* (2012) 117:100–11. doi: 10.1016/j.envres.2012.05.007
17. Eze IC, Hemkens LG, Bucher HC, Hoffmann B, Schindler C, Kunzli N, et al. Association between ambient air pollution and diabetes mellitus in Europe and North America: systematic review and meta-analysis. *Environ Health Perspect.* (2015) 123:381–9. doi: 10.1289/ehp.1307823
18. Kensara OA, Wootton SA, Phillips DI, Patel M, Jackson AA, Elia M, et al. Fetal programming of body composition: relation between birth weight and body composition measured with dual-energy X-ray absorptiometry and anthropometric methods in older Englishmen. *Am J Clin Nutr.* (2005) 82:980–7. doi: 10.1093/ajcn/82.5.980
19. Regnault N, Gillman MW, Rifas-Shiman SL, Eggleston E, Oken E. Sex-specific associations of gestational glucose tolerance with childhood body composition. *Diabetes Care* (2013) 36:3045–53. doi: 10.2337/dc13-0333
20. Ogden CL, Carroll MD, Lawman HG, Fryar CD, Kruszon-Moran D, Kit BK, et al. Trends in obesity prevalence among children and adolescents in the United States, 1988-1994 Through 2013-2014. *JAMA* (2016) 315:2292–9. doi: 10.1001/jama.2016.6361
21. Oken E, Baccarelli AA, Gold DR, Kleinman KP, Litonjua AA, De Meo D, et al. Cohort profile: project viva. *Int J Epidemiol.* (2015) 44:37–48. doi: 10.1093/ije/dyu008
22. Kloog I, Chudnovsky AA, Just AC, Nordio F, Koutrakis P, Coull BA, et al. A new hybrid spatio-temporal model for estimating daily multi-year PM2.5 concentrations across northeastern USA using high resolution aerosol optical depth data. *Atmos Environ.* (2014) 95:581–90. doi: 10.1016/j.atmosenv.2014.07.014
23. Gryparis A, Coull B, Schwartz J, Suh H. Semiparametric latent variable regression models for spatio-teomporal modeling of mobile source particles in the greater Boston area. *J R Stat Soc.* (2007) 56:183–209. doi: 10.1111/j.1467-9876.2007.00573.x
24. Rifas-Shiman SL, Rich-Edwards JW, Scanlon KS, Kleinman KP, Gillman MW. Misdiagnosis of overweight and underweight children younger than 2 years of age due to length measurement bias. *MedGenMed.* (2005) 7:56.
25. United States Census Bureau. US Census 2000: Summary File 3 (2000). Available onine at: http://www.census.gov/census2000/sumfile3.html (Accessed May 18, 2015).
26. Aris IM, Rifas-Shiman SL, Li LJ, Kleinman K, Coull BA, Gold DR, et al. Pre-, perinatal and parental predictors of body mass index trajectory milestones. *J Pediatr.* (2018) 201:69–77.e8. doi: 10.1016/j.jpeds.2018.05.041
27. Karner AA, Eisinger DS, Niemeier DA. Near-roadway air quality: synthesizing the findings from real-world data. *Environ Sci Technol.* (2010) 44:5334–44. doi: 10.1021/es100008x
28. Cole SR, Platt RW, Schisterman EF, Chu H, Westreich D, Richardson D, et al. Illustrating bias due to conditioning on a collider. *Int J Epidemiol.* (2010) 39:417–20. doi: 10.1093/ije/dyp334
29. Bertin M, Chevrier C, Serrano T, Monfort C, Cordier S, Viel JF. Sex-specific differences in fetal growth in newborns exposed prenatally to traffic-related air pollution in the PELAGIE mother-child cohort (Brittany, France). *Environ Res.* (2015) 142:680–7. doi: 10.1016/j.envres.2015.09.006
30. Lakshmanan A, Chiu YH, Coull BA, Just AC, Maxwell SL, Schwartz J, et al. Associations between prenatal traffic-related air pollution exposure and birth weight: modification by sex and maternal pre-pregnancy body mass index. *Environ Res.* (2015) 137:268–77. doi: 10.1016/j.envres.2014.10.035
31. *Environmental Protection Agency, Observational Data for Black Carbon* (2012). Available online at: https://yosemite.epa.gov/sab/sabproduct.nsf/0/

05011472499C2FB28525774A0074DADE/$File/BC+RTC+External+Peer+Review+Draft-opt.pdf (Accessed December 12, 2018).

32. Switkowski KM, Jacques PF, Must A, Kleinman KP, Gillman MW, Oken E. Maternal protein intake during pregnancy and linear growth in the offspring. *Am J Clin Nutr.* (2016) 104:1128–36. doi: 10.3945/ajcn.115.128421
33. Wright RJ, Cohen S, Carey V, Weiss ST, Gold DR. Parental stress as a predictor of wheezing in infancy: a prospective birth-cohort study. *Am J Respir Crit Care Med.* (2002) 165:358–65. doi: 10.1164/ajrccm.165.3.2102016
34. Dong GH, Qian ZM, Liu MM, Wang D, Ren WH, Bawa S, et al. Breastfeeding as a modifier of the respiratory effects of air pollution in children. *Epidemiology* (2013) 24:387–94. doi: 10.1097/EDE.0b013e3182877eb8
35. Khalili R, Bartell SM, Hu X, Liu Y, Chang HH, Belanoff C, et al. Early-life exposure to PM2.5 and risk of acute asthma clinical encounters among children in Massachusetts: a case-crossover analysis. *Environ Health* (2018) 17:20. doi: 10.1186/s12940-018-0361-6
36. Aris IM, Bernard JY, Chen LW, Tint MT, Pang WW, Lim WY, et al. Infant body mass index peak and early childhood cardio-metabolic risk markers in a multi-ethnic Asian birth cohort. *Int J Epidemiol.* (2017) 46:513–25. doi: 10.1093/ije/dyw232
37. Hughes AR, Sherriff A, Ness AR, Reilly JJ. Timing of adiposity rebound and adiposity in adolescence. *Pediatrics* (2014) 134:e1354–61. doi: 10.1542/peds.2014-1908
38. Mavanji V, Teske JA, Billington CJ, Kotz CM. Partial sleep deprivation by environmental noise increases food intake and body weight in obesity-resistant rats. *Obesity* (2013) 21:1396–405. doi: 10.1002/oby.20182
39. Obayashi K, Saeki K, Iwamoto J, Okamoto N, Tomioka K, Nezu S, et al. Exposure to light at night, nocturnal urinary melatonin excretion, and obesity/dyslipidemia in the elderly: a cross-sectional analysis of the HEIJO-KYO study. *J Clin Endocrinol Metab.* (2013) 98:337–44. doi: 10.1210/jc.2012-2874
40. Laurent O, Hu J, Li L, Kleeman MJ, Bartell SM, Cockburn M, et al. Low birth weight and air pollution in California: Which sources and components drive the risk? *Environ Int.* (2016) 92–93:471–7. doi: 10.1016/j.envint.2016.04.034

16

Metabolism Disrupting Chemicals and Alteration of Neuroendocrine Circuits Controlling Food Intake and Energy Metabolism

Marilena Marraudino [1,2], *Brigitta Bonaldo* [1,2], *Alice Farinetti* [1,2], *GianCarlo Panzica* [1,2*], *Giovanna Ponti* [1,3] *and Stefano Gotti* [1,2]

[1] *Neuroscience Institute Cavalieri Ottolenghi, Turin, Italy,* [2] *Department of Neuroscience "Rita Levi-Montalcini", University of Turin, Turin, Italy,* [3] *Department of Veterinary Sciences, University of Turin, Turin, Italy*

Correspondence:
GianCarlo Panzica
giancarlo.panzica@unito.it

The metabolism-disrupting chemicals (MDCs) are molecules (largely belonging to the category of endocrine disrupting chemicals, EDCs) that can cause important diseases as the metabolic syndrome, obesity, Type 2 Diabetes Mellitus or fatty liver. MDCs act on fat tissue and liver, may regulate gut functions (influencing absorption), but they may also alter the hypothalamic peptidergic circuits that control food intake and energy metabolism. These circuits are normally regulated by several factors, including estrogens, therefore those EDCs that are able to bind estrogen receptors may promote metabolic changes through their action on the same hypothalamic circuits. Here, we discuss data showing how the exposure to some MDCs can alter the expression of neuropeptides within the hypothalamic circuits involved in food intake and energy metabolism. In particular, in this review we have described the effects at hypothalamic level of three known EDCs: Genistein, an isoflavone (phytoestrogen) abundant in soy-based food (a possible new not-synthetic MDC), Bisphenol A (compound involved in the manufacturing of many consumer plastic products), and Tributyltin chloride (one of the most dangerous and toxic endocrine disruptor, used in antifouling paint for boats).

Keywords: metabolic disruptor, food intake, hypothalamus, estrogens, bisphenol A, tributyltin, genistein

THE HYPOTHALAMIC CONTROL OF FOOD-INTAKE AND ENERGY METABOLISM

The hypothalamus plays an essential role in controlling food intake and energetic status, mainly through two antagonistic neuronal populations of the hypothalamic arcuate nucleus (ARC): the orexigenic neurons (appetite-stimulating), characterized by the co-expression of agouti-related peptide (AgRP) and neuropeptide Y (NPY), and the anorexigenic neurons (appetite-suppressing) that co-express pro-opiomelanocortin (POMC) and cocaine- and amphetamine-regulated transcript (CART) (1–4) (**Figure 1**). These ARC neurons project to other hypothalamic nuclei, among which the Ventromedial hypothalamic (VMH), and the Paraventricular (PVN) nuclei (**Figure 1**). The latter one is the most important center of metabolic control: it integrates orexigenic and anorexigenic inputs from ARC and modulates energy expenditure through the hypothalamic pituitary adrenal (HPA)-axis (5), and the hypothalamic pituitary thyroid (HPT)-axis (6, 7).

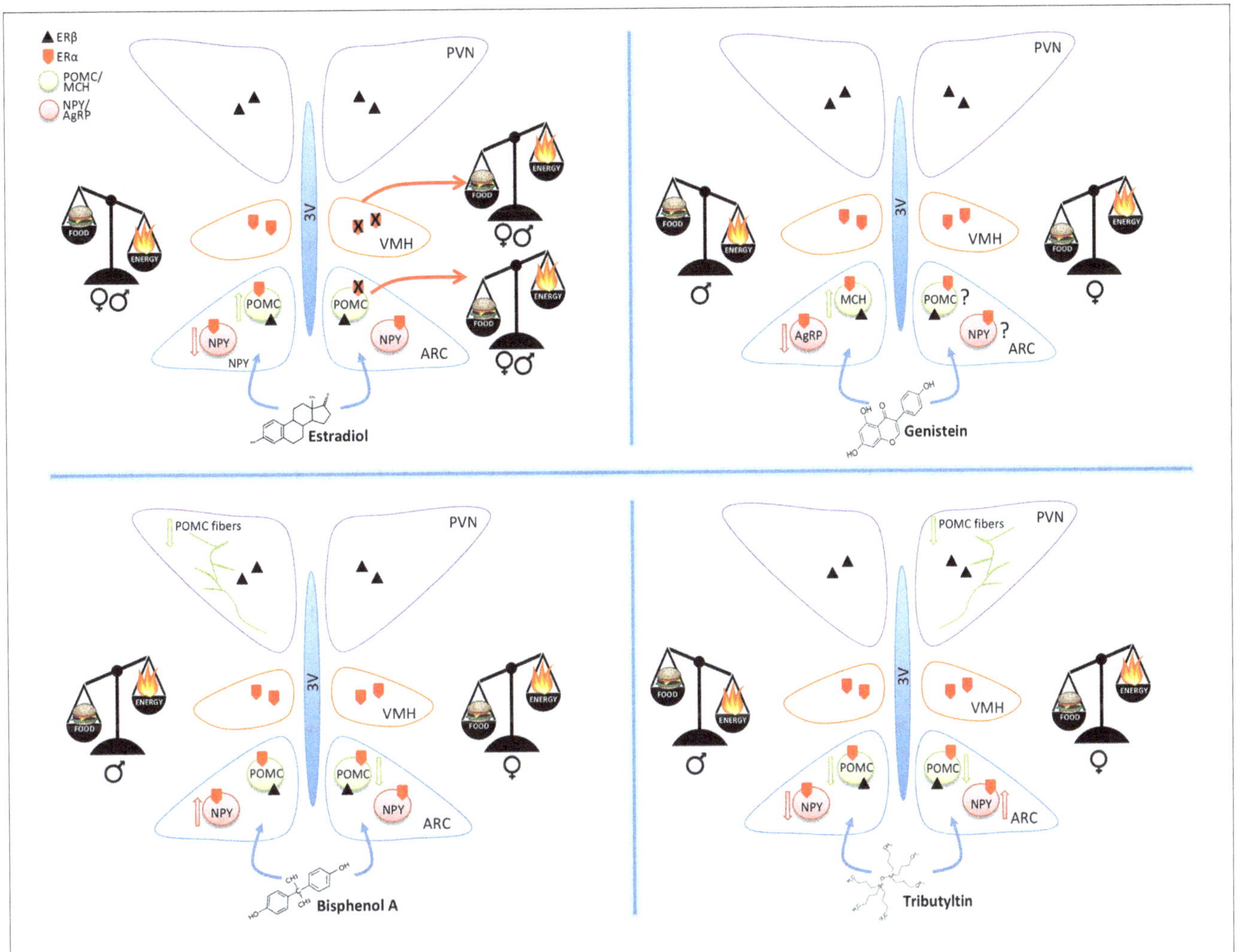

FIGURE 1 | Schematic drawings summarizing the effect of estradiol, genistein, bisphenol A, and tributyltin on the orexigenic (NPY/AgRP) and anorexigenic (POMC/MCH) neurons of the hypothalamic arcuate nucleus (ARC), projecting to the ventromedial (VMH) and paraventricular (PVN) nuclei. All these nuclei contain estrogen receptors α and β mediating the effects of estradiol and of the other substances. The exposure to different molecules induces an imbalance in food intake (food) or energy expenditure (energy). These effects may be similar in both sexes (estradiol), or different (the other MDC) and are mediated by effects on the two main populations of ARC (up arrow = increased expression, down arrows = decreased expression). POMC projections to PVN are also affected.

These systems are sensitive to peripheral signals of energetic balance (for example leptin, insulin, and GHrelin). Leptin blood levels depend on the size of fat stores (8) and acts as an anorexigenic factor to adjust energy requirements, fat reserves, and food intake (9). In contrast, GHrelin has an orexigenic role in the central control of appetite and metabolism (10). Moreover, also sexual hormones, thyroid hormones, and growth factors can modulate the hypothalamic circuits regulating appetite, satiety, and metabolism (11). In particular, in mammals, estradiol (E_2) has an important role on the regulation of food intake and metabolism with an appetite-suppressing effect (12, 13).

Several synthetic or natural molecules that are present in the environment may interact with the estrogen or androgen signaling chain (xenoestrogens, xenoandrogens) and have been classified as endocrine disrupting chemicals [EDCs, (14)]. In addition, many of these EDCs have been considered to belong to the category of metabolism disrupting chemicals (see below), however, little attention has been dedicated, until now, to their action of neural circuits controlling food intake and energy metabolism.

CENTRAL ACTION OF METABOLISM-DISRUPTING CHEMICALS (MDCS)

The metabolism-disrupting chemicals (MDCs) have been defined (Parma Consensus Statement, (15) as those endocrine disrupting chemicals (EDCs) that are able to promote metabolic changes that can result in obesity, Type 2 Diabetes Mellitus (T2DM) or fatty liver in animals including humans. The major targets for these compounds are the fat tissue and the liver (11), however, they may regulate nutrient ingestion and metabolism by altering intestinal transport, secretion of gut peptides, composition of the gut microbiota as well as the expression of hypothalamic neuropeptides that control food intake (11, 16). Several studies reported that MDCs can alter food intake, with different effects based on dose, timing, and exposure duration (17–19). In particular, exposure to MDCs during the perinatal period and/or adulthood modifies the cues that regulate energy homeostasis, such as serum levels of insulin, leptin, and fatty acids (20).

In this short review, we will describe the neuroendocrinological effects of a possible new, not-synthetic, MDC (Genistein), and of two synthetic identified MDCs (Bisphenol A and Tributyltin), (**Table 1**).

Genistein

Soy isoflavones, in particular Genistein (GEN), are very abundant in soy-based food (28) and are an important source of EDCs (29). GEN action requires both estrogen receptor (ER)α and ERβ (30), although, compared to E_2, GEN affinity is low for ERα, while it is similar for ERβ (31–33). ERα is required for GEN effect in females and ERβ, as well as PPARγ, in males (34, 35). Even if the sensitivity of the hypothalamus to GEN is well-acknowledged (36, 37), very little is known on neuronal circuits controlling energetic metabolism.

In vitro, GEN induces adipocytes' apoptosis, decreases lipid accumulation, and increases lipolysis. Moreover, GEN decreases leptin synthesis (38) and inhibits its secretion (39). *In vivo*, GEN effect depends on sex (40, 41) and on the administered dose (42). In females, an anti-obesogenic effect of GEN is reported for many obese mouse models (43, 44), in juvenile and adult ovariectomized (45, 46) and intact mice (34). This effect is dose dependent (42): GEN inhibits adipogenesis at low concentrations and enhances it at high concentrations (47, 48). GEN effect on fat pad weight is opposite in males, with an obesogenic effect at low doses (34, 35, 49) and an antiobesogenic effect at high doses (34). The effect of GEN during perinatal development may be very different: many studies report an obesogenic effect (50, 51), although only in females (52), while others report an anti-obesogenic effect in males (21, 53). GEN effect during development may be due to epigenetic modifications in the offsprings (54) or to an alteration of the development of estrogen sensitive circuits regulating energetic metabolism, as for other MDCs (11). In fact, GEN is able to affect neural circuits controlling animal welfare and fertility (36, 37), although little is known about its effects on neuronal circuits controlling energetic metabolism. A previous study (21) addressed the effect of soy phytoestrogens, daidzein, and genistein, on the hypothalamus of male mice, reporting that high phytoestrogens levels throughout embryonal and postnatal life decrease AgRP and increase MCH, orexin A and TRH mRNA levels, but it has no effect on NPY, POMC, and CART expression [(21), **Figure 1**]. While, our ongoing study in male and female mice demonstrates that early postnatal exposure to GEN, in a dose comparable to exposure level in babies fed with soy-based formula, determines an obesogenic phenotype in adult females and a long-term sex specific effects on hypothalamic kiss, POMC and Orexin systems (55). Early post-natal administration of GEN is also influencing the differentiation of other neural circuits in mice not directly related to the control of metabolism (i.e., nitrergic, vasopressinergic, and dopaminergic circuits, [(36), Ponti et al. submitted].

GEN effect on humans is not clear (56). GEN metabolism and bioavailability depends on gut microbioma (57) and GEN exposure may be highly affected by vegan/vegetarian diets (58). The use of soy-based meal replacement formula was effective in lowering body weight and fat mass and reducing LDL cholesterol in obese individuals and together with physical exercise has a beneficial effect on leptin levels in postmenopausal women (59). In contrast, healthy, normal-weight postmenopausal women did not show improvement in metabolic parameters when given high-dose isoflavones (60).

The complexity of the data on the animal and epidemiological studies on the regulation of energetic metabolism, as well as on other neuronal circuits indicate that GEN is a powerful natural compound which may have at the same time highly beneficial or detrimental effects (37) which are worth to be investigated in more detail. Moreover, the contradictory experimental data underline the importance of considering the timing of exposure, the dose/concentration, the sex, and the species-specificity when establishing safety recommendations for dietary GEN intake, especially if in early-life.

Bisphenol A

Since 1930s, Bisphenol A (BPA) has been involved in the manufacturing of many consumer products [e.g., plastics, PVC, food packaging, thermal papers, (61)]. Thanks to its structure, BPA interacts with a variety of hormone receptors (22): ERα, ERβ, GPR30, and estrogen-related receptor γ [ERRγ, (22)]. Moreover, BPA could also interact with androgen receptor (AR), peroxisome proliferator-activated receptor γ (PPARγ), glucocorticoid receptor (GR), and thyroid hormone receptors [THs, (22)]. These findings strongly suggest that BPA is a multi-target compound that can act on a wide range of hormone-sensitive elements. In fact, BPA has been described also as MDC and the evidences of its role in the alterations of the metabolic axis are increasing (11).

BPA potential obesogenic effects are related to alteration of peripheral parameters, such as weight gain, modifications of leptin or insulin plasma levels, or alterations in the adipose tissue [for a recent review see (62)]. Few studies investigated BPA effects on hypothalamic systems controlling food intake and energy homeostasis, and they are mainly focused on the perinatal exposure (18). BPA exposure of mice from gestational day 0 to Post Natal Day (PND) 21 through diet (1 or 20 μg BPA/kg diet) in combination with HFD had a sexually dimorphic effect on hypothalamic circuits: in males, it impairs glucose tolerance, reduces POMC fiber innervation in the PVN and, in combination with HFD, increases NPY and AgRP expression in the ARC. In females, BPA induces a weight gain, increases food intake, adiposity, and leptin blood levels, while in combination with HFD reduces POMC mRNA expression in the ARC (18). Taken together these data support the idea that BPA acts as a MDC in a sexually dimorphic way [(22), **Figure 1**].

Gestational BPA exposure (5 mg/L BPA through drinking water) of Sprague-Dawley rat dams increases the proliferation

TABLE 1 | Summary of the effects of genistein (GEN), bisphenol A (BPA), and tributyltin (TBT) on circuits controlling food intake and energetic status in rodent hypothalamus.

Compound	Experimental model	Administration	Dose	End point	Effects SNC	Peripheral effects	References
GEN	Male CD1 mice	Orally for 6 weeks to both parents before mating	Soy based food (~190 ppm GEN)	Adult males (3 and 6 months old)	↓ AgRP (mRNA) ↑ MCH (mRNA) ↑ Orexin-A (mRNA) ↑ TRH (mRNA) =NPY (mRNA) =POMC (mRNA) =CART (mRNA)	↓ body weight ↓ adiposity ↓ resistance to cold ↑ lipid oxydation ↑ locomotor activity ↑ muscle mass in males ↑ food intake in males	(21)
BPA	CD-1 mice	Perinatal (GD0 until weaning, PND21)	1 or 20 μg/kg diet	Adult males and females	**Females:** ↓ POMC mRNA in ARC (when combined with HFD) ↑ ERα+ POMC+ cells in ARC ↑ ERα in ARC **Males:** ↓ POMC fiber in PVN ↑ ERα+ POMC cells in ARC ↑ NPY and AgRP expression in ARC (when combined with HFD)	**Dams**: ≠ BW ≠ Food intake **Females:** ↑ in food intake ↑ weight adiposity ↑ leptin plasma level **Males:** ↑ energy expenditure ↑ leptin plasma level Impaired glucose tolerance	(18)
BPA	CD-1 mice	Perinatal (GD0 until weaning P21) (+GD12 BrdU)	20 μg/kg (0.02 ppm) diet	Males and females pups (PND2-8-10-16-21) + adult (PND130) for leptin measurements	↓ Density of POMC fiber in PVN	Leptin resistance Delayed postnatal leptin surges	(22)
BPA	Sprague-Dawley rats	Maternal and gestational exposure (2 weeks prior mating and throughout pregnancy)	5 mg/L in drinking water	Males pups at PND1 sacrificed to obtain NPCs + control NPCs treated *in vitro*.	***In vivo*:** ↑ hypothalamic NPCs proliferation and differentiation ↑ neuroproliferative (Hes1) and proneurogenic (Ngn3) protein expression ↑ AgRP/NPY expression ↓ POMC expression ***In vitro***: ↑ AgRP/NPY expression ↓ POMC expression ↑neuron/glia ratio ↑ LSD1		(23)
BPS	Swiss Albino mice	From PND21 for 10 weeks of treatment	0-25-50-100 μg/kg/day in drinking water	Adult males	↑AgRP mRNA ≠ POMC, CART and NPY mRNA ↓ APJ mRNA ≠ Apelin mRNA	↑ BW ↑ Food intake ↑ Feed efficiency	(24)
TBT	C57Bl/6	Acute in adult mice	10 mg/Kg of body weight	Adult males	↑ *c-fos* expression in ARC		(25)

(Continued)

TABLE 1 | Continued

Compound	Experimental model	Administration	Dose	End point	Effects SNC	Peripheral effects	References
TBT	C57Bl/6	Chronic in adult mice (from PND90 to PND120)	0.025 mg/Kg of body weight	Adult males and females	**Females:** ↑ NPY in VMH ↓ Y1 transgene expression in PVN and VMH **Males:** ↓ NPY in ARC, PVN and DMH ↓ Y1 transgene expression in ARC, PVN, DMH and VMH (p-value close to significance)	**Females:** ↓ circulating leptin level ↑ feed efficiency **Males:** ↓ circulating leptin level ↑ feed efficiency	(19)
TBT	CD-1 mice	Chronic in adult mice (from PND30 to PND65)	0.025 mg/Kg of body weight	Adult males and females	**Females:** ↓ POMC in ARC, DMH and PVN **Males:** ↓ POMC in PVN		(26)
TBT	Sprague-Dawley rats	Chronic in rats for 54 days	0.5 µg/Kg of body weight	Adult males and females	**Females:** ↑ NPY *mRNA* expression **Males:** ↓ POMC, CART and AgRP *mRNA* expression	**Females:** ↑ food intake	(27)

and differentiation of cultured primary hypothalamic neural progenitors (NPCs), as well as the expression of AgRP, while the expression of POMC is reduced (23). BPA is also acting on the kiss system in both rats (63) and mice (64), inducing sexually dimorphic alterations in the cell number of ARC and preoptic populations. Moreover, perinatal treatment with BPA decreases the percentage of kisspeptin-ir fibers in PVN during the postnatal development in female mice (65).

While studies on BPA effects are slowly increasing, only a few studies focus on BPA-analogs: postnatal exposure from PND21 for 10 weeks with 25-50-100 μg/kg BW/day of bisphenol S (BPS) in drinking water affects orexigenic hypothalamic systems resulting in a dose-dependent increase of AgRP mRNA level but not in NPY one or in anorexigenic neuropeptides [POMC, CART; (24)].

Considering the complex relationships between the different circuits involved in the control of food intake and energy homeostasis, further studies are needed to clarify all the effects related to the exposure to BPA and to its less described analogs. In fact, after recognizing the EDC's properties of BPA (66), the search for an appropriate substitute became a fundamental problem to solve. At present, more than 15 BP analogs have been synthesized (67, 68) but none is a real solution. The safety of two of the most used BPA substitutes, BPS and bisphenol F, still remain unclear: *in vitro* and *in vivo* studies, suggests that they share with BPA not only the endocrine-disrupting properties but also the metabolic disrupting ones (69–71).

Both GEN and BPA share a common xenoestrogenic activity, therefore it is possible that they may exert their action altering the estrogens' action on metabolism regulation. In fact, in mammals estradiol (E_2) has an important role on the regulation of food intake and metabolism with an appetite-suppressing effect (12, 13). In female rodents, ovariectomy (OVX) induces an increased body weight and hyper-adiposity, E_2 treatment can robustly inhibit food intake (72, 73). Similarly, in our species, women report a decrease in appetite during the periovulatory stage of ovarian cycle, when E_2 reach a maximal peak (12, 74), while, the development of obesity, type II diabetes and metabolic syndrome in menopause has been correlated with the low E_2 level (75, 76). These metabolic diseases are partially reverted by E_2 replacement therapy (77, 78).

E_2 action is mediated by ERs, in particular, the intracellular ERα, may affect different aspects of regulation of food intake and energy metabolism. This is confirmed by the observation that in rodents deletion of ERα gene cause obesity (79) and the blockage of the appetite-suppressing effect of E_2 treatment (73). In humans, the polymorphisms in the estrogen receptor alpha gene have been associated with body fat distribution (80). The suppression of ERα expression in VMH alters the anorexigenic effect of E_2 treatment, leading to obesity, hyperphagia, and reduced energy expenditure in female mice and rats [(81), **Figure 1**].

Moreover, in ARC and VMH, many neurons co-express ERα and the isoform b of leptin receptor (LepRb) (82). Leptin levels are correlated with E_2 fluctuation: a decrease of E_2 reduces leptin secretion, which can be restored by E_2 treatment (83). Furthermore, both gonadal hormones (84, 85) and leptin (86) modulate Kisspeptin (kiss) anorexigenic neurons. In fact, kiss peptide, co-localizes with ERα (87) and LepRb (88) in ARC. Reciprocal connections link kiss cells, NPY and POMC neurons (89): Kiss excites POMC system directly through the kiss receptor (GPR54) expressed by POMC neurons (90) and inhibits NPY neurons indirectly by enhancing GABA-mediated inhibitory synaptic tone (91). Therefore, hypothalamic kiss system may be a good target for E_2 in the regulation of food intake and energy metabolism along with the well-known control of reproduction.

Few studies analyzed sexual dimorphism on feeding circuits. The World Health Organization (WHO) reported that the obesity prevalently affects women, and it reaches at twice the rates of men in some regions of the world (92). E_2 has an important anorexigenic role also in males: the deletion of ERα in mice, (79, 93), as well as the mutation of ERα in men, causes obesity (94, 95) (**Figure 1**). Moreover, E_2 treatment in males reduces body weight (4, 96). Sexual dimorphism is reported also for NPY and POMC systems (97, 98) and for their receptors (99–101).

These data support the hypothesis that the metabolic disrupting properties of GEN and BPA as well as of other xenoestrogens are based on their ability in interfering with the estrogenic regulation of metabolism and food intake [reviewed in (11)].

Tributyltin

Organotin chemicals are compounds containing at least one bond between tin and carbon. The most studied is Tributyltin chloride (TBT), one of the most dangerous and toxic EDC presents in the environment acting as MDC at both peripheral (102) and central level [for recent reviews see (103–106)]. Due to its primarily use in antifouling paint for boats (94), TBT exerted toxicological effects on marine organisms. As a result, fish and fishery products are the main source of human exposure.

Unlike GEN and BPA, Tributyltin chloride (TBT) is an androgen agonist (it binds ARs), while it has no affinity for ERα (107). More recently, TBT has been identified as agonist ligand for RXR and PPARγ (108) and as a promoter of adipogenesis, favoring obesity (109). In fact, PPARγ and RXRγ are strongly express within hypothalamus (110) by nuclei interesting in metabolic and food intake control (as VMH, LH, PVN). Moreover, blocking with pharmacological antagonists or with shRNA the central endogenous activation of PPARγ led to negative energy balance, restored leptin-sensitivity in high-fat diet (HFD)-fed rats (111).

Acute exposure to TBT induced a significant increase of cell expressing c-fos in the ARC nucleus in adult mice (25), thus suggesting a direct action of TBT at the hypothalamic level. A few other studies confirmed this observation. In fact, a chronical exposure to TBT induced a diminution of NPY expression in adult male but not in female mice, a decrease of circulating leptin level, and a decrease of Y1 receptor transgene expression in both sexes (19). Also the POMC immunoreactive system was influenced (26) with a significant decrease of POMC-positive structures in female mice only (**Figure 1**).

In rats, TBT exposure increased significantly NPY expression in the female together with an increase of food intake, while male presented a decrease of AgRP and CART and appetite (27). Another interesting study in rats investigated whether TBT dependent metabolic disorders were correlated with abnormal hypothalamus-pituitary-gonadal (HPG) axis function, as well as kisspeptin action: after a chronic treatment with TBT, female showed metabolic dysfunctions and HPG axis abnormalities, providing evidence that TBT leads to toxic effects direct on the HPG axis and/or indirectly by abnormal metabolic regulation of the HPG axis (112). TBT has an action also on the hypothalamic-pituitary-adrenal (HPA) axis function (113): a recent study showed that, in female rats, TBT disrupts the morphophysiology of the HPA, leading to an increase in CRH mRNA expression, a decrease in ACTH release and an increase in corticosterone levels (114). Moreover, many studies *in vivo* and *in vitro* have shown TBT effects also on the thyroid morphophysiology and the homeostasis of hypothalamus-pituitary-thyroid axis. TBT may act altering T3 and T4 level (115, 116), down-regulating of thyroid peroxidase, and up-regulating of the thyroid-stimulating hormone receptor (117). TBT given to pregnant mice induces hypothyroidism in the progeny, and induces a dose-dependent increase of T3-independent TRH transcription levels in the hypothalamus of dams (118).

Experimental and epidemiological evidence suggest that the gut microbiota is responsible for significant immunologic, neuronal and endocrine changes that lead to obesity (119), and, recently, it was demonstrated that TBT affect the microbiota system in treated mice, inducing dyslipidemia (120).

In conclusion, TBT has strong effects on both the periphery, with its effects on the mechanisms promoting adipogenesis (121, 122) and the brain by altering the hypothalamic neuroendocrine centers regulating food intake and metabolism (19, 26, 105, 123). All data collected up to now strongly suggest that TBT is a potent MDC.

CONCLUSION

In recent years, obesity and metabolic syndromes are increased; even if it is necessary to consider the possible genetic predispositions, and the excessive food intake without appropriate physical exercise, probably the causes should be sought also in numerous natural or synthetic substances that pervade our environment, known as MDCs.

While the possible role as metabolic disruptors of these substances, in particular BPA and TBT, is widely recognized both at hypothalamic and peripheral level, the GEN effect remains controversial on a peripheral level and still unclear, on the hypothalamic neuroendocrine circuits involved in food intake. Therefore, more studies are needed to clarify the interference of these compounds on the complex neural circuit that controls food intake and metabolism.

AUTHOR CONTRIBUTIONS

All the authors searched the bibliography. MM wrote a first draft, all the other authors checked for specific part of the manuscript. SG and GCP coordinated the final manuscript.

FUNDING

This study was supported by Ministero dell'Istruzione, dell'Università e della Ricerca–MIUR project Dipartimenti di Eccellenza 2018–2022 to Department of Neuroscience Rita Levi Montalcini and Department of Veterinary Science; University of Torino, Ricerca locale to GP, GCP, SG, and Cavalieri-Ottolenghi Foundation, Orbassano, Italy. MM fellowship was generously granted by Prof. G.C. Bergui.

REFERENCES

1. Gropp E, Shanabrough M, Borok E, Xu AW, Janoschek R, Buch T, et al. Agouti-related peptide-expressing neurons are mandatory for feeding. *Nat Neurosci.* (2005) 8:1289–91. doi: 10.1038/nn1548
2. Balthasar N, Dalgaard LT, Lee CE, Yu J, Funahashi H, Williams T, et al. Divergence of melanocortin pathways in the control of food intake and energy expenditure. *Cell* (2005) 123 493–505. doi: 10.1016/j.cell.2005.08.035
3. Timper K, Bruning JC. Hypothalamic circuits regulating appetite and energy homeostasis: pathways to obesity. *Dis Model Mech.* (2017) 10:679–89. doi: 10.1242/dmm.026609
4. Gao Q, Horvath TL. Neurobiology of feeding and energy expenditure. *Annu Rev Neurosci.* (2007) 30:367–98. doi: 10.1146/annurev.neuro.30.051606.094324
5. van Swieten MM, Pandit R, Adan RA, van der Plasse G. The neuroanatomical function of leptin in the hypothalamus. *J Chem Neuroanat.* (2014) 61–62:207–20. doi: 10.1016/j.jchemneu.2014.05.004
6. Leibowitz SF, and Wortley KE, Hypothalamic control of energy balance: different peptides, different functions. *Peptides* (2004) 25:473–504. doi: 10.1016/j.peptides.2004.02.006
7. Lechan RM, Fekete C. Role of melanocortin signaling in the regulation of the hypothalamic-pituitary-thyroid (HPT) axis. *Peptides* (2006) 27:310–25. doi: 10.1016/j.peptides.2005.01.033
8. Halaas JL, Gajiwala KS, Maffei M, Cohen SL, Chait BT, Rabinowitz D, et al. Weight-reducing effects of the plasma protein encoded by the obese gene. *Science* (1995) 269:543–6. doi: 10.1126/science.7624777
9. Casanueva FF, Dieguez C. Neuroendocrine regulation and actions of leptin. *Front Neuroendocrinol.* (1999) 20:317–63. doi: 10.1006/frne.1999.0187
10. Solomou S, Korbonits M. The role of ghrelin in weight-regulation disorders: implications in clinical practice. *Hormones* (2014) 13:458–75. doi: 10.14310/horm.2002.1551
11. Heindel JJ, Blumberg B, Cave M, Machtinger R, Mantovani A, Mendez MA, et al. Metabolism disrupting chemicals and metabolic disorders. *Reprod Toxicol* (2017) 68:3-33. doi: 10.1016/j.reprotox.2016.10.001
12. Martinez de Morentin PB, Gonzalez-Garcia I, Martins L, Lage R, Fernandez-Mallo D, Martinez-Sanchez N, et al. Estradiol regulates brown adipose tissue thermogenesis via hypothalamic AMPK. *Cell Metab.* (2014) 20 41–53. doi: 10.1016/j.cmet.2014.03.031
13. Martinez de Morentin PB, Lage R, Gonzalez-Garcia I, Ruiz-Pino F, Martins L, Fernandez-Mallo D, et al. Pregnancy induces resistance to the anorectic effect of hypothalamic malonyl-CoA and the thermogenic effect of hypothalamic AMPK inhibition in female rats. *Endocrinology* (2015) 156:947–60. doi: 10.1210/en.2014-1611
14. Zoeller RT, Brown TR, Doan LL, Gore AC, Skakkebaek NE, Soto AM, et al. Endocrine-disrupting chemicals and public health protection: a statement of principles from The Endocrine Society. *Endocrinology* (2012) 153:4097–110. doi: 10.1210/en.2012-1422
15. Heindel JJ, Vom Saal FS, Blumberg B, Bovolin P, Calamandrei G, Ceresini G, et al. Parma consensus statement on metabolic disruptors. *Environ Health* (2015) 14:54. doi: 10.1186/s12940-015-0042-7
16. Nadal A, Quesada I, Tuduri E, Nogueiras R, Alonso-Magdalena P. Endocrine-disrupting chemicals and the regulation of energy balance. *Nat Rev Endocrinol.* (2017) 13:536–46. doi: 10.1038/nrendo.2017.51
17. Angle BM, Do RP, Ponzi D, Stahlhut RW, Drury BE, Nagel SC, et al. Metabolic disruption in male mice due to fetal exposure to low but not high doses of bisphenol A (BPA): evidence for effects on body weight, food intake, adipocytes, leptin, adiponectin, insulin and glucose regulation. *Reprod Toxicol.* (2013) 42:256–68. doi: 10.1016/j.reprotox.2013.07.017
18. Mackay H, Patterson ZR, Khazall R, Patel S, Tsirlin D, Abizaid A. Organizational effects of perinatal exposure to bisphenol-A and diethylstilbestrol on arcuate nucleus circuitry controlling food intake and energy expenditure in male and female CD-1 mice. *Endocrinology* (2013) 154:1465–75. doi: 10.1210/en.2012-2044
19. Bo E, Farinetti A, Marraudino M, Sterchele D, Eva C, Gotti S, et al. Adult exposure to tributyltin affects hypothalamic neuropeptide Y, Y1 receptor distribution, and circulating leptin in mice. *Andrology* (2016) 4:723–34. doi: 10.1111/andr.12222
20. Stern JH, Rutkowski JM, Scherer PE. Adiponectin, leptin, and fatty acids in the maintenance of metabolic homeostasis through adipose tissue crosstalk. *Cell Metab.* (2016) 23:770–84. doi: 10.1016/j.cmet.2016.04.011
21. Cederroth CR, Vinciguerra M, Kuhne F, Madani R, Doerge DR, Visser TJ, et al. A phytoestrogen-rich diet increases energy expenditure and decreases adiposity in mice. *Environ Health Perspect.* (2007) 115:1467–73. doi: 10.1289/ehp.10413
22. MacKay H, Patterson ZR, Abizaid A. Perinatal exposure to low-dose bisphenol-a disrupts the structural and functional development of the hypothalamic feeding circuitry. *Endocrinology* (2017) 158:768–77. doi: 10.1210/en.2016-1718
23. Desai M, Ferrini MG, Han G, Jellyman JK, Ross MG. *In vivo* maternal and *in vitro* BPA exposure effects on hypothalamic neurogenesis and appetite regulators. *Environ Res.* (2018) 164:45–52. doi: 10.1016/j.envres.2018.02.011
24. Rezg R, Abot A, Mornagui B, Aydi S, Knauf C. Effects of bisphenol S on hypothalamic neuropeptides regulating feeding behavior and apelin/APJ system in mice. *Ecotoxicol Environ Saf.* (2018) 161:459–66. doi: 10.1016/j.ecoenv.2018.06.001
25. Bo E, Viglietti-Panzica C, Panzica GC. Acute exposure to tributyltin induces c-fos activation in the hypothalamic arcuate nucleus of adult male mice. *Neurotoxicology* (2011) 32:277–80. doi: 10.1016/j.neuro.2010.12.011
26. Farinetti A, Marraudino M, Ponti G, Panzica G, Gotti S. Chronic treatment with tributyltin induces sexually dimorphic alterations in the hypothalamic POMC system of adult mice. *Cell Tissue Res.* (2018). 374:587–94 doi: 10.1007/s00441-018-2896-9
27. He K, Zhang J, Chen Z. Effect of tributyltin on the food intake and brain neuropeptide expression in rats. *Endokrynol Pol.* (2014) 65:485–90. doi: 10.5603/EP.2014.0068
28. Whitten PL, Patisaul HB. Cross-species and interassay comparisons of phytoestrogen action. *Environ Health Perspect.* (2001) 109 (Suppl. 1) 5–20. doi: 10.1289/ehp.01109s15
29. Thigpen JE, Setchell KD, Saunders HE, Haseman JK, Grant MG, Forsythe DB. Selecting the appropriate rodent diet for endocrine disruptor research and testing studies. *ILAR J.* (2004) 45:401-16. doi: 10.1093/ilar.45.4.401
30. Cooke PS, Naaz A. Effects of estrogens and the phytoestrogen genistein on adipogenesis and lipogenesis in males and females. *Birth Defects Res A Clin Mol Teratol.* (2005) 73 472–3. doi: 10.1002/bdra.20142
31. Kuiper GG, Lemmen JG, Carlsson B, Corton JC, Safe SH, van der Saag PT, et al. Interaction of estrogenic chemicals and phytoestrogens with estrogen receptor beta. *Endocrinology* (1998) 139:4252–63. doi: 10.1210/endo.139.10.6216
32. Morito K, Hirose T, Kinjo J, Hirakawa T, Okawa M, Nohara T, et al. Interaction of phytoestrogens with estrogen receptors alpha and beta. *Biol Pharm Bull.* (2001) 24:351–6. doi: 10.1248/bpb.24.351
33. Pettersson K, Delaunay F, Gustafsson JA. Estrogen receptor beta acts as a dominant regulator of estrogen signaling. *Oncogene* (2000) 19:4970–8. doi: 10.1038/sj.onc.1203828
34. Penza M, Montani C, Romani A, Vignolini P, Pampaloni B, Tanini A, et al. Genistein affects adipose tissue deposition in a dose-dependent

and gender-specific manner. *Endocrinology* (2006) 147:5740–51. doi: 10.1210/en.2006-0365
35. Zanella I, Marrazzo E, Biasiotto G, Penza M, Romani A, Vignolini P, et al. Soy and the soy isoflavone genistein promote adipose tissue development in male mice on a low-fat diet. *Eur J Nutr.* (2015) 54:1095–107. doi: 10.1007/s00394-014-0786-9
36. Ponti G, Rodriguez-Gomez A, Farinetti A, Marraudino M, Filice F, Foglio B, et al. Early postnatal genistein administration permanently affects nitrergic and vasopressinergic systems in a sex-specific way. *Neuroscience* (2017) 346:203–15. doi: 10.1016/j.neuroscience.2017.01.024
37. Patisaul HB. Endocrine disruption by dietary phyto-oestrogens: impact on dimorphic sexual systems and behaviours. *Proc Nutr Soc.* (2017) 76:130–44. doi: 10.1017/S0029665116000677
38. Phrakonkham P, Viengchareun S, Belloir C, Lombes M, Artur Y, Canivenc-Lavier MC. Dietary xenoestrogens differentially impair 3T3-L1 preadipocyte differentiation and persistently affect leptin synthesis. *J Steroid Biochem Mol Biol.* (2008) 110:95–103. doi: 10.1016/j.jsbmb.2008.02.006
39. Rayalam S, Della-Fera MA, Baile CA. Phytochemicals and regulation of the adipocyte life cycle. *J Nutr Biochem.* (2008) 19:717–26. doi: 10.1016/j.jnutbio.2007.12.007
40. Catmull S, Masood F, Schacht S, Dolan R, Stegman D, Leung L, et al. Dietary genistein rescues reduced basal chloride secretion in diabetic jejunum via sex-dependent mechanisms. *Cell Physiol Biochem.* (2016) 40:335–46. doi: 10.1159/000452549
41. Schacht S, Masood F, Catmull S, Dolan R, Altabtabaee R, Grow W, et al. Dietary genistein influences number of acetylcholine receptors in female diabetic jejunum. *J Diabetes Res.* (2017) 2017:3568146. doi: 10.1155/2017/3568146
42. Mosqueda-Solis A, Lasa A, Gomez-Zorita S, Eseberri I, Pico C, Portillo MP. Screening of potential anti-adipogenic effects of phenolic compounds showing different chemical structure in 3T3-L1 preadipocytes. *Food Funct.* (2017):3576–86. doi: 10.1039/C7FO00679A
43. Yang JY, Lee SJ, Park HW, Cha YS. Effect of genistein with carnitine administration on lipid parameters and obesity in C57Bl/6J mice fed a high-fat diet. *J Med Food* (2006) 9:459–67. doi: 10.1089/jmf.2006.9.459
44. Weigt C, Hertrampf T, Kluxen FM, Flenker U, Hulsemann F, Fritzemeier KH, et al. Molecular effects of ER alpha- and beta-selective agonists on regulation of energy homeostasis in obese female Wistar rats. *Mol Cell Endocrinol* (2013) 377:147–58. doi: 10.1016/j.mce.2013.07.007
45. Kim HK, Nelson-Dooley C, Della-Fera MA, Yang JY, Zhang W, Duan J, et al. Genistein decreases food intake, body weight, and fat pad weight and causes adipose tissue apoptosis in ovariectomized female mice. *J Nutr.* (2006) 136:409–14. doi: 10.1093/jn/136.2.409
46. Naaz A, Yellayi S, Zakroczymski MA, Bunick D, Doerge DR, Lubahn DB, et al. The soy isoflavone genistein decreases adipose deposition in mice. *Endocrinology* (2003) 144:3315–20. doi: 10.1210/en.2003-0076
47. Harmon AW, Harp JB. Differential effects of flavonoids on 3T3-L1 adipogenesis and lipolysis. *Am J Physiol Cell Physiol.* (2001) 280:C807–13. doi: 10.1152/ajpcell.2001.280.4.C807
48. Dang ZC, Audinot V, Papapoulos SE, Boutin JA, Löwik CW. Peroxisome proliferator-activated receptor gamma (PPARgamma) as a molecular target for the soy phytoestrogen genistein. *J Biol Chem.* (2003) 278:962–7.doi: 10.1074/jbc.M209483200
49. Lee YM, Choi JS, Kim MH, Jung MH, Lee YS, Song J. Effects of dietary genistein on hepatic lipid metabolism and mitochondrial function in mice fed high-fat diets. *Nutrition* (2006) 22:956–64. doi: 10.1016/j.nut.2005.12.014
50. Ruhlen RL, Howdeshell KL, Mao J, Taylor JA, Bronson FH, Newbold RR, et al. Low phytoestrogen levels in feed increase fetal serum estradiol resulting in the "fetal estrogenization syndrome" and obesity in CD-1 mice. *Environ Health Perspect.* (2008) 116:322–8. doi: 10.1289/ehp.10448
51. Newbold RR, Padilla-Banks E, Snyder RJ, Jefferson WN. Developmental exposure to estrogenic compounds and obesity. *Birth Defects Res A Clin Mol Teratol* (2005) 73:478–80. doi: 10.1002/bdra.20147
52. Strakovsky RS, Lezmi S, Flaws JA, Schantz SL, Pan YX, Helferich WG. Genistein exposure during the early postnatal period favors the development of obesity in female, but not male rats. *Toxicol Sci.* (2014) 138:161–74. doi: 10.1093/toxsci/kft331
53. Zhang YB, Yan JD, Yang SQ, Guo JP, Zhang X, Sun XX, et al. Maternal genistein intake can reduce body weight in male offspring. *Biomed Environ Sci.* (2015) 28:769–72.doi: 10.3967/bes2015.107
54. Dolinoy DC, Weidman JR, Waterland RA, Jirtle RL. Maternal genistein alters coat color and protects Avy mouse offspring from obesity by modifying the fetal epigenome. *Environ Health Perspect.* (2006) 114:567–72. doi: 10.1289/ehp.8700
55. Marraudino M, Ponti G, Farinetti A, Macchi E, Accornero P, Gotti S, et al. Early postnatal genistein administration has a sexually dimorphic obesogenic effect and organizational effects on hypothalamic neuroendocrine circuits in CD1 mice. In: Carrillo Urbano B, Pinos Sanchez H. editors. *2nd Int. Congress Psychobiology.* UNED: Ávila. (2017) pp. 133.
56. Amiot MJ, Riva C, Vinet A. Effects of dietary polyphenols on metabolic syndrome features in humans: a systematic review. *Obes Rev.* (2016) 17:573–86. doi: 10.1111/obr.12409
57. Nielsen IL, Williamson G. Review of the factors affecting bioavailability of soy isoflavones in humans. *Nutr Cancer* (2007) 57:1–10. doi: 10.1080/01635580701267677
58. Tordjman K, Grinshpan L, Novack L, Goen T, Segev D, Beacher L, et al. Exposure to endocrine disrupting chemicals among residents of a rural vegetarian/vegan community. *Environ Int.* (2016) 97:68–75. doi: 10.1016/j.envint.2016.10.018
59. Llaneza P, Gonzalez C, Fernandez-Inarrea J, Alonso A, Diaz F, Arnott I, et al. Soy isoflavones, diet and physical exercise modify serum cytokines in healthy obese postmenopausal women. *Phytomedicine* (2011) 18:245–50. doi: 10.1016/j.phymed.2010.07.011
60. Behloul N, Wu G. Genistein: a promising therapeutic agent for obesity and diabetes treatment. *Eur J Pharmacol.* (2013) 698:31–8. doi: 10.1016/j.ejphar.2012.11.013
61. Ribeiro E, Ladeira C, Viegas S. Occupational exposure to bisphenol A (BPA): a reality that still needs to be unveiled. Toxics (2017) 5:22. doi: 10.3390/toxics5030022
62. Legeay S, Faure S. Is bisphenol A an environmental obesogen? *Fundam Clin Pharmacol.* (2017) 31:594–609. doi: 10.1111/fcp.12300
63. Patisaul HB, Todd KL, Mickens JA, Adewale HB. Impact of neonatal exposure to the ERalpha agonist PPT, bisphenol-A or phytoestrogens on hypothalamic kisspeptin fiber density in male and female rats. *Neurotoxicology* (2009) 30:350–7. doi: 10.1016/j.neuro.2009.02.010
64. Panzica GC, Bo E, Martini MA, Miceli D, Mura E, Viglietti-Panzica C, et al. Neuropeptides and enzymes are targets for the action of endocrine disrupting chemicals in the vertebrate brain. *J Toxicol Environ Health B Crit Rev.* (2011) 14:449–72. doi: 10.1080/10937404.2011.578562
65. Marraudino M, Farinetti A, Troisi E, Miceli D, Gotti S, Panzica G. *Kisspeptin and Paraventricular Nucleus: Effects of Bisphenol A on CD1 Female Mice, XXV GISN Meeting.* Rome (2015). p. 16.
66. Rubin BS. Bisphenol A: an endocrine disruptor with widespread exposure and multiple effects. *J Steroid Biochem Mol Biol.* (2011) 127:27–34. doi: 10.1016/j.jsbmb.2011.05.002
67. Dhanjai, Sinha A, Wu L, Lu X, Chen J, Jain R. Advances in sensing and biosensing of bisphenols: a review. *Anal Chim Acta.* (2018) 998:1–27. doi: 10.1016/j.aca.2017.09.048
68. Dhanjai, Sinha A, Wu L, Lu X, Chen J, Jain R. Corrigendum to "advances in sensing and biosensing of bisphenols: a review" (ACA 998 (2018) 1-27). *Anal Chim Acta* (2018) 1029:125–9. doi: 10.1016/j.aca.2018.05.047
69. Ivry Del Moral L, Le Corre L, Poirier H, Niot I, Truntzer T, Merlin JF, et al. Obesogen effects after perinatal exposure of 4,4'-sulfonyldiphenol (Bisphenol S) in C57BL/6 mice. *Toxicology* (2016) 357–8:11–20. doi: 10.1016/j.tox.2016.05.023
70. Boucher JG, Gagne R, Rowan-Carroll A, Boudreau A, Yauk CL, Atlas E. Bisphenol A and Bisphenol S induce distinct transcriptional profiles in differentiating human primary preadipocytes. *PLoS ONE* (2016) 11:e0163318. doi: 10.1371/journal.pone.0163318
71. Boucher JG, Ahmed S, Atlas E. Bisphenol S induces adipogenesis in primary human preadipocytes from female donors. *Endocrinology* (2016) 157:1397–407. doi: 10.1210/en.2015-1872
72. Blaustein JD, Gentry RT, Roy EJ, Wade GN. Effects of ovariectomy and estradiol on body weight and food intake in gold thioglucose-treated mice. *Physiol Behav.* (1976) 17:1027–30. doi: 10.1016/0031-9384(76)90028-7

73. Geary N, Asarian L, Korach KS, Pfaff DW, Ogawa S. Deficits in E2-dependent control of feeding, weight gain, and cholecystokinin satiation in ER-alpha null mice. *Endocrinology* (2001) 142:4751–7. doi: 10.1210/endo.142.11.8504
74. Mauvais-Jarvis F, Clegg DJ, Hevener AL. The role of estrogens in control of energy balance and glucose homeostasis. *Endocr Rev* (2013) 34:309–38. doi: 10.1210/er.2012-1055
75. Allende-Vigo MZ. Women and the metabolic syndrome: an overview of its peculiarities. *P R Health Sci J.* (2008) 27:190–5. Available online at: http://prhsj.rcm.upr.edu/index.php/prhsj/article/view/67/51
76. Coyoy A, Guerra-Araiza C, Camacho-Arroyo I. Metabolism regulation by estrogens and their receptors in the central nervous system before and after menopause. *Horm Metab Res.* (2016) 48:489–96. doi: 10.1055/s-0042-110320
77. Hart-Unger S, Korach KS. Estrogens and obesity: is it all in our heads? *Cell Metab.* (2011) 14:435–6. doi: 10.1016/j.cmet.2011.09.003
78. Meirelles RM. Menopause and metabolic syndrome. *Arq Bras Endocrinol Metabol.* (2014) 58:91–6. doi: 10.1590/0004-2730000002909
79. Heine PA, Taylor JA, Iwamoto GA, Lubahn DB, Cooke PS. Increased adipose tissue in male and female estrogen receptor-alpha knockout mice. *Proc Natl Acad Sci USA.* (2000) 97:12729–34. doi: 10.1073/pnas.97.23.12729
80. Okura T, Koda M, Ando F, Niino N, Ohta S, Shimokata H. Association of polymorphisms in the estrogen receptor alpha gene with body fat distribution. *Int J Obes Relat Metab Disord.* (2003) 27:1020–7. doi: 10.1038/sj.ijo.0802378
81. Musatov S, Chen W, Pfaff DW, Mobbs CV, Yang XJ, Clegg DJ, et al. Silencing of estrogen receptor alpha in the ventromedial nucleus of hypothalamus leads to metabolic syndrome. *Proc Natl Acad Sci USA.* (2007) 104:2501–6. doi: 10.1073/pnas.0610787104
82. Diano S, Kalra SP, Sakamoto H, Horvath TL. Leptin receptors in estrogen receptor-containing neurons of the female rat hypothalamus. *Brain Res.* (1998) 812:256–9. doi: 10.1016/S0006-8993(98)00936-6
83. Clegg DJ, Brown LM, Woods SC, Benoit SC. Gonadal hormones determine sensitivity to central leptin and insulin. *Diabetes* (2006) 55:978–87. doi: 10.2337/diabetes.55.04.06.db05-1339
84. Marraudino M, Miceli D, Farinetti A, Ponti G, Panzica G, Gotti S. Kisspeptin innervation of the hypothalamic paraventricular nucleus: sexual dimorphism and effect of estrous cycle in female mice. *J Anat.* (2017) 230:775–86. doi: 10.1111/joa.12603
85. Marraudino M, Martini M, Trova S, Farinetti A, Ponti G, Gotti S, Panzica G. Kisspeptin system in ovariectomized mice: estradiol and progesterone regulation. *Brain Res.* (2018) 1688:8–14. doi: 10.1016/j.brainres.2018.03.014
86. Castellano JM, Tena-Sempere M. Metabolic control of female puberty: potential therapeutic targets. *Expert Opin Ther Targets* (2016) 20:1181–93. doi: 10.1080/14728222.2016.1212015
87. Burke MC, Letts PA, Krajewski SJ, Rance NE. Coexpression of dynorphin and neurokinin B immunoreactivity in the rat hypothalamus: morphologic evidence of interrelated function within the arcuate nucleus. *J Comp Neurol.* (2006) 498:712–26. doi: 10.1002/cne.21086
88. Smith JT, Clifton DK, Steiner RA. Regulation of the neuroendocrine reproductive axis by kisspeptin-GPR54 signaling. *Reproduction* (2006) 131:623–30. doi: 10.1530/rep.1.00368
89. Backholer K, Smith JT, Rao A, Pereira A, Iqbal J, Ogawa S, et al. Kisspeptin cells in the ewe brain respond to leptin and communicate with neuropeptide Y and proopiomelanocortin cells. *Endocrinology* (2010) 151:2233–43. doi: 10.1210/en.2009-1190
90. Higo S, Iijima N, Ozawa H. Characterisation of Kiss1r (Gpr54)-expressing neurones in the arcuate nucleus of the female rat hypothalamus. *J Neuroendocrinol.* (2017) 29. doi: 10.1111/jne.12452
91. Fu LY, van den Pol AN. Kisspeptin directly excites anorexigenic proopiomelanocortin neurons but inhibits orexigenic neuropeptide Y cells by an indirect synaptic mechanism. *J Neurosci.* (2010) 30:10205–19. doi: 10.1523/JNEUROSCI.2098-10.2010
92. WHO. *Fact Sheet: Obesity and Overweight.* WHO Fact Sheet 311 (2014).
93. Callewaert F, Venken K, Ophoff J, De Gendt K, Torcasio A, van Lenthe GH, et al. Differential regulation of bone and body composition in male mice with combined inactivation of androgen and estrogen receptor-alpha. *FASEB J.* (2009) 23:232–40. doi: 10.1096/fj.08-113456
94. Grumbach MM, Auchus RJ. Estrogen: consequences and implications of human mutations in synthesis and action. *J Clin Endocrinol Metab.* (1999) 84:4677–94. doi: 10.1210/jc.84.12.4677
95. Smith BK, York DA, Bray GA. Chronic cerebroventricular galanin does not induce sustained hyperphagia or obesity. *Peptides* (1994) 15:1267–72. doi: 10.1016/0196-9781(94)90152-X
96. Finan B, Yang B, Ottaway N, Stemmer K, Muller TD, Yi CX, et al. Targeted estrogen delivery reverses the metabolic syndrome. *Nat Med.* (2012) 18:1847–56. doi: 10.1038/nm.3009
97. Xu Y, Faulkner LD, Hill JW. Cross-Talk between metabolism and reproduction: the role of POMC and SF1 neurons. *Front Endocrinol.* (2011) 2:98. doi: 10.3389/fendo.2011.00098
98. Urban JH, Bauer-Dantoin AC, Levine JE. Neuropeptide Y gene expression in the arcuate nucleus: sexual dimorphism and modulation by testosterone. *Endocrinology* (1993) 132:139–45. doi: 10.1210/endo.132.1.8419120
99. Martini M, Sica M, Gotti S, Eva C, Panzica GC. Effects of estrous cycle and sex on the expression of neuropeptide Y Y1 receptor in discrete hypothalamic and limbic nuclei of transgenic mice. *Peptides* (2011) 32:1330–4. doi: 10.1016/j.peptides.2011.04.004
100. Qu F, Zhang D, Chen LT, Wang FF, Pan JX, Zhu YM, et al. Auricular acupressure reduces anxiety levels and improves outcomes of *in vitro* fertilization: a prospective, randomized and controlled study. *Sci Rep.* (2014) 4:5028. doi: 10.1038/srep05028
101. Gelez H, Poirier S, Facchinetti P, Allers KA, Wayman C, Bernabe J, et al. Neuroanatomical distribution of the melanocortin-4 receptors in male and female rodent brain. *J Chem Neuroanat.* (2010) 40:310–24. doi: 10.1016/j.jchemneu.2010.09.002
102. Grun F. The obesogen tributyltin. *Vitam Horm.* (2014) 94:277–325. doi: 10.1016/B978-0-12-800095-3.00011-0
103. Marques VB, Faria RA, Dos Santos L. Overview of the pathophysiological implications of organotins on the endocrine system. *Front Endocrinol.* (2018) 9:101. doi: 10.3389/fendo.2018.00101
104. Ferraz da Silva, Freitas-Lima LC, Graceli JB, Rodrigues LCM. Organotins in neuronal damage, brain function, and behavior: a short review. *Front Endocrinol.* (2017) 8:366. doi: 10.3389/fendo.2017.00366
105. Santos-Silva AP, Andrade MN, Pereira-Rodrigues P, Paiva-Melo FD, Soares P, Graceli JB, et al. Frontiers in endocrine disruption: Impacts of organotin on the hypothalamus-pituitary-thyroid axis. *Mol Cell Endocrinol.* (2018) 460:246–57. doi: 10.1016/j.mce.2017.07.038
106. Decherf S, Demeneix BA. The obesogen hypothesis: a shift of focus from the periphery to the hypothalamus. *J Toxicol Environ Health B Crit Rev.* (2011) 14:423–48. doi: 10.1080/10937404.2011.578561
107. Satoh K, Nagai F, Aoki N. Several environmental pollutants have binding affinities for both androgen receptor and estrogen receptor a. *J Health Sci.* (2001) 47:495–501. doi: 10.1248/jhs.47.495
108. Nakanishi T. Endocrine disruption induced by organotin compounds; organotins function as a powerful agonist for nuclear receptors rather than an aromatase inhibitor. *J Toxicol Sci.* (2008) 33:269–76. doi: 10.2131/jts.33.269
109. Grun F, Blumberg B. Endocrine disrupters as obesogens. *Mol Cell Endocrinol.* (2009) 304:19–29. doi: 10.1016/j.mce.2009.02.018
110. Moreno S, Farioli-Vecchioli S, Ceru MP. Immunolocalization of peroxisome proliferator-activated receptors and retinoid X receptors in the adult rat CNS. *Neuroscience* (2004) 123:131–45. doi: 10.1016/j.neuroscience.2003.08.064
111. Ryan KK, Li B, Grayson BE, Matter EK, Woods SC, Seeley RJ. A role for central nervous system PPAR-gamma in the regulation of energy balance. *Nat Med* (2011) 17:623–6. doi: 10.1038/nm.2349
112. Sena GC, Freitas-Lima LC, Merlo E, Podratz PL, de Araujo JF, Brandao PA, et al. Environmental obesogen tributyltin chloride leads to abnormal hypothalamic-pituitary-gonadal axis function by disruption in kisspeptin/leptin signaling in female rats. *Toxicol Appl Pharmacol.* (2017) 319:22–38. doi: 10.1016/j.taap.2017.01.021
113. Incollingo Rodriguez AC, Epel ES, White ML, Standen EC, Seckl JR, Tomiyama AJ. Hypothalamic-pituitary-adrenal axis dysregulation and cortisol activity in obesity: a systematic review. *Psychoneuroendocrinology* (2015) 62:301–18. doi: 10.1016/j.psyneuen.2015.08.014

114. Merlo E, Podratz PL, Sena GC, de Araujo JF, Lima LC, Alves IS, et al. The environmental pollutant tributyltin chloride disrupts the hypothalamic-pituitary-adrenal axis at different levels in female rats. *Endocrinology* (2016) 157:2978–95. doi: 10.1210/en.2015-1896
115. Adeeko A, Li D, Forsyth DS, Casey V, Cooke GM, Barthelemy J, et al. Effects of in utero tributyltin chloride exposure in the rat on pregnancy outcome. *Toxicol Sci.* (2003) 74:407–15. doi: 10.1093/toxsci/kfg131
116. Rodrigues-Pereira P, Palmero C, Medina de MAttos R, Gran da Silva DLS, Graceli JB, Santos-Silva AP, et al. Influence of organotin on thyroid morphophysiological status. *Environ Health Sci.* (2015) 1:1–7. doi: 10.15436/2378-6841.15.01815.018
117. Sharan S, Nikhil K, Roy P. Disruption of thyroid hormone functions by low dose exposure of tributyltin: an *in vitro* and *in vivo* approach. *Gen Comp Endocrinol.* (2014) 206:155–65. doi: 10.1016/j.ygcen.2014.07.027
118. Decherf S, Seugnet I, Fini JB, Clerget-Froidevaux MS, Demeneix BA. Disruption of thyroid hormone-dependent hypothalamic set-points by environmental contaminants. *Mol Cell Endocrinol.* (2010) 323:172–82. doi: 10.1016/j.mce.2010.04.010
119. Ochoa-Reparaz J, Kasper LH. The second brain: is the gut microbiota a link between obesity and central nervous system disorders? *Curr Obes Rep.* (2016) 5:51–64. doi: 10.1007/s13679-016-0191-1
120. Guo H, Yan H, Cheng D, Wei X, Kou R, Si J. Tributyltin exposure induces gut microbiome dysbiosis with increased body weight gain and dyslipidemia in mice. *Environ Toxicol Pharmacol.* (2018) 60:202–8. doi: 10.1016/j.etap.2018.04.020
121. Regnier SM, El-Hashani E, Kamau W, Zhang X, Massad NL, Sargis RM. Tributyltin differentially promotes development of a phenotypically distinct adipocyte. *Obesity* (2015) 23:1864–71. doi: 10.1002/oby.21174
122. Yanik SC, Baker AH, Mann KK, Schlezinger JJ. Organotins are potent activators of PPARgamma and adipocyte differentiation in bone marrow multipotent mesenchymal stromal cells. *Toxicol Sci* (2011) 122:476–88. doi: 10.1093/toxsci/kfr140
123. Decherf S, Seugnet I, Kouidhi S, Lopez-Juarez A, Clerget-Froidevaux MS, Demeneix BA. Thyroid hormone exerts negative feedback on hypothalamic type 4 melanocortin receptor expression. *Proc Natl Acad Sci USA.* (2010) 107:4471-6. doi: 10.1073/pnas.0905190107

17

Endocrine-Mediated Mechanisms of Metabolic Disruption and New Approaches to Examine the Public Health Threat

Christopher D. Kassotis* and Heather M. Stapleton

Nicholas School of the Environment, Duke University, Durham, NC, United States

***Correspondence:**
Christopher D. Kassotis
christopher.kassotis@duke.edu

Obesity and metabolic disorders are of great societal concern and generate substantial human health care costs globally. Interventions have resulted in only minimal impacts on disrupting this worsening health trend, increasing attention on putative environmental contributors. Exposure to numerous environmental contaminants have, over decades, been demonstrated to result in increased metabolic dysfunction and/or weight gain in cell and animal models, and in some cases, even in humans. There are numerous mechanisms through which environmental contaminants may contribute to metabolic dysfunction, though certain mechanisms, such as activation of the peroxisome proliferator activated receptor gamma or the retinoid x receptor, have received considerably more attention than less-studied mechanisms such as antagonism of the thyroid receptor, androgen receptor, or mitochondrial toxicity. As such, research on putative metabolic disruptors is growing rapidly, as is our understanding of molecular mechanisms underlying these effects. Concurrent with these advances, new research has evaluated current models of adipogenesis, and new models have been proposed. Only in the last several years have studies really begun to address complex mixtures of contaminants and how these mixtures may disrupt metabolic health in environmentally relevant exposure scenarios. Several studies have begun to assess environmental mixtures from various environments and study the mechanisms underlying their putative metabolic dysfunction; these studies hold real promise in highlighting crucial mechanisms driving observed organismal effects. In addition, high-throughput toxicity databases (ToxCast, etc.) may provide future benefits in prioritizing chemicals for *in vivo* testing, particularly once the causative molecular mechanisms promoting dysfunction are better understood and expert critiques are used to hone the databases. In this review, we will review the available literature linking metabolic disruption to endocrine-mediated molecular mechanisms, discuss the novel application of environmental mixtures and implications for *in vivo* metabolic health, and discuss the putative utility of applying high-throughput toxicity databases to answering complex organismal health outcome questions.

Keywords: endocrine disrupting chemicals, obesogen, diabetogen, adipogenesis, 3T3-L1, obesity, diabetes

ENDOCRINE DISRUPTORS AS CAUSATIVE FACTOR IN METABOLIC DISRUPTION

Endocrine disrupting chemicals (EDCs) have been demonstrated to directly modulate metabolism *in vivo* and/or triglyceride accumulation *in vitro* through various receptor-mediated pathways (1–5), suggesting a potential causative link between exposure to EDCs and the increasing global prevalence of metabolic disorders, including obesity (6). Chronic metabolic health conditions are rapidly increasing in prevalence and cost to society worldwide: in the US, 39.6 and 9.7% of adults aged 20 and older are currently classified as obese or have been diagnosed with diabetes, respectively, with increasing occurrence in younger age groups as well (7–10). These conditions contribute to a rising share of health care costs; in the US, >$600 million is directed to obesity-related and diabetes-related illnesses in adults (10, 11). These effects are mirrored in animal populations, with an analysis of >20,000 animals from 24 populations reporting increased weight gain in numerous species including monkeys, both laboratory and urban mice, cats, dogs, etc. (12). Notably, attempted interventions have yielded minimal effects, and analyses have determined that activity, caloric intake, and genetics are insufficient to explain the magnitude and speed of this change (13, 14). As fat cell development is driven and modulated by nuclear hormone receptor signaling (2, 15–17), EDCs that activate or inhibit these hormone pathways may be causative agents in promoting modulation of fat cell development, energy homeostasis, basal metabolic rate, hormonal control of appetite and satiety, and brain circuitry controlling food intake and energy expenditure and ultimately contributing to the development of Metabolic Syndrome (**Figure 1**) (18).

Numerous environmental toxicants have been demonstrated as metabolic disruptors *in vivo*, supporting EDCs as a causative factor in these adverse health trends (14). There is a rich literature demonstrating effects of antibiotics on weight gain in humans and diverse animal species. Experiments demonstrating their efficacy in promoting weight gain in agricultural species were published by the 1950's, presumably operating through effects on gut microbiota impacting the processing of carbohydrates in the diet (19, 20). More recent publications have demonstrated that several weeks of subtherapeutic antibiotics increase fat mass and weight, particularly when begun during gestation (21, 22), and human epidemiological studies have demonstrated increased risk of becoming overweight when children were exposed early in life (23, 24). Other notable examples include diethylstilbestrol (DES), a pharmaceutical provided to pregnant women in the 1940's through 1970's in the mistaken assumption it would reduce rates of abortion, miscarriage, and premature labor (25); it was later determined to induce a variety of adverse health effects in both males and females exposed during gestation (26–29). DES has been demonstrated to promote triglyceride accumulation *in vitro*, seemingly through an estrogen-receptor mediated mechanism (30), and both gestational and perinatal DES exposure increases body weight, body fat, and alters serum lipid profiles in rodent models throughout life (31–33). Increased risks of obesity in human adults exposed prenatally to DES have also been reported (34), delineating apparent translational effects.

Our lab has recently demonstrated that common chemicals and environmental mixtures associated with unconventional oil and gas (UOG) operations can activate the peroxisome proliferator activated receptor gamma (PPARγ) and promote triglyceride accumulation and pre-adipocyte proliferation *in vitro* (35), and that gestational exposure to a mixture of UOG chemicals resulted in increased body weights through weaning in a rodent model (36, 37). UOG development has also been associated with increased prevalence of low birth weight and small for gestational age births in the Northeast US (38), and decreased prevalence of low birth weights and increased risk of higher birth weight babies in Colorado (39); both low (40, 41) and high (42, 43) birth weights are associated with greater risks for obesity later in life.

As costs associated with *in vivo* screening of putative metabolism disruptors are prohibitively high, utilizing lower-order testing, and screening is essential to narrow higher-order testing to chemicals most likely to be active. Various pre-adipocyte and mesenchymal stem cell models (both rodent and human, primarily) have been utilized to assess putative *in vivo* metabolic disruptors *in vitro*; 3T3-L1 mouse pre-adipocytes have proven reliable as an *in vitro* screen for identifying likely obesogenic chemicals *in vivo*, and other models such as the OP9 mouse bone marrow-derived stromal pre-adipocyte cell line (44, 45) allow for assessments of varying molecular pathways important for the process of differentiation. Additionally, various multipotent mesenchymal cells and cell lines (46, 47) offer the additional ability to assess commitment to the adipocyte lineage as a distinct process from adipocyte differentiation (48). However, these assays are lengthy and their relative abilities to correctly identify chemicals may depend on both cell line and cell source. As such, there is a critical need to develop better methods for correctly predicting metabolic disruptors. Several high-throughput (HTP) screening programs now exist (Tox21, ToxCast) that report activity across mechanisms known to modulate metabolic health for thousands of chemicals. Harnessing these data sets to broadly assess high-scoring chemicals (across these molecular pathways) for more targeted *in vitro* and *in vivo* testing could provide a valuable tool for reducing research costs and more broadly assessing the tens of thousands of commercial chemicals for potential contributions to adverse health outcomes in humans and/or animals.

In addition to high-throughput screening, assessments of mixtures have become more commonplace in recent years. Tools to evaluate the chemical constituents and biological activities associated with complex environmental mixtures have vastly increased the capabilities within this sphere, though standard approaches to mixtures are still lacking in many respects, particularly in terms of relevance to human and animal exposure. One notable mixture that has received increasing attention is indoor house dust; our laboratory and others have collected and analytically characterized house dust from different environments around the world and routinely report numerous classes of EDCs (known to be hormonally active), including flame retardants, phthalates, pesticides, perfluoroalkyl substances (PFAS), and others that span a wide range of concentrations (49–51). Humans, and perhaps most importantly small children, are chronically

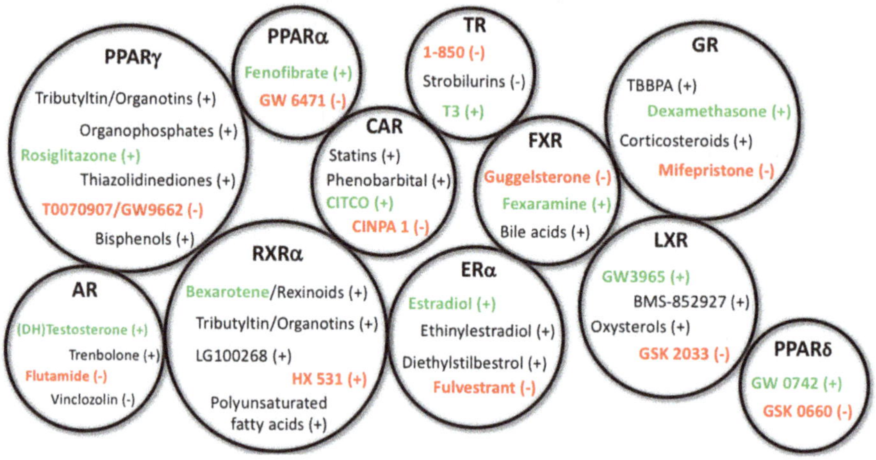

FIGURE 1 | Representative EDCs Capable of Affecting Adipogenesis. Representative endocrine disrupting chemicals (EDCs) capable of affecting adipogenesis and/or metabolic health through the specified nuclear receptor pathways listed above. Gross circle size intended to express a general sense of the reported research into assessing these varying mechanisms; for example, PPARγ, RXRα, and GR have previously received the bulk of the research, whereas others have received less. Agonists for the receptors are depicted with a (+) following the chemicals, whereas antagonists are denoted with the (−). Standard positive and negative control chemicals for each receptor (for evaluating these pathways) are bolded to distinguish from the other EDC examples. PPAR, peroxisome proliferator activated receptor; RXR, retinoid X receptor; AR, androgen receptor; ER, estrogen receptor; CAR, constitutive androstane receptor; TR, thyroid receptor; FXR, farnesoid X receptor; LXR, liver X receptor; GR, glucocorticoid receptor.

exposed to household dust, and thus receive exposure to EDCs present in the dust. The EPA estimates children ingest 60–100 mg of dust per day from indoor environments (52), contributing to chronic oral and inhalation exposures to EDCs (49, 53, 54), and compounded by other routes of exposure. Notably, numerous studies have demonstrated clear links between levels of indoor semi-volatile indoor contaminants (SVOCs) on hand wipes with levels in house dust (55, 56), with other studies demonstrating clear links with urinary and serum levels (55, 57, 58), providing evidence for this exposure route contributing to an increased body burden of specific chemicals. As such, environmental matrices such as this may represent a clear exposure route for humans and could provide critical information on biological effects of summed mixture exposures.

NUCLEAR RECEPTOR MECHANISMS MEDIATING METABOLIC DISRUPTION

While activation of the peroxisome proliferator activated receptor gamma (PPARγ) is likely the best-described mechanism through which adipogenesis is initiated/promoted, activation or inhibition of numerous other receptor systems have been described to directly or indirectly modulate adipocyte lineage commitment and/or differentiation of pre-adipocytes and subsequent accumulation of triglycerides, including thyroid receptor-beta (TRβ), glucocorticoid receptor (GR), estrogen receptor (ER), androgen receptor (AR), liver X receptor (LXR), retinoid X receptor (RXR), and others (59) (**Table 1**). Several studies have assessed the expression of nuclear receptors throughout the differentiation process, reporting that 30 nuclear receptors were expressed throughout the differentiation process to varying degrees and at varying timepoints (15, 60). Recent work by Chappell et al. demonstrated putative GR-mediated effects prior to PPARγ activation after exposure of 3T3-L1 cells to tetrabrominated bisphenol A (TBBPA) (61). Notably, EDCs capable of acting through each of these pathways have been described previously to modulate metabolic health *in vitro, in vivo*, or in human epidemiological studies; though importantly, certain molecular mechanisms have received far greater research attention than others (**Figure 2**).

Peroxisome Proliferator Activated Receptors (PPARs)

PPARγ is often considered the only nuclear receptor whose activation is necessary and sufficient to initiate adipogenesis (62, 63). Treatment of 3T3-L1 cells as well as other pre-adipocyte and/or other committed adipocyte lineage cells with PPARγ agonists induces a potent and efficacious increase in triglyceride accumulation, which has long been realized (64, 65); as such, PPARγ agonists such as rosiglitazone and/or troglitazone are routinely utilized as positive control ligands for these assays (63). Utilized as therapeutic agents to treat type 2 diabetes, these thiazolidinediones may act to improve insulin sensitivity via induction of PPARγ in diverse tissue types, proliferation of smaller adipocytes that are more insulin-sensitive, or via mediation of the tumor necrosis factor alpha (TNF-α), leptin, or fatty acid signaling pathways [reviewed in (66)]. To establish the necessity of this pathway to adipogenesis, Rosen et al. utilized embryonic stem cell and chimeric mouse models. They demonstrated that PPARγ-null cells tended to not generate adipocytes, suggesting an essential role for this receptor in their formation.

TABLE 1 | Major hormone receptor pathways capable of promoting adipogenesis.

Receptor	Activity	*In vitro* effects	*In vivo* effects	Epidemiological effects
PPARγ	Agonism	Promotes adipocyte differentiation, also some promotion of pre-adipocyte proliferation	Increased adipose fat deposition, body weights	Increased body weights, reverse hyperglycemia/treat diabetes
PPARβ/δ	Agonism	Promotes adipocyte differentiation	Activation improves lipid profiles, depletes lipid accumulation, increases resistance to diet-induced obesity	PPARβ/δ agonists reduce LDL cholesterol, triglycerides, insulin, and increase HDL cholesterol*
PPARα	Agonism	Promotes adipocyte differentiation	Activation improves hyperinsulinemia and hyperglycemia, reduces weight and adiposity	PPARα agonists reduce serum triglycerides and LDL cholesterol, increase HDL cholesterol
RXRα	Agonism	Promotes adipocyte lineage commitment, adipocyte differentiation	Ablated RXR mice are resistant to diet/chemical-induced obesity	RXR agonists increase plasma triglycerides, cholesterol, decreased thyroid hormones
GR	Agonism	Promotes adipocyte differentiation, pre-adipocyte proliferation	GR knock-down mice are resistant to diet-induced obesity, have improved insulin sensitivity and glucose tolerance, and increased energy expenditure	Excess glucocorticoids associated with increased weight, adiposity, and decreased glucose tolerance/insulin sensitivity
TR	Antagonism	Promotes adipocyte differentiation	TR null mice exhibit increased adipogenesis	Low thyroid hormone levels promote weight gain, high levels promote weight loss
ER	Agonism	Inhibits adipocyte differentiation, promotes pre-adipocyte proliferation	ERKO mice exhibit increased adiposity	Decreased estrogen in menopause associated with increased abdominal obesity
AR	Antagonism	Promotes adipocyte differentiation, no effect on pre-adipocyte proliferation	AR agonism has anti-adipogenic effects in rodents	Low androgen levels associated with increased abdominal obesity, reversed with supplementation
LXR	Agonism	Promotes adipocyte differentiation, pre-adipocyte proliferation	LXR knockout mice exhibit less adipose and are glucose-intolerant; agonist treatment reduces energy expenditure	LXR agonist treatments increase triglycerides, cholesterol, and other negative molecular markers
PXR	Agonism	Promotes adipocyte differentiation	PXR ablation inhibits diet-induced obesity, insulin resistance, and fatty liver disease; agonist treatment promotes adiposity in mice	PXR agonist treatments reported to induce hyperglycemia and increase diabetes risk
CAR	Agonism	Promotes adipocyte differentiation	CAR agonist treatment enhances insulin sensitivity, improves glucose and lipid metabolism, reverses diet-induced obesity	CAR agonist treatment decreases plasma glucose and improves insulin sensitivity
FXR	Agonism	Agonists induce adipocyte differentiation, antagonists reverse	FXR agonist induces weight gain and glucose intolerance in mice	FXR agonist treatments promote reduced lipid accumulation and increased glucose uptake, reduced HDL and increased LDL cholesterol, improved insulin sensitivity
InsR	Agonism	Promotes adipocyte differentiation, triglyceride accumulation	Increased weight gain and glucose intolerance	Insulin supplementation promote increased weight gain, cholesterol, and blood pressure
IGFR	Agonism	Promotes adipocyte differentiation, triglyceride accumulation	Increased weight gain and glucose intolerance	Increased weight gain, triglycerides

Descriptive effects for several major hormone receptor pathways that influence the process of adipogenesis and weight maintenance. Summarized evidence is provided for direction of effects, as well as in vitro, in vivo, and human epidemiological evidence. References and more detailed descriptions can be found within the relevant subsections of the manuscript, within section Nuclear Receptor Mechanisms Mediating Metabolic Disruption.

**Due to lack of specific, potent, and available ligands, there is minimal reported work in humans. Summarized work describes effects observed in monkey models following treatment with receptor-specific agonists.*

They further demonstrated gene dosage effects *in vitro*; cells lacking both copies of PPARγ could not be induced to differentiate, cells with one copy exhibited an intermediate degree of differentiation, and wild-type cells exhibited robust differentiation and efficacious expression of adipocyte-specific molecular markers (62). Clonal expansion and growth arrest occurs concurrently with expression of two proteins, PPARγ and the CCAAT enhancer binding protein alpha (C/EBPα), and these markers are both important for the differentiation of pre-adipocytes to adipocytes (63). Further experiments in this laboratory demonstrated that while C/EBPα is also a primary marker for the initiation of differentiation, it operates within a single initiating pathway with PPARγ (67). In cells deficient of PPARγ, C/EBPα was not capable of promoting adipogenesis by itself, suggesting an important but non-essential role in inducing and maintaining PPARγ expression, as well as an accessory role

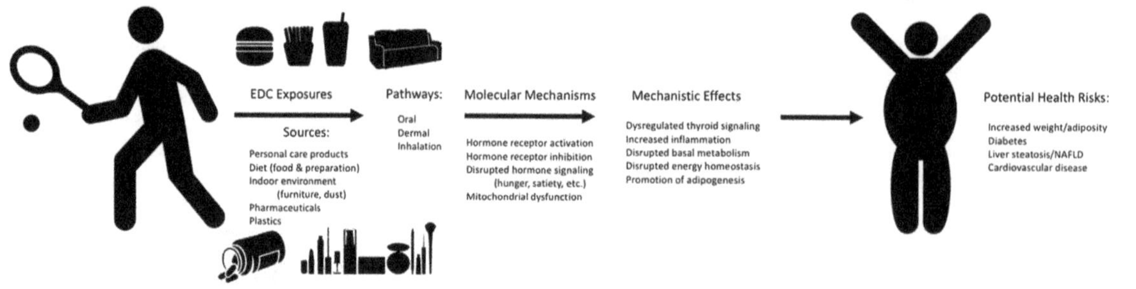

FIGURE 2 | Mechanisms of EDC Exposure and Potential Human Metabolic Health Effects. Graphical depiction of the potential sources and exposure pathways for humans to endocrine disrupting chemicals (EDCs), the molecular mechanisms related to metabolic health through which these EDCs may act to drive specific mechanistic effects, all of which may contribute to potential adverse health risks for humans. Effects reported are representative and are not comprehensive to all molecular mechanisms and mechanistic effects.

in mediating insulin sensitivity via direct induction of the insulin receptor (67).

The other PPAR isoforms, α and β/δ, have received considerably less attention as it relates to adipogenesis, though gain/loss-of-function experiments suggest putative roles. Experiments *in vitro* demonstrated that induction with a PPARβ/δ-specific ligand induced robust triglyceride accumulation in wild type cells (68) [and *in vivo* (69)], while PPARβ/δ-null cells differentiate and accumulate triglycerides less efficaciously following PPARγ-mediated induction (68). This suggests that while PPARβ/δ is not necessary for adipogenesis, the interplay of these isoforms is necessary to induce maximal differentiation and triglyceride accumulation in adipocytes. This was supported by other work reporting that PPARβ/δ activation promotes PPARγ expression, potentially bolstering adipogenesis, and providing a supportive role (70, 71). When examining the isoforms in isolation, Brun et al. reported that receptor isoform-specific activation via ligands failed to induce adipogenesis and triglyceride accumulation for PPARβ/δ, but did for PPARα, if to a lesser extent and over a longer time-course than via activation of PPARγ (72). RNA isolations on day five demonstrated that PPARα-treated cells had minimal or no induction of various adipocyte markers, relative to robust induction in the PPARγ-treated cells; however, both had robust expression by day seven post-induction, while PPARβ/δ exhibited only minimal expression at much later time points (72). Further experiments demonstrated that C/EBPα acted cooperatively with PPARγ to stimulate adipogenesis as expected, but not with PPARα or β/δ (72), suggesting distinct mechanisms. PPARβ/δ activation in mice has anti-adipogenic effects, improving lipid profiles, reducing lipid accumulation, and increasing resistance to diet-induced obesity (73, 74). PPARα activation in mice has similarly been demonstrated to result in anti-adipogenic effects, including improved hyperinsulinemia and hyperglycemia, lowered triglycerides, increased resistance to diet-induced obesity, and decreased weight and adiposity (75–77). Fenofibrates (PPARα agonists) administered to humans have similarly been demonstrated to decrease serum triglycerides and LDL cholesterol and increase HDL cholesterol (78, 79). While absence of good selective PPARβ/δ agonists has hindered human therapeutic examination, limited work with a selective and potent PPARβ/δ agonist in rhesus monkeys reported lowered LDL cholesterol, triglycerides, insulin, and increased HDL cholesterol (80).

Retinoid X Receptor (RXRα)

PPARγ functions as a heterodimer with RXR, suggesting that this receptor might also have dependent and/or independent roles in adipogenesis (62). Indeed, more than a decade ago, it was reported that organotins, potent activators of both PPARγ and RXRα, were also extremely potent inducers of adipogenesis (81, 82). Other studies have confirmed that receptor-specific activation of RXRα promotes both adipogenic differentiation and pre-adipocyte proliferation (60, 83, 84). Mechanistic experiments have further determined that of more than 5000 PPARγ:RXR DNA-binding sites in adipocytes, most are occupied by non-PPARγ:RXR heterodimers during the early stages of differentiation and transition to PPARγ:RXR in the later stages of differentiation (85). Mice with ablated adipocyte-RXRα are resistant to diet and chemical-induced obesity and exhibit impaired lipolysis during fasting (86); RXR agonists have also been demonstrated to sensitize diabetic and obese mice to insulin (87) and decrease hyperglycemia, hypertriglyceridemia, hyperinsulinemia, and both weight gain and food intake in several rodent models (87–89). More recent work from the Blumberg lab elegantly described RXR activation as an essential signal for commitment of mesenchymal stem cells to the adipocyte cell lineage, as well as separately promoting subsequent differentiation (48). Follow-up investigation determined that RXR activation-induced adipocyte differentiation created a functionally distinct adipocyte relative to those induced by PPARγ activation; RXR activation resulted in decreased glucose uptake, expression of adiponectin, and did not induce molecular pathways involved in adipocyte browning, suggesting a dysfunctional white adipose tissue that could potentially contribute to elevated obesity and/or diabetes risk (90). Therapeutic treatment by rexinoids in humans has reported increased plasma triglycerides, increased plasma cholesterol, and decreased thyroid hormones (91–93).

Liver X Receptor (LXR), Constitutive Androstane Receptor (CAR), Pregnane X Receptor (PXR), and Farnesoid X Receptor (FXR)

LXR, CAR, FXR, AND PXR are permissive binding partners with RXR, forming receptor heterodimers that can be activated by ligands for either receptor or both (potentially resulting in a synergistic effect), reviewed in Shulman et al. (94). LXRα is expressed primarily in the adipose, liver, intestine, and kidney, while the β isoform is ubiquitously expressed; LXRs mediate cholesterol transport, stimulating cholesterol efflux from macrophages, promoting transport in serum and uptake into liver, increase degradation of cholesterol into bile acids, inhibit absorption in the intestine, and synthesize fatty acids and triglycerides (94). Some disparate results have been reported *in vitro:* Hummasti et al. reported that LXR agonists failed to promote triglyceride accumulation and/or adipocyte differentiation in 3T3-L1 cells and 3T3-F442A cells, though did regulate adipocyte-specific gene expression (95). However, other studies have described LXR-mediated promotion of triglyceride accumulation, adipocyte differentiation, adipocyte-specific gene expression, and pre-adipocyte proliferation both *in vitro* and *in vivo* (60, 96, 97), potentially via activation of PPARγ (96, 97). These disparate results could be explained by cells lines and/or cell sources, as we previously reported different LXR expression and responsiveness in varying pre-adipocyte sources (60). Selective knockdown experiments have demonstrated LXRα as the primary regulator of lipolysis (98), with the β isoform more involved in cholesterol regulation (99). LXRβ-specific knockout mice have less adipose, but normal insulin sensitivity and adipocyte hormones; however, they are glucose-intolerant and accumulate lipid in pancreatic islets, putatively mediated by regulation of cholesterol transporters (99). Adipocytes have been demonstrated to be smaller in LXR deficient mice (97), and energy expenditure is increased, with reduced triglyceride accumulation in brown adipose (100); in parallel, energy expenditure is reduced in LXR agonist-treated wild type mice, and triglyceride accumulation was increased in brown adipose (100). In humans, LXR expression is higher in obese individuals, and receptor isoform polymorphisms have been associated with increased risks of obesity (101). Therapeutic treatment with LXR agonists resulted in increased plasma and hepatic triglycerides, cholesterol, and other negative metabolic markers in humans as well as primate and rodent models (102), despite some beneficial effects.

CAR and PXR are two closely-related liver-enriched receptors that have also been associated with metabolic function, and were reviewed in detail previously (103, 104). While originally appreciated as regulating xenobiotic metabolizing enzymes, they have also been demonstrated to help regulate energy homeostasis, immune function, lipid metabolism, and glucose homeostasis (103, 104). PXR appears to mediate effects through PPARγ, with PXR activation directly inducing PPARγ and other lipogenic gene expression such as Cd36, though potentially in a species-specific manner (104). CAR may promote effects on energy homeostasis through crosstalk with PPARα, or similarly to PXR, through activation of the free fatty acid uptake transporter Cd36 and inhibition of sterol regulatory element-binding protein (SREBP) (105). In animals, PXR ablation inhibits diet-induced obesity, insulin resistance, and fatty liver disease in various rodent models, suggesting PXR antagonism as a putative anti-obesogenic and anti-diabetic pathway (104, 106). PXR agonist treatment in mice promotes hepatic triglyceride accumulation, and constitutively active PXR mice exhibit enlarged and fatty liver disease, reviewed in (107). Treatment with CAR agonists, in contrast, enhances insulin sensitivity, improves glucose and lipid metabolism, and reverses diet-induced obesity in rodents, reviewed in (103). In humans, the CAR agonist phenobarbital has been reported to decrease plasma glucose levels and improve insulin sensitivity in patients with diabetes (103, 108, 109), and though PXR is particularly promiscuous, activation of PXR by rifampicin, statins, and other pharmaceuticals have been reported to induce hyperglycemia in patients and increase the risk of developing diabetes (106). While activation of CAR is seemingly more therapeutically beneficial relative to PXR, it also carries with it side effects such as liver hyperplasia and carcinogenesis (103), among other effects.

Modulation of FXR has also been assessed as it relates to adipogenesis and a potential therapeutic target in treating metabolic syndrome, reviewed in (110). Endogenously activated by bile acids, FXR regulates bile acid synthesis, enterohepatic circulation, lipid metabolism, and thus indirectly regulates other bile acid associated receptors, discussed in Prawitt et al. (111). Researchers have described that FXR is expressed in adipocytes from adult mice and in differentiated 3T3-L1 cells, but not in the undifferentiated pre-adipocytes (112). Treatment with an FXR agonist increased adipocyte differentiation in 3T3-L1 cells, whereas treatment with an FXR antagonist reversed this (112); FXR agonist treatment also enhanced insulin signaling and insulin-stimulated glucose uptake (113). Pro-apoptotic and anti-adipogenic effects of guggelsterone (FXR antagonist) have also been reported by other researchers (114). Treatment with an FXR agonist in mice with diet-induced obesity worsened weight gain and glucose intolerance, seemingly mediated through reduction of the bile acid pool size and energy expenditure (115). However, other research in mouse models suggests beneficial effects for FXR agonist (GW4064) treatment (111, 116). FXR knockout/deficient mice exhibit decreased adipose tissue, lower leptin concentrations, elevated plasma free fatty acids, resistance to rosiglitazone-induced obesity, and their embryonic fibroblasts are also resistant to rosiglitazone-induced triglyceride accumulation and differentiation due to increased lipolysis and decreased lipogenesis (113, 117, 118); despite these apparent positive metabolic effects, FXR deficient animals (both mice and rabbits) also exhibit impaired glucose tolerance and insulin resistance, which are corrected with FXR agonist supplementation (113, 119). FXR expression has also been demonstrated to be downregulated and/or dysfunctional in obese humans (110, 120), suggesting downregulation may play a potential role in human obesity. PXR mice exhibit FXR agonist therapeutic trials in humans have reported reduced liver lipid accumulation and increased glucose uptake [reviewed in (110)], reduced HDL cholesterol and increased LDL cholesterol, and improvements in insulin resistance [reviewed in (111)], suggesting that FXR antagonists and/or selective FXR receptor modulators might promote more beneficial effects in some tissues and for specific metabolic endpoints (116).

Thyroid Receptor (TR)

TR also forms a heterodimer with RXR, though in contrast to other receptors discussed above, it is considered a non-permissive heterodimer (can be activated only by thyroid receptor ligands and not RXR ligands), reviewed in Shulman et al. (94). While less frequently assessed as a contributory molecular pathway for adipogenesis, one of the defining characteristics of thyroid hormone action is maintenance of metabolic health and maintenance of lipid and carbohydrate metabolism, blood pressure, and body mass [reviewed in (94, 121)]. Hypothyroidism (low thyroxine (T4) and triiodothyronine (T3), high thyroid stimulating hormone (TSH)) is characterized by weight gain, while hyperthyroidism (high T4 and T3, low TSH) is characterized by weight loss (122, 123). As such, thyroid hormones are generally considered anti-obesogenic, and hypothyroid-associated adiposity can be reduced with supplementation (124–126). TRα primarily regulates thermogenesis and TRβ primarily regulates cholesterol metabolism and lipogenesis, as well as a number of genes and enzymes necessary for pre-adipocyte proliferation and adipocyte differentiation, either directly or via PPARγ [reviewed in (121)]. Studies have demonstrated some disparate findings regarding the role of TR in adipogenesis itself. For example, antagonism of TR has been demonstrated to efficaciously modulate adipocyte differentiation, purportedly via PPARγ, reviewed in (16); however, we've previously demonstrated that 3T3-L1 treatment with 1-850 (TR antagonist) resulted in efficacious triglyceride accumulation (60), and TR-null mice exhibit increased adipogenesis (127). Others, in contrast, have reported that treatment with triiodothyronine (T3; TR agonist) promoted adipocyte gene expression and decreased pre-adipocyte proliferation in Ob L771 mouse pre-adipocytes (128) or triglyceride accumulation and lipogenic gene expression in 3T3-L1 pre-adipocytes (60, 129). Other work suggested differing roles at varying levels of treatment; when 3T3-F442A cells were treated with hyperthyroid T3 levels, the proportion of adipocytes was increased but expression of lipogenic enzymes and triglyceride accumulation were decreased, whereas lower levels stimulated adipose conversion, expression of lipogenic enzymes, and pre-adipocyte proliferation (130).

Glucocorticoid Receptor (GR)

The GR is intimately connected to lipid metabolism, with a wealth of *in vitro*, *in vivo*, and human epidemiological evidence supporting its role in adipose formation and maintenance [reviewed in (131)]. Treatment with dexamethasone induces a potent and efficacious triglyceride accumulation and pre-adipocyte proliferation response in various mesenchymal and pre-adipocyte models, often to greater extents and at lower concentrations than through direct activation of PPARγ (60, 132), potentially mediated at least in part through activation of PPARγ (133), though in other cases without meaningful activation of PPARγ (134); in support, treatment with GR antagonists inhibits differentiation in various mesenchymal and pre-adipocyte models (135). Other studies have reported that glucocorticoids alone were insufficient to promote adipogenesis either in 3T3-L1 cells (136) or in other models (137), though stimulated robust differentiation in combination with insulin (137). As mentioned above, Chappell et al. demonstrated putative GR-mediated effects prior to PPARγ activation after exposure to tetrabrominated bisphenol A (TBBPA) (61), which may explain why isobutylmethylxanthine (IBMX; PPARγ ligand) treatment prior to dexamethasone (GR agonist) failed to induce significant differentiation using the same cell model in another lab, while dexamethasone treatment before IBMX promoted robust differentiation (138). The authors posited that glucocorticoid activation may be necessary for an intermediate commitment state prior to differentiation via PPARγ (138); however, this could also be due to differing responsiveness to PPARγ and GR ligands based on 3T3-L1 cell source, which we have reported on previously (60).

Other research has evaluated the putative role of the mineralocorticoid receptor (MR), an additional high-affinity binder of glucocorticoids; treatment of 3T3-F442A and 3T3-L1 cells with the mineralocorticoid agonist aldosterone promoted adipocyte differentiation, which appeared to be mediated through PPARγ activation; inhibition and knock-down of the MR inhibited adipogenesis, whereas knock-down of the GR did not (139). More recent work, however, demonstrated that silencing GR, but not MR, inhibited the pro-adipogenic activity of cortisol, and also decreased leptin and adiponectin, whereas MR knock-down actually increased leptin (140). Research in mice investigated knocking out local glucocorticoid action via 11β-hydroxysteroid dehydrogenase (glucocorticoid inactivator) overexpression exhibited resistance to diet-induced obesity/reduced fat accumulation, decreased food intake, improved insulin sensitivity and glucose tolerance, and increased energy expenditure (141). Glucocorticoid excess in mice in contrast resulted in decreased osteogenic gene expression and mineralization and increased expression of adipogenic genes (142). Cushing's syndrome (excess cortisol production) is associated with increased weight gain, hypertension, type 2 diabetes, and fatty tissue deposits (143, 144), suggesting a pro-adipogenic effect of glucocorticoids in humans as well. Further, prenatal/antenatal dexamethasone (GR agonist) is often utilized to promote development of lungs in infants at risk of being born premature (145, 146). Epidemiological studies have reported that dexamethasone treatment is associated with reduced birth weight in infants, even after correcting for weeks of gestation (145, 146), and exhibited hypertension and greater subsequent administration of insulin for hyperglycemia (146).

Estrogens and Androgens

Often considered opposing sex steroids, androgens, and estrogens have also been described to have opposing effects on adipogenesis, reviewed in Cooke and Naaz (147). Experiments comparing differentiation extent in rat pre-adipocytes determined no effects for either androgens or estrogens in promoting differentiation in male pre-adipocytes; however, estrogens elicited a pro-adipogenic effect (via pre-adipocyte proliferation) and androgens elicited an anti-androgenic effect in female cells, potentially mediated by modulation of insulin growth factor 1 receptor (IGF1R) and PPARγ expression (148). This promotion of pre-adipocyte proliferation by estrogens has been successfully replicated in both male and female omental pre-adipocytes (149), while the inhibitory effect of estrogens on differentiation/triglyceride accumulation may be dose-dependent (150). Related work has determined some of the inhibitory effects of estrogens on adipogenesis appear to occur through the G-protein-coupled estrogen receptor 1 (GPER) rather than the classical estrogen receptor itself (151), and that inhibitory effects on adipogenesis are concurrent with enhancement of osteogenesis (152). Interestingly, estrogen receptor knock-out (ERKO) mice exhibit increased fat pad weights, adipocyte size, and adipocyte numbers relative to wild type control animals, as well as insulin resistance and impaired glucose tolerance (153). This is mirrored in humans, as decreased estrogen levels at menopause are associated with increased abdominal obesity that is ameliorated with estrogen replacement therapy [reviewed in (154)], an effect also observed in ovariectomized female mice (155).

Androgens are generally considered anti-obesogenic [reviewed in (156, 157)], and treatment with androgens has been demonstrated to inhibit adipogenesis in adipose tissue samples from both sexes (158) and reduce fat mass in humans [reviewed in (159)]. Dihydrotestosterone inhibits triglyceride accumulation and adipocyte gene expression in human mesenchymal stem cells and pre-adipocytes from various depots, whereas anti-androgen co-treatment attenuated those effects, and had no apparent impact on pre-adipocyte proliferation in either model (160). Other research has replicated these findings, suggesting some of the effects occur through inhibition of the multipotent stem cell to pre-adipocyte commitment (161, 162). In contrast, anti-androgens have been suggested to act as obesogens; androgen receptor knock out (ARKO) mice exhibit increased obesity (163), flutamide has been demonstrated to modulate lipid profiles in women (164), and hypogonadism (characterized by testosterone deficiency) is associated with obesity, hypertension, dyslipidemia, insulin resistance, and other metabolic effects, which may be corrected with androgen supplementation (159).

Other Receptors

A variety of other receptors, from the nuclear receptor family, receptor tyrosine kinase family, and others, have described roles in adipogenesis and/or lipogenesis. For example, both the insulin and IGF-1 receptors have widely accepted roles in growth, tissue-specific hypertrophy, and weight maintenance (165–168). Many others, including the aryl hydrocarbon, retinoic acid, low density lipoprotein receptors, among others, have established roles in adipogenesis but could not be discussed in detail within the scope of this review. Importantly, while the bulk of study has assessed activation of PPARγ and RXR, numerous other receptor systems interplay to promote and maintain adipocytes, and must be taken into account when evaluating environmental mixtures.

MITOCHONDRIAL TOXICITY AS A CONTRIBUTORY FACTOR TO METABOLIC DISRUPTION

Mitochondria are the major location of fatty acid oxidation, making them essential in lipid metabolism; as such, dysfunction can contribute to numerous adverse metabolic health consequences, including altered lipid accumulation, metabolism, and insulin resistance (169, 170). Mitochondrial function is intimately connected with metabolic health, as it helps regulate energy expenditure, production of ATP, and removal of reactive oxygen species (ROS); ROS reduce oxygen consumption and inhibit fatty acid oxidation in adipocytes, promoting lipid accumulation [reviewed in (169)]. ROS production mainly occurs at complex I and III in mitochondria, and is increased when excess electrons are provided to the mitochondrial respiratory chains (when proton gradient is high and ATP demand is low), as described in Kim et al. (171). Excess electrons are transferred to oxygen, converted to superoxide, and subsequently to hydrogen peroxide; this ROS acts to damage proteins, DNA, and lipids, and activates pathways (via activation of serine kinases) that phosphorylate insulin receptor substrate proteins and inhibit insulin signaling, thus promoting insulin resistance and ultimately resulting in metabolic dysfunction (171, 172). Mitochondrial dysfunction and resultant lipid accumulation in accessory tissues is also capable of further impeding insulin signaling and glucose metabolism, promoting further dysfunction (173); indeed, maternal obesity during pregnancy in rodents contributes to a transgenerational mitochondrial dysfunction phenotype (inhibited insulin signaling for three generations) (174). Notably, chronic oxidative stress has been well-described in obese individuals, suggesting a link between ROS production/management and hyperplasia [reviewed in (175)]. To minimize damage from these ROS, cells require a balance between ATP synthesis through oxidative phosphorylation and dissipation of the proton gradient (169). Mitochondrial dysfunction can also directly contribute to cardiovascular disease, another hallmark disease of metabolic syndrome, and myocardial metabolic function is intimately connected to obesity, diabetes, and altered insulin signaling [reviewed in (176)]. Research suggests that decreases in ATP production due to inhibited mitochondrial respiration, increased oxidative stress, and inhibited calcium signaling can all contribute to diastolic dysfunction via reduced velocity of myocardial relaxation velocity and myocardial compliance (173, 176).

Adipocytes are capable of regulating metabolic insults by altering their number, morphology, as well as the intracellular mitochondrial distribution (169). Mitochondrial biogenesis is an essential component of adipogenesis, with mitochondrial numbers increasing markedly after initiation of pre-adipocyte differentiation and reaching a maximum toward the end; this can be noted via treatment with the PPARγ agonist rosiglitazone, wherein treated cells demonstrate increased mitochondrial content and function, with increased basal oxygen consumption, ATP respiration, and proton leak (173, 177, 178). ATP levels are naturally reduced with increasing degree of adipocyte differentiation, putatively due to increased ATP demands for lipogenesis (179), and reduced levels are further exacerbated when electron transport chain inhibition occurs (178). Reduced mitochondrial biogenesis, ATP levels, and dysfunctional mitochondrial electron transport have been reported in both humans and animals with metabolic syndrome (173, 179). PPARγ co-activator 1α (PGC-1α) is a master regulator of mitochondrial biogenesis and gene expression and is a potent co-activator of PPAR isoforms: expression in fat or muscle cells increases mtDNA content, expression of mitochondrial genes, and mitochondrial respiration (176). PGC-1α-stimulated biogenesis in the heart ultimately promotes overt heart failure, another mechanism through which metabolic dysfunction can lead to cardiac dysfunction (176). Biogenesis appears closely linked to adipocyte differentiation, as up-regulation of mitochondrial biogenesis is well-reported following induction of adipogenesis and for up to 10 days post-differentiation (177, 180), suggesting that mitochondria are needed to supply the substrates and factors necessary to support adipogenesis-driven lipogenesis. Mitochondria also have functionally distinct roles in white vs. brown adipose tissue. White adipose tissue is composed of numerous depots of large lipid droplet adipocytes throughout the body and is essential for maintenance of metabolic health. Brown adipose tissue, in contrast, is smaller and localized to the neck and upper-chest in adult humans, and is composed of adipocytes with large numbers of smaller lipid droplets and more numerous mitochondria [reviewed in (180)]. In brown adipose tissue, the heat derived from thermogenesis is produced primarily by the high mitochondrial content of these cells, via oxidation of fatty acids and other components (180). Uncoupling proteins (UCPs) play a key role in this process, serving to uncouple mitochondrial respiration from ATP generation by inducing a proton leak, which subsequently allows for energy dissipation as heat (180).

Numerous environmental toxicants have been demonstrated to promote mitochondrial dysfunction, and these contaminants may also advance metabolic dysfunction, leading to obesity, and diabetes. Certain mitochondrial disorders that are characterized by impaired oxidative phosphorylation are also associated with disrupted lipid homeostasis: myoclonic epilepsy with ragged red fibers is associated with triglyceride accumulation in muscles and multiple symmetrical lipomatosis, a condition characterized by abnormally small white adipocytes containing numerous small lipid droplets rather than the classical large central droplet that displaces the nucleus (170). Mitochondrial oxidative phosphorylation inhibitors and protein synthesis inhibitors impair mitochondrial respiration and promote triglyceride accumulation in 3T3-L1 cells, which retain their precursor fibroblastic morphology and do not express adipocyte-specific markers (170, 180). Previous research has demonstrated that treatment of 3T3-L1 cells with rotenone (a complex I inhibitor), antimycin A, stigmatellin, and myxothiazol (complex III inhibitors), and oligomycin (ATP synthase inhibitor) promoted triglyceride accumulation in a dose-dependent manner (170). Interestingly, these mitochondrial respiration inhibitors promoted triglyceride accumulation in numerous small lipid droplets, cells retained their fibroblastic morphology, and classical adipocyte-specific genes were not expressed in these cells (170), suggesting a differentiation-independent mechanism of triglyceride accumulation. Specifically, antimycin A, which inhibits complex III, induces triglyceride accumulation in pre-adipocytes via a putative differentiation-independent mechanism (170); these cells exhibit multi-vesicular lipid accumulation, reduced expression of standard differentiation markers (FABP4, C/EBP), and suppression of PPARγ and RXR, supporting other studies suggesting mitochondrial dysfunction may inhibit adipocyte differentiation (178).

We recently demonstrated a similar phenotype in experiments with pyraclostrobin, a strobilurin-class fungicide used on strawberries, spinach, and other produce items, with production of >2 million pounds per year (181, 182). Pyraclostrobin and other strobilurin fungicides have been demonstrated to inhibit complex III (183), suggesting a potential mechanism for metabolic disruption. We previously reported that pyraclostrobin, azoxystrobin, fluoxastrobin, and trifloxystrobin all induced both triglyceride accumulation and pre-adipocyte proliferation in 3T3-L1 cells (184). Previous research in 3T3-L1 cells and a human adipose-derived stem cell model suggested this did not occur through activation of PPARγ and that standard differentiation markers were lacking (47, 185), supporting the case for a differentiation-independent mechanism. Mechanism was further interrogated in our laboratory through co-exposure experiments in 3T3-L1 cells; we reported that PPARγ antagonists did not protect against pyraclostrobin-mediated triglyceride accumulation (177). Instead, pyraclostrobin promoted mitochondrial dysfunction, including reduced ATP, mitochondrial membrane potential, basal mitochondrial respiration, ATP-linked respiration, and spare respiratory capacity (177). In addition, pyraclostrobin-treated cells exhibited reduced expression of genes regulating glucose transport, glycolysis, fatty acid oxidation, and lipogenesis (177). Lastly, co-treatment with a cAMP responsive element binding protein (CREB) inhibitor reduced pyraclostrobin-mediated triglyceride accumulation (177). These results all suggest that toxicants capable of disrupting mitochondrial function may also have the potential to affect metabolic health, via modulation of lipogenesis and other metabolic processes.

Similarly, a recent study reported that several samples of oil sands process-affected water (OSPW), wastewater produced during the extraction of bitumen from oil sands, exhibited PPARγ agonist activity and promoted triglyceride accumulation in 3T3-L1 cells (186). Causative ligand characterization identified several hydroxylated/polyoxygenated carboxylic acids and hydroxylated sulfates as the major PPARγ ligands (186); naphthenic acids, a mixture of carboxylic acids and natural component of petroleum, are a major component of OSPW. Interestingly, while these are posited as promoting adipogenesis via PPARγ activation, a recent publication demonstrated that naphthenic acids isolated from oil sands water acted to uncouple oxidative phosphorylation, inhibit respiration, and increase the production of ROS (187). As noted above, these are mechanisms that can promote triglyceride accumulation in cells, suggesting that this may be an additional mechanism for the observed adipogenic effects of these waters in the previous publication (186). Notably, this occurred at environmentally-relevant concentrations for OSPW, suggesting that this or a combination of these mechanisms may promote the environmental sample-induced adipogenicity.

Mitochondrial ROS is produced by pre-adipocytes during and throughout differentiation, and its presence activates several early-stage differentiation markers, including C/EBP, PPAR, and CREB (63, 188). Direct impacts on adipogenesis appear less certain, which has been delineated in greater detail previously (189); research suggests that ROS may be essential for adipogenesis, but also may perturb the process. Some research has demonstrated that ROS promoted mitotic clonal expansion in 3T3-L1 cells (190), a necessary step prior to induction of differentiation. Other research has described inhibitory effects on differentiation, with ROS inhibiting both pre-adipocyte proliferation and adipocyte differentiation/triglyceride accumulation (180, 191, 192). Still other researchers, via co-treatment experiments utilizing antioxidants, demonstrated that ROS impacted differentiation but not pre-adipocyte proliferation: treatment with an antioxidant (reducing ROS) reduced lipid accumulation in mesenchymal stem cells (193). However, the varying cell models used for these experiments may mediate these apparent differences; all studies agree that ROS appear to modulate early-stage differentiation, though the mechanisms of this modulation appear to vary based on cell lines, sources, and experimental details.

Several mitochondrial toxicants have been demonstrated to promote insulin resistance and/or metabolic syndrome in epidemiological studies, reviewed in detail previously (172, 194), though this research area has as of yet received limited attention in the context of metabolic disruption. Several organochlorine pesticides have been implicated in metabolic effects via mitochondrial dysfunction. Specifically, atrazine has been demonstrated to directly inhibit complexes I and III, reducing oxygen consumption and leading to accumulation of superoxides; chronic exposure in rats has been demonstrated to decrease basal metabolic rate, and increase body weight, intra-abdominal fat, and promote insulin resistance independent of food intake or activity levels (172, 195). Much of the remaining literature has focused on the role of polychlorinated biphenyls (PCBs). Several congeners have been demonstrated to promote mitochondrial dysfunction *in vitro* (196, 197), exposure resulted in/exacerbated obesity, insulin resistance, and hyperinsulinemia in mice (198), and higher exposure to PCBs has been linked to increased risk of obesity, dyslipidemia, and/or insulin resistance in a number of epidemiological studies (199–202).

AVAILABLE *IN VITRO* MODELS OF ADIPOGENESIS AND METABOLIC DISRUPTION

Numerous *in vitro* models have been developed and utilized for the purpose of identifying potential metabolic disrupting chemicals, reviewed in detail previously (203, 204). Generally, these models can be described as assessing two key parameters of adipocyte development: commitment to the adipocyte lineage from multipotent precursor cells (generally through the use of mesenchymal stem cell (MSC) models) and differentiation into mature adipocytes (generally through the use of pre-adipocyte models). MSC models have the additional benefit of being capable of assessing both endpoints, though are seemingly less frequently utilized than the available pre-adipocyte models. In addition, several research groups have begun to report on the three-dimensional culture of pre-adipocytes, which may shed additional light on mechanisms in a more physiologically relevant system. All of these assays are lengthy and their relative abilities to correctly identify chemicals may depend on both cell line and cell source. As such, there is a critical need to develop better methods for correctly predicting metabolic disruptors. While murine models have historically been used preferentially, a growing number of species utilized and a growing movement toward utilization of human models may help expand our understanding of translational mechanisms and potential environmental contaminant impacts on human health.

Perhaps the best known pre-adipocyte model is the 3T3-L1 mouse cell line. First described in the 1970's, it has proven reliable as an *in vitro* screen over several decades for identifying likely obesogenic chemicals *in vivo* (205, 206). These cells are already committed to the adipocyte lineage and cannot develop into other cell types; however, they generally require activation of particular signaling pathways to promote further development. Following exposure to adipogenic chemicals, these cells differentiate into adipocytes, accumulate triglycerides, and come to resemble a mature human white fat cell (44, 46, 205, 206). While 3T3-L1 cells have seemingly come to be considered the de facto model of adipogenesis, some inherent concerns remain about their utility. As we have described recently (60), while this line has been well-characterized (207), it is somewhat unreliable in sourcing. For example, while we know much about the molecular mechanisms underpinning the development of mature adipocytes based on this cell line, nuclear receptor expression related to adipogenesis is markedly different between different lots and sources of this cell line (60). Moreover, on investigation into this apparent discord in source, we discovered that the American Type Culture Collection (ATCC) maintains five distinct lots of 3T3-L1 cells, which all seemingly have differing degrees of differentiation success. This issue with cell line integrity was highlighted in a recent paper (208), suggesting that these differences can contribute to real discrepancies in the ability to replicate findings across laboratories. As the current ATCC cells are meaningfully different in the expression of key adipogenic pathways from the Zenbio-sourced cells (which are sourced from the isolating laboratory), it is unclear whether our understanding of the mechanisms underlying adipogenesis are from the original cells, the ATCC cells, or where these research paths diverge. Care needs to be taken to assess reproducibility across stocks and between laboratories and carefully untangle where the research underlying this cell line belongs. Other pre-adipocyte models also exist, including the OP9 mouse bone marrow-derived stromal pre-adipocyte cell line (44, 45), a line that allows for considerably faster differentiation, though which we have demonstrated to exhibit different nuclear receptor expression and differing degrees of responsiveness to adipogenic chemicals (60). These varying pre-adipocyte models allow for assessments of varying molecular pathways important for the process of differentiation via both source of the cells and species [discussed further in (204)].

Various multipotent mesenchymal cells and cell lines (46, 47) offer the additional ability to assess commitment to the adipocyte lineage as a distinct process from adipocyte differentiation (48). MSC use and applicability in adipogenesis research has been reviewed in detail previously (209). The variability of these cell lines are reportedly lower than the pre-adipocyte models, they are purportedly easier to isolate and culture, and they have additional utility in that they can be utilized to assess both differentiation of adipocytes but also commitment to the adipocyte lineage vs. other cell lineages. For example, many researchers have utilized these cell lines to evaluate the interplay between commitment to the osteogenic vs. adipogenic lineages following exposure to specific environmental contaminants (210–213). Recent work elegantly described a novel protocol for evaluating both adipogenic lineage commitment and subsequent differentiation as distinct processes in primary MSCs (48), which has been described previously for the C3H10T1/2 stem cell model (214, 215). These advancements raise the utility of this model and warrants further investigation into replicability, reproducibility of this model across laboratories, and comparisons of translation to human health relative to the pre-adipocyte models currently utilized.

Lastly, a number of research labs have begun to describe spheroid cell cultures of adipocyte models (216–220), which may carry some inherent benefits over the standard adherent monolayer cultures. These studies have suggested that spheroid culture improves the efficiency, extent, and/or speed of differentiation (216–221), retains the multipotent potential of these cells (217, 222), and transcriptomic analyses have suggested a potentially more representative model of adipocyte gene expression relative to known *in vivo* mechanisms (216). These models may allow for a more comprehensive understanding of adipose physiology than was possible via interrogation of the monolayer cell cultures, and should be evaluated further for replicability and translation potential relative to the standard monolayer cultures.

METABOLIC DISRUPTION POTENTIAL OF ENVIRONMENTAL MIXTURES

As noted above, the assessments of environmental samples have proven an interesting new approach to evaluating potential mixture toxicity. With tens of thousands of chemicals in use and new chemicals regularly added, there are too many to characterize individually, and certainly no capabilities to assess all potential combinations of them (223, 224). Body burden studies have and continue to report human exposure to hundreds of chemicals on a regular basis (225, 226), demonstrating the problem of realistic mixture exposure studies. To add to the complexity, research has reported additive effects on several hormone receptors both *in vitro* and *in vivo* (227–231), demonstrating that mixtures can induce effects at levels below those induced by individual chemicals. From a toxicological perspective, evaluating whole environmental samples: wastewater, surface/groundwater, indoor house dust, air samples, etc. for biological activities has emerged as a promising tact to assess potential adverse health concerns from exposure to actual mixtures present in the environment, given that it can evaluate more realistic environmentally relevant exposures (**Figure 3**).

Numerous natural and exogenous contaminants can contribute to human exposure; as such, measuring the total receptor bioactivities has proven useful for assessing the total magnitude of potential effects (232–239). While analytical chemistry techniques and equipment have drastically improved, allowing for more precise measurements of contaminants at lower concentrations, recent research has suggested we lack complete information on all causative bioactive chemicals present in the environment (240, 241). While non-targeted analytical efforts have improved, we still lack sufficient software and comprehensive protocols to enable robust and reproducible non-targeted assessments of contaminants across laboratories. To address this need of addressing mixture toxicity without necessarily understanding the full chemical complexity, bioassays have been utilized to assess biological activities of actual environmental samples. Reporter gene assays are one such commonly-utilized tool, assessing total receptor activities (agonism and antagonism), and valued due to their low cost, ease of use, reliability, high sensitivity, and ease of adapting for multiple receptors (227–244). These assays provide the capability to assess the total receptor activity of potentially numerous low-concentration EDCs (without identifying each causative chemical) rather than assessing each constituent chemical individually.

Applying this method to human epidemiological research has shown great potential; a number of researchers have rigorously characterized how *in vivo* mixtures of contaminants correspond with total hormone receptor bioactivities of human and animal matrices (serum, tissues, etc.) (245–251). Moreover, some researchers have begun to utilize bioactivities directly to assess human health outcomes. For example, researchers have correlated the total placental estrogenic activity with increased reproductive malformations (252) and impaired motor development (253), total adipose estrogenic activity with increased risk for breast cancer (254), and placental estrogenic activity with increased birth weight in boys (255). Other research has failed to report significant associations, including a lack of any association between adipose estrogenic activity and risk for type-2 diabetes (256), potentially due to a greater role for other receptors in pathogenesis (257). These studies demonstrate the potential utility of this method, particularly when targeted based on a comprehensive understanding of etiology and molecular mechanisms.

Several studies have begun to apply these techniques to metabolic endpoints, assessing pertinent receptor bioactivities (GR, PPARγ, and others) as well as utilizing less high-throughput

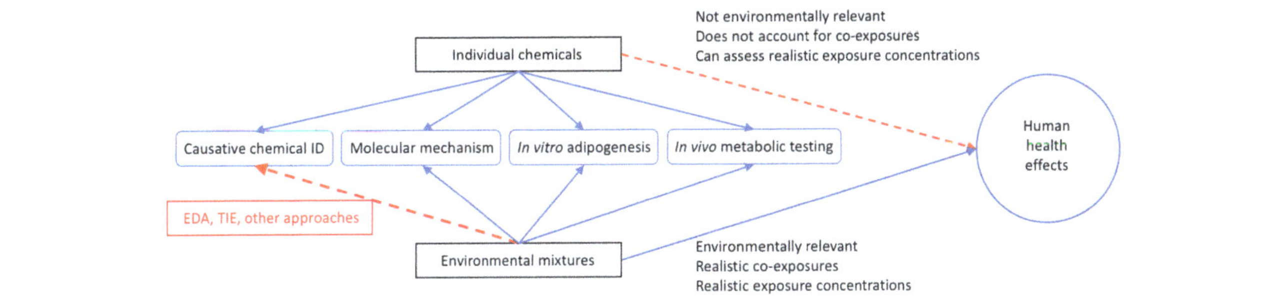

FIGURE 3 | Utility of Utilizing Environmental Mixtures for Human Health Assessments. Graphical depiction comparing individual chemicals and environmental mixtures for the assessment of potential human health effects. While environmental mixtures have less use in identifying causative chemicals in all cases (though tools like effect directed analysis (EDA) and toxicity identification evaluation (TIE) can be used to elucidate this), these mixtures are more relevant in reflecting the suite of chemicals that people are exposed to on a daily basis than utilizing single chemicals alone, and more often reflect actual environmental exposure concentrations. In this figure, the blue lines indicate positive relationships and the red lines indicate difficulty for single chemicals or mixtures in assessing the related outcome.

adipogenesis or other assays for predicting *in vivo* metabolic disruption potentials. Some of these environmental case studies are discussed in greater detail below:

Metabolic Disruption Potential of Indoor House Dust

As noted above, numerous studies have documented the detection of EDCs from diverse chemical classes in indoor house dust samples from a variety of sources. A number of studies have assessed the bioactivities for solvent-extracted house dust, reporting PPARγ, GR, and ER agonist activities as well as AR and TR antagonist activities, at concentrations $\geq$ 15 µg dust equivalence per mL (DEQ/mL, mass of extracted dust per volume of assay medium) (258–260). Our laboratory also assessed the modulation of PPARγ by house dust extracts, reporting that 21 of 24 examined indoor house dust extracts exhibited significant PPARγ binding at 3 mg DEQ/mL (120 µg dust per assay well) using a relative binding affinity assay (261) and 15 of 25 extracts activated PPARγ at $\leq$50% of the maximal positive control response at concentrations $\geq$100 µg DEQ/mL (4 µg/well) using a commercially-available reporter assay (262, 263). This work demonstrated activation of pathways known to regulate adipogenesis at very low concentrations, and subsequently informed our follow-up studies examining higher-order effects on adipogenesis.

We recently evaluated >40 common SVOCs that are routinely detected in indoor house dust samples for adipogenic activity in the 3T3-L1 murine pre-adipocyte cell model. We found that > two-thirds of these chemicals independently induced significant triglyceride accumulation and/or pre-adipocyte proliferation (184). Specifically, pyraclostrobin (strobilurin fungicide), dibutyl phthalate (DBP), tert-butyl-phenyl diphenyl phosphate (TBPDP), and the isopropylated triaryl phosphates (ITPs, mixture of isomers) exhibited near or supra-maximal triglyceride accumulation relative to the rosiglitazone (positive control)-induced maximum (184). We further assessed eleven house dust extracts collected from central North Carolina (NC), USA households; we found that ten of these 11 extracts exhibited significant triglyceride accumulation and/or pre-adipocyte proliferation at <20 µg of dust/well (184). This activity occurred at orders of magnitude lower concentrations than those the EPA estimates children to consume each day. As such, this raises concerns for potential impacts on *in vivo* metabolic health.

A recent follow-up to this study evaluated the adipogenic activity of 137 house dust extracts from central NC households and attempted to determine putative causative chemicals, molecular mechanisms, and potential impacts on human metabolic health (264). We reported that 90% of the dust extracts exhibited significant adipogenic activity, <60% via significant triglyceride accumulation, and >70% of samples via significant pre-adipocyte proliferation, with >40% of effects occurring at <10 µg dust/well (264). Increasing dust-induced triglyceride accumulation was positively correlated with serum thyroid stimulating hormone levels in adult residents, and negatively correlated with serum free triiodothyronine (T3) and thyroxine (T4) (264). Interestingly, proliferation tended to be positively correlated with residents' body mass index (BMI; $p < 0.10$), potentially suggesting adipogenic chemicals present in the dust are associated with the weights of residents, but further research with larger sample sizes are needed to substantiate this. We further assessed TR antagonism as a potential contributory causative mechanism in these effects, and found that TRβ antagonism of these extracts (265) was positively correlated with triglyceride accumulation (264). Both T3 co-treatment and siRNA knock-down of TR inhibited the dust-induced triglyceride accumulation of these extracts, supporting the role of TR antagonism as a contributory molecular mechanism.

Metabolic Disruption Potential of Oil and Gas-Associated Wastewaters

Three separate sets of studies have assessed different aspects of oil and gas operations and metabolic disruption, reporting *in vitro* and/or *in vivo* evidence of metabolic disruption by oil and gas associated environmental mixtures. The first assessed three replicate samples of oil sands process-affected water (OSPW), wastewater produced during the extraction of bitumen from oil sands (186). They reported that an OSPW sample activated PPARγ at concentrations as low as 0.025x relative water concentration (40-fold dilution relative to pure water). This sample was further fractionated, with the majority of PPARγ activity in fractions two and five (five fractions), and fractions three through five exhibited significant triglyceride accumulation and induction of adipogenic genes (fatty acid binding protein and lipoprotein lipase). A pull-down assay and chemical analysis was further utilized to identify the causative ligands present in fraction five that were inducing the adipogenic effects; this analysis revealed hydroxylated/polyoxygenated carboxylic acids and hydroxylated sulfates as the major PPARγ ligands inducing adipogenesis in these samples (186), though the small sample size requires further substantiation.

Another set of studies assessed the metabolic disruption potential of crude oil singly or mixed with Corexit oil dispersant mixture (266, 267). To distinguish these mixtures, they utilized several simpler mixtures in culture media, including: Corexit 9500 + MC252 oil, varying dilutions of MC252 oil, and varying dilutions of Corexit with corn oil; they found that the Corexit + oil treatments stimulated PPARγ, while the MC252 oil alone did not, suggesting a component of Corexit promoting the observed effects (267). The Corexit + oil mixture was further fractionated to determine causative ligands, with Tween 80 and dioctyl sodium sulfosuccinate (DOSS) identified as highly abundant chemicals in the active fraction (267). DOSS was further demonstrated to be active in PPAR response element-luciferase transgenic mice and stimulate triglyceride accumulation and expression of fatty acid binding protein (Fabp4) in 3T3-L1 cells (267). Follow-up work assessed the Corexit + oil mixture and Corexit alone for activation of RXRα, finding dose-dependent activation, presumably mediated by Corexit constituents (266). Constituent chemicals were further evaluated, and DOSS, Span 80, and Tween 80 all demonstrated some degree of RXRα activity, with Span 80 also stimulating triglyceride accumulation and adipocyte gene expression in 3T3-L1 cells. Interestingly, a combination of DOSS and Span 80 resulted in putative synergistic effects on adipocyte differentiation, potentially due to diverging molecular mechanisms (Span 80 exhibited a much more efficacious response for RXRα than PPARγ, while DOSS exhibited no RXRα activity but did activate PPARγ) (266).

The last set of studies, from our laboratory, evaluated unconventional oil and gas associated wastewater and chemicals. Our work on this topic began with receptor activity testing for 24 common hydraulic fracturing chemicals, reporting that 21 and 7 chemicals antagonized AR and TR in two cell-based assays, and that mixtures of these chemicals appeared to act synergistically for TR and additively for AR (36, 268). We further documented AR and TR antagonist activities in surface, ground, and/or drinking water near UOG operations in several regions, including CO, WY, WV, and ND [(268), Kassotis et al., in preparation, (269–271)], and evaluated a mixture of 23 common UOG chemicals via a gestational exposure experiment in C57 mice, reported putative metabolic effects (offspring exhibited increased body weights, among other effects) (36, 37). We further interrogated this by evaluating the ability of this 23-mix, several UOG wastewater samples, and several UOG wastewater-impacted surface water samples to stimulate adipogenesis in 3T3-L1 cells and activate PPARγ in a reporter gene assay (35). We demonstrated that UOG wastewater samples exhibited significant triglyceride accumulation and/or pre-adipocyte proliferation at relative water concentrations as low as 0.001x, UOG-impacted surface water extracts at concentrations as low as 0.04x, and the 23-mix at 1 μM; these effects co-occurred with PPARγ activation for some samples but not others (35), suggesting differing mechanisms. Related work demonstrated highly efficacious triglyceride accumulation for various non-ionic alkylphenol and alcohol polyethoxylates in the absence of PPARγ activation and potentially mediated by TR antagonism (272). These compounds are reportedly found at high concentrations in UOG wastewater (273–275) and may be responsible for some of the observed non-PPARγ-mediated effects observed in the UOG samples.

POTENTIAL UTILITY OF HIGH-THROUGHPUT DATABASES TO PREDICTING METABOLIC DISRUPTION

The costs and time investments associated with *in vivo* examination of putative metabolism disruptors are prohibitively high; as such, utilizing lower-order testing and screening is critical to target higher-order testing on chemicals most likely to be active. Application of numerous *in vitro* models for assessing putative "obesogens" or "metabolic disruptors" over the last several decades has revealed numerous contaminants capable of affecting metabolic health (18), with recent publications suggesting that these contaminants are likely common in indoor and outdoor environments (2, 184, 272). While these pre-adipocyte and mesenchymal stem cell models are useful in determining potential *in vivo* metabolic disruptors, they are also time and energy intensive and their relative abilities to correctly identify chemicals may depend on both cell line and source. Further, their mechanisms of assessing adipogenic commitment, adipocyte differentiation, adipocyte proliferation, and/or lipid accumulation may not capture the full spectrum of endpoints that compose metabolic dysfunction more broadly, particularly endpoints related to "diabetogens". As such, there is a critical need to develop better methods for correctly predicting metabolic disruptors, and while more simplistic models such as activation of PPARγ are often applied, the vast suite of mechanisms influencing this process (discussed above) require a more holistic approach to integrating causative molecular mechanisms. Several high-throughput (HTP) screening programs now exist (Tox21, ToxCast) that report activity across numerous molecular mechanisms for thousands of chemicals, many that are known to be relevant to metabolic health. Harnessing these data sets to broadly assess high-scoring chemicals (across relevant molecular pathways for select endpoints of interest) for more targeted higher-order testing may provide a valuable tool for reducing time and research costs and achieving a more broad assessment of the tens of thousands of commercial chemicals for potential contribution to adverse health outcomes in humans and/or animals.

This issue of utilizing HTP data in predictive models is not new and has been applied by a number of researchers to various *in vivo* endpoints, with varying degrees of success (276). Most of these methods have utilized ToxCast Phase I data, due to the more recent release (October 2015) of Phase II results, and as a result, some of the inherent issues reported by these studies have since been addressed. For example, Schwarzman et al. attempted to build a model to predict breast carcinogens, though had insufficient data on particular endpoints critical to altered mammary development (277). Many of the pathways missing, including prolactin, progesterone, and estrogen receptor beta effects, among others, are now pathways with associated assays in the Phase II database. Russell et al. applied a broad approach to predicting 60 *in vivo* endpoints, 56 of which were predicted at <55% accuracy (278), though notably did not aggregate assays to predict *in vivo* endpoints. Given that health outcomes are nearly always driven by overlapping molecular pathways, this is not altogether surprising. Other researchers utilized assay aggregation and were more successful in building predictive models that performed with promising accuracy (>70%). Martin et al. utilized a suite of ToxCast assays to develop a predictive model for rat reproductive toxicity, achieving ~75% accuracies for training and test sets (279). Notably, this model incorrectly predicted five of 21 external validation chemicals as predicted negatives, all of which reduced early offspring survival with limited accompanying effects on reproductive performance or reproductive tract development, suggesting a gap in assays targeting these endpoints. Another model applied ToxCast data to rat prenatal developmental toxicity, with >70% accuracy with species-specific models (280), and found that if they further refined this to more specific developmental outcomes, they got even better predictive success (80–90%). Liu et al. utilized both Phase I and Phase II data to predict hepatotoxicity (hypertrophy, injury, and proliferative lesions), and reported 53–61% accuracy using only Phase I data, but >80% when utilizing the expanded Phase II data (281).

Recently, Auerbach et al. presented predictive models of putative obesogenic and/or diabetogenic chemicals through analyzing ToxCast HTP results (282). The researchers, utilizing experts in a diversity of metabolic health disciplines, selected known molecular pathways that had been previously demonstrated to modulate metabolic health, and combined them into a combined score metric for predicting likely vs. less-likely metabolic disrupting chemicals. Janesick et al. recently tested a portion of this method, utilizing a suite of assays deemed relevant for adipocyte differentiation (16 assays across 8 molecular mechanisms) to assess 24 chemicals (11 with highest activation scores across the selected assays, 6 with medium activation scores, and 7 presumed negative controls with low activation scores) for activation of RXRα, PPARγ, and triglyceride accumulation in 3T3-L1 cells (47). They reported that 7 of 17 high and medium-scoring and 2 of 7 low-scoring chemicals were active in 3T3-L1 cells, suggesting poor predictivity (high rates of both false positives and false negatives). The authors suggested several potential hypotheses for the poor performance, including: poor performance of PPARγ assays, incorrect selection of assays for the predictive model, and improper weighting of endpoints (rather than based on mechanism importance) and assays within each endpoint (rather than based on assay performance).

We recently undertook an effort to improve the predictive utility of this model by expanding the pathways and attempting to incorporate some of the suggestions made by Janesick et al. (47). Among these, we expanded the outcome by performing a targeted literature search on all chemicals and any evidence of effects on metabolic health. This model performed best when used as a gross metabolic disruption prediction model, using literature searches to identify any *in vitro* or *in vivo* evidence of adipogenesis or disrupted metabolic health (weight gain, adipose development, insulin/glucose signaling, effects on appetite/satiety, etc.). When applied to a novel set of chemicals for which we had assessed adipogenic activities in 3T3-L1 cells (60, 184), the original prediction model performed well at predicting gross metabolic disruption; we observed low rates of both false negatives (7.9%) and false positives (7.9%), and an apparent accuracy of 84% (283).

We also attempted to bolster this model through inclusion of additional pathways known to modulate metabolic health, in hopes of reducing false negatives, though discovered that expanding the model to incorporate all of these pathways would produce an inappropriately large and unwieldy model with a considerably inflated false positive detection rate. Nonetheless, we determined that additional pathways could be incorporated into the model if there were a better method for de-selecting less important or artifactual pathways. Z score corrections were designed to address this by removing the bioactivities nearest cytotoxicity as presumed false negatives/non-specific effects. In our analysis, utilizing the cytotoxicity-derived z score values to remove putative cytotoxicity-impacted pathways was effective at reducing false positives, but at the expense of increasing false negatives. We determined that utilizing Z score corrections (even with a low threshold) was not an effective option to clarify important pathways and reduce false positives.

Results from these publications suggest that further improvements should focus on bolstering molecular pathways with poor-performing assays or where replicate experiments and/or assays are not available for a given endpoint within ToxCast. Ensuring data integrity and robustness is of profound importance to correct predictions. Efforts such as this have tremendous putative utility, as screening all chemicals and mixtures of chemicals for all endpoints is not feasible, and determining a screen of HTP assays could save tremendous time and cost and allow for a dramatically narrowed scope of testing *in vivo*. Further testing is required to substantiate this adipogenic prediction model for predicting *in vivo* metabolic disruption across a larger chemical space, but these preliminary results and success with other complex biological effects demonstrate a clear potential for implementation into predicting metabolic disruption and potentially helping reduce and better target *in vitro* and *in vivo* chemical assessments in the future.

AUTHOR CONTRIBUTIONS

CK and HS planned and outlined the proposed review. CK wrote the review, and HS read and bolstered the review via feedback and guidance.

FUNDING

Project supported by a grant (R01 ES016099) and a fellowship (F32 ES027320; CK) from the National Institute of Environmental Health Sciences.

REFERENCES

1. Chamorro-Garcia R, Sahu M, Abbey RJ, Laude J, Pham N, Blumberg B. Transgenerational inheritance of increased fat depot size, stem cell reprogramming, and hepatic steatosis elicited by prenatal exposure to the obesogen tributyltin in mice. *Environ Health Perspect.* (2013) 121:359–66. doi: 10.1289/ehp.1205701
2. Heindel JJ, vom Saal FS, Blumberg B, Bovolin P, Calamandrei G, Ceresini G, et al. Parma consensus statement on metabolic disruptors. *Environ Health* (2015) 14:54. doi: 10.1186/s12940-015-0042-7
3. Li X, Ycaza J, Blumberg B. The environmental obesogen tributyltin chloride acts via peroxisome proliferator activated receptor gamma to induce adipogenesis in murine 3T3-L1 preadipocytes. *J Steroid Biochem Mol Biol.* (2011) 127:9–15. doi: 10.1016/j.jsbmb.2011.03.012
4. Patisaul HB, Roberts SC, Mabrey N, McCaffrey KA, Gear RB, Braun J, et al. Accumulation and endocrine disrupting effects of the flame retardant mixture Firemaster(R) 550 in rats: an exploratory assessment. *J Biochem Mol Toxicol.* (2013) 27:124–36. doi: 10.1002/jbt.21439
5. Riu A, McCollum CW, Pinto CL, Grimaldi M, Hillenweck A, Perdu E, et al. Halogenated bisphenol-A analogs act as obesogens in zebrafish larvae (Danio rerio). *Toxicol Sci.* (2014) 139:48–58. doi: 10.1093/toxsci/kfu036
6. The Endocrine Disruption Exchange (TEDX). *TEDX List of Potential Endocrine Disruptors* (2018). Available online at: https://endocrinedisruption.org/interactive-tools/tedx-list-of-potential-endocrine-disruptors/search-the-tedx-list
7. Skinner AC, Ravanbakht SN, Skelton JA, Perrin EM, Armstrong SC. Prevalence of obesity and severe obesity in US children, 1999–2016. *Pediatrics* (2018) 24:1116–23. doi: 10.1542/peds.2017-3459
8. Hales CM, Carroll MD, Fryar CD, Ogden CL. *Prevalence of Obesity Among Adults and Youth: United States, 2015–2016.* Hyattsville, MD: National Center for Health Statistics (2017). Available online at: https://www.cdc.gov/nchs/data/databriefs/db288.pdf
9. Ruiz D, Becerra M, Jagai JS, Ard K, Sargis RM. Disparities in environmental exposures to endocrine-disrupting chemicals and diabetes risk in vulnerable populations. *Diabetes Care* (2018) 41:193–205. doi: 10.2337/dc16-2765
10. Yang W, Dall TM, Beronjia K, Lin J, Semilla AP, Chakrabarti R, et al. *Economic Costs of Diabetes in the U.S. in 2017. Diabetes Care* (2018) 41:917–28.
11. Biener A, Cawley J, Meyerhoefer C. The impact of obesity on medical care costs and labor market outcomes in the US. *Clin Chem.* (2018) 64:108–17. doi: 10.1373/clinchem.2017.272450
12. Klimentidis YC, Beasley TM, Lin HY, Murati G, Glass GE, Guyton M, et al. Canaries in the coal mine: a cross-species analysis of the plurality of obesity epidemics. *Proc Biol Sci.* (2011) 278:1626–32. doi: 10.1098/rspb.2010.1890
13. Brown TJ, Todd A, O'Malley C, Moore HJ, Husband AK, Bambra C, et al. Community pharmacy-delivered interventions for public health priorities: a systematic review of interventions for alcohol reduction, smoking cessation and weight management, including meta-analysis for smoking cessation. *BMJ Open* (2016) 6:e0 09828. doi: 10.1136/bmjopen-2015-009828
14. Baillie-Hamilton PF. Chemical toxins: a hypothesis to explain the global obesity epidemic. *J Altern Complement Med.* (2002) 8:185–92. doi: 10.1089/107555302317371479
15. Fu M, Sun T, Bookout AL, Downes M, Yu RT, Evans RM, et al. A nuclear receptor atlas: 3T3-L1 adipogenesis. *Mol Endocrinol.* (2005) 19:2437–50. doi: 10.1210/me.2004-0539
16. Lu C, Cheng SY. Thyroid hormone receptors regulate adipogenesis and carcinogenesis via crosstalk signaling with peroxisome proliferator-activated receptors. *J Mol Endocrinol.* (2010) 44:143–54. doi: 10.1677/JME-09-0107
17. Niemela SM, Miettinen S, Konttinen Y, Waris T, Kellomaki M, Ashammakhi NA, et al. Fat tissue: views on reconstruction and exploitation. *J Craniofac Surg.* (2007) 18:325–35. doi: 10.1097/scs.0b013e3180333b6a
18. Heindel JJ, Blumberg B, Cave M, Machtinger R, Mantovani A, Mendez MA, et al. Metabolism disrupting chemicals and metabolic disorders. *Reprod Toxicol.* (2017) 68:3–33. doi: 10.1016/j.reprotox.2016.10.001
19. Coates ME, Dickinson CD, Harrison GF, Kon SK, Cummins SH, Cuthbertson WF. Mode of action of antibiotics in stimulating growth of chicks. *Nature* (1951) 168:332. doi: 10.1038/168332a0
20. Barber RS, Braude R, Mitchell KG. Antibiotic and copper supplements for fattening pigs. *Br J Nutr.* (1955) 9:378–81. doi: 10.1079/BJN19550054
21. Cox LM, Yamanishi S, Sohn J, Alekseyenko AV, Leung JM, Cho I, et al. Altering the intestinal microbiota during a critical developmental window has lasting metabolic consequences. *Cell* (2014) 158:705–21. doi: 10.1016/j.cell.2014.05.052
22. Cho I, Yamanishi S, Cox L, Methe BA, Zavadil J, Li K, et al. Antibiotics in early life alter the murine colonic microbiome and adiposity. *Nature* (2012) 488:621–6. doi: 10.1038/nature11400
23. Ajslev TA, Andersen CS, Gamborg M, Sorensen TI, Jess T. Childhood overweight after establishment of the gut microbiota: the role of delivery mode, pre-pregnancy weight and early administration of antibiotics. *Int J Obes.* (2011) 35:522–9. doi: 10.1038/ijo.2011.27
24. Trasande L, Blustein J, Liu M, Corwin E, Cox LM, Blaser MJ. Infant antibiotic exposures and early-life body mass. *Int J Obes.* (2013) 37:16–23. doi: 10.1038/ijo.2012.132
25. Barnes AB, Colton T, Gundersen J, Noller KL, Tilley BC, Strama T, et al. Fertility and outcome of pregnancy in women exposed in utero to diethylstilbestrol. *N Engl J Med.* (1980) 302:5. doi: 10.1056/NEJM198003133021105
26. Herbst AL, Hubby MM, Blough RR, Azizi F. A comparison of pregnancy experience in DES-exposed and DES-unexposed daughters. *J Reprod Med.* (1980) 24:62–9. doi: 10.1097/00006254-198007000-00023
27. Herbst AL, Scully RE, Robboy SJ. Prenatal diethylstilbestrol exposure and human genital tract abnormalities. *Natl Cancer Inst Monogr.* (1979) 51:11.
28. Hoover RN, Hyer M, Pfeiffer RM, Adam E, Bond B, Cheville AL, et al. Adverse health outcomes in women exposed in utero to diethylstilbestrol. *N Engl J Med.* (2011) 365:1304–14. doi: 10.1056/NEJMoa1013961
29. Newbold RR, Bullock BC, Mc Lachlan JA. Exposure to diethylstilbestrol during pregnancy permanently alters the ovary and oviduct. *Biol Reprod.* (1983) 28:735–44. doi: 10.1095/biolreprod28.3.735
30. Hao CJ, Cheng XJ, Xia HF, Ma X. The endocrine disruptor diethylstilbestrol induces adipocyte differentiation and promotes obesity in mice. *Toxicol Appl Pharmacol.* (2012) 263:102–10. doi: 10.1016/j.taap.2012.06.003
31. Newbold RR, Padilla-Banks E, Jefferson WN. Environmental estrogens and obesity. *Mol Cell Endocrinol.* (2009) 304:84–9. doi: 10.1016/j.mce.2009.02.024
32. Newbold RR, Padilla-Banks E, Snyder RJ, Jefferson WN. Perinatal exposure to environmental estrogens and the development of obesity. *Mol Nutr Food Res.* (2007) 51:912–7. doi: 10.1002/mnfr.200600259
33. Newbold RR, Padilla-Banks E, Snyder RJ, Phillips TM, Jefferson WN. Developmental exposure to endocrine disruptors and the obesity epidemic. *Reprod Toxicol.* (2007) 23:290–6. doi: 10.1016/j.reprotox.2006.12.010
34. Hatch EE, Troisi R, Palmer JR, Wise LA, Titus L, Strohsnitter WC, et al. Prenatal diethylstilbestrol exposure and risk of obesity in adult women. *J Dev Orig Health Dis.* (2015) 6:201–7. doi: 10.1017/S2040174415000033
35. Kassotis CD, Nagel SC, Stapleton HM. Unconventional oil and gas chemicals and wastewater-impacted water samples promote adipogenesis via PPARγ-dependent and independent mechanisms in 3T3-L1 cells. *Sci Total Environ.* (2018) 640–1:1601–10. doi: 10.1016/j.scitotenv.2018.05.030

36. Kassotis CD, Bromfield JJ, Klemp KC, Meng CX, Wolfe A, Zoeller RT, et al. Adverse reproductive and developmental health outcomes following prenatal exposure to a hydraulic fracturing chemical mixture in female C57Bl/6 mice. *Endocrinology* (2016) 157:3469–81. doi: 10.1210/en.2016-1242
37. Kassotis CD, Klemp KC, Vu DC, Lin CH, Meng CX, Besch-Williford CL, et al. Endocrine-disrupting activity of hydraulic fracturing chemicals and adverse health outcomes after prenatal exposure in male mice. *Endocrinology* 156 (2015):4458–73. doi: 10.1210/en.2015-1375
38. Stacy SL, Brink LL, Larkin JC, Sadovsky Y, Goldstein BD, Pitt BR, et al. Perinatal outcomes and unconventional natural gas operations in southwest pennsylvania. *PLoS ONE* (2015) 10:e0126425. doi: 10.1371/journal.pone.0126425
39. McKenzie LM, Guo R, Witter RZ, Savitz DA, Newman LS, Adgate JL. Birth outcomes and maternal residential proximity to natural gas development in rural Colorado. *Environ Health Perspect.* (2014) 122:412–7. doi: 10.1289/ehp.1306722
40. Jornayvaz FR, Vollenweider P, Bochud M, Mooser V, Waeber G, Marques-Vidal P. Low birth weight leads to obesity, diabetes and increased leptin levels in adults: the CoLaus study. *Cardiovasc Diabetol.* (2016) 15:73. doi: 10.1186/s12933-016-0389-2
41. Curhan GC, Willett WC, Rimm EB, Spiegelman D, Ascherio AL, Stampfer MJ. Birth weight and adult hypertension, diabetes mellitus, and obesity in US men. *Circulation* (1996) 94:3246–50. doi: 10.1161/01.CIR.94.12.3246
42. Hirschler V, Bugna J, Roque M, Gilligan T, Gonzalez C. Does low birth weight predict obesity/overweight and metabolic syndrome in elementary school children? *Arch Med Res.* (2008) 39:796–802. doi: 10.1016/j.arcmed.2008.08.003
43. Danielzik S, Czerwinski-Mast M, Langnase K, Dilba B, Muller MJ. Parental overweight, socioeconomic status and high birth weight are the major determinants of overweight and obesity in 5–7 y-old children: baseline data of the Kiel Obesity Prevention Study (KOPS). *Int J Obes Relat Metab Disord.* (2004) 28:1494–502. doi: 10.1038/sj.ijo.0802756
44. Wolins NE, Quaynor BK, Skinner JR, Tzekov A, Park C, Choi K, et al. OP9 mouse stromal cells rapidly differentiate into adipocytes: characterization of a useful new model of adipogenesis. *J Lipid Res.* (2006) 47:450–60. doi: 10.1194/jlr.D500037-JLR200
45. Lane JM, Doyle JR, Fortin JP, Kopin AS, Ordovas JM. Development of an OP9 derived cell line as a robust model to rapidly study adipocyte differentiation. *PLoS ONE* (2014) 9:e112123. doi: 10.1371/journal.pone.0112123
46. Pillai HK, Fang M, Beglov D, Kozakov D, Vajda S, Stapleton HM, et al. Ligand binding and activation of PPARgamma by Firemaster(R) 550: effects on adipogenesis and osteogenesis in vitro. *Environ Health Perspect.* (2014) 122:1225–32. doi: 10.1289/ehp.1408111
47. Janesick AS, Dimastrogiovanni G, Vanek L, Boulos C, Chamorro-García R, Tang W, et al. On the utility of ToxCast and ToxPi as methods for identifying new obesogens. *Environ Health Perspect.* (2016) 124:1214–26. doi: 10.1289/ehp.1510352
48. Shoucri BM, Martinez ES, Abreo TJ, Hung VT, Moosova Z, Shioda T, et al. Retinoid X receptor activation alters the chromatin landscape to commit mesenchymal stem cells to the adipose lineage. *Endocrinology* (2017) 158:3109–25. doi: 10.1210/en.2017-00348
49. Rudel RA, Camann DE, Spengler JD, Korn LR, Brody JG. Phthalates, alkylphenols, pesticides, polybrominated diphenyl ethers, and other endocrine-disrupting compounds in indoor air and dust. *Environ Sci Technol.* (2003) 37:4543–53. doi: 10.1021/es0264596
50. Stapleton HM, Harner T, Shoeib M, Keller JM, Schantz MM, Leigh SD, et al. Determination of polybrominated diphenyl ethers in indoor dust standard reference materials. *Anal Bioanal Chem.* (2006) 384:791–800. doi: 10.1007/s00216-005-0227-y
51. Stapleton HM, Klosterhaus S, Eagle S, Fuh J, Meeker JD, Blum A, et al. Detection of organophosphate flame retardants in furniture foam and U.S. house dust. *Environ Sci Technol.* (2009) 43:7490–5. doi: 10.1021/es9014019
52. US Environmental Protection Agency (EPA). *Exposure Factors Handbook Chapter 5 (Update): Soil and Dust Ingestion.* Washington, DC: US EPA Office of Research and Development (2017).
53. Fraser AJ, Webster TF, Watkins DJ, Nelson JW, Stapleton HM, Calafat AM, et al. Polyfluorinated compounds in serum linked to indoor air in office environments. *Environ Sci Technol.* (2012) 46:1209–15. doi: 10.1021/es2038257
54. Watkins DJ, McClean MD, Fraser AJ, Weinberg J, Stapleton HM, Webster TF. Associations between PBDEs in office air, dust, and surface wipes. *Environ Int.* (2013) 59:124–32. doi: 10.1016/j.envint.2013.06.001
55. Hoffman K, Garantziotis S, Birnbaum LS, Stapleton HM. Monitoring indoor exposure to organophosphate flame retardants: hand wipes and house dust. *Environ Health Perspect.* (2015) 123:160–5. doi: 10.1289/ehp.1408669
56. Stapleton HM, Misenheimer J, Hoffman K, Webster TF. Flame retardant associations between children's handwipes and house dust. *Chemosphere* (2014) 116:54–60. doi: 10.1016/j.chemosphere.2013.12.100
57. Phillips AL, Hammel SC, Hoffman K, Lorenzo AM, Chen A, Webster TF, et al. Children's residential exposure to organophosphate ester flame retardants and plasticizers: Investigating exposure pathways in the TESIE study. *Environ Int.* (2018) 116:176–85. doi: 10.1016/j.envint.2018.04.013
58. Hoffman K, Webster TF, Sjodin A, Stapleton HM. Toddler's behavior and its impacts on exposure to polybrominated diphenyl ethers. *J Expo Sci Environ Epidemiol.* (2017) 27:193–7. doi: 10.1038/jes.2016.11
59. Niemelä S, Miettinen S, Sarkanen JR, Ashammakhi N. Adipose tissue and adipocyte differentiation: molecular and cellular aspects and tissue engineering applications. In: Ashammakhi N, Reis R, Chiellini F, editors. *Topics in Tissue Engineering* (2008). p. 1–26. Available online at: https://www.oulu.fi/spareparts/ebook_topics_in_t_e_vol4/
60. Kassotis CD, Masse L, Kim S, Schlezinger JJ, Webster TF, Stapleton HM. Characterization of adipogenic chemicals in three different cell culture systems: implications for reproducibility based on cell source and handling. *Sci Rep.* (2017) 7:42104. doi: 10.1038/srep42104
61. Chappell VA, Janesick A, Blumberg B, Fenton SE. Tetrabromobisphenol-A promotes early adipogenesis and lipogenesis in 3T3-L1 cells. *Toxicol Sci.* (2018) 166:332–44. doi: 10.1093/toxsci/kfy209
62. Rosen ED, Sarraf P, Troy AE, Bradwin G, Moore K, Milstone DS, et al. PPAR gamma is required for the differentiation of adipose tissue *in vivo* and *in vitro*. *Mol Cell* (1999) 4:611–7. doi: 10.1016/S1097-2765(00)80211-7
63. Rosen ED, Spiegelman BM. Molecular regulation of adipogenesis. *Annu Rev Cell Dev Biol.* (2000) 16:145–71. doi: 10.1146/annurev.cellbio.16.1.145
64. Chawla A, Schwarz EJ, Dimaculangan DD, Lazar MA. Peroxisome proliferator-activated receptor (PPAR) gamma: adipose-predominant expression and induction early in adipocyte differentiation. *Endocrinology* (1994) 135:798 800. doi: 10.1210/endo.135.2.8033830
65. Lehmann JM, Moore LB, Smith-Oliver TA, Wilkison WO, Willson TM, Kliewer SA. An antidiabetic thiazolidinedione is a high affinity ligand for peroxisome proliferator-activated receptor y (PPARy). *J Biol Chem.* (1995) 270:12953–6. doi: 10.1074/jbc.270.22.12953
66. Spiegelman BM. PPAR-gamma: adipogenic regulator and thiazolidinedione receptor. *Diabetes* (1998) 47:507–14. doi: 10.2337/diabetes.47.4.507
67. Rosen ED, C.-Hsu H, Wang X, Sakai S, Freeman MW, Gonzalez FJ, et al. C/EBP-alpha induces adipogenesis through PPAR-gamma: a unified pathway. *Genes Dev.* (2001) 16:22–6. doi: 10.1101/gad.948702
68. Matsusue K, Peters JM, Gonzalez FJ. PPARbeta/delta potentiates PPARgamma-stimulated adipocyte differentiation. *FASEB J.* (2004) 18:1477–9. doi: 10.1096/fj.04 1944fje
69. Schmuth M, Haqq CM, Cairns WJ, Holder JC, Dorsam S, Chang S, et al. Peroxisome proliferator-activated receptor (PPAR)-beta/delta stimulates differentiation and lipid accumulation in keratinocytes. *J Invest Dermatol.* (2004) 122:971–83. doi: 10.1111/j.0022-202X.2004.22412.x
70. Bastie C, Holst D, Gaillard D, Jehl-Pietri C, Grimaldi PA. Expression of peroxisome proliferator-activated receptor PPARdelta promotes induction of PPARgamma and adipocyte differentiation in 3T3C2 fibroblasts. *J Biol Chem.* (1999) 274:21920–5. doi: 10.1074/jbc.274.31.21920
71. Bastie C, Luquet S, Holst D, Jehl-Pietri C, Grimaldi PA. Alterations of peroxisome proliferator-activated receptor δ activity affect fatty acid-controlled adipose differentiation. *J Biol Chem.* (2000) 275:38768–73. doi: 10.1074/jbc.M006450200
72. Brun RP, Tontonoz P, Forman BM, Ellis R, Chen J, Evans RM, et al. Differential activation of adipogenesis by multiple PPAR isoforms. *Genes Dev.* (1996) 10:974–84. doi: 10.1101/gad.10.8.974

73. Wang YX, Lee CH, Tiep S, Yu RT, Ham J, Kang H, et al. Peroxisome-proliferator-activated receptor delta activates fat metabolism to prevent obesity. *Cell* (2003) 113:159–70. doi: 10.1016/S0092-8674(03)00269-1
74. Peters JM, Lee SS, Li W, Ward JM, Gavrilova O, Everett C, et al. Growth, adipose, brain, and skin alterations resulting from targeted disruption of the mouse peroxisome proliferator-activated receptor beta(delta). *Mol Cell Biol.* (2000) 20:5119–28. doi: 10.1128/MCB.20.14.5119-5128.2000
75. Guerre-Millo M, Gervois P, Raspe E, Madsen L, Poulain P, Derudas B, et al. Peroxisome proliferator-activated receptor alpha activators improve insulin sensitivity and reduce adiposity. *J Biol Chem.* (2000) 275:16638–42. doi: 10.1074/jbc.275.22.16638
76. Jeong S, Yoon M. Fenofibrate inhibits adipocyte hypertrophy and insulin resistance by activating adipose PPARalpha in high fat diet-induced obese mice. *Exp Mol Med.* (2009) 41:397–405. doi: 10.3858/emm.2009.41.6.045
77. Tsuchida A, Yamauchi T, Takekawa S, Hada Y, Ito Y, Maki T, et al. Peroxisome proliferator-activated receptor (PPAR)alpha activation increases adiponectin receptors and reduces obesity-related inflammation in adipose tissue: comparison of activation of PPARalpha, PPARgamma, and their combination. *Diabetes* (2005) 54:3358–70. doi: 10.2337/diabetes.54.12.3358
78. Das M, Irvin MR, Sha J, Aslibekyan S, Hidalgo B, Perry RT, et al. Lipid changes due to fenofibrate treatment are not associated with changes in DNA methylation patterns in the GOLDN study. *Front Genet.* (2015) 6:304. doi: 10.3389/fgene.2015.00304
79. Forcheron F, Cachefo A, Thevenon S, Pinteur C, Beylot M. Mechanisms of the triglyceride- and cholesterol-lowering effect of fenofibrate in hyperlipidemic type 2 diabetic patients. *Diabetes* (2002) 51:3486–91. doi: 10.2337/diabetes.51.12.3486
80. Oliver WR Jr, Shenk JL, Snaith MR, Russell CS, Plunket KD, Bodkin NL, Lewis MC, et al. A selective peroxisome proliferator-activated receptor delta agonist promotes reverse cholesterol transport. *Proc Nat Acad Sci USA.* (2001) 98:5306–11. doi: 10.1073/pnas.091021198
81. Kanayama T, Kobayashi N, Mamiya S, Nakanishi T, Nishikawa J. Organotin compounds promote adipocyte differentiation as agonists of the peroxisome proliferator-activated receptor gamma/retinoid X receptor pathway. *Mol Pharmacol.* (2005) 67:766–74. doi: 10.1124/mol.104.008409
82. Grun F, Watanabe H, Zamanian Z, Maeda L, Arima K, Cubacha R, et al. Endocrine-disrupting organotin compounds are potent inducers of adipogenesis in vertebrates. *Mol Endocrinol.* (2006) 20:2141–55. doi: 10.1210/me.2005-0367
83. Tontonoz P, Singer S, Forman BM, Sarraf P, Fletcher JA, Fletcher CD, et al. Terminal differentiation of human liposarcoma cells induced by ligands for peroxisome proliferator-activated receptor gamma and the retinoid X receptor. *Proc Nat Acad Sci USA.* (1997) 94:237–41. doi: 10.1073/pnas.94.1.237
84. Canan Koch SS, Dardashti LJ, Cesario RM, Croston GE, Boehm MF, Heyman RA, et al. Synthesis of retinoid X receptor-specific ligands that are potent inducers of adipogenesis in 3T3-L1 cells. *J Med Chem.* (1999) 42:742–50. doi: 10.1021/jm980621r
85. Nielsen R, Pedersen TA, Hagenbeek D, Moulos P, Siersbaek R, Megens E, et al. Genome-wide profiling of PPARgamma:RXR and RNA polymerase II occupancy reveals temporal activation of distinct metabolic pathways and changes in RXR dimer composition during adipogenesis. *Genes Dev.* (2008) 22:2953–67. doi: 10.1101/gad.501108
86. Imai T, Jiang M, Chambon P, Metzger D. Impaired adipogenesis and lipolysis in the mouse upon selective ablation of the retinoid X receptor alpha mediated by a tamoxifen-inducible chimeric Cre recombinase (Cre-ERT2) in adipocytes. *Proc Nat Acad Sci USA.* (2001) 98:224–8. doi: 10.1073/pnas.011528898
87. Mukherjee R, Davies PJ, Crombie DL, Bischoff ED, Cesario RM, Jow L, et al. Sensitization of diabetic and obese mice to insulin by retinoid X receptor agonists. *Nature* (1997) 386:407–10. doi: 10.1038/386407a0
88. Sadasivuni MK, Reddy BM, Singh J, Anup MO, Sunil V, Lakshmi MN, et al. CNX-013-B2, a unique pan tissue acting rexinoid, modulates several nuclear receptors and controls multiple risk factors of the metabolic syndrome without risk of hypertriglyceridemia, hepatomegaly and body weight gain in animal models. *Diabetol Metab Syndr.* (2014) 6:83. doi: 10.1186/1758-5996-6-83
89. Emilsson V, O'Dowd J, Wang S, Liu YL, Sennitt M, Heyman R, et al. The effects of rexinoids and rosiglitazone on body weight and uncoupling protein isoform expression in the Zucker fa/fa rat. *Metabolism* (2000) 49:1610–5. doi: 10.1053/meta.2000.18692
90. Shoucri BM, Hung VT, Chamorro-Garcia R, Shioda T, Blumberg B. Retinoid X receptor activation during adipogenesis of female mesenchymal stem cells programs a dysfunctional adipocyte. *Endocrinology* (2018) 159:2863–83. doi: 10.1210/en.2018-00056
91. Farol LT, Hymes KB. Bexarotene: a clinical review. *Expert Rev Anticancer Ther.* (2004) 4:180–8. doi: 10.1586/14737140.4.2.180
92. de Vries-van der Weij J, de Haan W, Hu L, Kuif M, Oei HL, van der Hoorn JW, et al. Bexarotene induces dyslipidemia by increased very low-density lipoprotein production and cholesteryl ester transfer protein-mediated reduction of high-density lipoprotein. *Endocrinology* (2009) 150:2368–75. doi: 10.1210/en.2008-1540
93. Pinaire JA, Reifel-Miller A. Therapeutic potential of retinoid x receptor modulators for the treatment of the metabolic syndrome. *PPAR Res.* (2007) 2007:94156. doi: 10.1155/2007/94156
94. Shulman AI, Mangelsdorf DJ. Retinoid x receptor heterodimers in the metabolic syndrome. *N Engl J Med.* (2005) 353:604–15. doi: 10.1056/NEJMra043590
95. Hummasti S, Laffitte BA, Watson MA, Galardi C, Chao LC, Ramamurthy L, et al. Liver X receptors are regulators of adipocyte gene expression but not differentiation: identification of apoD as a direct target. *J Lipid Res.* (2004) 45:616–25. doi: 10.1194/jlr.M300312-JLR200
96. Seo JB, Moon HM, Kim WS, Lee YS, Jeong HW, Yoo EJ, et al. Activated liver X receptors stimulate adipocyte differentiation through induction of peroxisome proliferator-activated receptor gamma expression. *Mol Cell Biol.* (2004) 24:3430–44. doi: 10.1128/MCB.24.8.3430-3444.2004
97. Juvet LK, Andresen SM, Schuster GU, Dalen KT, Tobin KA, Hollung K, et al. On the role of liver X receptors in lipid accumulation in adipocytes. *Mol Endocrinol.* (2003) 17:172–82. doi: 10.1210/me.2001-0210
98. Stenson BM, Ryden M, Venteclef N, Dahlman I, Pettersson AM, Mairal A, et al. Liver X receptor (LXR) regulates human adipocyte lipolysis. *J Biol Chem.* (2011) 286:370–9. doi: 10.1074/jbc.M110.179499
99. Gerin I, Dolinsky VW, Shackman JG, Kennedy RT, Chiang SH, Burant CF, et al. LXRbeta is required for adipocyte growth, glucose homeostasis, and beta cell function. *J Biol Chem.* (2005) 280:23024–31. doi: 10.1074/jbc.M412564200
100. Korach-Andre M, Archer A, Barros RP, Parini P, Gustafsson JA. Both liver-X receptor (LXR) isoforms control energy expenditure by regulating brown adipose tissue activity. *Proc Nat Acad Sci USA.* (2011) 108:403–8. doi: 10.1073/pnas.1017884108
101. Dahlman I, Nilsson M, Jiao H, Hoffstedt J, Lindgren CM, Humphreys K, et al. Liver X receptor gene polymorphisms and adipose tissue expression levels in obesity. *Pharmacogenet Genomics* (2006) 16:881–9. doi: 10.1097/01.fpc.0000236334.49422.48
102. Kirchgessner TG, Sleph P, Ostrowski J, Lupisella J, Ryan CS, Liu X, et al. Beneficial and adverse effects of an LXR agonist on human lipid and lipoprotein metabolism and circulating neutrophils. *Cell Metab.* (2016) 24:223–33. doi: 10.1016/j.cmet.2016.07.016
103. Gao J, Xie W. Targeting xenobiotic receptors PXR and CAR for metabolic diseases. *Trends Pharmacol Sci.* (2012) 33:552–8. doi: 10.1016/j.tips.2012.07.003
104. Moreau A, Vilarem MJ, Maurel P, Pascussi JM. Xenoreceptors CAR and PXR activation and consequences on lipid metabolism, glucose homeostasis, and inflammatory response. *Mol Pharm.* (2008) 5:35–41. doi: 10.1021/mp700103m
105. Zhou J, Febbraio M, Wada T, Zhai Y, Kuruba R, He J, et al. Hepatic fatty acid transporter Cd36 is a common target of LXR, PXR, and PPARgamma in promoting steatosis. *Gastroenterology* (2008) 134:556–67. doi: 10.1053/j.gastro.2007.11.037
106. He J, Gao J, Xu M, Ren S, Stefanovic-Racic M, O'Doherty RM, et al. PXR ablation alleviates diet-induced and genetic obesity and insulin resistance in mice. *Diabetes* (2013) 62:1876–87. doi: 10.2337/db12-1039
107. Wada T, Gao J, Xie W. PXR and CAR in energy metabolism. *Trends Endocrinol Metabol.* (2009) 20:273–9. doi: 10.1016/j.tem.2009.03.003

108. Lahtela JT, Arranto AJ, Sotaniemi EA. Enzyme inducers improve insulin sensitivity in non-insulin-dependent diabetic subjects. *Diabetes* (1985) 34:911–6. doi: 10.2337/diab.34.9.911
109. Sotaniemi EA, Karvonen I. Glucose tolerance and insulin response to glucose load before and after enzyme inducing therapy in subjects with glucose intolerance and patients with NIDDM having hyperinsulinemia or relative insulin deficiency. *Diabetes Res.* (1989) 11:131–9.
110. Jiao Y, Lu Y, Li XY. Farnesoid X receptor: a master regulator of hepatic triglyceride and glucose homeostasis. *Acta Pharmacol Sin.* (2015) 36:44–50. doi: 10.1038/aps.2014.116
111. Prawitt J, Caron S, Staels B. How to modulate FXR activity to treat the metabolic syndrome. *Drug Discov Today Dis Mech.* (2009) 6:e55–64. doi: 10.1016/j.ddmec.2010.05.002
112. Rizzo G, Disante M, Mencarelli A, Renga B, Gioiello A, Pellicciari R, et al. The farnesoid X receptor promotes adipocyte differentiation and regulates adipose cell function *in vivo*. *Mol Pharmacol.* (2006) 70:1164–73. doi: 10.1124/mol.106.023820
113. Cariou B, van Harmelen K, Duran-Sandoval D, van Dijk TH, Grefhorst A, Abdelkarim M, et al. The farnesoid X receptor modulates adiposity and peripheral insulin sensitivity in mice. *J Biol Chem.* (2006) 281:11039–49. doi: 10.1074/jbc.M510258200
114. Yang JY, Della-Fera MA, Baile CA. Guggulsterone inhibits adipocyte differentiation and induces apoptosis in 3T3-L1 cells. *Obesity* (2008) 16:16–22. doi: 10.1038/oby.2007.24
115. Watanabe M, Horai Y, Houten SM, Morimoto K, Sugizaki T, Arita E, et al. Lowering bile acid pool size with a synthetic farnesoid X receptor (FXR) agonist induces obesity and diabetes through reduced energy expenditure. *J Biol Chem.* (2011) 286:26913–20. doi: 10.1074/jbc.M111.248203
116. Rader DJ, Liver X. Receptor and farnesoid X receptor as therapeutic targets. *Am J Cardiol.* (2007) 100:15N–9N. doi: 10.1016/j.amjcard.2007.08.008
117. Abdelkarim M, Caron S, Duhem C, Prawitt J, Dumont J, Lucas A, et al. The farnesoid X receptor regulates adipocyte differentiation and function by promoting peroxisome proliferator-activated receptor-gamma and interfering with the Wnt/beta-catenin pathways. *J Biol Chem.* (2010) 285:36759–67. doi: 10.1074/jbc.M110.166231
118. Prawitt J, Abdelkarim M, Stroeve JH, Popescu I, Duez H, Velagapudi VR, et al. Farnesoid X receptor deficiency improves glucose homeostasis in mouse models of obesity. *Diabetes* (2011) 60:1861–71. doi: 10.2337/db11-0030
119. Maneschi E, Vignozzi L, Morelli A, Mello T, Filippi S, Cellai I, et al. FXR activation normalizes insulin sensitivity in visceral preadipocytes of a rabbit model of MetS. *J Endocr.* (2013) 218:215–31. doi: 10.1530/JOE-13-0109
120. Lu Y, Ma Z, Zhang Z, Xiong X, Wang X, Zhang H, et al. Yin Yang 1 promotes hepatic steatosis through repression of farnesoid X receptor in obese mice. *Gut* (2014) 63:170–8. doi: 10.1136/gutjnl-2012-303150
121. Obregon MJ. Thyroid hormone and adipocyte differentiation. *Thyroid* (2008) 18:185–95. doi: 10.1089/thy.2007.0254
122. Kolyvanos Naumann U, Furer J, Kaser L, Vetter W. Hypothyroidism. main symptoms: fatigue, weight gain, depression, myalgia, edema. *Praxis* (2007) 96:1411–7. doi: 10.1024/1661-8157.96.38.1411
123. Bratusch-Marrain P, Schmid P, Waldhausl W, Schlick W. Specific weight loss in hyperthyroidism. *Horm Metab Res.* (1978) 10:412–5. doi: 10.1055/s-0028-1093403
124. Bryzgalova G, Effendic S, Khan A, Rehnmark S, Barbounis P, Boulet J, et al. Anti-obesity, anti-diabetic, and lipid lowering effects of the thyroid receptor beta subtype selective agonist KB-141. *J Steroid Biochem Mole Biol.* (2008) 111:262–7. doi: 10.1016/j.jsbmb.2008.06.010
125. Dale J, Daykin J, Holder R, Sheppard MC, Franklyn JA. Weight gain following treatment of hyperthyroidism. *Clin Endocrinol.* (2001) 55:233–9. doi: 10.1046/j.1365-2265.2001.01329.x
126. Lonn L, Stenlof K, Ottosson M, Lindroos AK, Nystrom E, Sjostrom L. Body weight and body composition changes after treatment of hyperthyroidism. *J Clin Endocr Metabol.* (1998) 83:4269–73. doi: 10.1210/jc.83.12.4269
127. Kindblom JM, Gevers EF, Skrtic SM, Lindberg MK, Gothe S, Tornell J, et al. Increased adipogenesis in bone marrow but decreased bone mineral density in mice devoid of thyroid hormone receptors. *Bone* (2005) 36:607–16. doi: 10.1016/j.bone.2005.01.017
128. Darimont C, Gaillard D, Ailhaud G, Negrel R. Terminal differentiation of mouse preadipocyte cells: adipogenic and antimitogenic role of triiodothyronine. *Mol Cell Endocr.* (1993) 98:67–73. doi: 10.1016/0303-7207(93)90238-F
129. Jiang W, Miyamoto T, Kakizawa T, Sakuma T, Nishio S, Takeda T, et al. Expression of thyroid hormone receptor alpha in 3T3-L1 adipocytes; triiodothyronine increases the expression of lipogenic enzyme and triglyceride accumulation. *J Endocr.* (2004) 182:295–302. doi: 10.1677/joe.0.1820295
130. Flores-Delgado G, Marsch-Moreno M, Kuri-Harcuch W. Thyroid hormone stimulates adipocyte differentiation of 3T3 cells. *Mol Cell Biochem.* (1987) 76:35–43. doi: 10.1007/BF00219396
131. John K, Marino JS, Sanchez ER, Hinds TD, Jr. The glucocorticoid receptor: cause of or cure for obesity? *Am J Physiol. Endocr Metabol.* (2016) 310:E249–57. doi: 10.1152/ajpendo.00478.2015
132. Contador D, Ezquer F, Espinosa M, Arango-Rodriguez M, Puebla C, Sobrevia L, et al. Dexamethasone and rosiglitazone are sufficient and necessary for producing functional adipocytes from mesenchymal stem cells. *Exp Biol Med.* (2015) 240:1235–46. doi: 10.1177/1535370214566565
133. Vidal-Puig AJ, Considine RV, Jimenez-Linan M, Werman A, Pories WJ, Caro JF, et al. Peroxisome proliferator-activated receptor gene expression in human tissues. effects of obesity, weight loss, and regulation by insulin and glucocorticoids. *J Clin Invest* (1997) 99:2416–22. doi: 10.1172/JCI119424
134. Sargis RM, Johnson DN, Choudhury RA, Brady MJ. Environmental endocrine disruptors promote adipogenesis in the 3T3-L1 cell line through glucocorticoid receptor activation. *Obesity* (2010) 18:1283–8. doi: 10.1038/oby.2009.419
135. Asada M, Rauch A, Shimizu H, Maruyama H, Miyaki S, Shibamori M, et al. DNA binding-dependent glucocorticoid receptor activity promotes adipogenesis via Kruppel-like factor 15 gene expression. *Lab Invest.* (2011) 91:203–15. doi: 10.1038/labinvest.2010.170
136. Greenberger JS. Corticosteroid-dependent differentiation of human marrow preadipocytes *in vitro*. *in vitro* (1979) 15:823–8. doi: 10.1007/BF02618309
137. Hauner H, Schmid P, Pfeiffer EF. Glucocorticoids and insulin promote the differentiation of human adipocyte precursor cells into fat cells. *J Clin Endocrinol Metabol.* (1987) 64:832–5. doi: 10.1210/jcem-64-4-832
138. Pantoja C, Huff JT, Yamamoto KR. Glucocorticoid signaling defines a novel commitment state during adipogenesis *in vitro*. *Mol Biol Cell.* (2008) 19:4032–41. doi: 10.1091/mbc.e08-04-0420
139. Caprio M, Feve B, Claes A, Viengchareun S, Lombes M, Zennaro MC. Pivotal role of the mineralocorticoid receptor in corticosteroid-induced adipogenesis. *FASEB J.* (2007) 21:2185–94. doi: 10.1096/fj.06-7970com
140. Lee MJ, Fried SK. The glucocorticoid receptor, not the mineralocorticoid receptor, plays the dominant role in adipogenesis and adipokine production in human adipocytes. *Int J Obes.* (2014) 38:1228–33. doi: 10.1038/ijo.2014.6
141. Kershaw EE, Morton NM, Dhillon H, Ramage L, Seckl JR, Flier JS. Adipocyte-specific glucocorticoid inactivation protects against diet-induced obesity. *Diabetes* (2005) 54:1023–31. doi: 10.2337/diabetes.54.4.1023
142. Yao W, Cheng Z, Busse C, Pham A, Nakamura MC, Lane NE. Glucocorticoid excess in mice results in early activation of osteoclastogenesis and adipogenesis and prolonged suppression of osteogenesis: a longitudinal study of gene expression in bone tissue from glucocorticoid-treated mice. *Arthritis Rheum.* (2008) 58:1674–86. doi: 10.1002/art.23454
143. Nieman LK, Biller BM, Findling JW, Newell-Price J, Savage MO, Stewart PM, et al. The diagnosis of cushing's syndrome: an endocrine society clinical practice guideline. *J Clin Endocr Metabol.* (2008) 93:1526–40. doi: 10.1210/jc.2008-0125
144. Krotkiewski M, Blohme B, Lindholm N, Bjorntorp P. The effects of adrenal corticosteroids on regional adipocyte size in man. *J Clin Endocr Metabol.* (1976) 42:91–7. doi: 10.1210/jcem-42-1-91
145. Bloom SL, Sheffield JS, McIntire DD, Leveno KJ. Antenatal dexamethasone and decreased birth weight. *Obstetr Gynecol.* (2001) 97:485–90. Available online at: https://journals.lww.com/greenjournal/Fulltext/2001/04000/Antenatal_Dexamethasone_and_Decreased_Birth_Weight.1.aspx
146. Halliday H. Adverse effects of early dexamethasone treatment in extremely-low-birth-weight infants. *J Pediatr.* (2001) 139:163–4. doi: 10.1056/NEJM200101113440203
147. Cooke PS, Naaz A. Role of estrogens in adipocyte development and function. *Exp Biol Med.* (2004) 229:1127–35. doi: 10.1177/153537020422901107

148. Dieudonne MN, Pecquery R, Leneveu MC, Giudicelli Y. Opposite effects of androgens and estrogens on adipogenesis in rat preadipocytes: evidence for sex and site-related specificities and possible involvement of insulin-like growth factor 1 receptor and peroxisome proliferator-activated receptor gamma2. *Endocrinology* (2000) 141:649–56. doi: 10.1210/endo.141.2.7293
149. Roncari DA, Van RL. Promotion of human adipocyte precursor replication by 17beta-estradiol in culture. *J Clin Invest.* (1978) 62:503–8. doi: 10.1172/JCI109153
150. Hong L, Colpan A, Peptan IA. Modulations of 17-beta estradiol on osteogenic and adipogenic differentiations of human mesenchymal stem cells. *Tissue Eng.* (2006) 12:2747–53. doi: 10.1089/ten.2006.12.2747
151. Zhu P, Yuen JM, Sham KW, Cheng CH. GPER mediates the inhibitory actions of estrogen on adipogenesis in 3T3-L1 cells through perturbation of mitotic clonal expansion. *General Comp Endocrinol.* (2013) 193:19–26. doi: 10.1016/j.ygcen.2013.07.004
152. Okazaki R, Inoue D, Shibata M, Saika M, Kido S, Ooka H, et al. Estrogen promotes early osteoblast differentiation and inhibits adipocyte differentiation in mouse bone marrow stromal cell lines that express estrogen receptor (ER) alpha or beta. *Endocrinology* (2002) 143:2349–56. doi: 10.1210/endo.143.6.8854
153. Heine PA, Taylor JA, Iwamoto GA, Lubahn DB, Cooke PS. Increased adipose tissue in male and female estrogen receptor-alpha knockout mice. *Proc Nat Acad Sci USA.* (2000) 97:12729–34. doi: 10.1073/pnas.97.23.12729
154. Davis SR, Castelo-Branco C, Chedraui P, Lumsden MA, Nappi RE, Shah D, et al. Understanding weight gain at menopause. *Climacteric* (2012) 15:419–429. doi: 10.3109/13697137.2012.707385
155. Stubbins RE, Holcomb VB, Hong J, Nunez NP. Estrogen modulates abdominal adiposity and protects female mice from obesity and impaired glucose tolerance. *Eur J Nutr.* (2012) 51:861–70. doi: 10.1007/s00394-011-0266-4
156. Blouin K, Boivin A, Tchernof A. Androgens and body fat distribution. *J Steroid Biochem Mol Biol.* (2008) 108:272–80. doi: 10.1016/j.jsbmb.2007.09.001
157. O'Reilly MW, House PJ, Tomlinson JW. Understanding androgen action in adipose tissue. *J Steroid Biochem Mol Biol.* (2014) 143:277–84. doi: 10.1016/j.jsbmb.2014.04.008
158. Blouin K, Nadeau M, Perreault M, Veilleux A, Drolet R, Marceau P, et al. Effects of androgens on adipocyte differentiation and adipose tissue explant metabolism in men and women. *Clin Endocrinol.* (2010) 72:176–88. doi: 10.1111/j.1365-2265.2009.03645.x
159. Mammi C, Calanchini M, Antelmi A, Cinti F, Rosano GM, Lenzi A, et al. Androgens and adipose tissue in males: a complex and reciprocal interplay. *Int J Endocrinol.* (2012) 2012:789653. doi: 10.1155/2012/789653
160. Gupta V, Bhasin S, Guo W, Singh R, Miki R, Chauhan P, et al. Effects of dihydrotestosterone on differentiation and proliferation of human mesenchymal stem cells and preadipocytes. *Mol Cel Endocrinol.* (2008) 296:32–40. doi: 10.1016/j.mce.2008.08.019
161. Chazenbalk G, Singh P, Irge D, Shah A, Abbott DH, Dumesic DA. Androgens inhibit adipogenesis during human adipose stem cell commitment to preadipocyte formation. *Steroids* (2013) 78:920–6. doi: 10.1016/j.steroids.2013.05.001
162. Singh R, Artaza JN, Taylor WE, Gonzalez-Cadavid NF, Bhasin S. Androgens stimulate myogenic differentiation and inhibit adipogenesis in C3H 10T1/2 pluripotent cells through an androgen receptor-mediated pathway. *Endocrinology* (2003) 144:5081–8. doi: 10.1210/en.2003-0741
163. Sato T, Matsumoto T, Yamada T, Watanabe T, Kawano H, Kato S. Late onset of obesity in male androgen receptor-deficient (AR KO) mice. *Biochem Biophys Res Commun.* (2003) 300:167–71. doi: 10.1016/S0006-291X(02)02774-2
164. Diamanti-Kandarakis E, Mitrakou A, Raptis S, Tolis G, Duleba AJ. The effect of a pure antiandrogen receptor blocker, flutamide, on the lipid profile in the polycystic ovary syndrome. *J Clin Endocrinol Metabol.* (1998) 83:2699–705. doi: 10.1210/jcem.83.8.5041
165. Cusin I, Sainsbury A, Doyle P, Rohner-Jeanrenaud F, Jeanrenaud B. The ob gene and insulin. a relationship leading to clues to the understanding of obesity. *Diabetes* (1995) 44:1467–70. doi: 10.2337/diab.44.12.1467
166. Cusin I, Rohner-Jeanrenaud F, Terrettaz J, Jeanrenaud B. Hyperinsulinemia and its impact on obesity and insulin resistance. *Int J Obes Relat Metab Disord.* (1992) 16 (Suppl. 4):S1–11.
167. Jeanrenaud B. Insulin and obesity. *Diabetologia* (1979) 17:133–8. doi: 10.1007/BF01219738
168. Garten A, Schuster S, Kiess W. The insulin-like growth factors in adipogenesis and obesity. *Endocrinol Metab Clin North Am.* (2012) 41:283–95. doi: 10.1016/j.ecl.2012.04.011
169. Bournat JC, Brown CW. Mitochondrial dysfunction in obesity. *Curr Opin Endocrinol Diabet Obes.* (2010) 17:446–52. doi: 10.1097/MED.0b013e32833c3026
170. Vankoningsloo S, Piens M, Lecocq C, Gilson A, De Pauw A, Renard P, et al. Mitochondrial dysfunction induces triglyceride accumulation in 3T3-L1 cells: role of fatty acid beta-oxidation and glucose. *J Lipid Res.* (2005) 46:1133–49. doi: 10.1194/jlr.M400464-JLR200
171. Kim JA, Wei Y, Sowers JR. Role of mitochondrial dysfunction in insulin resistance. *Circul Res.* (2008) 102:401–14. doi: 10.1161/CIRCRESAHA.107.165472
172. Lim S, Cho YM, Park KS, Lee HK. Persistent organic pollutants, mitochondrial dysfunction, and metabolic syndrome. *Ann NY Acad Sci.* (2010) 1201:166–76. doi: 10.1111/j.1749-6632.2010.05622.x
173. Ren J, Pulakat L, Whaley-Connell A, Sowers JR. Mitochondrial biogenesis in the metabolic syndrome and cardiovascular disease. *J Mol Med.* (2010) 88:993–1001. doi: 10.1007/s00109-010-0663-9
174. Saben JL, Boudoures AL, Asghar Z, Thompson A, Drury A, Zhang W, et al. Maternal metabolic syndrome programs mitochondrial dysfunction via germline changes across three generations. *Cell Rep.* (2016) 16:1–8. doi: 10.1016/j.celrep.2016.05.065
175. De Pauw A, Tejerina S, Raes M, Keijer J, Arnould T. Mitochondrial (dys)function in adipocyte (de)differentiation and systemic metabolic alterations. *Am J Pathol.* (2009) 175:927–39. doi: 10.2353/ajpath.2009.081155
176. Bugger H, Abel ED. Molecular mechanisms for myocardial mitochondrial dysfunction in the metabolic syndrome. *Clin Sci.* (2008) 114:195–210. doi: 10.1042/CS20070166
177. Luz AL, Kassotis CD, Stapleton HM, Meyer JN. The high-production volume fungicide pyraclostrobin induces triglyceride accumulation associated with mitochondrial dysfunction, and promotes adipocyte differentiation independent of PPARgamma activation, in 3T3-L1 cells. *Toxicol.* (2018) 393:150–9. doi: 10.1016/j.tox.2017.11.010
178. Lu RH, Ji H, Chang ZG, Su SS, Yang GS. Mitochondrial development and the influence of its dysfunction during rat adipocyte differentiation. *Mol Biol Rep.* (2010) 37:2173–82. doi: 10.1007/s11033-009-9695-z
179. Kusminski CM, Scherer PE. Mitochondrial dysfunction in white adipose tissue. *Trends Endocrinol Metabol.* (2012) 23:435–43. doi: 10.1016/j.tem.2012.06.004
180. Medina-Gomez G. Mitochondria and endocrine function of adipose tissue. *Best Prac Res. Clin. Endocrinol Metabol.* (2012) 26:791–804. doi: 10.1016/j.beem.2012.06.002
181. U. Survey SG. Estimated annual agricultural pesticide use - pyraclostrobin. In: U.S.D.o. Interior, editor. *Pesticide National Synthesis Project* (2016). Available online at: https://water.usgs.gov/nawqa/pnsp/usage/maps/show_map.php?year=2016&map=PYRACLOSTROBIN&hilo=L
182. Pearson BL, Simon JM, McCoy ES, Salazar G, Fragola G, Zylka MJ. Identification of chemicals that mimic transcriptional changes associated with autism, brain aging and neurodegeneration. *Nature Commun.* (2016) 7:11173. doi: 10.1038/ncomms11173
183. Bartlett DW, Clough JM, Godwin JR, Hall AA, Hamer M, Parr-Dobrzanski B. The strobilurin fungicides. *Pest Manag Sci.* (2002) 58:649–62. doi: 10.1002/ps.520
184. Kassotis CD, Hoffman K, Stapleton HM. Characterization of adipogenic activity of semi-volatile indoor contaminants and house dust. *Environ Sci Technol In* (2017) 51:8735–45. doi: 10.1021/acs.est.7b01788
185. Foley B, Doheny DL, Black MB, Pendse SN, Wetmore BA, Clewell RA, et al. Screening toxcast prioritized chemicals for PPARG function in a human adipose-derived stem cell model of adipogenesis. *Toxicol Sci.* (2017) 155:85–100. doi: 10.1093/toxsci/kfw186
186. Peng H, Sun J, Alharbi HA, Jones PD, Giesy JP, Wiseman S. Peroxisome proliferator-activated receptor γ is a sensitive target for oil sands

process-affected water: effects on adipogenesis and identification of ligands. *Environ Sci Technol.* (2016) 50:7816–24. doi: 10.1021/acs.est.6b 01890
187. Rundle K, Sharaf M, Stevens D, Kamunde C, Van Den Heuvel MR. Oil sands-derived naphthenic acids are oxidative uncouplers and impair electron transport in isolated mitochondria. *Environ Sci Technol.* (2018) 52:10803–11. doi: 10.1021/acs.est.8b02638
188. Tormos KV, Anso E, Hamanaka RB, Eisenbart J, Joseph J, Kalyanaraman B, et al. Mitochondrial complex III ROS regulate adipocyte differentiation. *Cell Metab.* (2011) 14:537–44. doi: 10.1016/j.cmet.2011.08.007
189. Wang X, Hai C. Redox modulation of adipocyte differentiation: hypothesis of "Redox Chain" and novel insights into intervention of adipogenesis and obesity. *Free Radic Biol Med.* (2015) 89:99–125. doi: 10.1016/j.freeradbiomed.2015.07.012
190. Lee H, Lee YJ, Choi H, Ko EH, Kim JW. Reactive oxygen species facilitate adipocyte differentiation by accelerating mitotic clonal expansion. *J Biol Chem.* (2009) 284:10601–9. doi: 10.1074/jbc.M808742200
191. Carriere A, Carmona MC, Fernandez Y, Rigoulet M, Wenger RH, Penicaud L, et al. Mitochondrial reactive oxygen species control the transcription factor CHOP-10/GADD153 and adipocyte differentiation: a mechanism for hypoxia-dependent effect. *J Biol Chem.* (2004) 279:40462–9. doi: 10.1074/jbc.M407258200
192. Carriere A, Fernandez Y, Rigoulet M, Penicaud L, Casteilla L. Inhibition of preadipocyte proliferation by mitochondrial reactive oxygen species. *FEBS Lett.* (2003) 550:163–7. doi: 10.1016/S0014-5793(03) 00862-7
193. Kanda Y, Hinata T, Kang SW, Watanabe Y. Reactive oxygen species mediate adipocyte differentiation in mesenchymal stem cells. *Life Sci.* (2011) 89:250–8. doi: 10.1016/j.lfs.2011.06.007
194. Lee HK, Cho YM, Kwak SH, Lim S, Park KS, Shim EB. Mitochondrial dysfunction and metabolic syndrome-looking for environmental factors. *Biochim Biophys Acta* (2010) 1800:282–9. doi: 10.1016/j.bbagen.2009.11.010
195. Lim S, Ahn SY, Song IC, Chung MH, Jang HC, Park KS, et al. Chronic exposure to the herbicide, atrazine, causes mitochondrial dysfunction and insulin resistance. *PLoS ONE* (2009) 4:e5186. doi: 10.1371/journal.pone.0005186
196. Shen K, Shen C, Yu J, Yu C, Chen L, Shi D, et al. PCB congeners induced mitochondrial dysfunction in Vero cells. *J Hazard Mater.* (2011) 185:24–8. doi: 10.1016/j.jhazmat.2010.08.061
197. Aly HA, Domenech O. Aroclor 1254 induced cytotoxicity and mitochondrial dysfunction in isolated rat hepatocytes. *Toxicology* (2009) 262:175–83. doi: 10.1016/j.tox.2009.05.018
198. Gray SL, Shaw AC, Gagne AX, Chan HM. Chronic exposure to PCBs (Aroclor 1254) exacerbates obesity-induced insulin resistance and hyperinsulinemia in mice. *J Toxicol Environ Health. Part A* (2013) 76:701–15. doi: 10.1080/15287394.2013.796503
199. Donat-Vargas C, Gea A, Sayon-Orea C, Carlos S, Martinez-Gonzalez MA, Bes-Rastrollo M. Association between dietary intakes of PCBs and the risk of obesity: the SUN project. *J Epidemiol Commun Health* (2014) 68:834–41. doi: 10.1136/jech-2013-203752
200. Lee DH, Steffes MW, Sjodin A, Jones RS, Needham LL, Jacobs DR Jr. Low dose organochlorine pesticides and polychlorinated biphenyls predict obesity, dyslipidemia, and insulin resistance among people free of diabetes. *PLoS ONE* (2011) 6:e15977. doi: 10.1371/journal.pone.0015977
201. Tanaka T, Morita A, Kato M, Hirai T, Mizoue T, Terauchi Y, et al. Congener-specific polychlorinated biphenyls and the prevalence of diabetes in the Saku Control Obesity Program (SCOP). *Endocr J.* (2011) 58:589–96. doi: 10.1507/endocrj.K10E-361
202. Dirinck E, Jorens PG, Covaci A, Geens T, Roosens L, Neels H, et al. Obesity and persistent organic pollutants: possible obesogenic effect of organochlorine pesticides and polychlorinated biphenyls. *Obesity* (2011) 19:709–14. doi: 10.1038/oby.2010.133
203. Poulos SP, Dodson MV, Hausman GJ. Cell line models for differentiation: preadipocytes and adipocytes. *Exp Biol Med.* (2010) 235:1185–93. doi: 10.1258/ebm.2010.010063
204. Ruiz-Ojeda FJ, Ruperez AI, Gomez-Llorente C, Gil A, Aguilera CM. Cell models and their application for studying adipogenic differentiation in relation to obesity: a review. *Int J Mol Sci.* (2016) 17:E1040. doi: 10.3390/ijms17071040
205. Green H, Kehinde O. An established preadipose cell line and its differentiation in culture. II. Factors affecting the adipose conversion. *Cell* (1975) 5:19–27. doi: 10.1016/0092-8674(75)90087-2
206. Green H, Meuth M. An established pre-adipose cell line and its differentiation in culture. *Cell* (1974) 3:127–33. doi: 10.1016/0092-8674(74)90116-0
207. Guo X, Liao K. Analysis of gene expression profile during 3T3-L1 preadipocyte differentiation. *Gene* (2000) 251:45–53. doi: 10.1016/S0378-1119(00)00192-X
208. Kleensang A, Vantangoli MM, Odwin-DaCosta S, Andersen ME, Boekelheide K, Bouhifd M, et al. Genetic variability in a frozen batch of MCF-7 cells invisible in routine authentication affecting cell function. *Sci Rep.* (2016) 6:28994. doi: 10.1038/srep28994
209. Janderova L, McNeil M, Murrell AN, Mynatt RL, Smith SR. Human mesenchymal stem cells as an in vitro model for human adipogenesis. *Obes Res.* (2003) 11:65–74. doi: 10.1038/oby.2003.11
210. Muruganandan S, Roman AA, Sinal CJ. Adipocyte differentiation of bone marrow-derived mesenchymal stem cells: cross talk with the osteoblastogenic program. *Cel Mol Life Sci.* (2009) 66:236–53. doi: 10.1007/s00018-008-8429-z
211. Yue R, Zhou BO, Shimada IS, Zhao Z, Morrison SJ. Leptin receptor promotes adipogenesis and reduces osteogenesis by regulating mesenchymal stromal cells in adult bone marrow. *Cell Stem Cell* (2016) 18:782–96. doi: 10.1016/j.stem.2016.02.015
212. Csaki C, Matis U, Mobasheri A, Ye H, Shakibaei M. Chondrogenesis, osteogenesis and adipogenesis of canine mesenchymal stem cells: a biochemical, morphological and ultrastructural study. *Histochem Cell Biol.* (2007) 128:507–20. doi: 10.1007/s00418-007-0337-z
213. Kim S, Li A, Monti S, Schlezinger JJ. Tributyltin induces a transcriptional response without a brite adipocyte signature in adipocyte models. *Arch Toxicol.* (2018) 92:2859–74. doi: 10.1007/s00204-018-2268-y
214. Tang QQ, Otto TC, Lane MD. Commitment of C3H10T1/2 pluripotent stem cells to the adipocyte lineage. *Proc Nat Acad Sci USA.* (2004) 101:9607–11. doi: 10.1073/pnas.0403100101
215. Katagiri T, Yamaguchi A, Ikeda T, Yoshiki S, Wozney JM, Rosen V, et al. The non-osteogenic mouse pluripotent cell line, C3H10T1/2, is induced to differentiate into osteoblastic cells by recombinant human bone morphogenetic protein 2. *Biochem Biophys Res Commun* (1990) 172:295–9. doi: 10.1016/S0006-291X(05)80208-6
216. Wang W, Itaka K, Ohba S, Nishiyama N, Chung UI, Yamasaki Y, et al. 3D spheroid culture system on micropatterned substrates for improved differentiation efficiency of multipotent mesenchymal stem cells. *Biomaterials* (2009) 30:2705–15. doi: 10.1016/j.biomaterials.2009.01.030
217. Baraniak PR, McDevitt TC. Scaffold-free culture of mesenchymal stem cell spheroids in suspension preserves multilineage potential. *Cell Tissue Res.* (2012) 347:701–11. doi: 10.1007/s00441-011-1215-5
218. Cheng NC, Wang S, Young TH. The influence of spheroid formation of human adipose-derived stem cells on chitosan films on stemness and differentiation capabilities. *Biomaterials* (2012) 33:1748–58. doi: 10.1016/j.biomaterials.2011.11.049
219. Turner PA, Gurumurthy B, Bailey JL, Elks CM, Janorkar AV. Adipogenic differentiation of human adipose-derived stem cells grown as spheroids. *Process Biochem.* (2017) 59:312–20. doi: 10.1016/j.procbio.2017.02.003
220. Turner PA, Harris LM, Purser CA, Baker RC, Janorkar AV. A surface-tethered spheroid model for functional evaluation of 3T3-L1 adipocytes. *Biotechnol Bioeng.* (2014) 111:174–83. doi: 10.1002/bit.25099
221. Miyagawa Y, Okita H, Hiroyama M, Sakamoto R, Kobayashi M, Nakajima H, et al. A microfabricated scaffold induces the spheroid formation of human bone marrow-derived mesenchymal progenitor cells and promotes efficient adipogenic differentiation. *Tissue Eng Part A.* (2011) 17:513–21. doi: 10.1089/ten.tea.2009.0810
222. Kapur SK, Wang X, Shang H, Yun S, Li X, Feng G, et al. Human adipose stem cells maintain proliferative, synthetic and multipotential properties when suspension cultured as self-assembling spheroids. *Biofabrication* (2012) 4:025004. doi: 10.1088/1758-5082/4/2/025004

223. Saxton D. *Toxic Substances Control Act Inventory.* US Environmental Protection Agency (2014).
224. Markell D. An overview of TSCA, its history and key underlying assumptions, and its place in environmental regulation. *Washington Univ J Law Pol.* (2010) 32:42. Available online at: https://openscholarship.wustl.edu/law_journal_law_policy/vol32/iss1/11/
225. D.o.H.a.Services H. *National Report on Human Exposure to Environmental Chemicals.* Centers for Disease Control and Prevention (2015).
226. Houlihan J, Kropp T, Wiles R, Gray S, Campbell C. *BodyBurden: The Pollution in Newborns.* Environmental Working Group (2005).
227. Silva E, Rajapakse N, Kortenkamp A. Something from "nothing"–eight weak estrogenic chemicals combined at concentrations below NOECs produce significant mixture effects. *Environ Sci Technol.* (2002) 36:1751–6. doi: 10.1021/es0101227
228. Rajapakse N, Silva E, Kortenkamp A. Combining xenoestrogens at levels below individual no-observed-effect concentrations dramatically enhances steroid hormone action. *Environ Health Perspect.* (2002) 110:917–21. doi: 10.1289/ehp.02110917
229. Christiansen S, Scholze M, Axelstad M, Boberg J, Kortenkamp A, Hass U. Combined exposure to anti-androgens causes markedly increased frequencies of hypospadias in the rat. *Int J Androl.* (2008) 31:241–8. doi: 10.1111/j.1365-2605.2008.00866.x
230. Orton F, Rosivatz E, Scholze M, Kortenkamp A. Competitive androgen receptor antagonism as a factor determining the predictability of cumulative antiandrogenic effects of widely used pesticides. *Environ Health Perspect.* (2012) 120:1578–84. doi: 10.1289/ehp.1205391
231. Thrupp TJ, Runnalls TJ, Scholze M, Kugathas S, Kortenkamp A, Sumpter JP. The consequences of exposure to mixtures of chemicals: Something from 'nothing' and 'a lot from a little' when fish are exposed to steroid hormones. *Sci Total Environ.* (2018) 619–20:1482–92. doi: 10.1016/j.scitotenv.2017.11.081
232. Zhao LJ, Ying GG, Yang B, Liu SL, Zhou J, Chen FZ, et al. Screening of multiple hormonal activities in surface water and sediment from the Pearl River system, South China, using effect-directed in vitro bioassays. *Environ Toxicol Chem.* (2011) 30:2208–15. doi: 10.1002/etc.625
233. Soto AM, Calabro JM, Prechtl NV, Yau AY, Orlando EF, Daxenberger A, et al. Androgenic and estrogenic activity in water bodies receiving cattle feedlot effluent in Eastern Nebraska, USA. Environ Health Perspect. (2003) 112:346–52. doi: 10.1289/ehp.6590
234. Pawlowski S, Ternes TA, Bonerz M, Rastall AC, Erdinger L, Braunbeck T. Estrogenicity of solid phase-extracted water samples from two municipal sewage treatment plant effluents and river Rhine water using the yeast estrogen screen. *Toxicol in vitro* (2004) 18:129–38. doi: 10.1016/j.tiv.2003.08.006
235. Shi W, Hu X, Zhang F, Hu G, Hao Y, Zhang X, et al. Occurrence of thyroid hormone activities in drinking water from eastern China: contributions of phthalate esters. *Environ Sci Technol.* (2012) 46:1811–8. doi: 10.1021/es202625r
236. Schriks M, Van Leerdam JASC, Van Der Linden B, Van Der Burg, Van Wezel AP, De Voogt P. High-resolution mass spectrometric identification and quantification of glucocorticoid compounds in various Wastewaters in The Netherlands. *Environ Sci Technol.* (2010) 44:4766–74. doi: 10.1021/es100013x
237. Van der Linden SC, Heringa MB, Man HY, Sonneveld E, Puijker LM, Brouwer A, et al. Detection of multiple hormonal activities in wastewater effluents and surface water, using a panel of steroid receptor CALUX bioassays. *Environ Sci Technol.* (2008) 42:5814–20. doi: 10.1021/es702897y
238. Stavreva DA, George AA, Klausmeyer P, Varticovski L, Sack D, Voss TC, et al. Prevalent glucocorticoid and androgen activity in US water sources. *Sci Rep.* (2012) 2:937. doi: 10.1038/srep00937
239. Liu S, Ying GG, Zhou LJ, Zhang RQ, Chen ZF, Lai HJ. Steroids in a typical swine farm and their release into the environment. *Water Res.* (2012) 46:3754–68. doi: 10.1016/j.watres.2012.04.006
240. Rostkowski P, Horwood J, Shears JA, Lange A, Oladapo FO, Besselink HT, et al. Bioassay-Directed identification of novel antiandrogenic compounds in bile of fish exposed to wastewater effluents. *Environ Sci Technol.* (2011) 45:10660–7. doi: 10.1021/es202966c
241. Kortenkamp A, Scholze M, Ermler S. Mind the gap: can we explain declining male reproductive health with known antiandrogens? *Reproduction* (2014) 147:515–27. doi: 10.1530/REP-13-0440
242. Office of Prevention, Toxic Substances. *OPPTS 890.1300: Estrogen Receptor Transcriptional Activation (Human Cell Line (HeLa-9903))* (2009). p. 23.
243. Naylor LH. Reporter gene technology: the future looks bright. *Biochem Pharmacol.* (1999) 58:749–57. doi: 10.1016/S0006-2952(99)00096-9
244. Soto AM, Maffini MV, Schaeberle CM, Sonnenschein C. Strengths and weaknesses of *in vitro* assays for estrogenic and androgenic activity. *Best Pract Res Clin Endocrinol Metabol.* (2006) 20:15–33. doi: 10.1016/j.beem.2005.09.001
245. Kruger T, Hjelmborg PS, Jonsson BA, Hagmar L, Giwercman A, Manicardi GC, et al. Xenoandrogenic activity in serum differs across European and Inuit populations. *Environ Health Perspect.* (2007) 115 (Suppl. 1):21–7. doi: 10.1289/ehp.9353
246. Lopez-Espinosa MJ, Silva E, Granada A, Molina-Molina JM, Fernandez MF, Aguilar-Garduno C, et al. Assessment of the total effective xenoestrogen burden in extracts of human placentas. *Biomarkers* (2009) 14:271–7. doi: 10.1080/13547500902893744
247. Fernandez MF, Aguilar-Garduno C, Molina-Molina JM, Arrebola JP, Olea N. The total effective xenoestrogen burden, a biomarker of exposure to xenoestrogen mixtures, is predicted by the (anti)estrogenicity of its components. *Reprod Toxicol.* (2008) 26:8–12. doi: 10.1016/j.reprotox.2008.06.002
248. Arrebola JP, Fernandez MF, Molina-Molina JM, Martin-Olmedo P, Exposito J, Olea N. Predictors of the total effective xenoestrogen burden (TEXB) in human adipose tissue. A pilot study. *Reprod Toxicol.* (2012) 33:45–52. doi: 10.1016/j.reprotox.2011.10.015
249. Fernandez MF, Molina-Molina JM, Lopez-Espinosa MJ, Freire C, Campoy C, Ibarluzea J, et al. Biomonitoring of environmental estrogens in human tissues. *Int J Hyg Environ Health* (2007) 210:429–32. doi: 10.1016/j.ijheh.2007.01.014
250. Fernandez MF, Santa-Marina L, Ibarluzea JM, Exposito J, Aurrekoetxea JJ, Torne P, et al. Analysis of population characteristics related to the total effective xenoestrogen burden: a biomarker of xenoestrogen exposure in breast cancer. *Eur J Cancer* (2007) 43:1290–9. doi: 10.1016/j.ejca.2007.03.010
251. Yordy JE, Mollenhauer MA, Wilson RM, Wells RS, Hohn A, Sweeney J, et al. Complex contaminant exposure in cetaceans: a comparative E-Screen analysis of bottlenose dolphin blubber and mixtures of four persistent organic pollutants. *Environ Toxicol Chem.* (2010) 29:2143–53. doi: 10.1002/etc.279
252. Fernandez MF, Olmos B, Granada A, Lopez-Espinosa MJ, Molina-Molina JM, Fernandez JM, et al. Human exposure to endocrine-disrupting chemicals and prenatal risk factors for cryptorchidism and hypospadias: a nested case-control study. *Environ Health Perspect.* (2007) 115 (Suppl. 1):8–14. doi: 10.1289/ehp.9351
253. Vilahur N, Fernandez MF, Bustamante M, Ramos R, Forns J, Ballester F, et al. In utero exposure to mixtures of xenoestrogens and child neuropsychological development. *Environ Res.* (2014) 134C:98–104. doi: 10.1016/j.envres.2014.07.002
254. Ibarluzea Jm J, Fernandez MF, Santa-Marina L, Olea-Serrano MF, Rivas AM, Aurrekoetxea JJ, et al. Breast cancer risk and the combined effect of environmental estrogens. *Cancer Causes Control* (2004) 15:591–600. doi: 10.1023/B:CACO.0000036167.51236.86
255. Vilahur N, Molina-Molina JM, Bustamante M, Murcia M, Arrebola JP, Ballester F, et al. Male specific association between xenoestrogen levels in placenta and birthweight. *Environ Int.* (2013) 51:174–81. doi: 10.1016/j.envint.2012.10.004
256. Arrebola JP, Pumarega J, Gasull M, Fernandez MF, Martin-Olmedo P, Molina-Molina JM, et al. Adipose tissue concentrations of persistent organic pollutants and prevalence of type 2 diabetes in adults from Southern Spain. *Environ Res.* (2013) 122:31–7. doi: 10.1016/j.envres.2012.12.001
257. Ruzzin J, Lee DH, Carpenter DO, Jacobs DR, Jr. Reconsidering metabolic diseases: the impacts of persistent organic pollutants. *Atherosclerosis* (2012) 224:1–3. doi: 10.1016/j.atherosclerosis.2012.02.039
258. Chou HP, Lee HC, Ko CF, Lin JY, Kawanishi M, Yagi T, et al. Detection of hormone-like and genotoxic activities in indoor dust from taiwan using

a battery of in vitro bioassays. *Aerosol Air Qual Res.* (2015) 15:1412–21. doi: 10.4209/aaqr.2015.06.0404
259. Suzuki G, Takigami H, Nose K, Takahashi S, Asari M, Sakai S. Dioxin-like and transthyretin-binding compounds in indoor dusts collected from Japan: average daily dose and possible implications for children. *Environ Sci Technol.* (2007) 41:1487–93. doi: 10.1021/es061907l
260. Suzuki G, Tue NM, Malarvannan G, Sudaryanto A, Takahashi S, Tanabe S, et al. Similarities in the endocrine-disrupting potencies of indoor dust and flame retardants by using human osteosarcoma (U2OS) cell-based reporter gene assays. *Environm Sci Technol.* (2013) 47:2898–908. doi: 10.1021/es304691a
261. Fang M, Webster TF, Ferguson PL, Stapleton HM. Characterizing the peroxisome proliferator-activated receptor (PPARgamma) ligand binding potential of several major flame retardants, their metabolites, and chemical mixtures in house dust. *Environ Health Perspect.* (2015) 123:166–72. doi: 10.1289/ehp.1408522
262. Fang M, Webster TF, Stapleton HM. Activation of human peroxisome proliferator-activated nuclear receptors (PPARgamma1) by semi-volatile compounds (SVOCs) and chemical mixtures in indoor dust. *Environ Sci Technol.* (2015) 49:10057–64. doi: 10.1021/acs.est.5b01523
263. Fang M, Webster TF, Stapleton HM. Effect-directed analysis of human peroxisome proliferator-activated nuclear receptors (PPARgamma1) ligands in indoor dust. *Environ Sci Technol.* (2015) 49:10065–73. doi: 10.1021/acs.est.5b01524
264. Kassotis, CD, Kollitz, EM, Hoffman, K, Sosa, JA, and Stapleton, HM. Thyroid receptor antagonism as a contributory mechanism for adipogenesis induced by environmental mixtures in 3T3-L1 cells. (in press).
265. Kollitz EM, Kassotis CD, Hoffman K, Ferguson PL, Sosa JA, Stapleton HM. Chemical mixtures isolated from house dust disrupt thyroid receptor β (TRβ) signaling. *Environ Sci Technol.* (2018) 52:11857–64. doi: 10.1021/acs.est.8b03283
266. Bowers RR, Temkin AM, Guillette LJ, Baatz JE, Spyropoulos DD. The commonly used nonionic surfactant Span 80 has RXRalpha transactivation activity, which likely increases the obesogenic potential of oil dispersants and food emulsifiers. *General Comparat Endocrinol.* (2016) 238:61–8. doi: 10.1016/j.ygcen.2016.04.029
267. Temkin AM, Bowers RR, Magaletta ME, Holshouser S, Maggi A, Ciana P, et al. Effects of crude oil/dispersant mixture and dispersant components on ppargamma activity and : identification of dioctyl sodium sulfosuccinate (DOSS; CAS #577–11–7) as a probable obesogen. *Environ Health Perspect.* (2015) 124:112–19. doi: 10.1289/ehp.1409672
268. Kassotis CD, Tillitt DE, Davis JW, Hormann AM, Nagel SC. Estrogen and androgen receptor activities of hydraulic fracturing chemicals and surface and ground water in a drilling-dense region. *Endocrinology* (2014) 155:897–907. doi: 10.1210/en.2013-1697
269. Kassotis CD, Iwanowicz LR, Akob DM, Cozzarelli IM, Mumford AC, Orem WH, et al. Endocrine disrupting activities of surface water associated with a West Virginia oil and gas industry wastewater disposal site. *Sci Total Environ.* (2016) 557–8:901–10. doi: 10.1016/j.scitotenv.2016.03.113
270. Kassotis CD, Vu DC, Vo PH, Lin HC, Cornelius-Green JN, Patton S, et al. Endocrine disrupting activities and organic contaminants associated with oil and gas operations in wyoming groundwater. *Arch Environ Contamin Toxicol.* (2018) 75:247–58. doi: 10.1007/s00244-018-0521-2
271. Cozzarelli IM, Skalak KJ, Kent DB, Engle MA, Benthem A, Mumford AC, et al. Environmental signatures and effects of an oil and gas wastewater spill in the Williston Basin, North Dakota. *Sci Total Environ.* (2017) 579:1781–93. doi: 10.1016/j.scitotenv.2016.11.157
272. Kassotis CD, Kollitz EM, Ferguson PL, Stapleton HM. Nonionic ethoxylated surfactants induce adipogenesis in 3T3-L1 cells. *Toxicol Sci.* (2018) 162:124–36. doi: 10.1093/toxsci/kfx234
273. Getzinger GJ, O'Connor MP, Hoelzer K, Drollette BD, Karatum O, Deshusses MA, et al. Natural gas residual fluids: sources, endpoints, and organic chemical composition after centralized waste treatment in Pennsylvania. *Environ Sci Technol.* (2015) 49:8347–55. doi: 10.1021/acs.est.5b00471
274. Ferrer I, Thurman EM. Chemical constituents and analytical approaches for hydraulic fracturing waters. *Trends Environ Anal Chem.* (2015) 5:18–25. doi: 10.1016/j.teac.2015.01.003
275. Thurman EM, Ferrer I, Blotevogel J, Borch T. Analysis of hydraulic fracturing flowback and produced waters using accurate mass: identification of ethoxylated surfactants. *Anal Chem.* (2014) 86:9653–61. doi: 10.1021/ac502163k
276. Knudsen TB, Keller DA, Sander M, Carney EW, Doerrer NG, Eaton DL, et al. FutureTox II: *in vitro* data and in silico models for predictive toxicology. *Toxicol Sci.* (2015) 143:256–67. doi: 10.1093/toxsci/kfu234
277. Schwarzman MR, Ackerman JM, Dairkee SH, Fenton SE, Johnson D, Navarro KM, et al. Screening for chemical contributions to breast cancer risk: a case study for chemical safety evaluation. *Environ Health Perspect.* (2015) 123:1255–64. doi: 10.1289/ehp.1408337
278. Thomas RS, Black MB, Li L, Healy E, Chu TM, Bao W, et al. A comprehensive statistical analysis of predicting in vivo hazard using high-throughput in vitro screening. *Toxicol Sci.* (2012) 128:398–417. doi: 10.1093/toxsci/kfs159
279. Martin MT, Knudsen TB, Reif DM, Houck KA, Judson RS, Kavlock RJ, et al. Predictive model of rat reproductive toxicity from ToxCast high throughput screening. *Biol Reprod.* (2011) 85:327–39. doi: 10.1095/biolreprod.111.090977
280. Sipes NS, Martin MT, Reif DM, Kleinstreuer NC, Judson RS, Singh AV, et al. Predictive models of prenatal developmental toxicity from ToxCast high-throughput screening data. *Toxicol Sci.* (2011) 124:109–27. doi: 10.1093/toxsci/kfr220
281. Liu J, Mansouri K, Judson RS, Martin MT, Hong H, Chen M, et al. Predicting hepatotoxicity using ToxCast in vitro bioactivity and chemical structure. *Chem Res Toxicol.* (2015) 28:738–51. doi: 10.1021/tx500501h
282. Auerbach S, Filer D, Reif D, Walker V, Holloway AC, Schlezinger J, et al. Prioritizing environmental chemicals for obesity and diabetes outcomes research: a screening approach using toxcast high-throughput data. *Environ Health Perspect.* (2016) 124:1141–54. doi: 10.1289/ehp.1510456
283. Kassotis CD, Hoffman K, Filer D, Stapleton HM. Building a Predictive Model with ToxCast Data to Evaluate Potential Metabolic Disruption by Environmental Chemicals. (in press).

18

Interventions to Address Environmental Metabolism-Disrupting Chemicals: Changing the Narrative to Empower Action to Restore Metabolic Health

Robert M. Sargis*[1]*, Jerrold J. Heindel[2] and Vasantha Padmanabhan[3]

[1] Department of Medicine, University of Illinois at Chicago, Chicago, IL, United States, [2] Program on Endocrine Disruption Strategies, Commonweal, Bolinas, CA, United States, [3] Department of Pediatrics, University of Michigan, Ann Arbor, MI, United States

***Correspondence:**
Robert M. Sargis
rsargis@uic.edu

Metabolic disease rates have increased dramatically over the last four decades. Classic understanding of metabolic physiology has attributed these global trends to decreased physical activity and caloric excess; however, these traditional risk factors insufficiently explain the magnitude and rapidity of metabolic health deterioration. Recently, the novel contribution of environmental metabolism-disrupting chemicals (MDCs) to various metabolic diseases (including obesity, diabetes, and non-alcoholic fatty liver disease) is becoming recognized. As this burgeoning body of evidence has matured, various organic and inorganic pollutants of human and natural origin have emerged as metabolic disease risk factors based on population-level and experimental data. Recognition of these heretofore underappreciated metabolic stressors now mandates that efforts to mitigate the devastating consequences of metabolic disease include dedicated efforts to address environmental drivers of disease risk; however, there have not been adequate recommendations to reduce exposures or to mitigate the effects of exposures on disease outcomes. To address this knowledge gap and advance the clinical translation of MDC science, herein discussed are behaviors that increase exposures to MDCs, interventional studies to reduce those exposures, and small-scale clinical trials to reduce the body burden of MDCs. Also, we discuss evidence from cell-based and animal studies that provide insights into MDC mechanisms of action, the influence of modifiable dietary factors on MDC toxicity, and factors that modulate MDC transplacental carriage as well as their impact on metabolic homeostasis. A particular emphasis of this discussion is on critical developmental windows during which short-term MDC exposure can elicit long-term disruptions in metabolic health with potential inter- and transgenerational effects. While data gaps remain and further studies are needed, the current state of evidence regarding interventions to address MDC exposures illuminates approaches to address environmental drivers of metabolic disease risk. It is now incumbent on clinicians and public health agencies to incorporate this knowledge into comprehensive strategies to address the metabolic disease pandemic.

Keywords: diabetes, endocrine disruptor, non-alcoholic fatty liver disease, intervention, metabolism, obesity, metabolism-disrupting chemical

CHANGING THE NARRATIVE OF ENVIRONMENTAL HEALTH

The desire to live a healthy, disease-free life is universal; however, this goal is sadly unattainable for most of us. Diseases occur across the lifespan, often without warning. While patients' goals are to achieve a quick cure for their disease, chronic conditions requiring life-long therapy in which the clinical approach is to "manage" the disease often plague patients. While appropriate and timely treatment can stave off many of the complications of these chronic medical problems, the individual and societal costs of this treatment strategy are staggering. A better approach, indeed the holy grail for addressing the current plague of chronic disease, is to focus on disease prevention, which better ensures long term health with attendant economic benefits. Thus, what is needed is a narrative change that shifts the focus from management to prevention.

Such efforts, however, require an understanding of the factors driving chronic disease pathogenesis as well as validated strategies for addressing those risk factors. There is overwhelming evidence linking environmental factors such as chemicals, diet, stress, drugs, and lifestyle to the etiology of many chronic diseases. Thus, there is a desperate need to include improvements in our environment as part of comprehensive efforts to reduce the burden of chronic disease. To this end, this review focuses on one essential aspect of environmentally-driven disease, namely exposure to environmental toxicants and approaches to mitigate their impact on disease susceptibility and development. Specifically, we focus on one category of environmental pollutants, those that cause metabolic disease (metabolism-disrupting chemicals, MDCs). These MDCs represent a subset of environmental endocrine-disrupting chemicals (EDCs) that have been shown to disrupt metabolic physiology or are associated with metabolic disorders in cell-based, animal, or epidemiological studies (1). This discussion of MDCs provides valuable proof-of-principle for developing comprehensive approaches to reduce environmentally-mediated disease. Importantly, the approaches described herein have universal applicability for reducing the impact of myriad environmental chemicals on human health and disease.

This discussion comes at a crucial time. Recent analyses focusing on a subset of MDCs suggest that these toxicants are significant contributors to the societal burden of metabolic diseases and their attendant healthcare costs (2). Furthermore, these analyses likely underestimate the total contribution of MDCs to metabolic disease burden as they were restricted to a small subset of suspected MDCs and do not take into account potential additive or synergistic effects resulting from combinatorial exposures. In addition, many patients are increasingly aware of the potential role environmental toxicants play in disease development; however, it is clear that knowledge gaps exist regarding the potential health impacts of environmental toxicants in a given individual. Moreover, there is a lack of comprehensive clinical guidance to empower patients to address their environmental risk. Improving approaches to environmental health requires an ability to explain the dangers imposed by exposure, which may not become apparent for decades, against the (in)conveniences of lifestyle and policy changes necessary to reduce those exposures. We hope this review will contribute to changing the narrative by focusing the attention of scientists, physicians/health professionals, policy makers, and families on the available evidence to reduce disease-inducing exposures while also stimulating research to enhance our capacity to prevent the environmental contribution to the devastating individual and societal burden of metabolic disease.

THE CONFLUENCE OF ENVIRONMENT AND METABOLIC HEALTH

Over the last several decades, there has been a staggering increase in the prevalence of metabolic diseases across the globe. According to the World Health Organization (WHO), obesity rates have tripled since 1975 (3), and non-alcoholic fatty liver disease is now a leading cause of liver failure (4). Diabetes currently afflicts 9.2% of the global population with an estimated 629 million individuals predicted to suffer from the disease by the year 2045 (5). Perhaps even more concerning is the fact that these diseases are emerging at ever younger ages, transforming obesity, fatty liver disease, and diabetes from diseases of adulthood into common pediatric conditions (6–9). While it is without question that genetic susceptibility challenged by caloric excess and physical inactivity are central drivers of this epidemic, these factors insufficiently account for the rapidity and magnitude of the metabolic disease pandemic. Thus, identifying and addressing other contributors is essential for improving public health.

Endocrine disrupting chemicals (EDCs), defined as "an exogenous chemical, or mixtures of chemicals, that interfere with any aspect of hormone action" (10), are emerging as additional contributors to this pandemic. Approximately 1,000 EDCs have been identified (11). These chemicals have been linked to a variety of diseases, especially when the exposure occurs during development (10, 12, 13). In 2006 the term "obesogen" was coined by the Blumberg Laboratory (14) to describe a subclass of EDCs that cause obesity, a theretofore poorly appreciated consequence of environmental exposures. Data began to be assimilated showing how toxicants were also associated with other metabolic diseases, including diabetes (15), and soon a new word "diabesogen" was coined to describe a chemical that could induce type 2 diabetes and obesity (16). Over the ensuing years, it became clear that some chemicals could cause obesity, type 2 diabetes, or non-alcoholic fatty liver disease, while also leading to the metabolic syndrome (1, 17–19). In 2017, Heindel et al. proposed the term "Metabolism-Disrupting Chemicals" (MDCs) or "Metabolism Disruptors" for this subclass of EDCs to simplify the nomenclature (1). Thus, while obesogens are a subclass of MDCs, MDCs are a subclass of the more general EDCs; furthermore, these data suggest that MDCs as a class have a potentially broader role in the pathophysiology of many metabolic diseases.

Indeed, cellular, animal, and human evidence now implicates diverse classes of environmental toxicants as MDCs, including but not limited to bisphenol A (BPA), phthalates, chemical constituents of air pollution, antifouling agents, polychlorinated biphenyls (PCBs), various pesticides, perfluoroalkyl substances (PFAS), nicotine, and toxic metals (1, 18, 20, 21). Importantly, the rapidly advancing science in this area has moved from identifying associations to ascribing specific molecular mechanisms to the metabolism-disrupting properties of many of these toxicants (19, 22–24). While the strength of evidence linking any given chemical to metabolic dysfunction varies, the expansion and maturation of the field has solidified environmental exposures as relevant contributors to metabolic disease risk. Furthermore, as the field has earned greater attention, patients are increasingly concerned about how their environment impacts their health and are desperate for clinical guidance on how to reduce their exposure risk. Evidence is now beginning to coalesce that will empower physicians and public health officials to translate MDC science into action to improve health.

WINDOWS OF SUSCEPTIBILITY TO MDCS

To effectively focus on disease prevention via specific interventions, it is essential to understand the most sensitive times during which interventions are likely to have the most significant impact. Endocrine and metabolic signaling exert activational effects across the lifespan; during critical developmental windows, however, these signaling events also exert organizational effects that lead to permanent changes in tissue assembly. While metabolic regulation is sensitive to activational perturbations by MDCs across the lifespan, an emerging body of literature has specifically implicated MDC exposures during critical organizational windows of development in the pathogenesis of metabolic disease later in life (**Figure 1**). Known as the Developmental Origins of Health and Disease (DOHaD), this field has expanded from nutritional stressors to those imposed by toxicant exposures (13, 25, 26). While programming events occurring during development are likely essential for adapting to the external milieu, this process of "adaptation" may be corrupted when developmental programs and the external milieu are mismatched, creating a disease-promoting interaction between intrinsic and extrinsic risk factors (27). Indeed, exposure to several MDCs across developmental windows in early life (e.g., *in utero* and early postnatal [reviewed in *ref.* (1)]) are now implicated in the misprogramming of metabolic homeostasis. While the most sensitive window of exposure is during fetal development and the first years of life (i.e., the periods during which tissues are organizing), other sensitive periods, including preconception, pregnancy, and peripuberty, might also be sensitive to the deleterious effects of MDCs (28–30). Perhaps most disturbing are data from animal models showing that exposure to MDCs during development results in disease susceptibility that can be transmitted across generations (31, 32). Thus, reducing developmental exposures and antagonizing MDC effects are of paramount importance for preserving metabolic health across generations.

While the underlying mechanisms responsible for the sensitivity of a particular developmental window to the adverse effects of MDCs remain incompletely understood, epigenetic alterations are a likely culprit (13). Thus, mitigating exposures during early windows of susceptibility that induce epigenetic modifications is expected to have the most significant impact for preventing diseases arising from MDC exposure. It is clear, however, that eliminating exposures across the lifespan will also be essential to reduce activational effects of EDCs to lessen the severity of metabolic disease phenotypes. Thus, strategies to comprehensively address the impact of environmental toxicants on metabolic health must eliminate exposures that induce organizational effects to prevent disease as well as activational effects to lessen the severity of metabolic dysfunction.

STRATEGIES TO MITIGATE THE IMPACT OF ENVIRONMENTAL MDCS

It is clear that reductions in the industrial production, use, and environmental dissemination of MDCs are an essential part of any strategy to limit the impact of this modifiable risk factor. However, additional approaches are required to bridge the gaps created by delays in the adoption of "green" chemistry or recalcitrance in moving to a "first do no harm" approach to economic development. There are three general categories of interventions necessary to protect human metabolic health: (1) strategies to empower individuals to reduce their exposures to MDCs; (2) interventions to reduce the burden of persistent pollutants that bioaccumulate; and (3) therapeutic/dietary approaches to antagonize the deleterious effects of exposures. Current evidence suggests that paradigmatic approaches are evolving in each of these core areas. This new information should provide the impetus to include environmental management strategies as essential pillars of clinical care plans to comprehensively address the individual and societal burden of metabolic diseases. This is a vital step as most clinical practice guidelines are entirely blind to the role of environmental toxicants as mediators of metabolic risk (33–35). Importantly, efforts to incorporate environmental toxicology into clinical practice are not meant to suggest an usurpation of lifestyle interventions to address metabolic disease risk; rather, we propose adaptations to comprehensive frameworks to address the pandemic of metabolic disease that include adjunctive initiatives to address environmental contributors to disease risk.

Reducing Exposures to MDCs

There are two ways to minimize exposure to MDCs: (1) reduce actual exposure to the chemicals themselves, or (2) reduce their post-exposure accumulation in the body. Understanding the sources of human exposure is key to clinical guidance to reduce exposure to MDCs. There are a variety of resources available that provide information on the origins of MDCs and how to limit contact with them. The Endocrine Disruptor Exchange (TEDx) (11), the Environmental Working Group (36), and the new Because Health (37) websites offer excellent examples of exposure reduction strategies. Information on air quality is also publicly available at AirNow.gov (38). There are also mobile apps to help reduce exposures and help find toxin-free food, cosmetics, and household products as well as to gain knowledge about air quality

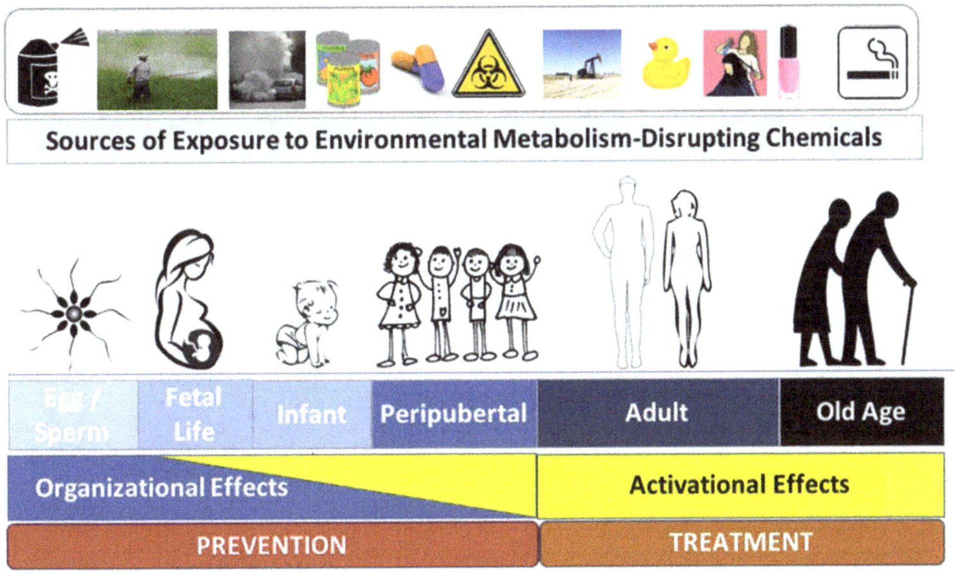

FIGURE 1 | Metabolism-Disrupting Chemicals (MDCs) across the Lifespan. Exposure to MDCs can exert adverse effects across the lifespan. Later in life the effects of MDCs are principally activational; however, early in life, MDCs can exert organizational effects that program increased long-term risk to metabolic diseases. Interventions to prevent adverse metabolic effects from environmental toxicants include efforts aimed at disease prevention (to principally address potential organizational effects) and disease treatment (to principally address activational effects). Images from pixabay.com and openclipart.org.

conditions (39–45). In addition, we have recently developed a concise Healthcare Provider Guide to empower practitioners to discuss exposure reduction strategies with their patients (46). The American Academy of Pediatrics (47) provides further guidance. **Table 1** shows examples of prudent measures that can reduce exposures to MDCs. These measures are relevant across the lifespan from fetal life through childhood, puberty, adulthood, and aging.

To understand which interventions are likely to reduce exposures, it is instructive to examine those practices that increase contact with MDCs. Indeed, data from several studies demonstrate that behavioral choices impact MDC exposure. For example, phthalate levels are positively correlated with consumption of fast food (48, 49). Use of polycarbonate water bottles increases BPA levels (50), as does canned soup consumption (51). Because phthalates and BPA are non-persistent, individuals should recognize and limit their contact with potential sources in order to lower their burden of exposure.

Indeed, several clinical studies have attempted to test this supposition. In an intervention among Latina girls that focused on reducing exposure to personal care products, investigators showed reductions in mono-ethyl phthalate, methyl and propyl parabens, triclosan, and benzophenone (52). Similarly, restricting diets to foods with limited packaging decreased levels of BPA and diethylhexyl phthalate (DEHP) (53). Furthermore, a study in Taiwanese children showed that attention to handwashing coupled with reducing consumption of beverages from plastic cups decreased phthalate levels (54). These data support the conjecture that behavioral change can lower levels of non-persistent toxicants, including those linked to metabolic dysfunction. Such approaches to reduce MDC contact can, therefore, be employed across the lifespan, especially in pregnancy during which there is the potential to impact the metabolic health of multiple generations.

Air pollution is another significant source of MDCs. For example, residents of rural Michigan who were exposed to urban air for only 4–5 hours daily for 5 days exhibited an increase in the homeostatic model assessment of insulin resistance (HOMA-IR) for each 10 $\mu g/m^3$ increase in particulate matter 2.5 μm in size or smaller ($PM_{2.5}$) (55). Among individuals with the metabolic syndrome living in Beijing, China, increases in $PM_{2.5}$ and black carbon correlated with increases in insulin resistance (56). In a small study of individuals with preexisting diabetes, vascular dynamics were shown to be adversely affected by increases in $PM_{2.5}$ (57). These data suggest that the relationship between metabolic function and air quality are, in fact, dynamic. As such, efforts to improve air quality are likely to have salutary effects on population level metabolic health. On an individual level, avoidance of exposures (e.g., by avoiding heavily-traveled streets during commutes or while exercising) may be beneficial. Similarly, avoiding outdoor activities during periods of poor air quality are also likely necessary, as is cessation of practices that worsen local air quality such as burning organic matter, using gasoline-powered lawn care equipment, smoking indoors, and using household chemicals. Patients can be empowered to consider air quality when making choices about outdoor activities through publicly-available websites such as AirNow (38) (**Table 1**).

Despite such encouraging avenues to reduce exposure by behavioral changes, some critical questions remain regarding

TABLE 1 | Interventions and resources to address exposures to metabolism-disrupting chemicals.

Personal care and hygiene	1. Wash your hands regularly using soaps without fragrances and antibiotics. Ensure you have clean hands before preparing and eating food. 2. Minimize handling of receipts and thermal paper. 3. Read labels and avoid products that contain phthalates and parabens. 4. Avoid use of phthalate- and BPA-containing products; recognize that "phthalate-free" and "BPA-free" products may contain other replacement chemicals of concern. 5. Avoid fragrances and opt for cosmetics labeled as "no synthetic fragrance," "scented only with essential oils," or "phthalate-free." 6. Avoid all cosmetics containing lead.
Children	1. Encourage your local school council to reduce school bus emissions, including idling. 2. Avoid hand-me-down plastic toys. 3. Utilize glass alternatives for infant formula bottles. Recognize toys that are labeled "BPA-free" may contain other replacement chemicals of concern.
During pregnancy	1. Ensure adequate intake of calcium, iron, and iodine. 2. Consult guides on the safe intake of fish and seafood.
Food and beverage	1. Eat a diversified diet with plenty of variety. 2. Eat fresh and frozen foods, and reduce consumption of canned and processed foods. 3. Prepare more meals at home with an emphasis on fresh ingredients. 4. Wash fruits and vegetables before consuming them. 5. If possible, purchase organic produce, meat, and dairy products. 6. Choose foods grown and raised locally. 7. Consider using a water filter. This is especially important for those using well water in areas in which arsenic contaminates groundwater as well as for those living in old houses with lead pipes. 8. Store food in glass, stainless steel, or porcelain whenever possible, especially for hot liquids and foods. 9. Avoid plastic containers, especially those designated #3, #6, and #7. 10. Don't microwave foods and beverages in plastic containers. 11. Trim fat from meat and the skin from fish. Cook meat and fish on a rack to let them drain. 12. Consult local guidance regarding which sport fish are safe to consume. 13. Eliminate consumption of sugar-sweetened beverages. 14. Eat a diet that is high in fiber.
Exercise and activity	1. Exercise! But choose times and places with better air quality. For instance, avoid exercise in high traffic areas if possible. Opt for routes away from busy roads. 2. Avoid outdoor activities when air pollution levels are high.
At home	1. Forbid smoking indoors. 2. Do not burn trash. 3. Using a damp cloth, regularly clean your floors and remove dust. 4. Replace old fluorescent bulbs and deteriorating construction materials from older buildings. 5. For those using well water supplied by a submersible pump, if you notice an oily film or fuel odor in your water, determine whether the pump has failed and replace it if necessary. Contact your local Department of Public Health for information on how to clean the well. 6. Choose electrical appliances to limit indoor air pollution. 7. Opt for paints that are low in volatile organic chemicals (VOCs). 8. Limit use of household chemicals, including cleaning supplies, pesticides, and solvents.
In the garden	1. Plant trees and preserve forests to filter air and reduce the "heat island effect". 2. Plant native species of plants and trees. 3. Do not burn leaf litter and wood. 4. Use hand-powered or electric lawn care equipment and eliminate use of gas-powered equipment. 5. Eliminate use of all pesticides.
Getting around	1. Use public transit whenever possible. 2. Choose travel times and routes that limit idling. 3. Walk or bicycle while using safe routes that limit exposure to air pollution. 4. Avoid places that allow smoking.
Advocate	1. Encourage funding for public transportation options as well as safe bicycling paths. 2. Advocate for sustainable development that maximizes energy efficiency, preserves natural spaces, and encourages walkability. Encourage the development of municipal codes that mandate the use of green roofs, cladding buildings in plants such as ivy, and planting trees. 3. Demand energy from renewable sources and infrastructure to support electric vehicles. 4. Promote efforts to expand walking and bicycle paths. 5. Encourage efforts to make public spaces tobacco-free, including restaurants and bars. 6. Demand that municipalities, park districts, and golf courses eliminate the use of pesticides. 7. Advocate for federal legislation to improve labeling of products so that consumers are adequately informed of their exposures.

(Continued)

TABLE 1 | Continued

Sources and additional resources to identify and reduce exposures	1. The Endocrine Disruptor Exchange (TEDx) [https://endocrinedisruption.org] 2. Environmental Work Group (EWG) [https://www.ewg.org] 3. EWG's Skin Deep Guide to Cosmetics [https://www.ewg.org/skindeep/] 4. EWG's Guide to Sunscreens [https://www.ewg.org/sunscreen/] 5. Because Health [https://www.becausehealth.org] 6. AirNow [https://www.airnow.gov] 7. American Academy of Pediatrics [https://www.aap.org/en-us/Pages/Default.aspx] 8. American College of Obstetrics and Gynecology [https://www.acog.org/Clinical-Guidance-and-Publications/Committee-Opinions/Committee-on-Health-Care-for-Underserved-Women/Exposure-to-Toxic-Environmental-Agents] 9. Ruiz et al. *Diabetes Care*, 2018 [(46) as well as supplement and references therein].

the scalability and persistence of these types of interventions and the state of our knowledge regarding the impact of MDC exposure during different developmental windows. In a 3-day study of pregnant women, provision of a diet consisting mostly of fresh, organic foods for 3 days did not lower phthalate levels, perhaps due to the short study time (58). Furthermore, additional concerns regarding the efficacy of behavioral interventions were dramatically raised by a study that sought to lower phthalate levels through the substitution of all meals with organic alternatives. This study did not only fail to reduce phthalate levels, but levels of DEHP *rose* markedly (59). Further, examination revealed a concentrated source of phthalates in the organic alternatives: ground coriander and milk. This study underscores one of the central challenges in providing individuals with clinical guidance on exposure reduction strategies. Current laws regulating the labeling of foods, personal care products, and other goods are woefully inadequate when it comes to providing consumers with knowledge about the chemicals that they contain. In addition to closing these gaps in exposure knowledge, further studies are also required to unequivocally show that interventions that lower exposure levels also meaningfully improve metabolic health.

Addressing MDC Exposure During Critical Developmental Windows

Developmental periods during early life are especially sensitive windows during which exposure to MDCs increases long-term disease susceptibility. Thus, it is important to prioritize exposure reduction during pregnancy and early childhood, the periods during which metabolic tissues are organizing and therefore exquisitely sensitive to misprogramming events that augment later life metabolic disease risk. Many of the same methods that are useful to reduce exposures in adults are also helpful during pregnancy. In addition, since misprogramming may result from altered epigenetic regulation, which is potentially heritable, interventions that antagonize toxicant-induced epigenetic changes may represent viable approaches for mitigating the developmental origins of metabolic dysfunction induced by MDCs across generations. Indeed, there are data showing proof-of-principle for strategies that can prevent epigenetic misprogramming. In seminal work, the MDC BPA was shown to shift coat color in A^{vy} mice via DNA hypomethylation; diets supplemented with methyl donors, including betaine, choline, folic acid, and vitamin B12 antagonized this effect (60). Interestingly, this impact of methyl donors may be relevant in humans as well. In a cross-sectional study of couples undergoing assisted reproductive interventions, high maternal folate intake attenuated the negative association between BPA levels and *in vitro* fertilization success (61). Whether these benefits arise from changes in DNA methylation or are dependent on other factors requires further study, but taken together, these data suggest that interventions to support one-carbon metabolism may modulate some of the adverse effects of some developmental MDC exposures.

This premise is, however, not a clear panacea. In a mouse model of developmental arsenic exposure, folate supplementation lowered the burden of arsenic in maternal livers but did not prevent toxicant-induced reductions in fetal body weight and increases in hepatic S-adenosylmethionine and S-adenosylhomocysteine levels (62). Moreover, this study showed that coordinate exposure to folate and arsenic led to marked changes in DNA methylation, including adverse effects on genes regulating fetal development, suggesting that combined high folate intake in the context of arsenic exposure may *augment* fetal risk (62). In contrast, maternal folate and B12 supplementation reversed the effects of prenatal arsenic exposure on fasting hyperglycemia and insulin resistance in the male offspring of dams maintained on a diet adequate for folate and vitamin B12 (63). Importantly, there were no global hepatic DNA methylation changes associated with the effects of arsenic on glucose homeostasis (63). These data raise important questions about the potential to prevent adverse effects of MDCs on metabolic programming by modulating the epigenetic machinery. While the possibility to meaningfully intervene exists in some contexts, it remains unclear how specific the intervention is to the insult. In other words, the ability to target epigenetic interventions to the defects induced by MDC exposures may lack the specificity to achieve the desired effect. Moreover, in the worst case, as with folate supplementation with arsenic, the intervention may worsen outcomes. Nonetheless, as knowledge of epigenetic programming expands and specific alterations in epigenetic marks and gene expression are defined as biomarkers of exposure, it is likely that this area will become a focus of future intervention strategies.

Therapeutic Approaches to Antagonize the Deleterious Effects of MDCs

As knowledge and understanding of MDCs has evolved, an emerging field of interest focuses on reducing adverse MDC effects by directly targeting their mechanisms of toxicity. To date, there are a limited number of studies in this area to suggest that some interventions may mitigate the adverse metabolic impact of MDCs. For example, the natural plant phenol resveratrol has been shown to antagonize PCB-induced impairments in adipocytic insulin signaling *in vitro* and *in vivo* with attendant improvements in systemic glucose tolerance and insulin sensitivity (64). *N*-acetylcysteine (NAC) is an FDA-approved medication used to treat acetaminophen (paracetamol) toxicity, to address respiratory secretions for those with lung diseases, as well as in other conditions. The benefits of NAC in protecting against acetaminophen-induced hepatic injury are thought to arise through elevations in the antioxidant glutathione. In rat models, NAC has been shown to reduce PCB-induced hepatic steatosis (65) and to prevent glucose intolerance resulting from acute exposure to arsenic (66). NAC has also been shown to antagonize arsenic-induced alterations in glucose homeostasis in mice, potentially by protecting pancreatic β-cells (67). When used in conjunction with monoisoamyl dimercaptosuccinic acid (DMSA), NAC restored liver glutathione levels and protected against chronic arsenic poisoning in guinea pigs (68). Pretreatment with NAC also attenuated arsenic-induced hepatic injury and mitochondrial dysfunction (69). In another study of combinatorial interventions, co-treatment with NAC and *meso*-2,3-DMSA reduced hepatic oxidative damage to a greater extent than either agent alone (70). In rats, NAC protected against arsenic-induced liver toxicity, and coadministration of zinc potentiated this effect (71). In a separate study, however, zinc was shown to have limited capacity to mitigate or prevent PCB-induced liver toxicity in rats despite known disruptions in zinc metabolism stemming from PCB exposure (72). These data provide tantalizing evidence that interventions during adulthood have the capacity to mitigate the deleterious effects of some MDCs on tissues regulating metabolic homesostasis by targeting the mechanisms and downstream effectors of MDC action. However, further data are required to better understand how applicable these interventions are to other MDCs as well as whether they are safe and effective interventions in human populations, especially pregnant women and children.

There are also approaches that focus on pathways common to many environmental chemicals, namely oxidative stress and/or inflammation. A "healthy" diet can itself reduce the risk of chronic inflammation, thus reducing the effects of some MDCs (73). Foods rich in fruits and vegetables, green tea, and omega-3 fatty acids can reduce inflammation and oxidative stress via the upregulation of antioxidant enzymes; this can reduce MDC effects, including cardiovascular toxicity (74–76). For example, broccoli sprouts contain chemicals that generate sulforaphane, which induces antioxidant enzymes; consumption of a broccoli sprout beverage providing 600 μmol glucoraphanin and 40 μmol sulforaphane daily for 12 weeks increased excretion of conjugates of the toxicants benzene and acrolein (77).

Several vitamin and mineral deficiencies during pregnancy have been shown to promote metabolic dysfunction in offspring later in life, which could interact with MDCs to increase disease manifestation and severity. These include deficiencies in vitamin B12 (78), chromium (79), and zinc (80). The similarity of outcomes resulting from such deficiencies and MDC exposures raise several fundamental questions. First, do MDCs that alter metabolic programming elicit their effects in whole or in part by altering vitamin and mineral metabolism? Second, does repletion or supplementation with these vitamins and minerals antagonize or rescue the adverse impact of MDCs on metabolic function? Understanding the commonalities and differences across classes of developmental stressors that potentiate long-term metabolic disease risk are likely to offer practitioners insights into interventions to protect the health of pregnant women and children. While this area of nutritional intervention is still in its infancy, these data suggest the potential for dietary interventions to be an effective and safe approach to reducing the toxicities of MDCs as well as other EDCs.

Growing evidence points to EDCs such as arsenic, lead, and nanoparticles affecting the gut microbiome (81–83). In turn, gut microbiota may modulate environmental chemical toxicity (84, 85). For instance, a study conducted in mice found that exposure to BPA from periconception through weaning resulted in sex-specific and generational differences in the gut microbiome and metabolic pathways related to metabolic dysfunction (86). Considering that gut microbiota play a role in metabolizing MDCs and have the potential to alter their toxicodynamics as well as their detrimental effects, the therapeutic utility of microbiome manipulation via probiotic supplementation is a fertile avenue for investigating future therapeutic interventions.

Effective Interventions in the Context of Non-MDC Developmental Stressors

In the search for effective interventions for developmental MDC exposures, manipulations that antagonize the adverse metabolic effects of other types of environmental stressors may be helpful. For example, inducing stress in dams during the last week of pregnancy by repeated restraint results in alterations in hippocampal glucocorticoid receptors in adult offspring; blocking maternal corticosterone production blunted this effect (87). In a study of rats, early post-natal handling was able to mitigate some of the adverse effects of prenatal stress on programming of the hypothalamic-pituitary-adrenal (HPA) axis (88). Because HPA hyperactivation promotes metabolic dysfunction due to excessive production and/or action of glucocorticoids, these data suggest that *in utero* or early post-natal interventions to address HPA programming may have beneficial effects on metabolism. Although the extent to which HPA programming contributes to the action of MDCs remains to be clarified, the centrality of this endocrine axis to metabolic fate suggests that interventions that prevent the hyperactivation of HPA signaling may help antagonize metabolic disruptions induced by some MDCs.

In utero nutritional status has been linked to metabolic dysfunction later in life. A study using rats selectively bred to develop diet-induced obesity showed that rearing pups in large litters vs. normal litters (16 vs. 10 pups/dam) resulted in an attenuation of diet-induced obesity with attendant changes in leptin signaling (89). In another intriguing study, provision of a running wheel to rats sensitive to diet-induced obesity at 36 days of age resulted in reduced adiposity and increased thermogenesis relative to sedentary controls; furthermore, only 3 weeks of exercise was sufficient to reduce long-term weight gain (90). These data suggest that, at least in rats, early post-natal interventions may reprogram some metabolic parameters to favor *improved* metabolic health. How these interventions may work in negating the impact of developmental MDC exposures in humans and especially pregnant women and children remains to be explored.

Reducing the Legacy of Persistent Pollutants

Among environmental toxicants linked to metabolic dysfunction, some of the best characterized are persistent organic pollutants (POPs). These include such legacy contaminants as polychlorinated biphenyls (PCBs) and dioxins as well as organochlorine pesticides such as dichlorodiphenyltrichloroethane (DDT). While production of many of these toxicants has been banned or significantly restricted, their biological and environmental persistence ensures they are, and will continue to be, relevant from an environmental perspective for many years to come. Persistent pollutants are passed down from generation to generation across the placenta or through lactation (91, 92), which underscores their continued importance. Thus, interventions are required to reduce the body burden of these toxicants to avoid transmitting their risk to future generations.

One approach to eliminate POPs leverages the fact that many of these toxicants undergo enterohepatic circulation. The non-absorbable fat olestra (Olean™) is not a substrate for pancreatic lipases; as such, it is excreted unchanged in feces. It was commercialized in the 1990s in a variety of processed foods as a means to provide the qualities of fatty foods without the attendant caloric content. In high quantities, however, olestra induces steatorrhea. For this reason, as well the loss of fat soluble vitamins due to reduced fat absorption, olestra was removed from the market. While deleterious in the context of vitamin metabolism, the capacity of olestra to facilitate passage of fat soluble molecules from the gastrointestinal tract has the potential to clear MDCs that undergo enterohepatic circulation. The capacity of olestra to remove POPs was examined in a series of small studies. In two patients with chloracne (eruption of blackheads, cysts, and pustules resulting from over-exposure to certain halogenated aromatic compounds), olestra was shown to accelerate the fecal excretion of 2,3,7,8-tetrachlorodibenzo-*p*-dioxin (TCDD) (93). In a case of organochlorine toxicity, namely contamination with the PCB mixture Arochlor 1254, treatment for 2 years with olestra (~16 g/day) led to weight loss with concordant improvements in the subject's diabetes and dyslipidemia (94). In a randomized, year-long trial of residents with elevated serum PCB levels in Anniston, Alabama, elimination of 37 coplanar PCBs was accelerated in the olestra group (15 g/day), but not among those receiving vegetable oil (95). The context of the intervention may be important, however. Weight loss increases circulating levels of POPs (96–100). In one study, replacement of 33% of dietary fat with olestra reduced β-hexachlorocyclohexane concentrations, but did not attenuate the expected weight loss-induced rise in other organochlorines (101). While not necessarily conclusive, these data provide critical evidence that approaches to promote excretion of lipophilic compounds may be useful to reduce levels of POPs linked to metabolic dysfunction. In another study, treatment of 15 healthy women with 1,000 mg per day of vitamin C for 2 months also reduced levels of six PCBs and two organochlorines pesticides; however, levels of polybrominated diphenyl ethers (PBDEs) were unaffected (102).

While these studies demonstrate the potential to lower lipophilic MDC levels, several issues remain. Many of these studies were either small or case reports. Furthermore, except for one case study, the metabolic impact of actively reducing POP levels has not been shown. More extensive studies examining MDC elimination with metabolic phenotyping will be necessary for supporting such interventions. A second concern is that the side effects that led to olestra's removal from the commercial marketplace are likely to lead to poor patient adherence as part of any clinical intervention. As such, alternative approaches with a better risk profile are needed. Indeed, reasonable FDA-approved alternatives may already exist. Bile acid sequestrants are used to lower plasma cholesterol levels by facilitating fecal excretion of bile acids, which leads to the upregulation of the low-density lipoprotein receptor (LDL-R) in the liver and consequential clearance of LDL and its attendant cholesterol from the circulation. In addition to removing bile acids, these pharmaceutical agents also facilitate excretion of other molecules from the body. For example, the bile acid sequestrant cholestyramine is used as an adjunctive therapy in the treatment of thyrotoxicosis due to its ability to disrupt the enterohepatic circulation of thyroid hormone by facilitating its fecal excretion (103). Interestingly, in work published over 25 years ago, cholestyramine was shown to augment fecal excretion of PCBs in rats (104). In a clinical study of individuals from the Yucheng Cohort, combination treatment with cholestyramine and rice bran fiber augmented excretion of PCBs and polychlorinated dibenzofuran with some inter-individual variation in effectiveness (105). The question of whether cholestyramine can augment excretion of stored POPs in less highly exposed individuals warrants testing. It is also essential to determine whether this approach is broadly applicable to other lipophilic POPs. The fact that the bile acid sequestrant colesevelam has been shown to improve glucose homeostasis (106) underscores the importance of such a study. While this has been presumed to result from alterations in bile acid signaling, removal of glucose-raising POPs remains a plausible additional mechanism for colesevelam's beneficial metabolic effects.

Pharmacological agents that inhibit fat absorption may also promote excretion of POPs similar to olestra. Orlistat (Xenical™, Alli™), an inhibitor of pancreatic lipase, is FDA-approved for the treatment of obesity. While part of orlistat's weight loss effect is likely a consequence of behavioral changes to avoid fat consumption to limit adverse gastrointestinal side effects from fat malabsorption (e.g., steatorrhea, flatulence, and fecal incontinence), use of this agent on a low fat diet may yet facilitate clearance of fat soluble POPs by increasing fecal fat loss and is worth investigating. Of course, the risks of malabsorption, including the loss of fat soluble vitamins and essential fatty acids will need to be taken into account for any approach employing fecal fat loss.

One area of longstanding interest for removing PCBs and other legacy chemicals is dietary fiber. For instance, the dietary fibers pectin and konjac mannan attenuated the PCB-induced elevations in serum protein, high density lipoprotein-cholesterol, triglycerides, and liver lipids in rats (107). In another study, a chitosan-supplemented diet increased fecal excretion of PCBs when compared to fiber-free diets (108). Interestingly, compared to diets with water-insoluble fiber, fermentable fibers (polydextrose, indigestible dextrin, and soy polysaccharides) increased urinary PCB excretion (108). In a small study of nine Japanese couples followed for 2 years, consumption of fermented brown rice with *Aspergillus oryzae* (7.5–10.5 g immediately after each meal for 2 years) augmented elimination of polychlorinated dibenzo-*p*-dioxins and polychlorinated dibenzofurans (109).

The precise impact of fiber on MDCs are likely influenced by both the specific fiber as well as the MDC of interest. In an *in vitro* study, dietary fibers were shown to bind several polycyclic hydrocarbons; however, rice bran fiber and pulp lignin produced stronger effects than other types of fiber, including corn, wheat bran, and spinach among others (110). Indeed, in rat studies, wheat bran has complicated effects on PCB absorption and excretion. For example, compared to placebo, the addition of wheat bran to the diet augmented fecal excretion of dietary PCBs. Furthermore, switching from a control diet to a wheat bran-enriched diet enhanced excretion of previously absorbed PCBs; however, the impact of the wheat bran diet did not significantly lower adipose and hepatic PCB levels (111). In a follow-up study, wheat bran-enriched diets relative to a cellulose-based placebo during PCB exposure enhanced fecal excretion of PCBs; however, upon cessation of PCB exposure, wheat bran had a minimal impact on excretion of accumulated PCBs (112). Moreover, the effect of wheat bran on total body PCB accumulation and retention was determined to be minimal in both studies (111, 112). It appears that the chemical structure of the toxicant influences its ability to bind to fiber (110), suggesting that the potential benefit of dietary fiber interventions may be dependent on the specific MDC studied. Importantly, there do not appear to be any studies that have examined the impact of dietary fiber on non-persistent pollutants such as bisphenols and phthalates.

Weight Loss as Opportunity and Threat

Weight loss is a frequent intervention to reduce the risk of metabolic disease; however, weight loss has paradoxical effects on circulating levels of lipid-soluble EDCs. For example, a weight loss intervention among obese participants resulted in elevated levels of serum organohalogenated contaminants and their hydroxylated metabolites (96). In a study of 45 obese women who either received dietary counseling or underwent bariatric surgery, serum PCB levels were higher among those who lost weight; moreover, in the dietary intervention group, the rise in PCB levels were more pronounced among those who lost relatively more of the metabolically deleterious visceral adipose tissue (97). This finding is consistent with studies showing increases in plasma organochlorine levels proportional to the extent of weight loss (98) and increases in plasma PCBs and organochlorine pesticides after gastroplasty (99). The concentrations of POPs in breast milk is also associated with maternal weight loss (113). Bariatric surgery in 71 obese subjects resulted in significant weight loss, increased serum POP levels, and a 15% reduction in total PCB burden (100). In this study serum POP concentrations correlated with liver dysfunction although liver function and other metabolic parameters improved with weight loss (100). Another study also showed that the increase in PCB levels following weight loss did not attenuate the metabolic benefits of weight loss (114). Weight loss is known to lower basal metabolic rates and decrease levels of triiodothyronine (113, 114); whether increased PCB levels augment expected reductions in metabolic rates via known PCB-induced disruptions in the thyroid hormone axis requires further study (10). In general, these data indicate that, despite increases in blood levels of organochlorines, standard weight loss interventions remain an essential tool for addressing MDC-associated metabolic dysfunction. Moreover, weight loss-mediated mobilization of stored POPs may facilitate whole body elimination through complementary approaches, such as olestra, cholestyramine, dietary fiber, and other techniques.

The Impact of Diet as Insight and Intervention

An increasing number of studies have begun to examine the coordinate effects of diets and MDCs on metabolic physiology. The most common hypothesis explored in these studies is that dietary parameters, most often a high fat or high fat plus high sucrose ("Western") diet, will unmask or potentiate the adverse effects of MDCs on energy homeostasis. Developmental exposure to MDCs likely increases metabolic disease susceptibility. Thus, it is likely that a second hit, such as high fat/sugar diets or lack of exercise, will unmask latent disease susceptibility. There are now a few studies that explore the idea that MDCs add to, or synergize with, widely accepted risk factors that promote metabolic disease development. For example, female mice perinatally exposed to DDT were shown to develop glucose intolerance, hyperinsulinemia, and dyslipidemia with alterations in thermogenesis (115). In mouse models of perinatal exposure, high fat feeding amplified the adverse effects of BPA on glucose metabolism in adulthood in some (116), but not all studies (117). In a rat model, paternal exposure to BPA amplified the deleterious effects of a high fat diet on adult offspring (118). In adult exposure models, male mice exposed to BPA in the context of a high fat diet exhibited glucose intolerance with concordant impairments in skeletal muscle insulin signaling (119). Rats exposed to nonylphenol in the context of a high fat, high sucrose diet exhibited elevated blood glucose levels (120). Also, nonylphenol was shown to promote NAFLD in the context of this dietary manipulation with associated lipid accumulation and inflammatory changes (121). Chronic exposure to TCDD in the context of a high fat diet promoted weight gain with sexually dimorphic effects on fat distribution and hepatic steatosis with females exhibiting increases in liver lipid content (122). In a transgenerational study tributyltin (TBT) exposure in the F0 generation increased the sensitivity of mice in the F4 generation to a high fat diet (32). These mice exhibited normal weight gain until exposure to the high fat diet, which triggered accelerated weight gain and impaired weight loss upon switching back to a low fat diet. Finally, rats exposed gestationally and lactationally to BPA exhibited increased liver lipid accumulation and inflammation on a high fat diet after weaning (123). While some of these studies did not directly compare high fat diets (or high fat, high sucrose diets) to control diets, there is a suggestion that MDCs may augment the adverse effects of a metabolically stressful diet. A critical issue is how diets enriched in fat augment absorption of lipophilic MDCs when diet and exposures are both manipulated. In contrast, when dietary manipulation is dissociated from developmental exposure, data suggest a priming of metabolic dysfunction induced by developmental exposure to MDCs that is induced later in life. These findings broadly support standard clinical interventions to address metabolic dysfunction by restricting caloric consumption and limiting consumption of excess fats and sugars.

Interestingly, the impact of an MDC on specific metabolic outcomes may be dependent on the precise dietary intervention studied. On a standard rodent chow, exposure to the phenylsulfamide fungicide tolylfluanid promoted weight gain, increased fat mass, glucose intolerance, insulin resistance, and a disruption in circadian rhythms of feeding behavior (124). The same exposure in the context of a high fat plus high sucrose diet vs. a high sucrose diet alone yielded divergent effects on key metabolic outcomes. In the context of a high fat plus high sucrose diet, tolylfluanid did not appreciably affect weight gain, reduced adipose content modestly, but markedly exacerbated glucose intolerance with no effect on insulin sensitivity (125). In contrast, when incorporated into a high sucrose diet alone, tolylfluanid reduced weight gain while augmenting fat accumulation without any appreciable change in glucose tolerance or insulin sensitivity (125). These data strongly suggest that the impact of MDCs on metabolism may be dependent on both the dietary stressor as well as the metabolic outcome. Moreover, these data indicate that dietary sugars are modulators of MDC effects. This is important because many studies focus on high fat diets alone, even though increased sugar and refined carbohydrate intake tightly correlate with the onset of the metabolic disease pandemic in the last half century (126).

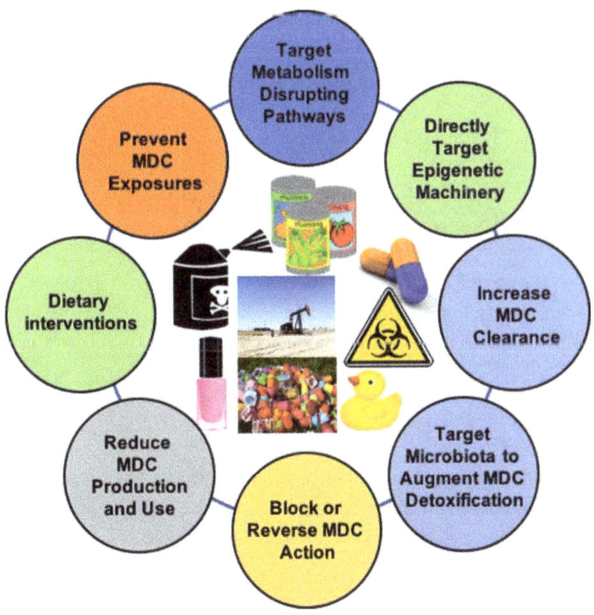

FIGURE 2 | Interventions to Address Exposure to Metabolism-Disrupting Chemicals (MDCs). The diversity of MDCs and their effects require comprehensive approaches to address this underappreciated metabolic disease risk factor. Images from pixabay.com and openclipart.org.

On the flip side, data suggesting that high fat, high sucrose, or Western diets potentiate the adverse metabolic effects of MDCs underscore the importance of dietary interventions in the treatment and prevention of metabolic diseases. In other words, reductions in caloric intake and dietary sugar, as well as saturated and *trans* fats, may be doubly beneficial by addressing both diet-associated disease risk as well as by reducing the impact of environmental toxicants. It will be fascinating to see whether nutritional interventions can elicit metabolic improvements among individuals with known exposures. Given the marked salutary metabolic effects of the "Mediterranean Diet" on human health (127, 128), it is essential to determine whether exposures to MDCs will affect the positive effects of this diet. In this regard, a recent 2 year randomized clinical trial that compared four common diets showed no difference in the extent of weight loss by diet type; however, participants with a higher level of PFAS had augmented weight regain, which was associated with a greater decline in basal metabolic rate during weight loss and less increase in basal metabolic rate during weight regain (129).

One exciting implication from these dietary studies is the potential to gain insights from cross-cultural comparisons of MDC effects. Comparisons of MDC effects across countries may leverage inherent differences in diets to identify those dietary components that modulate the impact of MDCs on metabolic health. Uncovering those protective dietary factors among populations less likely to suffer the adverse effects of MDCs may provide practitioners with valuable knowledge for advising patients on how to reduce their risk of MDC-induced/amplified disease.

While reducing exposure to MDCs is the primary and most effective strategy to reduce the toxic effects of these chemicals, a complimentary approach involves the activation of metabolizing systems to reduce the level of the active chemicals post-exposure (130). Specific dietary constituents may provide such an effect. *Brassica* crops (e.g., cabbage, broccoli, cauliflower, kale, collards, and brussel sprouts) contain chemicals that release sulforaphane upon hydrolysis. Sulphoraphane has been shown to help reduce obesity (131), improve glucose tolerance (132), and restore leptin sensitivity in high fat-sucrose diet fed obese mice (133). Sulforaphane functions by protecting against oxidative stress via activation of the Nrf2-ARE pathway in multiple tissues (134, 135). Also, sulforaphane has anticancer activity stemming from its effects on DNA methyltransferases and histone deacetyltransferaces as well as its epigenetic reactivation of Nrf2 (136). It is important to explore whether sulforaphane

TABLE 2 | Potential intervention strategies to reduce the deleterious effects of metabolism-disrupting chemicals.

Strategy	Chemical class(es)	Interventions	Models	Reference(s)
Employ existing resources that have compiled exposure sources and modify individual behaviors to reduce contact with those chemicals.	Various	Various	Humans (proposed)	(11, 36–47)
Identify and discontinue behaviors shown to *increase* exposure	Phthalates	Reducing fast food consumption	Humans	(48, 49)
	Bisphenol A	Avoiding use of polycarbonate water bottles	Humans	(50)
	Bisphenol A	Reducing canned soup consumption	Humans	(51)
	Air pollutants	Reducing contact with polluted urban air	Humans	(55–57)
Adopt practices shown to *decrease* exposures	Phthalates, parabens, triclosan, and benzophenone	Reducing use of personal care products	Humans	(52)
	Bisphenol A and phthalates	Consuming foods with limited packaging	Humans	(53)
	Phthalates	Washing hands and reducing use of plastic cups for beverages	Humans	(54)
Employ supplements to mitigate the adverse programming effects of exposures during development*	Bisphenol A	Supplement diets with methyl donors, including betaine, choline, folic acid, and vitamin B12	Rodents	(60)
	Bisphenol A	Maternal folate intake	Humans	(61)
	Arsenic	Maternal folate and B12 supplementation	Rodents	(63)
Discontinue supplements shown to potentiate the adverse developmental effects of MDCs*	Arsenic	Maternal folate supplementation	Rodents	(62)
Employ supplements that antagonize the mechanisms of MDC action	PCBs	Supplement with resveratrol	Rodents	(64)
	PCBs, arsenic	Supplement with N-acetylcysteine	Rodents	(65, 66, 69)
	Arsenic	Supplement with N-acetylcysteine and monoisoamyl dimercaptosuccinic acid	Rodents	(68, 70)
	Arsenic	Supplement with N-acetylcysteine + zinc	Rodents	(71)
Consume healthful diets	PCBs	Diets rich in fruits and vegetables	Humans	(73)
	PCBs	Green tea-containing diets	Rodents	(76)
	Benzene and acrolein	Broccoli sprout beverage containing glucoraphanin and sulforaphane	Humans	(77)
Facilitate excretion of persistent organic pollutants	TCDD, PCBs, β-hexachlorocyclohexane	Treatment with the non-digestible fat olestra (Olean^{TM})	Humans	(93–95, 101)
	PCBs, DDT, DDE	Supplementation with 1,000 mg/day ascorbic acid (vitamin D)	Humans	(102)
	PCBs	Treatment with cholestyramine	Rodents	(104)
	PCBs and polychlorinated dibenzofuran	Treatment with cholestyramine	Humans	(105)
	PCBs	Diets supplemented with chitosan	Rodents	(108)
	PCBs	Diets enriched in fermentable fibers (polydextrose, indigestible dextrin, and soy polysaccharides)	Rodents	(108)
	Polychlorinated dibenzo-*p*-dioxins, Polychlorinated dibenzofurans	Consumption of fermented brown rice with *Aspergillus oryzae* after each meal	Humans	(109)
	PCBs	Consumption of wheat bran-enriched diets	Rodents	(111, 112)
Avoid diets that amplify the adverse effects of MDCs	DDT, BPA	Perinatal exposure coupled with later-life high fat diet	Rodents	(115, 116, 118, 123)
	BPA, nonylphenol, TCDD	Concurrent exposure with high fat or high fat-high sucrose diet	Rodents	(119–122)
	TBT	TBT exposure in F0 generation with high fat diet in F4 generation	Rodents	(32)
	Tolylfluanid	Concurrent exposure to tolylfluanid and either a high fat-high sucrose diet or a high sucrose diet alone	Rodents	(125)

(Continued)

TABLE 2 | Continued

Strategy	Chemical class(es)	Interventions	Models	Reference(s)
Employ supplements that impair the activating metabolism of toxicants	Benzo(a)pyrene	Administration of resveratrol impaired benzo(a)pyrene metabolism and markers of colon cancer	Rodents	(137)
Address vitamin and mineral deficiencies that augment exposure to environmental toxicants	Mercury	Nutrients from fish are associated with protection against neurotoxicity	Humans	(138)
	Lead	Iron deficiency augments lead absorption while iron-enriched diets reduce transplacental transfer of lead	Humans	(139–141)
	Lead	Higher calcium intake and calcium supplementation reduces exposure among fetuses and infants	Humans	(142–144)
Consider supplementation with dietary adjuncts that antagonize mechanisms of toxicity in non-metabolic models that may also be related to metabolic disruption	Arsenic	Various interventions employing ascorbic acid and tocopherol; plant extracts; flavonoids and polyphenols; and selenium	Cell-Based, Rodents, and Humans	(147–162)
Employ supplements that reduce transmission of toxicants via breast milk	Dioxins	Supplementation with *Chlorella pyrenoidosa* extract during pregnancy reduced total toxic equivalents in breast milk	Humans	(161)

**Denotes an area in which both beneficial and harmful outcomes have been reported for the same intervention.*

can protect against MDC action in humans. It is essential to recognize, however, that in some cases the metabolites of an MDC may be more toxic than the parent compound. One such example is benzo(*a*)pyrene. In this case, resveratrol-mediated *impairments* in benzo(*a*)pyrene metabolism were shown to reduce colon cancer incidence and tumor size in a rat model by lowering DNA adduct formation, an essential mechanism in cancer initiation (137). Thus, while dietary or pharmacological induction of MDC metabolism pathways may hold promise, more work is needed to discern which MDCs are more likely to be detoxified by such an approach.

Merging Mechanisms of Action to Modes of Toxicity

As scientific advances in the field illuminate modes of metabolic toxicity, new opportunities will arise to individualize disease management plans. Over the course of the last decade, there have been significant advances in our pharmaceutical armamentarium for treating individuals with obesity, diabetes, NAFLD, and other metabolic conditions. Importantly, this includes entirely new classes of medications that address pathophysiological defects inherent to metabolic diseases. Recently, several signaling cascades have emerged as being critical for disease development. In diabetes, two examples are the sodium-glucose co-transporter 2 system in the kidney and gut-derived incretin hormones (33). The importance of these systems as well as our clinical capacity to modulate their activity raise three fundamental questions for the field. First, we must understand whether MDCs modulate these newly uncovered pathways. This understanding is especially salient for MDCs for which mechanisms of metabolic toxicity remain poorly delineated. Thus, emerging knowledge of disease processes should expand hypotheses regarding the modes by which MDCs induce or amplify metabolic dysfunction. Secondly, our rapidly increasing capacity to tailor medical therapy to the individual opens up unique opportunities to address the impact of known exposures. Indeed, a significant focus in diabetes care, as well as in other areas of medicine, is on the individualization of treatment (33). For patients with known exposures that cannot be meaningfully reduced or eliminated, incorporation of exposure assessment with consideration of MDC-associated mechanisms of toxicity offers another opportunity to individualize pharmacological management of their metabolic disease. For us to incorporate exposures into clinical decision making, data gaps need to be filled. There are many combinations of exposures in humans, which creates challenges to understanding the importance of MDCs as well as in devising targeted interventions. Regardless, the opportunities to leverage this knowledge have never been better. Third and finally, there are prospects for exposure science to drive drug development and disease treatment. Where environmental exposures have been linked with disease, examining metabolic toxicity using unbiased approaches may lead to new mechanisms of action that could be relevant to disease development more generally; moreover, these new pathways may be potentially druggable. In this way, MDCs may be used as molecular tools to uncover new biology that has the potential to improve human health.

Improving Resilience During Pregnancy

In addition to interventions meant to address the epigenetic alterations induced by MDC exposure, other interventions have been shown to protect against several environmental toxicants in the context of non-metabolic diseases. For example, some fish nutrients have been posited to protect children from the deleterious neurodevelopmental effects of mercury (138).

Iron deficiency augments lead absorption (139, 140), while iron-enriched diets appear to reduce transplacental transfer of lead (141). Similarly, higher dietary calcium intake and calcium supplementation during pregnancy and lactation may also minimize lead exposure of fetuses and infants (142, 143); however, this effect may be dependent on baseline calcium intake (144). In the context of arsenic exposure, several interventions have been shown to attenuate toxicity of this known MDC, including ascorbic acid and tocopherol (145–150); plants extracts, flavonoids, and polyphenols (151–154); and selenium (155–160). Finally, pregnant women instructed to take supplements of *Chlorella pyrenoidosa* (an algal extract; 6 g/day for 6 months) demonstrated 30% lower total toxic equivalents in breast milk relative to controls (161). While some of these interventions may be specific to the environmental toxicant studied, they suggest that targeted maternal interventions may reduce fetal and infant exposures resulting in a reduction in long-term, environmentally-mediated metabolic risk. Further work is needed, however, to ascertain whether these interventions meaningfully impact energy homeostasis.

COLLISION OF EXPOSURE SCIENCE, MEDICAL ETHICS, AND PATIENT CARE

Importantly, the gap in our knowledge of MDC sources has a unique extension into the field of clinical medicine, namely exposures arising from medical treatments. This creates novel ethical concerns for providers. Our modern healthcare system is built upon central tenets of medical ethics that guide the provision of care to patients. These principles include respect for autonomy, beneficence, non-maleficence, and justice (162). Related and critically important extensions of these ethical concepts include patient's rights to disclosure and for medical decisions to be made through a process of informed consent. While clinicians often do an excellent job of discussing the risks and benefits of specific pharmacological therapies, rarely (if ever) discussed are the potential impacts of "inactive" ingredients included in particular drug formulations. Undoubtedly, this is partially attributable to a lack of physician awareness and knowledge; however, the consequence is that patients are not appropriately informed of treatment risks and potential alternatives, violating the central tenet of autonomy. This is relevant to the current discussion because some medications are formulated with phthalates (163–165) and other synthetic polymers (166), making iatrogenesis a potentially significant source of phthalate and additional MDC exposure. Indeed, pharmaceuticals can be a potential source of dibutyl phthalate, a compound with known adverse reproductive and developmental effects (163). The positive association between current use of polymer-containing drugs and high rates of poor semen quality in men provide further evidence for this premise (167). Iatrogenic risk can be imposed by other physician-initiated practices as well, including infusion systems. In one study, switching from DEHP-plasticized polyvinylchloride (PVC) infusions systems to PVC-free lines for total parenteral nutrition (TPN) led to a marked reduction in TPN-associated cholestasis (168). This case illustrates both the importance of unappreciated and clinically significant risk associated with some exposures as well as the profound opportunity to reduce adverse outcomes by choosing delivery systems that avoid disease-associated exposures. Importantly, it also emphasizes the need for physicians to address fundamental knowledge gaps in this realm in order to empower their patients to make informed decisions about their care.

CONCLUSIONS

Increasing evidence implicates MDCs as contributors to the burgeoning global pandemic of metabolic disease. Addressing these novel risk factors requires the implementation of multifactorial intervention strategies across the lifespan (**Figure 2**). While more data are needed, the potential benefits of these approaches are now supported by a variety of proof-of-concept studies in animal models and humans (**Table 2**). Given the importance of developmental programming in metabolic outcomes, efforts to reduce maternal MDC exposure, prevent transplacental and lactational transmission of MDCs, and inhibit deleterious epigenetic alterations induced by MDCs offer unique opportunities to impact health across generations. The best studies in this area focus on interventions to reduce maternal-fetal transmission of specific MDCs, such as lead. Whether similar approaches will work for other common MDCs remains to be determined. Efforts to address metabolic programming through manipulation of one-carbon metabolism in order to affect DNA methylation or interventions to reverse altered programming *per se* may hold promise, but fundamental questions remain regarding whether such interventions are sufficiently specific to address MDC action while minimizing off-target epigenetic programming events. Resolving these challenges is critical as interventions targeting pregnancy and early life development have the potential to reduce long-term disease susceptibility, potentially across generations.

Importantly, many of the same interventions to reduce levels of MDCs and their adverse effects during pregnancy are useful across the lifespan. These include behavioral efforts to reduce exposures to known MDCs and providing consumers with the information essential for making informed choices. Indeed, these are likely the types of interventions that are most likely to have a clinically significant impact, especially for those MDCs that are non-persistent. Additionally, efforts to specifically antagonize the mechanisms by which MDCs induce metabolic dysfunction have shown some promise; however, this area needs more work. Unfortunately, some of the most comprehensively characterized MDCs are persistent pollutants with long biological half-lives that are less amenable to behavioral interventions. Thus, addressing these MDCs is especially challenging; however, some evidence suggests that disrupting the enterohepatic circulation of lipophilic MDCs may lead to meaningful reductions in the overall body burden of these toxicants. Unfortunately, most data exist for treatments with relatively noxious adverse effects; therefore, alternative approaches are needed for facilitating elimination of POPs. Where known exposures are linked to clear molecular mechanisms of metabolic dysfunction, use of pharmacological therapies specifically targeting MDC mechanisms of action may allow individualized treatment regimens that address the precise origins of a patient's metabolic dysfunction. Finally, avoidance of diets that amplify the deleterious effects of MDCs in favor of those that antagonize their effects is essential, while standard clinical advice to exercise and lose weight are equally necessary components for addressing the threat of environmental toxicants to metabolic health. As we gain a greater appreciation for how the diverse array of intrinsic and extrinsic risk factors that promote metabolic disease development interact with each other (27, 169), new interventions are likely to emerge.

In the end, however, any effective strategy must include comprehensive and sustained efforts to reduce exposures wherever and whenever possible. Current federal environmental policies do not account for metabolic disease risk, as recently discussed for diabetes (170). Incorporating metabolic health as a relevant outcome in local, regional, national, and international policy has the potential to transform risk assessment to support legislation that is likely to reduce exposures. In the end, reducing exposures is at the core of any effective intervention to address the adverse effects of a toxic environment on our health. To realize these preventive strategies, we need to change the narrative from a focus on managing chronic diseases to eliminating those factors that drive disease pathogenesis, including exposure to MDCs. To do so, clinicians must begin to appreciate the contribution of environmental toxicants to metabolic disease risk and begin to incorporate this knowledge into clinical practice. In the end, however, meaningful change on this front must occur at all levels from individuals to families, to clinicians, and ultimately to policy makers. The time to begin these efforts is now as the benefits of such an approach for both the individual and society are potentially enormous.

AUTHOR CONTRIBUTIONS

RS and VP conceived the manuscript. RS, JH, and VP all wrote and edited the manuscript.

FUNDING

This work was supported by the National Institute of Environmental Health Sciences (R01 ES028879 and P30 ES027792 to RS and P01 ES022844 and P30 ES017885 to VP) as well as the American Diabetes Association (17-JDF-033 to RS).

REFERENCES

1. Heindel JJ, Blumberg B, Cave M, Machtinger R, Mantovani A, Mendez MA, et al. Metabolism disrupting chemicals and metabolic disorders. *Reprod Toxicol.* (2017) 68:3–33. doi: 10.1016/j.reprotox.2016.10.001
2. Trasande L, Zoeller RT, Hass U, Kortenkamp A, Grandjean P, Myers JP, et al. Estimating burden and disease costs of exposure to endocrine disrupting chemicals in the European union. *J Clin Endocrinol Metabol.* (2015) 100:1245–55. doi: 10.1210/jc.2014-4324
3. World Health Organization. *Obesity and Overweight: World Health Organization.* (2018). Available online at: www.who.int/news-room/fact-sheets/detail/obesity-and-overweight
4. Cholankeril G, Wong RJ, Hu M, Perumpail RB, Yoo ER, Puri P, et al. Liver transplantation for nonalcoholic steatohepatitis in the US: temporal trends and outcomes. *Dig Dis Sci.* (2017) 62:2915–22. doi: 10.1007/s10620-017-4684-x
5. International Diabetes Federation. *IDF Diabetes Atlas, 8th Edition: International Diabetes Federation.* (2017). Available online at: https://www.idf.org/e-library/epidemiology-research/diabetes-atlas/134-idf-diabetes-atlas-8th-edition.html
6. Mayer-Davis EJ, Lawrence JM, Dabelea D, Divers J, Isom S, Dolan L, et al. Incidence trends of type 1 and type 2 diabetes among youths, 2002-2012. *N Engl J Med.* (2017) 376:1419–29. doi: 10.1056/NEJMoa1610187
7. Skinner AC, Ravanbakht SN, Skelton JA, Perrin EM, Armstrong SC. Prevalence of obesity and severe obesity in US Children, 1999-2016. *Pediatrics.* (2018) 24:1116–23. doi: 10.1542/peds.2017-3459
8. Welsh JA, Karpen S, Vos MB. Increasing prevalence of nonalcoholic fatty liver disease among United States adolescents, 1988-1994 to 2007-2010. *J Pediatr.* (2013) 162:496–500 e1. doi: 10.1016/j.jpeds.2012.08.043
9. Alisi A, Feldstein AE, Villani A, Raponi M, Nobili V. Pediatric nonalcoholic fatty liver disease: a multidisciplinary approach. *Nat Rev Gastroenterol Hepatol.* (2012) 9:152–61. doi: 10.1038/nrgastro.2011.273
10. Gore AC, Chappell VA, Fenton SE, Flaws JA, Nadal A, Prins GS, et al. EDC-2: The Endocrine Society's Second Scientific Statement on Endocrine-Disrupting Chemicals. *Endocr Rev.* (2015) 36:E1–150. doi: 10.1210/er.2015-1093
11. The Endocrine Disruption Exchange. *TEDx: The Endocrine Disruption Exchange Eckert, CO.* (2018). Available online at: https://endocrinedisruption.org
12. Heindel JJ, Skalla LA, Joubert BR, Dilworth CH, Gray KA. Review of developmental origins of health and disease publications in environmental epidemiology. *Reprod Toxicol.* (2017) 68:34–48. doi: 10.1016/j.reprotox.2016.11.011
13. Barouki R, Gluckman PD, Grandjean P, Hanson M, Heindel JJ. Developmental origins of non-communicable disease: implications for research and public health. *Environ Health* (2012) 11:42. doi: 10.1186/1476-069X-11-42
14. Grun F, Blumberg B. Environmental obesogens: organotins and endocrine disruption via nuclear receptor signaling. *Endocrinology* (2006) 147(6 Suppl):S50–5. doi: 10.1210/en.2005-1129
15. Neel BA, Sargis RM. The paradox of progress: environmental disruption of metabolism and the diabetes epidemic. *Diabetes* (2011) 60:1838–48. doi: 10.2337/db11-0153
16. Alonso-Magdalena P, Quesada I, Nadal A. Prenatal exposure to BPA and offspring outcomes: the diabesogenic behavior of BPA. *Dose Response* (2015) 13:1559325815590395. doi: 10.1177/1559325815590395
17. Heindel JJ, Vom Saal FS, Blumberg B, Bovolin P, Calamandrei G, Ceresini G, et al. Parma consensus statement on metabolic disruptors. *Environ Health* (2015) 14:54. doi: 10.1186/s12940-015-0042-7
18. Mimoto MS, Nadal A, Sargis RM. Polluted pathways: mechanisms of metabolic disruption by endocrine disrupting chemicals. *Curr Environ Health Rep.* (2017) 4:208–22. doi: 10.1007/s40572-017-0137-0
19. Sargis RM. The hijacking of cellular signaling and the diabetes epidemic: mechanisms of environmental disruption of insulin action and glucose homeostasis. *Diabet Metabol J.* (2014) 38:13-24. doi: 10.4093/dmj.2014.38.1.13
20. Darbre PD. Endocrine disruptors and obesity. *Curr Obes Rep.* (2017) 6:18–27. doi: 10.1007/s13679-017-0240-4
21. De Long NE, Holloway AC. Early-life chemical exposures and risk of metabolic syndrome. *Diabet Metab Syndr Obes.* (2017) 10:101–9. doi: 10.2147/DMSO.S95296

22. Foulds CE, Trevino LS, York B, Walker CL. Endocrine-disrupting chemicals and fatty liver disease. *Nat Rev Endocrinol.* (2017) 13:445–57. doi: 10.1038/nrendo.2017.42
23. Heindel JJ, Blumberg B. Environmental obesogens: mechanisms and controversies. *Annu Rev Pharmacol Toxicol.* (2018) 59:89–106. doi: 10.1146/annurev-pharmtox-010818-021304
24. Veiga-Lopez A, Pu Y, Gingrich J, Padmanabhan V. Obesogenic endocrine disrupting chemicals: identifying knowledge gaps. *Trends Endocrinol Metab.* (2018) 29:607–25. doi: 10.1016/j.tem.2018.06.003
25. Hanson MA, Gluckman PD. Developmental origins of health and disease–global public health implications. *Best Pract Res Clin Obstet Gynaecol.* (2015) 29:24–31. doi: 10.1016/j.bpobgyn.2014.06.007
26. Heindel JJ, Balbus J, Birnbaum L, Brune-Drisse MN, Grandjean P, Gray K, et al. Developmental origins of health and disease: integrating environmental influences. *Endocrinology* (2015) 156:3416–21. doi: 10.1210/EN.2015-1394
27. McHale CM, Osborne G, Morello-Frosch R, Salmon AG, Sandy MS, Solomon G, et al. Assessing health risks from multiple environmental stressors: moving from GxE to IxE. *Mutat Res.* (2018) 775:11–20. doi: 10.1016/j.mrrev.2017.11.003
28. Braun JM, Messerlian C, Hauser R. Fathers matter: why it's time to consider the impact of paternal environmental exposures on children's health. *Curr Epidemiol Rep.* (2017) 4:46–55. doi: 10.1007/s40471-017-0098-8
29. Soubry A. Epigenetics as a driver of developmental origins of health and disease: did we forget the fathers? *Bioessays* (2018) 40:201700113. doi: 10.1002/bies.201700113
30. Alonso-Magdalena P, Garcia-Arevalo M, Quesada I, Nadal A. Bisphenol-A treatment during pregnancy in mice: a new window of susceptibility for the development of diabetes in mothers later in life. *Endocrinology* (2015) 156:1659–70. doi: 10.1210/en.2014-1952
31. Skinner MK. Endocrine disruptors in 2015: epigenetic transgenerational inheritance. *Nat Rev Endocrinol.* (2016) 12:68–70. doi: 10.1038/nrendo.2015.206
32. Chamorro-Garcia R, Diaz-Castillo C, Shoucri BM, Kach H, Leavitt R, Shioda T, et al. Ancestral perinatal obesogen exposure results in a transgenerational thrifty phenotype in mice. *Nat Commun.* (2017) 8:2012. doi: 10.1038/s41467-017-01944-z
33. American Diabetes Association. Standards of Medical Care in Diabetes-2018. *Diabetes Care* (2018) 41(Suppl 1):S1–153. doi: 10.2337/dc18-Sint01
34. Blond E, Disse E, Cuerq C, Drai J, Valette PJ, Laville M, et al. EASL-EASD-EASO clinical practice guidelines for the management of non-alcoholic fatty liver disease in severely obese people: do they lead to over-referral? *Diabetologia* (2017) 60:1218–22. doi: 10.1007/s00125-017-4264-9
35. Gonzalez-Campoy JM, St Jeor ST, Castorino K, Ebrahim A, Hurley D, Jovanovic L, et al. Clinical practice guidelines for healthy eating for the prevention and treatment of metabolic and endocrine diseases in adults: cosponsored by the American Association of Clinical Endocrinologists/the American College of Endocrinology and the Obesity Society. *Endocr Pract.* (2013) 19(Suppl 3):1–82. doi: 10.4158/EP13155.GL
36. Environmental Working Group. *Environmental Working Group Washington, DC.* (2018). Available online at: https://www.ewg.org/
37. Because Health. *Because Health Bolinas, CA: Collaborative on Health and the Environment.* (2018). Available online at: https://www.becausehealth.org/
38. AirNow. *AirNow Washington, DC: Environmental Protection Agency.* (2018). Available online at: https://www.airnow.gov/
39. Dirty Dozen. *Dirty Dozen Washington, DC: Environmental Working Group.* (2018). Available online at: https://itunes.apple.com/us/app/dirty-dozen/id312336368?mt=8
40. Cosmetifique. *Cosmetifique.* (2018). Available online at: http://cosmetifique.com
41. GoodGuide. *GoodGuide.* (2018). Available online at: https://www.goodguide.com/
42. Thnk Dirty. *Think Dirty.* (2018). Available online at: www.thinkdirtyapp.com
43. Detox Me. *Detox Me Newton, MA: Silent Spring Institute.* (2018). Available online at: https://silentspring.org/detoxme/
44. Environmental Working Group. *Healthy Living App Washington, DC: Environmental Working Group.* (2018). Available online at: https://www.ewg.org/apps/
45. Air Matters. *Air Matters.* (2018). Available online at: https://itunes.apple.com/us/app/air-matters/id477700080?mt=8
46. Ruiz D, Becerra M, Jagai JS, Ard K, Sargis RM. Disparities in environmental exposures to endocrine-disrupting chemicals and diabetes risk in vulnerable populations. *Diabetes Care* (2018) 41:193–205. doi: 10.2337/dc16-2765
47. American Academy of Pediatrics. *Council on Environmental Health.* (2018). Available online at: https://www.aap.org/en-us/about-the-aap/Councils/Council-on-Environmental-Health/Pages/COEH.aspx
48. Zota AR, Phillips CA, Mitro SD. Recent fast food consumption and Bisphenol A and phthalates exposures among the U.S. population in NHANES, 2003-2010. *Environ Health Perspect.* (2016) 124:1521–8. doi: 10.1289/ehp.1510803
49. Watkins DJ, Eliot M, Sathyanarayana S, Calafat AM, Yolton K, Lanphear BP, et al. Variability and predictors of urinary concentrations of phthalate metabolites during early childhood. *Environ Sci Technol.* (2014) 48:8881–90. doi: 10.1021/es501744v
50. Makris KC, Andra SS, Jia A, Herrick L, Christophi CA, Snyder SA, et al. Association between water consumption from polycarbonate containers and bisphenol A intake during harsh environmental conditions in summer. *Environ Sci Technol.* (2013) 47:3333–43. doi: 10.1021/es304038k
51. Carwile JL, Ye X, Zhou X, Calafat AM, Michels KB. Canned soup consumption and urinary bisphenol A: a randomized crossover trial. *JAMA* (2011) 306:2218–20. doi: 10.1001/jama.2011.1721
52. Harley KG, Kogut K, Madrigal DS, Cardenas M, Vera IA, Meza-Alfaro G, et al. Reducing phthalate, paraben, and phenol exposure from personal care products in adolescent girls: findings from the HERMOSA intervention study. *Environ Health Perspect.* (2016) 124:1600–7. doi: 10.1289/ehp.1510514
53. Rudel RA, Gray JM, Engel CL, Rawsthorne TW, Dodson RE, Ackerman JM, et al. Food packaging and bisphenol A and bis(2-ethyhexyl) phthalate exposure: findings from a dietary intervention. *Environ Health Perspect.* (2011) 119:914–20. doi: 10.1289/ehp.1003170
54. Chen C-Y, Chou Y-Y, Lin S-J, Lee C-C. Developing an intervention strategy to reduce phthalate exposure in Taiwanese girls. *Sci Total Environ.* (2015) 517:125–31. doi: 10.1016/j.scitotenv.2015.02.021
55. Brook RD, Xu X, Bard RL, Dvonch JT, Morishita M, Kaciroti N, et al. Reduced metabolic insulin sensitivity following sub-acute exposures to low levels of ambient fine particulate matter air pollution. *Sci Total Environ.* (2013) 448:66–71. doi: 10.1016/j.scitotenv.2012.07.034
56. Brook RD, Sun Z, Brook JR, Zhao X, Ruan Y, Yan J, et al. Extreme air pollution conditions adversely affect blood pressure and insulin resistance the air pollution and cardiometabolic disease study. *Hypertension* (2016) 67:77–85. doi: 10.1161/HYPERTENSIONAHA.115.06237
57. Schneider A, Neas L, Herbst MC, Case M, Williams RW, Cascio W, et al. Endothelial dysfunction: associations with exposure to ambient fine particles in diabetic individuals. *Environ Health Perspect.* (2008) 116:1666–74. doi: 10.1289/ehp.11666
58. Barrett ES, Velez M, Qiu X, Chen SR. Reducing prenatal phthalate exposure through maternal dietary changes: results from a pilot study. *Matern Child Health J.* (2015) 19:1936–42. doi: 10.1007/s10995-015-1707-0
59. Sathyanarayana S, Alcedo G, Saelens BE, Zhou C, Dills RL, Yu J, et al. Unexpected results in a randomized dietary trial to reduce phthalate and bisphenol A exposures. *J Expo Sci Environ Epidemiol.* (2013) 23:378–84. doi: 10.1038/jes.2013.9
60. Dolinoy DC, Huang D, Jirtle RL. Maternal nutrient supplementation counteracts bisphenol A-induced DNA hypomethylation in early development. *Proc Natl Acad Sci USA.* (2007) 104:13056–61. doi: 10.1073/pnas.0703739104
61. Minguez-Alarcon L, Gaskins AJ, Chiu YH, Souter I, Williams PL, Calafat AM, et al. Dietary folate intake and modification of the association of urinary bisphenol A concentrations with *in vitro* fertilization outcomes among women from a fertility clinic. *Reprod Toxicol.* (2016) 65:104–12. doi: 10.1016/j.reprotox.2016.07.012
62. Tsang V, Fry RC, Niculescu MD, Rager JE, Saunders J, Paul DS, et al. The epigenetic effects of a high prenatal folate intake in male mouse fetuses

exposed *in utero* to arsenic. *Toxicol Appl Pharmacol.* (2012) 264:439–50. doi: 10.1016/j.taap.2012.08.022
63. Huang MC, Douillet C, Dover EN, Styblo M. Prenatal arsenic exposure and dietary folate and methylcobalamin supplementation alter the metabolic phenotype of C57BL/6J mice in a sex-specific manner. *Arch Toxicol.* (2018) 92:1925–37. doi: 10.1007/s00204-018-2206-z
64. Baker NA, English V, Sunkara M, Morris AJ, Pearson KJ, Cassis LA. Resveratrol protects against polychlorinated biphenyl-mediated impairment of glucose homeostasis in adipocytes. *J Nutr Biochem.* (2013) 24:2168–74. doi: 10.1016/j.jnutbio.2013.08.009
65. Lai IK, Dhakal K, Gadupudi GS, Li M, Ludewig G, Robertson LW, et al. N-acetylcysteine (NAC) diminishes the severity of PCB 126-induced fatty liver in male rodents. *Toxicology* (2012) 302:25–33. doi: 10.1016/j.tox.2012.07.007
66. Rezaei M, Khodayar MJ, Seydi E, Soheila A, Parsi IK. Acute, but not chronic, exposure to arsenic provokes glucose intolerance in rats: possible roles for oxidative stress and the adrenergic pathway. *Can J Diabet.* (2017) 41:273–80. doi: 10.1016/j.jcjd.2016.10.008
67. Lu TH, Su CC, Chen YW, Yang CY, Wu CC, Hung DZ, et al. Arsenic induces pancreatic beta-cell apoptosis via the oxidative stress-regulated mitochondria-dependent and endoplasmic reticulum stress-triggered signaling pathways. *Toxicol Lett.* (2011) 201:15–26. doi: 10.1016/j.toxlet.2010.11.019
68. Kannan GM, Flora SJ. Combined administration of N-acetylcysteine and monoisoamyl DMSA on tissue oxidative stress during arsenic chelation therapy. *Biol Trace Elem Res.* (2006) 110:43–59. doi: 10.1385/BTER:110:1:43
69. Santra A, Chowdhury A, Ghatak S, Biswas A, Dhali GK. Arsenic induces apoptosis in mouse liver is mitochondria dependent and is abrogated by N-acetylcysteine. *Toxicol Appl Pharmacol.* (2007) 220:146–55. doi: 10.1016/j.taap.2006.12.029
70. Abu El-Saad AM, Al-Kahtani MA, Abdel-Moneim AM. N-acetylcysteine and meso-2,3-dimercaptosuccinic acid alleviate oxidative stress and hepatic dysfunction induced by sodium arsenite in male rats. *Drug Des Devel Ther.* (2016) 10:3425–34. doi: 10.2147/DDDT.S115339
71. Modi M, Kaul RK, Kannan GM, Flora SJ. Co-administration of zinc and n-acetylcysteine prevents arsenic-induced tissue oxidative stress in male rats. *J Trace Elem Med Biol.* (2006) 20:197–204. doi: 10.1016/j.jtemb.2006.02.002
72. Klaren WD, Gibson-Corley KN, Wels B, Simmons DL, McCormick ML, Spitz DR, et al. Assessment of the mitigative capacity of dietary zinc on PCB126 hepatotoxicity and the contribution of zinc to toxicity. *Chem Res Toxicol.* (2016) 29:851–9. doi: 10.1021/acs.chemrestox.6b00022
73. Hofe CR, Feng L, Zephyr D, Stromberg AJ, Hennig B, Gaetke LM. Fruit and vegetable intake, as reflected by serum carotenoid concentrations, predicts reduced probability of polychlorinated biphenyl-associated risk for type 2 diabetes: National Health and Nutrition Examination Survey 2003-2004. *Nutr Res.* (2014) 34:285–93. doi: 10.1016/j.nutres.2014.02.001
74. Hoffman JB, Hennig B. Protective influence of healthful nutrition on mechanisms of environmental pollutant toxicity and disease risks. *Ann N Y Acad Sci.* (2017) 1398:99–107. doi: 10.1111/nyas.13365
75. Hennig B, Petriello MC, Gamble MV, Surh YJ, Kresty LA, Frank N, et al. The role of nutrition in influencing mechanisms involved in environmentally mediated diseases. *Rev Environ Health* (2018) 33:87–97. doi: 10.1515/reveh-2017-0038
76. Newsome BJ, Petriello MC, Han SG, Murphy MO, Eske KE, Sunkara M, et al. Green tea diet decreases PCB 126-induced oxidative stress in mice by up-regulating antioxidant enzymes. *J Nutr Biochem.* (2014) 25:126–35. doi: 10.1016/j.jnutbio.2013.10.003
77. Egner PA, Chen JG, Zarth AT, Ng DK, Wang JB, Kensler KH, et al. Rapid and sustainable detoxication of airborne pollutants by broccoli sprout beverage: results of a randomized clinical trial in China. *Cancer Prev Res.* (2014) 7:813–23. doi: 10.1158/1940-6207.CAPR-14-0103
78. Yajnik CS, Deshpande SS, Jackson AA, Refsum H, Rao S, Fisher DJ, et al. Vitamin B12 and folate concentrations during pregnancy and insulin resistance in the offspring: the Pune Maternal Nutrition Study. *Diabetologia* (2008) 51:29–38. doi: 10.1007/s00125-007-0793-y
79. Padmavathi IJ, Rao KR, Venu L, Ganeshan M, Kumar KA, Rao Ch N, et al. Chronic maternal dietary chromium restriction modulates visceral adiposity: probable underlying mechanisms. *Diabetes* (2010) 59:98–104. doi: 10.2337/db09-0779
80. Jou MY, Philipps AF, Lonnerdal B. Maternal zinc deficiency in rats affects growth and glucose metabolism in the offspring by inducing insulin resistance postnatally. *J Nutr.* (2010) 140:1621–7. doi: 10.3945/jn.109.119677
81. Lu K, Abo RP, Schlieper KA, Graffam ME, Levine S, Wishnok JS, et al. Arsenic exposure perturbs the gut microbiome and its metabolic profile in mice: an integrated metagenomics and metabolomics analysis. *Environ Health Perspect.* (2014) 122:284–91. doi: 10.1289/ehp.1307429
82. Wu J, Wen XW, Faulk C, Boehnke K, Zhang H, Dolinoy DC, et al. Perinatal lead exposure alters gut microbiota composition and results in sex-specific bodyweight increases in adult mice. *Toxicol Sci.* (2016) 151:324–33. doi: 10.1093/toxsci/kfw046
83. Williams K, Milner J, Boudreau MD, Gokulan K, Cerniglia CE, Khare S. Effects of subchronic exposure of silver nanoparticles on intestinal microbiota and gut-associated immune responses in the ileum of Sprague-Dawley rats. *Nanotoxicology* (2015) 9:279–89. doi: 10.3109/17435390.2014.921346
84. Velmurugan G, Ramprasath T, Gilles M, Swaminathan K, Ramasamy S. Gut microbiota, endocrine-disrupting chemicals, and the diabetes epidemic. *Trends Endocrinol Metab.* (2017) 28:612–25. doi: 10.1016/j.tem.2017.05.001
85. Rosenfeld CS. Gut dysbiosis in animals due to environmental chemical exposures. *Front Cell Infect Microbiol.* (2017) 7:396. doi: 10.3389/fcimb.2017.00396
86. Javurek AB, Spollen WG, Johnson SA, Bivens NJ, Bromert KH, Givan SA, et al. Effects of exposure to bisphenol A and ethinyl estradiol on the gut microbiota of parents and their offspring in a rodent model. *Gut Microbes* (2016) 7:471–85. doi: 10.1080/19490976.2016.1234657
87. Barbazanges A, Piazza PV, Le Moal M, Maccari S. Maternal glucocorticoid secretion mediates long-term effects of prenatal stress. *J Neurosci.* (1996) 16:3943–9. doi: 10.1523/JNEUROSCI.16-12-03943.1996
88. Smythe JW, McCormick CM, Meaney MJ. Median eminence corticotrophin-releasing hormone content following prenatal stress and neonatal handling. *Brain Res Bull.* (1996) 40:195–9. doi: 10.1016/0361-9230(95)02146-9
89. Patterson CM, Bouret SG, Park S, Irani BG, Dunn-Meynell AA, Levin BE. Large litter rearing enhances leptin sensitivity and protects selectively bred diet-induced obese rats from becoming obese. *Endocrinology* (2010) 151:4270–9. doi: 10.1210/en.2010-0401
90. Patterson CM, Dunn-Meynell AA, Levin BE. Three weeks of early-onset exercise prolongs obesity resistance in DIO rats after exercise cessation. *Am J Physiol Regul Integr Comp Physiol.* (2008) 294:R290–301. doi: 10.1152/ajpregu.00661.2007
91. Pirsaheb M, Limoee M, Namdari F, Khamutian R. Organochlorine pesticides residue in breast milk: a systematic review. *Med J Islam Repub Iran* (2015) 29:228.
92. Cariou R, Veyrand B, Yamada A, Berrebi A, Zalko D, Durand S, et al. Perfluoroalkyl acid (PFAA) levels and profiles in breast milk, maternal and cord serum of French women and their newborns. *Environ Int.* (2015) 84:71–81. doi: 10.1016/j.envint.2015.07.014
93. Geusau A, Tschachler E, Meixner M, Sandermann S, Papke O, Wolf C, et al. Olestra increases faecal excretion of 2,3,7,8-tetrachlorodibenzo-*p*-dioxin. *Lancet* (1999) 354:1266–7. doi: 10.1016/S0140-6736(99)04271-3
94. Redgrave TG, Wallace P, Jandacek RJ, Tso P. Treatment with a dietary fat substitute decreased Arochlor 1254 contamination in an obese diabetic male. *J Nutr Biochem.* (2005) 16:383–4. doi: 10.1016/j.jnutbio.2004.12.014
95. Jandacek RJ, Heubi JE, Buckley DD, Khoury JC, Turner WE, Sjodin A, et al. Reduction of the body burden of PCBs and DDE by dietary intervention in a randomized trial. *J Nutr Biochem.* (2014) 25:483–8. doi: 10.1016/j.jnutbio.2014.01.002
96. Dirtu AC, Dirinck E, Malarvannan G, Neels H, Van Gaal L, Jorens PG, et al. Dynamics of organohalogenated contaminants in human serum from obese individuals during one year of weight loss treatment. *Environ Sci Technol.* (2013) 47:12441–9. doi: 10.1021/es400657t
97. Dirinck E, Dirtu AC, Jorens PG, Malarvannan G, Covaci A, Van Gaal LF. Pivotal role for the visceral fat compartment in the release of persistent organic pollutants during weight loss. *J Clin Endocrinol Metab.* (2015) 100:4463–71. doi: 10.1210/jc.2015-2571

98. Hue O, Marcotte J, Berrigan F, Simoneau M, Dore J, Marceau P, et al. Increased plasma levels of toxic pollutants accompanying weight loss induced by hypocaloric diet or by bariatric surgery. *Obes Surg.* (2006) 16:1145–54. doi: 10.1381/096089206778392356
99. Charlier C, Desaive C, Plomteux G. Human exposure to endocrine disrupters: consequences of gastroplasty on plasma concentration of toxic pollutants. *Int J Obes Relat Metab Disord.* (2002) 26:1465–8. doi: 10.1038/sj.ijo.0802144
100. Kim MJ, Marchand P, Henegar C, Antignac JP, Alili R, Poitou C, et al. Fate and complex pathogenic effects of dioxins and polychlorinated biphenyls in obese subjects before and after drastic weight loss. *Environ Health Perspect.* (2011) 119:377–83. doi: 10.1289/ehp.1002848
101. Arguin H, Sanchez M, Bray GA, Lovejoy JC, Peters JC, Jandacek RJ, et al. Impact of adopting a vegan diet or an olestra supplementation on plasma organochlorine concentrations: results from two pilot studies. *Br J Nutr.* (2010) 103:1433–41. doi: 10.1017/S000711450999331X
102. Guo W, Huen K, Park JS, Petreas M, Crispo Smith S, Block G, et al. Vitamin C intervention may lower the levels of persistent organic pollutants in blood of healthy women - a pilot study. *Food Chem Toxicol.* (2016) 92:197–204. doi: 10.1016/j.fct.2016.04.006
103. Nayak B, Burman K. Thyrotoxicosis and thyroid storm. *Endocrinol Metab Clin North Am.* (2006) 35:663–86, vii. doi: 10.1016/j.ecl.2006.09.008
104. Takenaka S, Morita K, Tokiwa H, Takahashi K. Effects of rice bran fibre and cholestyramine on the faecal excretion of Kanechlor 600 (PCB) in rats. *Xenobiotica* (1991) 21:351–7. doi: 10.3109/00498259109039475
105. Iida T, Nakagawa R, Hirakawa H, Matsueda T, Morita K, Hamamura K, et al. Clinical trial of a combination of rice bran fiber and cholestyramine for promotion of fecal excretion of retained polychlorinated dibenzofuran and polychlorinated biphenyl in Yu-Cheng patients. *Fukuoka Igaku Zasshi* (1995) 86:226–33.
106. Rosenstock J, Rigby SP, Ford DM, Tao B, Chou HS. The glucose and lipid effects of colesevelam as monotherapy in drug-naive type 2 diabetes. *Horm Metab Res.* (2014) 46:348–53. doi: 10.1055/s-0033-1358759
107. Quazi S, Yokogoshi H, Yoshida A. Effect of dietary fiber on hypercholesterolemia induced by dietary PCB or cholesterol in rats. *J Nutr.* (1983) 113:1109–18. doi: 10.1093/jn/113.6.1109
108. Kimura Y, Nagata Y, Buddington RK. Some dietary fibers increase elimination of orally administered polychlorinated biphenyls but not that of retinol in mice. *J Nutr.* (2004) 134:135–42. doi: 10.1093/jn/134.1.135
109. Takasuga T, Senthilkumar K, Takemori H, Ohi E, Tsuji H, Nagayama J. Impact of FEBRA (fermented brown rice with Aspergillus oryzae) intake and concentrations of PCDDs, PCDFs and PCBs in blood of humans from Japan. *Chemosphere* (2004) 57:1409–26. doi: 10.1016/j.chemosphere.2004.08.082
110. Sera N, Morita K, Nagasoe M, Tokieda H, Kitaura T, Tokiwa H. Binding effect of polychlorinated compounds and environmental carcinogens on rice bran fiber. *J Nutr Biochem.* (2005) 16:50–8. doi: 10.1016/j.jnutbio.2004.09.005
111. De Vos S, De Schrijver R. Polychlorinated biphenyl distribution and faecal excretion in rats fed wheat bran. *Chemosphere* (2005) 61:374–82. doi: 10.1016/j.chemosphere.2005.02.086
112. Vermeylen W, De Vos S, De Schrijver R. Effects of dietary wheat bran on absorption and accumulation of PCBs in rats. *Chemosphere* (2008) 71:277–83. doi: 10.1016/j.chemosphere.2007.09.026
113. Lignell S, Winkvist A, Bertz F, Rasmussen KM, Glynn A, Aune M, et al. Environmental organic pollutants in human milk before and after weight loss. *Chemosphere* (2016) 159:96–102. doi: 10.1016/j.chemosphere.2016.05.077
114. Dirinck EL, Dirtu AC, Govindan M, Covaci A, Jorens PG, Van Gaal LF. Endocrine-disrupting polychlorinated biphenyls in metabolically healthy and unhealthy obese subjects before and after weight loss: difference at the start but not at the finish. *Am J Clin Nutr.* (2016) 103:989–98. doi: 10.3945/ajcn.115.119081
115. La Merrill M, Karey E, Moshier E, Lindtner C, La Frano MR, Newman JW, et al. Perinatal exposure of mice to the pesticide DDT impairs energy expenditure and metabolism in adult female offspring. *PLoS ONE* (2014) 9:e103337. doi: 10.1371/journal.pone.0103337
116. Wei J, Lin Y, Li Y, Ying C, Chen J, Song L, et al. Perinatal exposure to bisphenol A at reference dose predisposes offspring to metabolic syndrome in adult rats on a high-fat diet. *Endocrinology* (2011) 152:3049–61. doi: 10.1210/en.2011-0045
117. Patel BB, Di Iorio M, Chalifour LE. Metabolic response to chronic bisphenol A exposure in C57bl/6n mice. *Toxicol Rep.* (2014) 1:522–32. doi: 10.1016/j.toxrep.2014.07.012
118. Ding S, Fan Y, Zhao N, Yang H, Ye X, He D, et al. High-fat diet aggravates glucose homeostasis disorder caused by chronic exposure to bisphenol A. *J Endocrinol.* (2014) 221:167–79. doi: 10.1530/JOE-13-0386
119. Moon MK, Jeong IK, Jung Oh T, Ahn HY, Kim HH, Park YJ, et al. Long-term oral exposure to bisphenol A induces glucose intolerance and insulin resistance. *J Endocrinol.* (2015) 226:35–42. doi: 10.1530/JOE-14-0714
120. Yu J, Yang J, Luo Y, Mengxue Y, Li W, Yang Y, et al. The adverse effects of chronic low-dose exposure to nonylphenol on type 2 diabetes mellitus in high sucrose-high fat diet-treated rats. *Islets* (2018) 10:1–9. doi: 10.1080/19382014.2017.1404211
121. Yu J, Yang X, Yang X, Yang M, Wang P, Yang Y, et al. Nonylphenol aggravates non-alcoholic fatty liver disease in high sucrose-high fat diet-treated rats. *Sci Rep.* (2018) 8:3232. doi: 10.1038/s41598-018-21725-y
122. Brulport A, Le Corre L, Chagnon MC. Chronic exposure of 2,3,7,8-tetrachlorodibenzo-*p*-dioxin (TCDD) induces an obesogenic effect in C57BL/6J mice fed a high fat diet. *Toxicology* (2017) 390:43–52. doi: 10.1016/j.tox.2017.07.017
123. Wei J, Sun X, Chen Y, Li Y, Song L, Zhou Z, et al. Perinatal exposure to bisphenol A exacerbates nonalcoholic steatohepatitis-like phenotype in male rat offspring fed on a high-fat diet. *J Endocrinol.* (2014) 222:313–25. doi: 10.1530/JOE-14-0356
124. Regnier SM, Kirkley AG, Ye H, El-Hashani E, Zhang X, Neel BA, et al. Dietary exposure to the endocrine disruptor tolylfluanid promotes global metabolic dysfunction in male mice. *Endocrinology* (2015) 156:896–910. doi: 10.1210/en.2014-1668
125. Regnier SM, Kirkley AG, Ruiz D, Kamau W, Wu Q, Kannan K, et al. Diet-dependence of metabolic perturbations mediated by the endocrine disruptor tolylfluanid. *Endocr Connect.* (2018) 7:159–68. doi: 10.1530/EC-17-0320
126. Gross LS, Li L, Ford ES, Liu S. Increased consumption of refined carbohydrates and the epidemic of type 2 diabetes in the United States: an ecologic assessment. *Am J Clin Nutr.* (2004) 79:774–9. doi: 10.1093/ajcn/79.5.774
127. Shai I, Schwarzfuchs D, Henkin Y, Shahar DR, Witkow S, Greenberg I, et al. Weight loss with a low-carbohydrate, Mediterranean, or low-fat diet. *N Engl J Med.* (2008) 359:229–41. doi: 10.1056/NEJMoa0708681
128. Estruch R, Ros E, Salas-Salvado J, Covas MI, Corella D, Aros F, et al. Primary prevention of cardiovascular disease with a mediterranean diet supplemented with extra-virgin olive oil or nuts. *N Engl J Med.* (2018) 378:e34. doi: 10.1056/NEJMoa1800389
129. Liu G, Dhana K, Furtado JD, Rood J, Zong G, Liang L, et al. Perfluoroalkyl substances and changes in body weight and resting metabolic rate in response to weight-loss diets: a prospective study. *PLoS Med.* (2018) 15:e1002502. doi: 10.1371/journal.pmed.1002502
130. Yang CS. Influences of dietary and other factors on xenobiotic metabolism and carcinogenesis-a review article in memory of Dr. Allan H. Conney (1930-2013). *Nutr Cancer* (2015) 67:1207–13. doi: 10.1080/01635581.2015.1081010
131. Martins T, Colaco B, Venancio C, Pires MJ, Oliveira PA, Rosa E, et al. Potential effects of sulforaphane to fight obesity. *J Sci Food Agric.* (2018) 98:2837–44. doi: 10.1002/jsfa.8898
132. Xu Y, Fu JF, Chen JH, Zhang ZW, Zou ZQ, Han LY, et al. Sulforaphane ameliorates glucose intolerance in obese mice via the upregulation of the insulin signaling pathway. *Food Funct.* (2018) 9:4695–701. doi: 10.1039/c8fo00763b
133. Shawky NM, Segar L. Sulforaphane improves leptin responsiveness in high-fat high-sucrose diet-fed obese mice. *Eur J Pharmacol.* (2018) 835:108–14. doi: 10.1016/j.ejphar.2018.07.050
134. Yang SH, Yu LH, Li L, Guo Y, Zhang Y, Long M, et al. Protective mechanism of sulforaphane on cadmium-induced sertoli cell injury in mice testis via Nrf2/ARE signaling pathway. *Molecules* (2018) 23:23071774. doi: 10.3390/molecules23071774
135. Sohel MMH, Amin A, Prastowo S, Linares-Otoya L, Hoelker M, Schellander K, et al. Sulforaphane protects granulosa cells against oxidative stress via activation of NRF2-ARE pathway. *Cell Tissue Res.* (2018) 374:629–41. doi: 10.1007/s00441-018-2877-z..
136. Su X, Jiang X, Meng L, Dong X, Shen Y, Xin Y. Anticancer activity of sulforaphane: the epigenetic mechanisms and the Nrf2 signaling pathway. *Oxid Med Cell Longev.* (2018) 2018:5438179. doi: 10.1155/2018/5438179

137. Huderson AC, Rekha Devi PV, Niaz MS, Adunyah SE, Ramesh A. Alteration of benzo(a)pyrene biotransformation by resveratrol in Apc (Min/+) mouse model of colon carcinogenesis. *Invest New Drugs* (2018) 22:9. doi: 10.1007/s10637-018-0622-9
138. Myers GJ, Davidson PW, Strain JJ. Nutrient and methyl mercury exposure from consuming fish. *J Nutr.* (2007) 137:2805–8. doi: 10.1093/jn/137.12.2805
139. Wright RO, Tsaih SW, Schwartz J, Wright RJ, Hu H. Association between iron deficiency and blood lead level in a longitudinal analysis of children followed in an urban primary care clinic. *J Pediatr.* (2003) 142:9–14. doi: 10.1067/mpd.2003.mpd0344
140. Bradman A, Eskenazi B, Sutton P, Athanasoulis M, Goldman LR. Iron deficiency associated with higher blood lead in children living in contaminated environments. *Environ Health Perspect.* (2001) 109:1079–84. doi: 10.1289/ehp.011091079
141. Schell LM, Denham M, Stark AD, Gomez M, Ravenscroft J, Parsons PJ, et al. Maternal blood lead concentration, diet during pregnancy, and anthropometry predict neonatal blood lead in a socioeconomically disadvantaged population. *Environ Health Perspect.* (2003) 111:195–200. doi: 10.1289/ehp.5592
142. Hertz-Picciotto I, Schramm M, Watt-Morse M, Chantala K, Anderson J, Osterloh J. Patterns and determinants of blood lead during pregnancy. *Am J Epidemiol.* (2000) 152:829–37. doi: 10.1093/aje/152.9.829
143. Sargent JD, Dalton MA, O'Connor GT, Olmstead EM, Klein RZ. Randomized trial of calcium glycerophosphate-supplemented infant formula to prevent lead absorption. *Am J Clin Nutr.* (1999) 69:1224–30. doi: 10.1093/ajcn/69.6.1224
144. Markowitz ME, Sinnett M, Rosen JF. A randomized trial of calcium supplementation for childhood lead poisoning. *Pediatrics* (2004) 113(1 Pt 1):e34–9. doi: 10.1542/peds.113.1.e34
145. Ramanathan K, Anusuyadevi M, Shila S, Panneerselvam C. Ascorbic acid and alpha-tocopherol as potent modulators of apoptosis on arsenic induced toxicity in rats. *Toxicol Lett.* (2005) 156:297–306. doi: 10.1016/j.toxlet.2004.12.003
146. Ramanathan K, Shila S, Kumaran S, Panneerselvam C. Ascorbic acid and alpha-tocopherol as potent modulators on arsenic induced toxicity in mitochondria. *J Nutr Biochem.* (2003) 14:416–20. doi: 10.1016/S0955-2863(03)00076-7
147. Sohini, Rana SV. Protective effect of ascorbic acid against oxidative stress induced by inorganic arsenic in liver and kidney of rat. *Indian J Exp Biol.* (2007) 45:371–5.
148. Garcia-Chavez E, Jimenez I, Segura B, Del Razo LM. Lipid oxidative damage and distribution of inorganic arsenic and its metabolites in the rat nervous system after arsenite exposure: influence of alpha tocopherol supplementation. *Neurotoxicology* (2006) 27:1024–31. doi: 10.1016/j.neuro.2006.05.001
149. Wei M, Arnold L, Cano M, Cohen SM. Effects of co-administration of antioxidants and arsenicals on the rat urinary bladder epithelium. *Toxicol Sci.* (2005) 83:237–45. doi: 10.1093/toxsci/kfi033
150. Chattopadhyay S, Bhaumik S, Purkayastha M, Basu S, Nag Chaudhuri A, Das Gupta S. Apoptosis and necrosis in developing brain cells due to arsenic toxicity and protection with antioxidants. *Toxicol Lett.* (2002) 136:65–76. doi: 10.1016/S0378-4274(02)00282-5
151. Bongiovanni GA, Soria EA, Eynard AR. Effects of the plant flavonoids silymarin and quercetin on arsenite-induced oxidative stress in CHO-K1 cells. *Food Chem Toxicol.* (2007) 45:971–6. doi: 10.1016/j.fct.2006.12.002
152. Gupta R, Dubey DK, Kannan GM, Flora SJ. Concomitant administration of Moringa oleifera seed powder in the remediation of arsenic-induced oxidative stress in mouse. *Cell Biol Int.* (2007) 31:44–56. doi: 10.1016/j.cellbi.2006.09.007
153. Mandal AK, Das S, Basu MK, Chakrabarti RN, Das N. Hepatoprotective activity of liposomal flavonoid against arsenite-induced liver fibrosis. *J Pharmacol Exp Ther.* (2007) 320:994–1001. doi: 10.1124/jpet.106.114215
154. Sharma A, Sharma MK, Kumar M. Protective effect of Mentha piperita against arsenic-induced toxicity in liver of Swiss albino mice. *Basic Clin Pharmacol Toxicol.* (2007) 100:249–57. doi: 10.1111/j.1742-7843.2006.00030.x
155. Rabbani GH, Saha SK, Akhtar M, Marni F, Mitra AK, Ahmed S, et al. Antioxidants in detoxification of arsenic-induced oxidative injury in rabbits: preliminary results. *J Environ Sci Health A Tox Hazard Subst Environ Eng* (2003) 38:273–87. doi: 10.1081/ESE-120016894
156. Kibriya MG, Jasmine F, Argos M, Verret WJ, Rakibuz-Zaman M, Ahmed A, et al. Changes in gene expression profiles in response to selenium supplementation among individuals with arsenic-induced pre-malignant skin lesions. *Toxicol Lett.* (2007) 169:162–76. doi: 10.1016/j.toxlet.2007.01.006
157. Zeng H, Uthus EO, Combs GF Jr. Mechanistic aspects of the interaction between selenium and arsenic. *J Inorg Biochem.* (2005) 99:1269–74. doi: 10.1016/j.jinorgbio.2005.03.006
158. Hartwig A, Blessing H, Schwerdtle T, Walter I. Modulation of DNA repair processes by arsenic and selenium compounds. *Toxicology* (2003) 193:161–9. doi: 10.1016/j.tox.2003.08.004
159. Chattopadhyay S, Pal Ghosh S, Ghosh D, Debnath J. Effect of dietary co-administration of sodium selenite on sodium arsenite-induced ovarian and uterine disorders in mature albino rats. *Toxicol Sci.* (2003) 75:412–22. doi: 10.1093/toxsci/kfg194
160. Styblo M, Thomas DJ. Selenium modifies the metabolism and toxicity of arsenic in primary rat hepatocytes. *Toxicol Appl Pharmacol.* (2001) 172:52–61. doi: 10.1006/taap.2001.9134
161. Nakano S, Noguchi T, Takekoshi H, Suzuki G, Nakano M. Maternal-fetal distribution and transfer of dioxins in pregnant women in Japan, and attempts to reduce maternal transfer with Chlorella (Chlorella pyrenoidosa) supplements. *Chemosphere* (2005) 61:1244–55. doi: 10.1016/j.chemosphere.2005.03.080
162. Beauchamp TL, Childress JF. *Principles of Biomedical Ethics. 6th ed.* New York, NY: Oxford University Press (2009). p. 417.
163. Hernandez-Diaz S, Mitchell AA, Kelley KE, Calafat AM, Hauser R. Medications as a potential source of exposure to phthalates in the U.S. population. *Environ Health Perspect.* (2009) 117:185–9. doi: 10.1289/ehp.11766
164. Hernandez-Diaz S, Su YC, Mitchell AA, Kelley KE, Calafat AM, Hauser R. Medications as a potential source of exposure to phthalates among women of childbearing age. *Reprod Toxicol.* (2013) 37:1–5. doi: 10.1016/j.reprotox.2013.01.001
165. Kelley KE, Hernandez-Diaz S, Chaplin EL, Hauser R, Mitchell AA. Identification of phthalates in medications and dietary supplement formulations in the United States and Canada. *Environ Health Perspect.* (2012) 120:379–84. doi: 10.1289/ehp.1103998
166. Broe A, Ennis ZN, Pottegard A, Hallas J, Ahern T, Damkier P. Population exposure to phthalate-containing drugs. *Basic Clin Pharmacol Toxicol.* (2017) 121:153–8. doi: 10.1111/bcpt.12781
167. Broe A, Pottegard A, Hallas J, Ahern TP, Fedder J, Damkier P. Association between use of phthalate-containing medication and semen quality among men in couples referred for assisted reproduction. *Hum Reprod.* (2018) 33:503–11. doi: 10.1093/humrep/dey009
168. von Rettberg H, Hannman T, Subotic U, Brade J, Schaible T, Waag KL, et al. Use of di(2-ethylhexyl)phthalate-containing infusion systems increases the risk for cholestasis. *Pediatrics* (2009) 124:710–6. doi: 10.1542/peds.2008-1765
169. Sargis RM. Metabolic Disruption in context: clinical avenues for synergistic perturbations in energy homeostasis by endocrine disrupting chemicals. *Endocr Disrupt.* (2015) 3:e1080788. doi: 10.1080/23273747.2015.1080788
170. Shaikh S, Jagai JS, Ashley C, Zhou S, Sargis RM. Underutilized and under threat: environmental policy as a tool to address diabetes risk. *Curr Diab Rep.* (2018) 18:25. doi: 10.1007/s11892-018-0993-5

19

Endocrine Disrupting Chemicals: An Occult Mediator of Metabolic Disease

*Olga Papalou[1], Eleni A. Kandaraki[1], George Papadakis[2] and Evanthia Diamanti-Kandarakis[1]**

[1] Department of Endocrinology & Diabetes, Hygeia Hospital, Athens, Greece, [2] STEPS Stoffwechselzentrum, Biel/Bienne, Switzerland

***Correspondence:**
Evanthia Diamanti-Kandarakis
e.diamanti.kandarakis@gmail.com

Endocrine disrupting chemicals (EDCs), a heterogeneous group of exogenous chemicals that can interfere with any aspect of endogenous hormones, represent an emerging global threat for human metabolism. There is now considerable evidence that the observed upsurge of metabolic disease cannot be fully attributed to increased caloric intake, physical inactivity, sleep deficit, and ageing. Among environmental factors implicated in the global deterioration of metabolic health, EDCs have drawn the biggest attention of scientific community, and not unjustifiably. EDCs unleash a coordinated attack toward multiple components of human metabolism, including crucial, metabolically-active organs such as hypothalamus, adipose tissue, pancreatic beta cells, skeletal muscle, and liver. Specifically, EDCs' impact during critical developmental windows can promote the disruption of individual or multiple systems involved in metabolism, via inducing epigenetic changes that can permanently alter the epigenome in the germline, enabling changes to be transmitted to the subsequent generations. The clear effect of this multifaceted attack is the manifestation of metabolic disease, clinically expressed as obesity, metabolic syndrome, diabetes mellitus, and non-alcoholic fatty liver disease. Although limitations of EDCs research do exist, there is no doubt that EDCs constitute a crucial parameter of the global deterioration of metabolic health we currently encounter.

Keywords: obesity, insulin resistance, human metabolism, endocrine disrupting chemical (EDC), environmental contaminants, obesogens, enviromental chemicals, diabetes mellitus

INTRODUCTION

During the last 50 years, the global rates of obesity, diabetes, and metabolic disease have increased exponentially (1). Based on the data from the *International Diabetes Federation*, ~415 million people worldwide were estimated to have diabetes in 2015, a percentage that will rise to 642 million people by 2040 (2), while, simultaneously, in 2016, the *World Health Organization* estimated that 650 million people are obese and ~2 billion people are overweight worldwide (3). When these numbers are translated to individual morbidity and mortality, the calculated societal and financial burden we are facing is hugely disappointing (4–6). Thus, in order to tackle this burgeoning metabolic disease epidemic, we have to identify the underlying pathogenetic factors and mitigate their deleterious impact.

Genetic background, increased caloric intake, physical inactivity, sleep deficit, and aging have been recognized by medical community as major pathogenetic parameters in metabolic disease (7). However, existing bibliography suggests that the observed upsurge of metabolic disease cannot be fully attributed to the above-mentioned risk factors. In fact, individuals nowadays tend to weigh more than they did 20–30 years ago even when the amount of activity and caloric intake are the same (8).

Among environmental factors involved in the worldwide deterioration of metabolic health, endocrine disrupting chemicals (EDCs) have drawn the biggest attention of scientific community, and not unjustifiably (9). In fact, the documented increase of obesity and metabolic disease correlates and coincides chronically with an upsurge in EDCs generation and widespread use (10, 11). While emerging epidemiological data are highlighting the close association between EDCs and metabolic disease epidemic, experimental data, and animal models have postulated multiple potent pathways by which EDCs alter hormonal milieu and promote metabolic disease, mandating immediate action and policy-making.

In this review, we will present evidence of how environmental contaminants can perturb human metabolism, through interfering with control of energy metabolism and targeting multiple metabolically crucial organs, causing ultimately an altered balance toward obesity and dysmetabolism and contributing to this global metabolic emergency.

ENDOCRINE-DISRUPTING CHEMICALS (EDCS): HAVE WE OPENED THE PANDORA'S BOX?

Overview of Endocrine-Disrupting Chemicals–Historical Data

Endocrine-disrupting chemicals (EDCs) are defined as exogenous chemicals or mixtures of chemicals that interfere with any aspect of endogenous hormonal signaling, affecting not only production, release, and transport of hormones, but also their cellular metabolism, binding action, and elimination (9, 12). It is a heterogeneous, rapidly growing group of natural or man-made chemical compounds, including synthetic chemicals used as industrial solvents, plastics, plasticizers, fungicides, pesticides, heavy metals, and pharmaceutical agents (12, 13).

While scientific community was slowly gaining knowledge regarding environmental contaminants, it was in 1991 that the term "endocrine-disrupter" was firstly introduced (14).

In 2006, researchers at the University of California, Irvine, highlighted the role of EDCs in the global obesity epidemic and coined the term "obesogen" (15). Obesogens were defined as environmental agents that have the ability to promote obesity via inducing an increment in the number of fat cells and/or the storage of fat in adipocytes, as well as via shifting metabolism toward a mode of caloric storage (16). As the list of obesogenic chemicals is continuously growing, the obesogen field has broadened in recognizing chemicals that are linked with diabetes and other metabolic diseases (17). Thus, in 2015, the Parma consensus statement proposed the term "metabolism-disrupting chemicals (MDCs)" to describe the EDCs that can promote diabetes, obesity, and fatty liver, through perturbing metabolism at multiple cellular levels (18).

Overall, EDCs have ascended as a global health priority and organizations such as Endocrine Society and the WHO/UNEP have issued official statements regarding the putative health risks posed by EDCs, describing the plethora of diseases EDCs are related to, including reproduction, neurodevelopment, thyroid, metabolism, and hormone-related cancers (9, 19). Although we have made a considerable progress in understanding EDCs, we are still looking at the "tip of the iceberg" and there are much more to be learned (**Figure 1**).

EDCs Characteristics and Unique Properties

Over 1,000 synthesized chemical compounds are considered to be EDCs, such as plastics (bisphenol A), plasticizers (phthalates), industrial solvents/lubricants, and their byproducts (polychlorinated biphenyls, polybrominated biphenyls, dioxins), pesticides (methoxychlor, chlorpyrifos, dichlorodiphenyltrichloroethane), fungicides (vinclozolin), and pharmaceutical agents (diethylstilbestrol) (20). There are multiple routes of exposure to the above EDCs, including air, water, food, and consumer products. Some of them have low accumulation in human body (BPA, phthalates), while others are very lipophilic, accumulating easily in the food chain and the adipose tissue (persistent organic pollutants - POPs) (**Table 1**) (21). EDCs can also be found in various biological fluids, including sera, urine, amniotic fluid, and breast milk (22).

Although EDCs are characterized as a group of compounds with high heterogeneity, there are some key characteristics that define them and enable us to better understand their mechanism of action and their consequences.

- EDCs, just like hormones, may promote disrupting effects even in very low levels of exposure, particularly if exposure takes place in a critical developmental period. In fact, EDCs display a non-monotonic (U-shaped or biphasic) response, which means that low doses may have a much stronger impact in human body than higher doses (23, 24).
- EDCs usually display a much lower affinity for hormone receptors, compared to natural ligands. For instance, the affinity of the estrogen receptors (ER), ER-a and ER-b, for one of the most widespread EDCs, bisphenol-A (BPA) is 1,000–10,000 fold lower than for 17b-estradiol (E2) (25). Nevertheless, EDCs, even under these circumstances, can have detrimental effects in several human tissues.
- Time of exposure is critical in EDCs' effects. EDC exposure during sensitive developmental periods, such as fetal life, infancy, puberty, pregnancy, and menopause, can detrimentally affect individuals and predispose them to a multitude of diseases (26, 27).
- There is a lag between the time of exposure to EDCs and the clinical expression of a disease, suggesting that the repercussions of EDCs exposure may not be directly

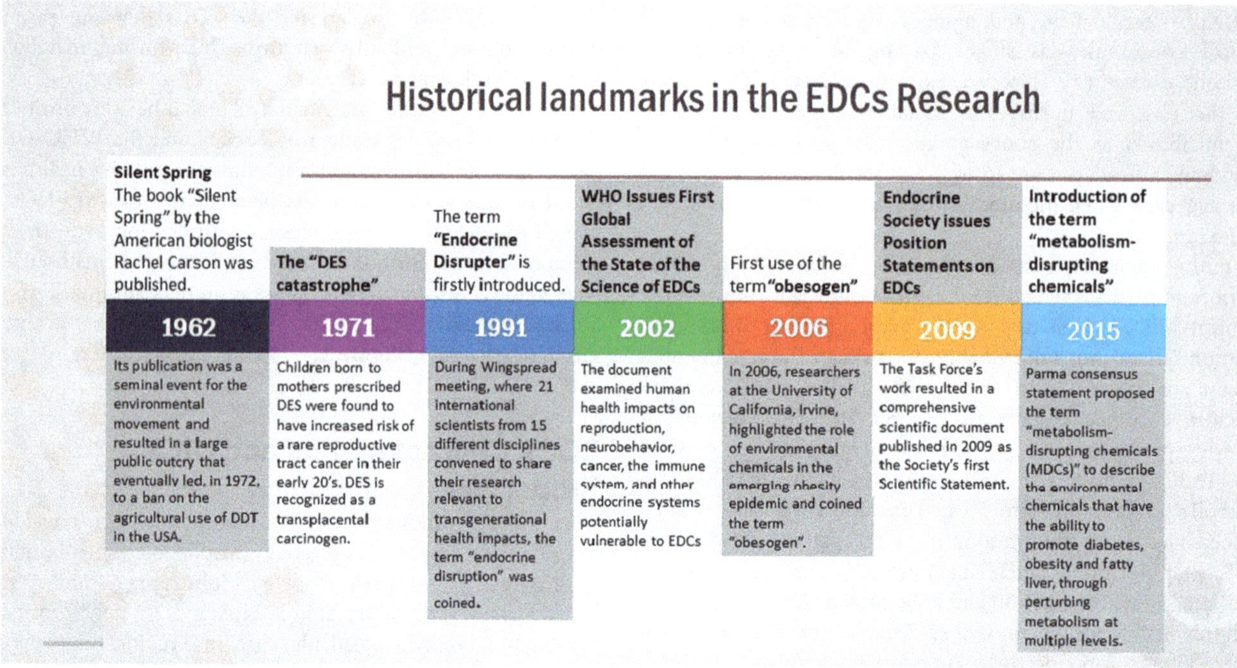

FIGURE 1 | Historical landmarks in the field of EDCs Research.

evident, but may be ultimately manifested many years after the exposure (12).

- Since environmental pollution is not caused by a single compound, it is rather reasonable that humans are constantly exposed not to one, but to a cocktail of EDCs. In a mixture, the different classes of EDCs interact in an either additive or synergistic way, making even more difficult not only to predict the net effect they provoke, but also to evince a cause-and-effect association between a specific EDC and an associated effect-disease (28).

Vulnerable Windows of Susceptibility–Developmental Programming and Transgenerational Effects of EDCs

The "Developmental origins of health and diseases" (DOHaD) hypothesis, initially expressed by David Barker, has introduced the concept that early life growth and development is vulnerable to environmental disruptors, which can determine the risk for health and disease (29). In other words, environmental disruption during critical developmental windows is capable of promoting subtle changes in gene expression and biological molecular processes, which, ultimately, alter permanently the developmental trajectory and lead to long-lasting dysfunction.

Nutrition has been introduced as a powerful environmental stimulus that can promote intrauterine modifications, manifesting later in life as increased vulnerability to obesity and dysmetabolism. More analytically, undernutrition *in utero* and low-birth weight, combined with early catch-up growth during infancy, was shown to be correlated with augmented risk for impaired metabolism, cardiovascular disease and reproductive deregulation in adulthood (30–32). Analogously, maternal obesity or obesogenic maternal diet during gestation, was associated with increased oxidative stress in the offspring, making them sensitive to diabetogenic effects (33, 34).

Apart from nutrition, EDCs also hold a special position in the DOHaD hypothesis. The "Diethylstilbestrol (DES) catastrophe" provided the original proof regarding the ability of EDCs to perturb developmental processes and predispose to certain diseases. Back in 1940–1970, prescription of DES to numerous women, in order to prevent miscarriage, led to reproductive tract anomalies and substantially increased the incidence of mammary cancer in their offspring (35). Nowadays, accumulating data support that EDCs impact during critical developmental windows can be disruptive for multiple systems involved in human metabolism. For example, both in animal and human studies, developmental exposure to DES, led to increased weight gain and adipocyte hyperplasia in the offspring, predisposing them to obesity during adulthood (36, 37). Likewise, EDCs acting during fetal or perinatal period, can permanently perturb adipose tissue function, via altering the programming of mesenchymal stem cells (38).

One of the main mechanisms, via which EDCs alter programming of cell and tissue differentiation, is by inducing epigenetic changes (9, 39). Epigenetic changes are defined as heritable alterations in gene expression, without any structural change in DNA sequence, which can be transmitted through mitosis and/or meiosis. There are several mechanisms, by which epigenetics can modulate gene expression and modify gene

TABLE 1 | Endocrine disruptors (EDCs) with documented metabolism-disrupting effects.

Endocrine disrupters (EDCs)	Description and characteristics
PERSISTENT ORGANIC POLLUTANTS (POPS)	
Dichlorodiphenyltrichloroethane (DDT)	A synthetic insecticide with a long half-life, extensive use, and lipophilic nature. The United States banned DDT in 1972 due to its effects on the environment and human health. DDT and its metabolites seem to contribute to the manifestation of endocrine-related diseases, including diabetes mellitus.
Dioxins	Dioxins are mainly by-products of industrial processes but can also result from natural processes, such as volcanic eruptions and forest fires. Their half-life in the body is estimated to be 7 to 11 years. They accumulate in food chain and in the adipose tissue of human body. The most harmful dioxin is 2,3,7,8-tetrachlorodibenzo -p-dioxin (TCDD).
Polychlorinated biphenyls (PCBs)	Man-made synthetic chemical mixtures, widely used in electrical equipment, ink solvents and especially plasticizers until the late 1970s, after which time they were banned. Their use has been associated with the obesity epidemic.
Perfluorinated compounds (PFCs)	PFCs have been detected in food packaging, furniture, clothes, cookware, and non-stick surfaces in order to repel grease and oil. They have been linked with obesity and adipose tissue dysfunction.
Polybrominated flame retardants	They have been used in a variety of materials, such as furniture, electronics, and construction materials, as flame retardants. Via accumulating in the environment and human fat tissue, these man-made chemicals have been linked with adverse health outcomes, including obesity.
NON-PERSISTENT EDCS	
Bishenol A (BPA)	A synthetic organic compound, mainly used as plasticizer, is commonly detected in water bottles, food containers, and metal-based cans. The magnitude of human exposure to this EDC is depicted to the observation that ~93% of Americans have measurable urine levels of BPA. It is characterized by a rapid metabolization to its non-bioactive forms and a short half-life (4–5 h in adult humans).
Phthalates	Pthalates have been widely used in the manufacture of polyvinyl chloride plastics and vinyl products. As a result, they have been detected in multiple household products, including pacifiers, children's toys, food packaging, medical devices, and furnishings. Animal models have displayed a close interrelationship between phthalates and metabolic disease.
Tributyltin	An organotin commonly used as a heat stabilizer and as fungicide. It can also be found in house dust. Although data on human exposures are scarce, it has been detected in human liver and blood.

transcription, including methylation of cytosine residues on DNA, post-translational modification of histones, and altered microRNA expression (40, 41).

Adult exposure to EDCs is likely a potential factor of adverse health outcomes. However, when this exposure takes place in early life development, EDCs-induced epigenetic alterations permanently affect the epigenome in the germline, enabling changes to be transmitted to the next generations (42). This transgenerational component of EDCs' can be applied only when exposure occurs during development. As soon as a pregnant female (F0) is exposed to an EDC, germline cells of her fetus (F1) are also exposed to it. These germline cells of the exposed F1 will be the gametes of the F2 generation, resulting in the direct exposure of the F2 generation to this EDC. F3 generation will be the first generation that has not been directly exposed to the EDC (43). Therefore, if the effects of the EDC persist in F3 generation, they considered to be transgenerational. (**Figure 2**).

Transgenerational sequelae of EDCs have been best studied in BPA and vinclozolin. Specifically, in animal models, prenatal exposure to BPA led to alterations in the prostate epigenome, affecting genes that are interrelated with prostate cancer (44, 45), while ancestral environmental exposure to vinclozolin in rodents was shown to be associated with transgenerational effects on the development of physiological, neural, and behavioral phenotypes in adulthood in the F3 generation(46, 47).

Regarding metabolism, experimental data about potential transgenerational effects of EDCs are now emerging. For example, prenatal TBT exposure via drinking water of pregnant F0 animals led to increased most white adipose tissue (WAT) depot weights, adipocyte size, and adipocyte number, and reprogrammed MSCs toward the adipocyte lineage at the expense of bone in all three subsequent generations(48). Skinner et al. have shown that a mixture of plastic derived compounds, BPA and phthalates, can promote epigenetic transgenerational alterations that predispose offspring in the F3 generation to obesity (49).

Overall, although the precise molecular mechanisms of how EDCs promote epigenetic changes remain unclear and cause and effect data are lacking, it is very likely that these chemicals have a more deleterious impact in human endocrine system than robust data can support so far. Even if we manage to annihilate environmental contaminants today, the impact of their disruptive effects to the next generations would be probably an after event documentation.

HUMAN METABOLISM: A PRECISE HORMONAL INTERPLAY BETWEEN TISSUES

Energy homeostasis involves the coordinated homeostatic regulation of food intake (energy inflow) and energy expenditure (energy outflow). A precise orchestration of the actions of metabolically-active, such as liver, pancreas, adipose tissue, brain, gut, and thyroid, stands in the core of human energy homeostasis

Hypothalamus has a critical role in regulating energy intake and appetite, decoding neural influences arising from other sites of the brain as well as hormonal signals. There are two different neural populations that coexist in the arcuate nucleus (ARC)

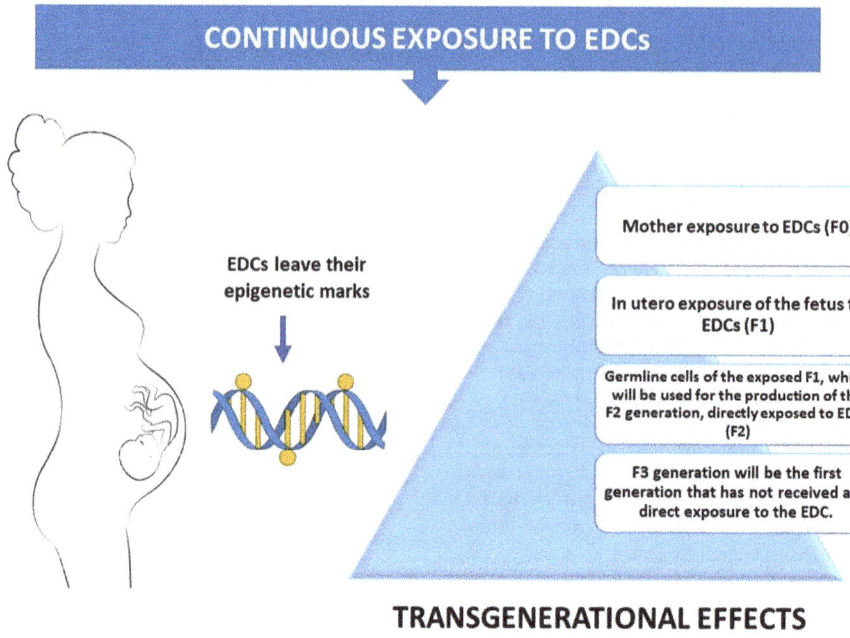

FIGURE 2 | A pregnant mother's exposure to the environment can inadvertently introduce EDCs into the exquisitely calibrated hormonal milieu of the embryo.

of hypothalamus and exert antagonistic effects: neuropeptide Y (NPY) and agouti-related protein (AgRP)-expressing neurons with orexigenic actions, whereas anorexigenic effects are expressed by proopiomelanocortin (POMC), cocaine expressing neurons and amphetamine-regulated transcript protein (CART)-expressing neurons (50).

More importantly, the gastrointestinal (GI) tract and particularly GI regulatory peptides, constitutes another benchmark for the regulation of energy homeostasis (51). Nutrient ingestion triggers gut peptides secretion, such as cholecystokinin (CCK), glucagon-like peptide-1 (GLP-1), and peptide YY (PYY), which via either activation of local neuronal circuits or endocrine signaling directly in the CNS, establishes a gut–brain axis (52, 53). Simultaneously, accumulating evidence suggests that any alteration in the microbiota composition can lead to an imbalanced production of metabolites and substances involved in the performance of physiological functions, and ultimately promote metabolic diseases, such as obesity and diabetes (54).

Adipose tissue constitutes one of the key regulators of energy homeostasis. As an endocrine gland with central role in nutrient metabolism, adipose tissue dysfunction stands in the pathophysiological "heart" of metabolic disease (55, 56). Adipocytes, the primary cells of adipose tissue, derive from mesenchymal stem cells (MSCs). Transformation of an MSC into an adipocyte requires initial commitment to the adipose lineage, followed by terminal differentiation into a mature adipocyte, where PPAR-γ pathway constitutes the master regulator of adipogenesis (57). Apart from mature adipocytes, the balance and the stage of receptor profile of other cell types in adipose tissue, including stem cells, preadipocytes, macrophages, neutrophils, lymphocytes, and endothelial cells, has a pivotal role in maintaining the control of energy homeostasis (58–60).

Via its multiple hormones, mainly glucagon and insulin, pancreas is the key regulator of glucose homeostasis. Increased exogenous glucose levels, after a meal, stimulate insulin secretion in β-cells. Specifically, glucose taken up by beta cells undergoes intermediary metabolism, promoting an increase in the ATP/ADP ratio and the closure of plasma membrane ATP-sensitive K+(KATP) channels. This induced cellular depolarization promotes insulin release from the cells, which enters the circulation and interacts with receptors in target-organs, initiating the insulin-mediated glucose disposal (61). Impairment of any of the above stages can lead to inadequate glucose-mediated insulin release and ultimately lead to diabetes. Apart from its central role in glucose regulation, strong evidence suggests that insulin, together with leptin, can influence hypothalamic control of energy homeostasis. However, the extent and nature of this co-interaction has to be further clarified (62). Converse to the actions of insulin, glucagon is secreted in response to low levels of blood glucose, in order to increase glucose production by stimulating glycogenolysis and gluconeogenesis by the liver. Glucagon seems to be also implicated in food intake and satiety. Preliminary data has shown that glucagon administration ameliorates the sense of hunger and diminishes food intake in humans and rats, confirming that glucagon specifically decreases meal size owing to increased satiation (63).

Skeletal muscle can be described as the traffic controller of the metabolic circulation. Via regulating about 80% of post-prandial insulin-stimulated glucose disposal skeletal muscle constitutes the starting point of energy production (64). As a pure energy-producing organ, it is full of mitochondria that also have a regulative role in energy homeostasis. Glucose transport in skeletal muscle is mediated through insulin, which triggers the recruitment of the glucose transporter GLUT4 to the plasma membrane. Insulin also activates the necessary enzymes (hexokinase and glycogen synthase) to enhance glycogen synthesis. When calorie intake exceeds energy expenditure, ample concentrations of energy substrates accumulate intracellularly in skeletal muscle. Increased glucose entry results in augmented glycolytic flux and glucose oxidation, leading ultimately to increased oxidative stress and metabolic deregulation (65).

Finally, liver constitutes the main glucose storage of human body, playing an important role both in anabolism and catabolism. It also stands in the heart of the metabolic interconnection of key organs, including skeletal muscle and adipose tissue (63). During fasting, liver is responsible for generating glucose as a fuel for the human body. After an increase in the pancreatic hormone glucagon, the cascade of kinase action that releases glucose from the stored glycogen via glycogenolysis is initiated in liver. As soon as glycogen is depleted, *de novo* glucose synthesis from lactate or glycerol undertakes the major role for the generation of glucose as a fuel for other tissues (66–68).

HUMAN METABOLISM UNDER ATTACK—EFFECT OF EDCS IN METABOLICALLY-ACTIVE ORGANS

Hypothalamus

EDCs may have a modulatory role in disrupting normal feeding behavior through interfering with the hypothalamic—hindbrain circuits and by directly interacting with steroid and nuclear receptors. Particularly, when EDC exposure begins early in life, *in utero* or perinatally, when the formation of these brain circuits takes place, the EDCs metabolic impact may be much greater for the feeding behavior (52).

BPA, a well-known EDC with estrogenic properties, has been highlighted as a potent disrupter of hypothalamic feeding circuitry, via multiple mechanisms. Firstly, acting *in utero*, neonatal exposure of female rats to BPA led to downregulation of hypothalamic ARC ER-a protein levels, known to exert anorexigenic effects (53). In another experimental model, perinatal exposure to BPA was found to adversely modulate the development of POMC system in the ARC in a sexually differentiated way. Specifically, early-life exposure to the obesogen BPA altered the expression of the genes encoding ER, NPY, POMC, and AgRP and decreased POMC fiber density in the paraventricular nucleus during adulthood, when offspring followed a high-fat diet, demonstrating that BPA can make them more vulnerable to manifesting diet-induced obesity and metabolic dysfunction (69). The same research group has also shown that perinatal exposure of mice to BPA or diethylstilbestrol (DES) at environmentally relevant doses can also perturb leptin actions to hypothalamus. In fact, mice exposed to these EDCs were more resistant to leptin-induced suppression of food intake, body weight loss, and hypothalamic pro-opiomelanocortin (POMC) upregulation, permanently altering the neurobiology of metabolic homeostasis (70).

Furthermore, data in bibliography suggest that *in utero* exposure to BPA can affect offspring not only during adulthood but can also lead to transgenerational effects, through inducing epigenetic changes in gene expression and DNA methylation of imprinted genes in the brain (71). Finally, BPA can also alter energy intake through inducing compulsive eating behavior. In this context, Sullivan et al. have shown that perinatal exposure of primates to BPA led to a significant change in the number of tyrosine hydroxylase-immunoreactive neurons in brain regions, supporting the hypothesis that BPA alters affective behaviors and hedonic feeding (58).

Among other EDCs, TCDD exposure during adulthood in a rodent model resulted in reduced food and water intake and altered macronutrient preference, via changes in the hypothalamic-pituitary-adrenal axis, the melanocortin neurocircuitry, and the neuropeptides that control fluid intake (59). Chronic exposure of pregnant mice to TBBPA inhibited the transcriptional activity of TSH-releasing hormone and melanocortin receptor 4 (MC4R) in the hypothalamus, which is a major regulator of energy homeostasis, with its mutations causing obesity (60). Finally, adult exposure to TBT in mice promoted profound alteration of the leptin-NPY-NPY-Y1 receptor system (72).

Recently, disruption of circadian rhythm, not only in hypothalamus but also in other tissues such as liver, has been identified as novel metabolic risk factor, with EDCs emerging as contributors to disease risk in this area (73). For example, tolyfluanid was shown to negatively affect normal circadian feeding patterns in mice (74), while studies in male zebrafish demonstrated that BPA can alter circadian activity (75).

Concluding, although data are still indicatory and sometimes controversial, we do have sufficient evidence regarding the involvement of EDCs in the regulation of food behavior in the brain that warrants further investigation by the scientific community.

Adipose Tissue

In view of the emerging epidemiological data linking EDCs exposure with obesity, experimental studies have focused on adipose tissue. In fact, adipose tissue can accumulate lipophillic EDCs and become the principal target tissue of obesogens. A variety of compounds has been shown to modulate adipocyte physiology, including insulin action and adipokine secretion, alter adipocyte differentiation and induce chronic inflammation. This EDCs-induced adipocyte dysfunction may be a contributing factor to the epidemic of metabolic disease (76).

Firstly, EDCs can promote adipogenesis, via disrupting fat cell differentiation and development. One of the first studies demonstrating it included an animal model of male C57BL/6 mice exposed to TBT, which displayed enhanced gene expression of the adipogenic markers CCAAT enhancer binding protein-β (C/EBPβ) and sterol regulatory element-binding protein-1 (Srebp1). In utero exposure to TBT resulted in augmented adipose mass in 10-week old males (66). Similarly, in another experimental model, PCBs—exposed adult male C57BL/6 mice exhibited increased body weight gain. This effect was found to be dependent on the aryl hydrocarbon receptor (AhR), as AhR-null mice did not show the same PCB-induced increase in body weight (66). Apart from the above, BPA, lead, PCB-126, atrazine, the fungicide triflumizole and organophosphate insecticides have also been incriminated as potent promoters of weight gain and adiposity in various animal models with variable levels of exposure (67).

PPARγ pathway disruption has been highlighted as one of the well-studied mechanisms by which EDCs promote adipogenesis. MSC up-regulation and preadipocyte differentiation into adipocytes have been shown to be triggered by numerous EDCs, such as DDT, BPA, phthalates, and PCBs [reviewed in (67)]. However, all the above EDCs differ structurally, indicating that their effects in adipocyte differentiation are potentiated through distinct pathways. A respectable share of EDCs elicits their adipogenic effects, through targeting PPARγ. EDCs can lead to enhanced adipogenesis either via directly binding and activating downstream cascades, or via increasing PPARγ expression, they allow for a lower threshold [reviewed in (68)]. Perinatal exposure to 4-nonylphenol (4-NP) resulted in an increase in PPARγ gene expression and sterol regulatory element-binding factor 1 (SREBF-1) expression in adipose tissue, affecting ultimately adipogenesis (77).

Another nuclear hormone receptor with a catalytic role in adipogenesis is the glucocorticoid receptor (GR). In an experimental model by Sargis RM, various EDCs were evaluated regarding their ability to stimulate the GR and drive adipogenesis in the 3T3-L1 cell lines. Among them, BPA, phthalates, and tolylfluanid (TF) were found to promote 3T3-L1 differentiation, through GR activation (78). Specifically, TF has been highlighted as a "structurally unique environmental glucocorticoid" actively implicated in GR signaling, as this fungicide has the ability to displace radiolabeled glucocorticoid from the GR (79). Finally, apart from the direct stimulation of the receptor, glucocorticoid signaling is also controlled by the interconversion of glucocorticoids between active and inactive states through the enzymatic action of 11β-hydroxysteroid dehydrogenase type 1 and 2 (11β-HSD-1/2). EDCs can act at this level, as well. For example, BPA also promotes GR-mediated indirect effects by increasing mRNA expression and enzymatic activity of 11β-HSD1 (80).

Apart from the effects in the adipocyte differentiation, EDCs can induce alterations in adipocyte endocrine function, via interfering with the mechanisms of action of key metabolic hormones. For example, TF exposure can attenuate insulin signal transduction via especially down-regulating insulin receptor substrate-1 (IRS-1) levels (81), while, simultaneously, it can imitate the binding of corticosterone to the GR and enhance insulin-induced lipogenesis (79). Furthermore, multiple experimental and animal models have shown that EDCs can modulate the synthesis and release of adipokines. For example, BPA can increase levels of leptin (82), decrease adiponectin secretion *in vitro* (83) and levels of adiponectin in mice offspring after *in utero* exposure (84), and enhance the release of IL-6 and TNF from human adipocytes (85). This disruption in the release of multiple signaling molecules can negatively affect local and systemic energy homeostasis, leading to inflammation, insulin resistance, dyslipidemia, and ultimately to metabolic dysfunction.

Pancreas

Environmental contaminants can negatively affect multiple aspects of β-cell physiology, including beta cell function and survival, insulin release, and glucose disposal. Dioxin exposure, mainly TCDD, was one of the first to be linked with metabolic alterations in multiple experimental studies. Specifically, TCDD was demonstrated to decrease glucose uptake in pancreas and impair insulin secretion (86). Through promoting continuous insulin release, TCDD exposure led to the consumption of cellular insulin reservoir and ultimately β-cell "exhaustion" (87), suggesting that insulin deficiency may ensue after sustained exposure to this compound. The adverse metabolic impact of TCDD has been also documented in human observational studies. In a longitudinal study of veterans exposed to TCDD during the Vietnam War, serum TCDD exposure was clearly interrelated with the prevalence of T2DM and insulin resistance in this population (88).

Among other EDCs, oral administration of TBT was shown to inhibit the proliferation and induce the apoptosis of islet cells via multiple pathways, causing a decrease of relative islet area in the animals treated for 60 days, which could result in a disruption of glucose homeostasis (89). Arsenic, another environmental pollutant that contaminates drinking water, can also impair insulin secretion, via downregulating insulin gene expression (90) and interfering with calpain-10-mediated proteolysis and activation of SNAP-25, a key step in insulin granule exocytosis (91). Indeed, epidemiological studies have confirmed the link between arsenic exposure and diabetes, with arsenic being correlated specifically with indices of β-cell dysfunction or decreased insulin secretion, more powerfully than with indices of insulin resistance (92).

BPA has also been investigated as a potent disrupter of beta cell function. Starting from *in utero*, an experimental model showed that pregnant mice treated with the BPA during gestation, at environmentally relevant doses, exhibit profound glucose intolerance and altered insulin sensitivity as well as increased body weight several months after delivery, mainly through impairments in beta-cell function and mass (93). Furthermore, *in vivo* experiments suggest that BPA exposure augments insulin release and glucose stimulated insulin secretion, in an estrogen receptor-a (ERa) dependent manner (94). Sex steroids, except for their primary reproductive role, exert key effects on metabolic target tissues, including pancreas, controlling β-cell insulin secretion in both cGMP-dependent and independent pathways. Thus, BPA can exert part of its metabolic effects in pancreas via estrogen-dependent pathways (95). In accordance with all the above, urinary BPA concentration in US adults were shown to be correlated with augmented β-cell function hyperinsulinemia and insulin resistance, particularly in men (96).

Recently, oxidative and endoplasmatic reticulum (ER) stress have been highlighted as crucial pathogenetic mechanisms of diabetes (97). In an experiment by Maechier P et al., β-cells exposed to hydrogen peroxide activated the production of p21 cyclin-dependent kinase inhibitor and decreased insulin mRNA, ATP and calcium flux reductions in mitochondria and cytosol (98). Furthermore, as shown by Tiedge et al. β-cells are lower in antioxidant enzymes levels (superoxide dismutase, catalase and glutathione peroxidase) and more sensitive to ROS adverse actions (99). Oxidative stress can significantly compromise β cell function, as pancreatic β cells are innately more sensitive. Several EDCs including BPA, arsenic and DEHP can disrupt β-cell function via promoting oxidative stress (68). For instance, rats exposed to phenolic compounds octylphenol, nonylphenol, and BPA displayed disrupted islet morphology and β-cell function, mainly via alterations in mitochondrial architecture and gene expression (100). Analogously, long-term exposure to BPA triggered spontaneous insulinitis in non-obese diabetic (NOD) mice, a model of immune-mediated diabetes, suggesting that BPA can accelerate the exhaustion of β-cell reserve via immune modulations in pancreatic islets. As it becomes obvious, the immunomodulatory effects of BPA in this animal model suggest that EDCs might also possibly contribute to the increasing T1DM prevalence (101).

Skeletal Muscle

In addition to data demonstrating that EDCs disrupt insulin production and beta cell function, an increasing body of evidence suggests that peripheral insulin action is also compromised. In fact, human exposure to various EDCs has been causally correlated with insulin resistance, such as BPA, TCDD, and phthalates (68). EDCs can disrupt insulin action via altering the expression or impairing the activity of multiple insulin signaling intermediates, including the insulin receptor, insulin receptors substrates, phosphatidylinositol-3-kinase (PI3k) - Protein kinase B (Akt) pathway and glucose transporters (102). For instance, BPA exposed rodents displayed glucose intolerance and global insulin resistance, due to disrupted insulin signaling, via defects in phosphorylation of both the insulin receptor and Akt (102, 103).

Liver

Except for skeletal muscle, liver is equally critical in orchestrating peripheral insulin actions and, therefore, for predicting metabolic risk. Among the environmental parameters that can have an adverse impact in the liver, EDCs have been widely highlighted, as they can catalytically perturb hepatic function. More analytically, EDCs have the ability to affect liver physiology and metabolism either indirectly, via the peripheral effects of adipose tissue dysfunction and pancreatic insulin release, or directly via autonomous effects in liver cells. The net effect of both of these actions is promoting lipogenesis, liver steatosis and ultimately non-alcoholic fatty liver disease (NAFLD) (104).

In pancreatic β cells, EDCs might increase or decrease insulin production, affecting indirectly hepatic lipogenesis, via down- or upregulating, through SREBP1C, the gene expression of various lipogenic enzymes. (105). Simultaneously, once an EDC enters the liver, it can bind to specific nuclear hormone receptors in liver cells (106). After EDC binding to these receptors, co-regulator proteins (either co-activators or co-repressors) are recruited and modulate gene expression of proteins involved in lipid homeostasis and/or the reprogramming of the epigenome. In the literature, various animal models have investigated the effect of EDC exposure in liver physiology, leading to the conclusion that EDCs can directly promote increased hepatic lipid accumulation and NAFLD (107–109).

Novel Players in the Metabolism Disruption by EDCs (Microbiota-Immune System)

There is a bidirectional relationship between microbiota and EDCs and since they both have been implicated in metabolic disease pathophysiology, we can assume that this interrelationship is not innocent (54). On the one hand, the GI bacteria with their catalytic enzymatic properties have the ability to metabolize numerous EDCs and, hence, either augmenting or diminishing their toxic effects to the mammalian host, while, on the other hand, EDCs may disrupt the composition and the physiological functions of the GI microbiota, triggering adverse metabolic effects (110). Although we currently do not know the exact underlying mechanisms, it is certain that GI microbiome is a novel regulator of the overall toxicity of EDCs in metabolism.

The role of the immune system in metabolic health has recently drawn the attention of the scientific society. Experimental data are demonstrating that both innate and adaptive immune reactions can crucially affect metabolic disease progression. Since immune cells and cytokine production are physiologically observed in the key organs of metabolism, it is believed that there is sustained co-interaction between the immune system and metabolic tissues (111). Thus, any immune dysfunction can adversely influence metabolic regulation. Simultaneously, experimental data suggest that EDCs can have immunomodulatory properties. For instance, in an experimental model of pregnant female rodents, it was shown that perinatal BPA exposure was accompanied by an imbalance in proinflammatory and anti-inflammatory immune responses, which longitudinally can affect their propensity to disease in adulthood (112). Furthermore, BPA and phthalates can alter cytokine levels, via their estrogen-like properties. Miao et al. showed that rats exposed to BPA displayed reduced expression of ER-a in islets, associated with increased proinflammatory cytokine levels in pancreatic lysates (113). Overall, although data are still indicative, immune dysfunction is highlighted as another unifying mechanism underlying the EDC-associated metabolic disease (114).

Sex-Dependent Effects of EDCs in the Sexually Dimorphic Metabolism

Human metabolism is characterized by important sex-specific asymmetries. Since the first observation that males and females differ in how they utilize and accumulate fat, a huge progress has been made in the effects of gonadal hormones in metabolic regulation (115). In fact, we currently know that even the central control of energy balance display sex dimorphic traits (116). For example, female POMC system is more responsive to leptin and less responsive to insulin, compared to males, an effect that is mediated through sex steroids (117). Similarly, peripheral metabolic organs, such as liver and adipose tissue, are equipped with estrogen and androgen receptors, which have the ability to alter metabolic signaling pathways in a sexually- dependent way (118, 119).

Apart from the human metabolism itself, EDCs also exert sexually dimorphic effects in metabolism regulation, via direct agonism or antagonism with sex hormone receptors. There is literature evidence that developmental EDC exposure, including BPA, results in altered neurodevelopment as early as fetal life, with sex specific effects observed throughout the brain even before puberty, indicating that the brain, the central regulator of energy homeostasis, is vulnerable to the sex-specific effects of EDCs(120). Furthermore, EDCs have the ability to masculinize or feminize metabolic traits, depending upon their dose and exposure duration. For example, in experimental models, BPA and DES were shown to induce increased body weight in female rodents and decreased or not altered body weight was observed in male ones (121, 122). Finally, in another study it was highlighted that female mice developmentally exposed to BPA exhibited decreased motivation to engage in voluntary physical activity and altered metabolism of carbohydrates, in comparison to males where none of these effects were observed (123).

EXTRAPOLATING CELLULAR MECHANISMS AND EFFECTS TO METABOLIC DISEASE PATHOPHYSIOLOGY

EDCs exert deleterious effects toward multiple critical components of human metabolism (**Figure 3**), leading to the manifestation of metabolic disease, clinically expressed as obesity, metabolic syndrome, diabetes mellitus, and NAFLD.

a. **Obesity:** A subset of EDCs, called "obesogens," promote adiposity by altering programming of fat cell development, increasing energy storage in fat tissue, and interfering with neuroendocrine control of appetite and satiety. Approximately 20 environmental chemicals are already known to exert obesogenic actions. Although the "obesogen hypothesis" was recently established, the body of evidence we have is enough to better comprehend obesity pathophysiology, in order to proceed to preventive measures. Reducing caloric intake and encouraging physical activity are key factors in tackling obesity. However, limiting EDC exposure, particularly during sensitive, developmental life stages, can be analogously beneficial in limiting the incidence of this burgeoning health problem (124).
b. **Insulin Resistance—Metabolic syndrome—Diabetes Mellitus:** Parma Consensus in 2015 has also introduced the "metabolic disruptor" hypothesis, according to which

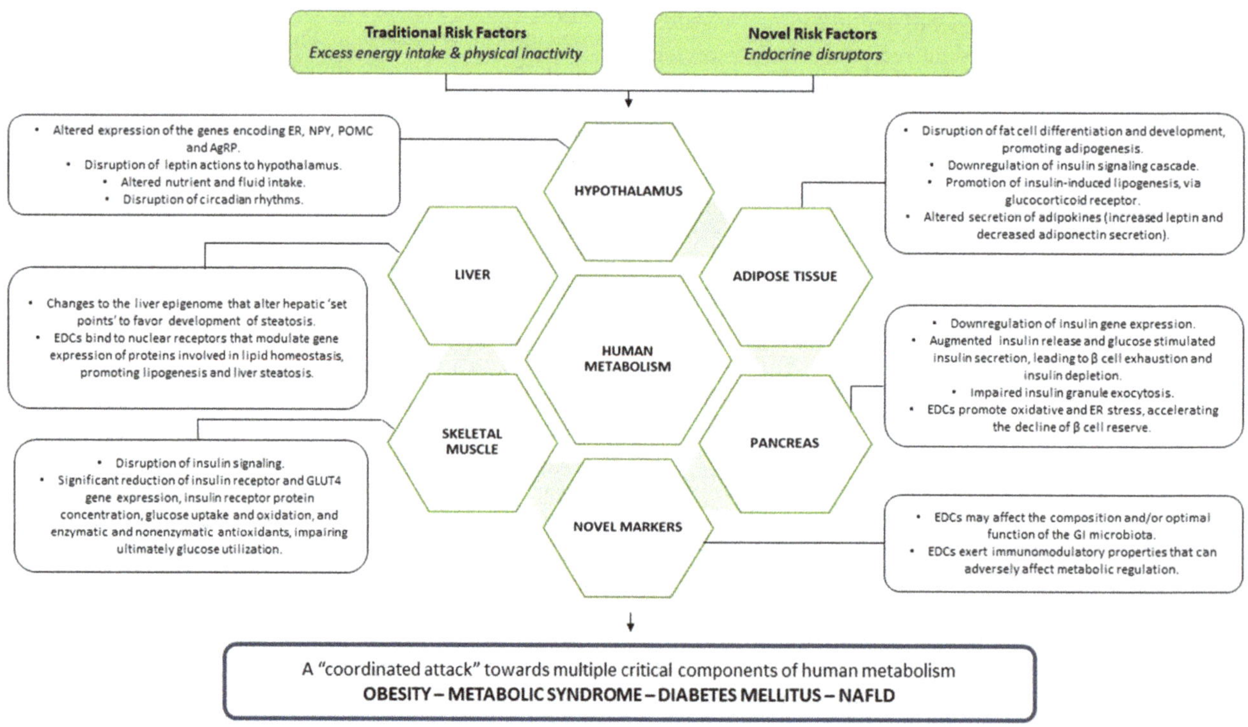

FIGURE 3 | EDCs, acting in parallel with traditional metabolic risk factors, unleash a coordinated attack toward every crucial component of human metabolism, leading ultimately to the manifestation of metabolic disease.

"environmental chemicals can act during development and/or other sensitive time periods across the lifespan to control adipose tissue development and/or by altering food intake and metabolism via specific effects on the brain, pancreas, adipose tissue, liver, GI tract, and muscle individually or in combination"(18). Susceptibility to metabolic disease may originate solely from the EDC exposure. However, in some cases, a second "hit" (e.g., high fat diet, stress) may be necessary for the EDCs effects to be clinically expressed. Either way, current scientific data are indicative that EDCs are implicated in metabolic disease pathogenesis and should be used as a solid ground not only for further research, but also for preventive strategies.

c. **Non-alcoholic fatty liver disease (NAFLD).** NAFLD represents one of the most rapidly rising and most prevalent liver disease worldwide. Its close association with metabolic syndrome and diabetes mellitus has urged scientific community to better understand its pathogenesis (125). EDCs, as mentioned above can promote NAFLD manifestation via directly or indirectly interfering with liver lipogenesis. In addition, developmental EDC exposure can promote epigenetic alterations, inducing metabolic reprogramming of genes that are involved in hepatic lipid homeostasis toward a metabolic set point that promotes NAFLD (104).

LIMITATIONS OF EDCS RESEARCH—FUTURE DIRECTIONS FOR SCIENTIFIC COMMUNITY

There is no doubt that scientific community has made a huge progress in EDCs research so far. However, there are still several challenging questions to address, in order to establish solid conclusions regarding the effect of EDCs in metabolic health and disease.

In fact, several systematic reviews and meta-analyses, published during the last decade, have tried to investigate the real magnitude of adverse effects of EDCs in humans. However, the majority of them have failed to reach definite conclusions and establish clear causal links between EDCs and disease (126–128). For example, reviews concerning the effects of BPA in pubertal development and metabolic disease reported conflicting results (129, 130), unable to substantiate any causal link. Inconclusive studies, in humans, are hammering the current position regarding phthalates and obesity (128), triclosan in various health outcomes (127), as well as EDCs and male reproductive disorders (126).

Therefore, the vital question arises: why we cannot still prove the harmful effects of EDCs in humans, despite that there is a plethora of experimental data? Among the answers the methodological one appears to be one of the most complex ones, since human studies of EDCs are methodologically a topic of challenging scientific research, where key limitations are preventing us from properly interpreting the findings and properly designing optimal human studies (131, 132). These key limitations involve low reliability of exposure assessment of EDCs with short half-lives, EDC mixtures, possibility of non-monotonic dose-response relationships, non-existence of an unexposed group, difficulties in measuring exposure during critical periods, and interactions with established risk factors (131).

So how can we override these research limitations, in order to reproduce human models of EDCs exposure? The answer is that we do not know yet. Among the above limitations, mixtures of EDCs are the most complicated issue. During the past decade, studies relating body exposures of multiple EDCs to endocrine disease have been published. For example, concerning metabolism, in an animal model by Ruzzin et al., rat exposure to a mixture of POPs led to the manifestation of insulin resistance, abdominal obesity, and hepatosteatosis, via a robust inhibition of insulin action and promotion of lipogenesis (133). However, further investigating EDC mixtures may contain pitfalls, particularly in the design of a "representative" EDC mixture that would be comparable to environmentally human exposures. Furthermore, taking into account that every human has a unique exposome, it is hardly possible to predict the net effect of EDCs mixture at the individual level in humans (28).

Furthermore, as we mentioned above, EDCs are commonly characterized by non-monotonic dose responses (NMDR), implying that EDCs actions at one dosage do not necessarily predict effects at another. In NMDR curves, increasing EDC dose is not accompanied by increased disease risk, but, on the contrary, disease risk reaches a plateau or even decreases. The underlying mechanisms of these dose-responses can be multiple, including antagonistic effects induced by receptors differing in their affinity, receptor desensitization, negative feedback with increasing doses, or dose-dependent metabolism modulation (23, 134).

Overall, despite the limitations we face in the design of experimental studies of EDCs and the caution required in deducing causality from epidemiological work in humans, most studies do underpin an interrelationship between EDCs exposure and adverse health outcomes.

In this context, we have the duty to continue exploring the effects of EDCs in human body, always with a multidisciplinary approach, as basic, translational, and clinical scientists' co-interaction can be paramount in translating research into clinical knowledge.

Finally, apart from setting research goals, scientific society should also focus on the social impact of EDCs. Familiarizing society with EDCs' harmful properties should be one of the primary focuses of scientific community. Through awakening general public, it might be easier for scientific and international organizations to draw the attention of politicians, who have a legislative role, as well as of regulatory agencies that evaluate EDCs, in order to promote changes in public health policies.

In the future, if we manage to improve research strategies and amplify social vigilance regarding EDCs, we are confident that through the accumulating evidence we will be able to promote greater regulation, more precaution and gradual restriction of the EDCs industrial uses, offering to our offspring a cleaner environment.

CONCLUSIONS

EDCs represent an emerging global threat for human's metabolic health. Scientific data published during the last 10 years have made an exponential progress in better understanding how environmental chemicals spherically attack metabolism, via interfering with every metabolically active organ of our body. Considering the fact that over 1,000 synthesized chemical compounds have been acknowledged as EDCs, it is clear that human metabolism is under a constant and coordinated attack. Although limitations of EDCs research do exist, there is no doubt that it is high time we took action. Improving research strategies, promoting public knowledge, and initiating preventive measures in EDCs industrial uses and applications can be key factors in tackling the global deterioration of metabolic health we currently encounter. The health of future generations is under attack, suggesting that if we don't further explore this scientific area, our children could be affected in decades to come.

AUTHOR CONTRIBUTIONS

ED-K designed and supervised the project, devising the main conceptual ideas and proof outline. OP, EK, and GP contributed to the implementation of the project and to the writing of the manuscript. All authors contributed to the final version of the manuscript.

REFERENCES

1. Ogden CL, Carroll MD, Kit BK, Flegal KM. Prevalence of childhood and adult obesity in the United States, 2011–2012. *J Am Med Assoc.* (2014) 311:806–14. doi: 10.1001/jama.2014.732
2. *IDF Diabetes Atlas. 8th Ed* (2017). Available online at: https://www.idf.org/e-library/epidemiology-research/diabetes-atlas.html
3. *WHO Global Status Report on Noncommunicable Diseases* (2016) Available online at: http://apps.who.int/iris/bitstream/handle/10665/148114/9789241564854_eng.pdf;jsessionid=3E13236F60C0D3C3275B85E0E927F96B?sequence=1
4. American Diabetes. Economic costs of diabetes in the US. in 2017. *Diabetes care.* (2018) 41:917–28. doi: 10.2337/dci18-0007
5. Lehnert T, Sonntag D, Konnopka A, Riedel-Heller S, Konig HH. Economic costs of overweight and obesity. *Best Pract Res Clin Endocrinol Metab.* (2013) 27:105–15. doi: 10.1016/j.beem.2013.01.002
6. Huang ES, Laiteerapong N, Liu JY, John PM, Moffet HH, Karter AJ. Rates of complications and mortality in older patients with diabetes mellitus: the diabetes and aging study. *JAMA Int Med.* (2014) 174:251–8. doi: 10.1001/jamainternmed.2013.12956
7. Schwartz MW, Seeley RJ, Zeltser LM, Drewnowski A, Ravussin E, Redman LM, et al. Obesity pathogenesis: an endocrine society scientific statement. *Endocr Rev.* (2017) 38:267–96. doi: 10.1210/er.2017-00111
8. Brown RE, Sharma AM, Ardern CI, Mirdamadi P, Mirdamadi P, Kuk JL. Secular differences in the association between caloric intake, macronutrient intake, and physical activity with obesity. *Obes Res Clin Prac.* (2016) 10:243–55. doi: 10.1016/j.orcp.2015.08.007
9. Gore AC, Chappell VA, Fenton SE, Flaws JA, Nadal A, Prins GS, et al. EDC-2: The endocrine society's second scientific statement on endocrine-disrupting chemicals. *Endocr Rev.* (2015) 36:E1–50. doi: 10.1210/er.2015-1093
10. Neel BA, Sargis RM. The paradox of progress: environmental disruption of metabolism and the diabetes epidemic. *Diabetes* (2011) 60:1838–48. doi: 10.2337/db11-0153
11. Baillie-Hamilton PF. Chemical toxins: a hypothesis to explain the global obesity epidemic. *J Alternat Compl Med.* (2002) 8:185–92. doi: 10.1089/107555302317371479
12. Diamanti-Kandarakis E, Bourguignon JP, Giudice LC, Hauser R, Prins GS, Soto AM, et al. Endocrine-disrupting chemicals: an Endocrine Society scientific statement. *Endocr Rev.* (2009) 30:293–342. doi: 10.1210/er.2009-0002
13. Zoeller RT, Brown TR, Doan LL, Gore AC, Skakkebaek NE, Soto AM, et al. Endocrine-disrupting chemicals and public health protection: a statement of principles from the endocrine society. *Endocrinology.* (2012) 153:4097–110. doi: 10.1210/en.2012-1422
14. Colborn T, vom Saal FS, Soto AM. Developmental effects of endocrine-disrupting chemicals in wildlife and humans. *Environ Health Perspect.* (1993) 101:378–84. doi: 10.1289/ehp.93101378
15. Grun F, Blumberg B. Environmental obesogens: organotins and endocrine disruption via nuclear receptor signaling. *Endocrinology.* (2006) 147:S50–5. doi: 10.1210/en.2005-1129
16. Janesick A, Blumberg B. Obesogens, stem cells and the developmental programming of obesity. *Int J Androl.* (2012) 35:437–48. doi: 10.1111/j.1365-2605.2012.01247.x
17. Heindel JJ, Blumberg B, Cave M, Machtinger R, Mantovani A, Mendez MA, et al. Metabolism disrupting chemicals and metabolic disorders. *Reprod Toxicol.* (2017) 68:3–33. doi: 10.1016/j.reprotox.2016.10.001
18. Heindel JJ, Vom Saal FS, Blumberg B, Bovolin P, Calamandrei G, Ceresini G, et al. Parma consensus statement on metabolic disruptors. *Environ Health.* (2015) 14:54. doi: 10.1186/s12940-015-0042-7
19. *World Health Organisation State of the Science of Endocrine Disrupting Chemicals - 2012* Available online at: http://apps.who.int/iris/bitstream/handle/10665/78102/WHO_HSE_PHE_IHE_2013.1_eng.pdf?sequence=1
20. Bergman A, Heindel JJ, Kasten T, Kidd KA, Jobling S, Neira M, et al. The impact of endocrine disruption: a consensus statement on the state of the science. *Environ Health Perspect.* (2013) 121:A104–6. doi: 10.1289/ehp.1205448
21. Cho MR, Shin JY, Hwang JH, Jacobs DR, Jr, Kim SY, Lee DH. Associations of fat mass and lean mass with bone mineral density differ by levels of persistent organic pollutants: national health and nutrition examination survey 1999–2004. *Chemosphere.* (2011) 82:1268–76. doi: 10.1016/j.chemosphere.2010.12.031
22. Koch CA, Diamanti-Kandarakis E. Introduction to endocrine disrupting chemicals–is it time to act? *Rev Endocr Metabol Disord.* (2015) 16:269–70. doi: 10.1007/s11154-016-9338-3
23. Rhomberg LR, Goodman JE. Low-dose effects and nonmonotonic dose-responses of endocrine disrupting chemicals: has the case been made? *Regulat Toxicol Pharmacol.* (2012) 64:130–3. doi: 10.1016/j.yrtph.2012.06.015
24. Vandenberg LN, Colborn T, Hayes TB, Heindel JJ, Jacobs DR, Jr., Lee DH, et al. Hormones and endocrine-disrupting chemicals: low-dose effects and nonmonotonic dose responses. *Endocr Rev.* (2012) 33:378–455. doi: 10.1210/er.2011-1050
25. Rochester JR. Bisphenol A and human health: a review of the literature. *Reproduct Toxicol.* (2013) 42:132–55. doi: 10.1016/j.reprotox.2013.08.008
26. Tabb MM, Blumberg B. New modes of action for endocrine-disrupting chemicals. *Mol Endocrinol.* (2006) 20:475–82. doi: 10.1210/me.2004-0513
27. Schug TT, Janesick A, Blumberg B, Heindel JJ. Endocrine disrupting chemicals and disease susceptibility. *J Steroid Biochem Mol Biol.* (2011) 127:204–15. doi: 10.1016/j.jsbmb.2011.08.007
28. Ribeiro E, Ladeira C, Viegas S. EDCs Mixtures: a stealthy hazard for human health? *Toxics.* (2017) 5:5. doi: 10.3390/toxics5010005
29. Barker DJ. The origins of the developmental origins theory. *J Int Med.* (2007) 261:412–7. doi: 10.1111/j.1365-2796.2007.01809.x
30. Barker DJ, Winter PD, Osmond C, Margetts B, Simmonds SJ. Weight in infancy and death from ischaemic heart disease. *Lancet.* (1989) 2:577–80. doi: 10.1016/S0140-6736(89)90710-1
31. Barker DJ, Osmond C, Golding J, Kuh D, Wadsworth ME. Growth *in utero*, blood pressure in childhood and adult life, and mortality from cardiovascular disease. *BMJ.* (1989) 298:564–7. doi: 10.1136/bmj.298.6673.564

32. Barker DJ. Maternal nutrition, fetal nutrition, and disease in later life. *Nutrition.* (1997) 13:807–13. doi: 10.1016/S0899-9007(97)00193-7
33. Saad MI, Abdelkhalek TM, Haiba MM, Saleh MM, Hanafi MY, Tawfik SH, et al. Maternal obesity and malnourishment exacerbate perinatal oxidative stress resulting in diabetogenic programming in F1 offspring. *J Endocrinol Invest.* (2015) 39:643–55. doi: 10.1007/s40618-015-0413-5.
34. Fetoui H, Garoui M, Zeghal N. Protein restriction in pregnant- and lactating rats-induced oxidative stress and hypohomocysteinaemia in their offspring. *J Anim Physiol Anim Nutr.* (2009) 93:263–70. doi: 10.1111/j.1439-0396.2008.00812.x
35. Newbold RR. Lessons learned from perinatal exposure to diethylstilbestrol. *Toxicol Appl Pharmacol.* (2004) 199:142–50. doi: 10.1016/j.taap.2003.11.033
36. Newbold RR, Padilla-Banks E, Jefferson WN. Environmental estrogens and obesity. *Mol Cell Endocrinol.* (2009) 304:84–9. doi: 10.1016/j.mce.2009.02.024
37. Hatch EE, Troisi R, Palmer JR, Wise LA, Titus L, Strohsnitter WC, et al. Prenatal diethylstilbestrol exposure and risk of obesity in adult women. *J Devel Orig Health Dis.* (2015) 6:201–7. doi: 10.1017/S2040174415000033
38. Blumberg B. Obesogens, stem cells and the maternal programming of obesity. *J Dev Orig Health Dis.* (2011) 2:3–8. doi: 10.1017/S2040174410000589
39. Rissman EF, Adli M. Minireview: transgenerational epigenetic inheritance: focus on endocrine disrupting compounds. *Endocrinology.* (2014) 155:2770–80. doi: 10.1210/en.2014-1123
40. Fleisch AF, Wright RO, Baccarelli AA. Environmental epigenetics: a role in endocrine disease? *J Mol Endocrinol.* (2012) 49:R61–7. doi: 10.1530/JME-12-0066
41. Ho SM, Johnson A, Tarapore P, Janakiram V, Zhang X, Leung YK. Environmental epigenetics and its implication on disease risk and health outcomes. *ILAR J.* (2012) 53:289–305. doi: 10.1093/ilar.53.3-4.289
42. Crews D, McLachlan JA. Epigenetics, evolution, endocrine disruption, health, and disease. *Endocrinology.* (2006) 147:S4–10. doi: 10.1210/en.2005-1122
43. Skinner MK. What is an epigenetic transgenerational phenotype? F3 or F2. *Reprod Toxicol.* (2008) 25:2–6. doi: 10.1016/j.reprotox.2007.09.001
44. Ho SM, Tang WY, Belmonte de Frausto J, Prins GS. Developmental exposure to estradiol and bisphenol A increases susceptibility to prostate carcinogenesis and epigenetically regulates phosphodiesterase type 4 variant 4. *Cancer Res.* (2006) 66:5624–32. doi: 10.1158/0008-5472.CAN-06-0516
45. Tang WY, Morey LM, Cheung YY, Birch L, Prins GS, Ho SM. Neonatal exposure to estradiol/bisphenol A alters promoter methylation and expression of Nsbp1 and Hpcal1 genes and transcriptional programs of Dnmt3a/b and Mbd2/4 in the rat prostate gland throughout life. *Endocrinology.* (2012) 153:42–55. doi: 10.1210/en.2011-1308
46. Gillette R, Miller-Crews I, Nilsson EE, Skinner MK, Gore AC, Crews D. Sexually dimorphic effects of ancestral exposure to vinclozolin on stress reactivity in rats. *Endocrinology.* (2014) 155:3853–66. doi: 10.1210/en.2014-1253
47. Crews D, Gillette R, Scarpino SV, Manikkam M, Savenkova MI, Skinner MK. Epigenetic transgenerational inheritance of altered stress responses. *Proc Nat Acad Sci USA.* (2012) 109:9143–8. doi: 10.1073/pnas.1118514109
48. Chamorro-Garcia R, Sahu M, Abbey RJ, Laude J, Pham N, Blumberg B. Transgenerational inheritance of increased fat depot size, stem cell reprogramming, and hepatic steatosis elicited by prenatal exposure to the obesogen tributyltin in mice. *Environ Health Perspect.* (2013) 121:359–66. doi: 10.1289/ehp.1205701
49. Manikkam M, Tracey R, Guerrero-Bosagna C, Skinner MK. Plastics derived endocrine disruptors (BPA, DEHP and DBP) induce epigenetic transgenerational inheritance of obesity, reproductive disease and sperm epimutations. *PLoS ONE.* (2013) 8:e55387. doi: 10.1371/journal.pone.0055387
50. Morton GJ, Meek TH, Schwartz MW. Neurobiology of food intake in health and disease. *Nat Rev Neurosci.* (2014) 15:367–78. doi: 10.1038/nrn3745
51. Duca FA, Lam TK. Gut microbiota, nutrient sensing and energy balance. *Diab Obes Metabol.* (2014) 16 (Suppl 1):68–76. doi: 10.1111/dom.12340
52. Walley SN, Roepke TA. Perinatal exposure to endocrine disrupting compounds and the control of feeding behavior-an overview. *Hormon Behav.* (2018) 101:22–28. doi: 10.1016/j.yhbeh.2017.10.017
53. Monje L, Varayoud J, Munoz-de-Toro M, Luque EH, Ramos JG. Exposure of neonatal female rats to bisphenol A disrupts hypothalamic LHRH pre-mRNA processing and estrogen receptor alpha expression in nuclei controlling estrous cyclicity. *Reproduct Toxicol.* (2010) 30:625–34. doi: 10.1016/j.reprotox.2010.08.004
54. Pascale, Marchesi N, Marelli C, Coppola A, Luzi L, Govoni S, et al. Microbiota and metabolic diseases. *Endocrine.* (2018) 61:357–71 doi: 10.1007/s12020-018-1605-5
55. Smorlesi, Frontini A, Giordano A, Cinti S. The adipose organ: white-brown adipocyte plasticity and metabolic inflammation. *Obes Rev.* (2012) 13 (Suppl 2):83–96. doi: 10.1111/j.1467-789X.2012.01039.x
56. Rosen ED. Two paths to fat. *Nature Cell Biol.* (2015) 17:360–1. doi: 10.1038/ncb3133
57. Rosen ED, MacDougald OA. Adipocyte differentiation from the inside out. *Nat Rev Mol Cell Biol.* (2006) 7:885–96. doi: 10.1038/nrm2066
58. Sullivan AW, Beach EC, Stetzik LA, Perry A, D'Addezio AS, Cushing BS, et al. A novel model for neuroendocrine toxicology: neurobehavioral effects of BPA exposure in a prosocial species, the prairie vole (Microtus ochrogaster). *Endocrinology.* (2014) 155:3867–81. doi: 10.1210/en.2014-1379
59. van Esterik JC, Verharen HW, Hodemaekers HM, Gremmer ER, Nagarajah B, Kamstra JH, et al. Compound- and sex-specific effects on programming of energy and immune homeostasis in adult C57BL/6JxFVB mice after perinatal TCDD and PCB 153. *Toxicol Appl Pharmacol.* (2015) 289:262–75. doi: 10.1016/j.taap.2015.09.017
60. Decherf S, Seugnet I, Fini JB, Clerget-Froidevaux MS, Demeneix BA. Disruption of thyroid hormone-dependent hypothalamic set-points by environmental contaminants. *Mol Cell Endocrinol.* (2010) 323:172–82. doi: 10.1016/j.mce.2010.04.010
61. Roder PV, Wu B, Liu Y, Han W. Pancreatic regulation of glucose homeostasis. *Exp Mol Med.* (2016) 48:e219. doi: 10.1038/emm.2016.6
62. Flier JS. Obesity wars: molecular progress confronts an expanding epidemic. *Cell.* (2004) 116:337–50. doi: 10.1016/S0092-8674(03)01081-X
63. Habegger KM, Heppner KM, Geary N, Bartness TJ, DiMarchi R, Tschop MH. The metabolic actions of glucagon revisited. *Nat Rev Endocrinol.* (2010) 6:689–97. doi: 10.1038/nrendo.2010.187
64. DeFronzo RA, Gunnarsson R, Bjorkman O, Olsson M, Wahren J. Effects of insulin on peripheral and splanchnic glucose metabolism in noninsulin-dependent (type II) diabetes mellitus. *J Clin Invest.* (1985) 76:149–55. doi: 10.1172/JCI111938
65. Ceriello, Motz E. Is oxidative stress the pathogenic mechanism underlying insulin resistance, diabetes, and cardiovascular disease? The common soil hypothesis revisited. *Arterioscler Thromb Vasc Biol* (2004) 24:816–23. doi: 10.1161/01.ATV.0000122852.22604.78
66. Grun F, Watanabe H, Zamanian Z, Maeda L, Arima K, Cubacha R, et al. Endocrine-disrupting organotin compounds are potent inducers of adipogenesis in vertebrates. *Mol Endocrinol.* (2006) 20:2141–55. doi: 10.1210/me.2005-0367
67. Bateman ME, Strong AL, McLachlan JA, Burow ME, Bunnell BA. The effects of endocrine disruptors on adipogenesis and osteogenesis in mesenchymal stem cells: a review. *Front Endocrinol.* (2016) 7:171. doi: 10.3389/fendo.2016.00171
68. Mimoto MS, Nadal A, Sargis RM. Polluted pathways: mechanisms of metabolic disruption by endocrine disrupting chemicals. *Curr Environ Health Rep.* (2017) 4:208–222. doi: 10.1007/s40572-017-0137-0
69. Mackay H, Patterson ZR, Khazall R, Patel S, Tsirlin D, Abizaid A. Organizational effects of perinatal exposure to bisphenol-A and diethylstilbestrol on arcuate nucleus circuitry controlling food intake and energy expenditure in male and female CD-1 mice. *Endocrinology.* (2013) 154:1465–75. doi: 10.1210/en.2012-2044
70. MacKay H, Patterson ZR, Abizaid A. Perinatal exposure to low-dose bisphenol-a disrupts the structural and functional development of the hypothalamic feeding circuitry. *Endocrinology.* (2017) 158:768–777. doi: 10.1210/en.2016-1718
71. Drobna Z, Henriksen AD, Wolstenholme JT, Montiel C, Lambeth PS, Shang S, et al. Transgenerational effects of Bisphenol A on gene expression and DNA methylation of imprinted genes in brain. *Endocrinology.* (2018) 159:132–44. doi: 10.1210/en.2017-00730

72. Bo E, Farinetti A, Marraudino M, Sterchele D, Eva C, Gotti S, et al. Adult exposure to tributyltin affects hypothalamic neuropeptide Y, Y1 receptor distribution, and circulating leptin in mice. *Andrology.* (2016) 4:723–34. doi: 10.1111/andr.12222
73. Longo VD, Panda S. Fasting, circadian rhythms, and time-restricted feeding in healthy lifespan. *Cell Metabol.* (2016) 23:1048–59. doi: 10.1016/j.cmet.2016.06.001
74. Regnier SM, Kirkley AG, Ye H, El-Hashani E, Zhang X, Neel BA, et al. Dietary exposure to the endocrine disruptor tolylfluanid promotes global metabolic dysfunction in male mice. *Endocrinology.* (2015) 156:896–910. doi: 10.1210/en.2014-1668
75. Weber DN, Hoffmann RG, Hoke ES, Tanguay RL. Bisphenol A exposure during early development induces sex-specific changes in adult zebrafish social interactions. *J Toxicol Environ Health. Part A.* (2015) 78:50–66. doi: 10.1080/15287394.2015.958419
76. Regnier SM, Sargis RM. Adipocytes under assault: environmental disruption of adipose physiology. *Biochim et Biophys Acta.* (2014) 1842:520–33. doi: 10.1016/j.bbadis.2013.05.028
77. Zhang HY, Xue WY, Li YY, Ma Y, Zhu YS, Huo WQ, et al. Perinatal exposure to 4-nonylphenol affects adipogenesis in first and second generation rats offspring. *Toxicol Lett.* (2014) 225:325–32. doi: 10.1016/j.toxlet.2013.12.011
78. Sargis RM, Johnson DN, Choudhury RA, Brady MJ. Environmental endocrine disruptors promote adipogenesis in the 3T3-L1 cell line through glucocorticoid receptor activation. *Obesity.* (2010) 18:1283–8. doi: 10.1038/oby.2009.419
79. Neel BA, Brady MJ, Sargis RM. The endocrine disrupting chemical tolylfluanid alters adipocyte metabolism via glucocorticoid receptor activation. *Mol Endocrinol.* (2013) 27:394–406. doi: 10.1210/me.2012-1270
80. Wang J, Sun B, Hou M, Pan X, Li X. The environmental obesogen bisphenol A promotes adipogenesis by increasing the amount of 11beta-hydroxysteroid dehydrogenase type 1 in the adipose tissue of children. *Int J Obes.* (2013) 37:999–1005. doi: 10.1038/ijo.2012.173
81. Sargis RM, Neel BA, Brock CO, Lin Y, Hickey AT, Carlton DA, et al. The novel endocrine disruptor tolylfluanid impairs insulin signaling in primary rodent and human adipocytes through a reduction in insulin receptor substrate-1 levels. *Biochim et Biophys Acta.* (2012) 1822:952–60. doi: 10.1016/j.bbadis.2012.02.015
82. Miyawaki J, Sakayama K, Kato H, Yamamoto H, Masuno H. Perinatal and postnatal exposure to bisphenol a increases adipose tissue mass and serum cholesterol level in mice. *J Atheroscler Thrombosis.* (2007) 14:245–52. doi: 10.5551/jat.E486
83. Hugo ER, Brandebourg TD, Woo JG, Loftus J, Alexander JW, Ben-Jonathan N. Bisphenol A at environmentally relevant doses inhibits adiponectin release from human adipose tissue explants and adipocytes. *Environ Health Perspect.* (2008) 116:1642–7. doi: 10.1289/ehp.11537
84. Angle BM, Do RP, Ponzi D, Stahlhut RW, Drury BE, Nagel SC, et al. Metabolic disruption in male mice due to fetal exposure to low but not high doses of bisphenol A (BPA): evidence for effects on body weight, food intake, adipocytes, leptin, adiponectin, insulin and glucose regulation. *Reprod Toxicol.* (2013) 42:256–68. doi: 10.1016/j.reprotox.2013.07.017
85. Valentino R, D'Esposito V, Passaretti F, Liotti A, Cabaro S, Longo M, et al. Bisphenol-A impairs insulin action and up-regulates inflammatory pathways in human subcutaneous adipocytes and 3T3-L1 cells. *PLoS ONE.* (2013) 8:e82099. doi: 10.1371/journal.pone.0082099
86. Enan E, Liu PC. Matsumura F. 2,3,7,8-Tetrachlorodibenzo-p-dioxin causes reduction of glucose transporting activities in the plasma membranes of adipose tissue and pancreas from the guinea pig. *J Biolo Chem.* (1992) 267:19785–91.
87. Kim YH, Shim YJ, Shin YJ, Sul D, Lee E, Min BH. 2,3,7,8-tetrachlorodibenzo-p-dioxin (TCDD) induces calcium influx through T-type calcium channel and enhances lysosomal exocytosis and insulin secretion in INS-1 cells. *Int J Toxicol.* (2009) 28:151–61. doi: 10.1177/1091581809336885
88. Michalek JE, Pavuk M. Diabetes and cancer in veterans of operation ranch Hand after adjustment for calendar period, days of spraying, and time spent in Southeast Asia. *J Occupat Environ Med.* (2008) 50:330–40. doi: 10.1097/JOM.0b013e31815f889b
89. Zuo Z, Wu T, Lin M, Zhang S, Yan F, Yang Z, et al. Chronic exposure to tributyltin chloride induces pancreatic islet cell apoptosis and disrupts glucose homeostasis in male mice. *Environ Sci Technol.* (2014) 48:5179–86. doi: 10.1021/es404729p
90. Diaz-Villasenor A, Sanchez-Soto MC, Cebrian ME, Ostrosky-Wegman P, Hiriart M. Sodium arsenite impairs insulin secretion and transcription in pancreatic beta-cells. *Toxicol Appl Pharmacol.* (2006) 214:30–4. doi: 10.1016/j.taap.2005.11.015
91. Diaz-Villasenor A, Burns AL, Salazar AM, Sordo M, Hiriart M, Cebrian ME, et al, Arsenite reduces insulin secretion in rat pancreatic beta-cells by decreasing the calcium-dependent calpain-10 proteolysis of SNAP-25. *Toxicol Appl Pharmacol.* (2008) 231:291–9. doi: 10.1016/j.taap.2008
92. Rhee SY, Hwang YC, Woo JT, Chin SO, Chon S, Kim YS. Arsenic exposure and prevalence of diabetes mellitus in Korean adults. *J Kor Med Sci.* (2013) 28:861–8. doi: 10.3346/jkms.2013.28.6.861
93. Alonso-Magdalena P, Garcia-Arevalo M, Quesada I, Nadal A. Bisphenol-A treatment during pregnancy in mice: a new window of susceptibility for the development of diabetes in mothers later in life. *Endocrinology.* (2015) 156:1659–70. doi: 10.1210/en.2014-1952
94. Alonso-Magdalena P, Morimoto S, Ripoll C, Fuentes E, Nadal A. The estrogenic effect of bisphenol A disrupts pancreatic beta-cell function *in vivo* and induces insulin resistance. *Environ Health Perspect.* (2006) 114:106–12. doi: 10.1289/ehp.8451
95. Nadal, Alonso-Magdalena P, Soriano S, Quesada I, Ropero AB. The pancreatic beta-cell as a target of estrogens and xenoestrogens: implications for blood glucose homeostasis and diabetes. *Mol Cell Endocrinol.* (2009) 304:63–8. doi: 10.1016/j.mce.2009.02.016
96. Beydoun HA, Khanal S, Zonderman AB, Beydoun MA. Sex differences in the association of urinary bisphenol-A concentration with selected indices of glucose homeostasis among U.S. adults. *Ann Epidemiol.* (2014) 24:90–7. doi: 10.1016/j.annepidem.2013.07.014
97. Hasnain SZ, Prins JB, McGuckin MA. Oxidative and endoplasmic reticulum stress in beta-cell dysfunction in diabetes. *J Mol Endocrinol.* (2016) 56: R33–54. doi: 10.1530/JME-15-0232
98. Maechler P, Jornot L, Wollheim CB. Hydrogen peroxide alters mitochondrial activation and insulin secretion in pancreatic beta cells. *J Biol Chem.* (1999) 274:27905–13. doi: 10.1074/jbc.274.39.27905
99. Tiedge M, Lortz S, Drinkgern J, Lenzen S. Relation between antioxidant enzyme gene expression and antioxidative defense status of insulin-producing cells. *Diabetes.* (1997) 46:1733–42. doi: 10.2337/diab.46.11.1733
100. Song L, Xia W, Zhou Z, Li Y, Lin Y, Wei J, et al. Low-level phenolic estrogen pollutants impair islet morphology and beta-cell function in isolated rat islets. *J Endocrinol.* (2012) 215:303–11. doi: 10.1530/JOE-12-0219
101. Bodin J, Bolling AK, Samuelsen M, Becher R, Lovik M, Nygaard UC. Long-term bisphenol A exposure accelerates insulitis development in diabetes-prone NOD mice. *Immunopharmacol Immunotoxicol.* (2013) 35:349–58. doi: 10.3109/08923973.2013.772195
102. Batista TM, Alonso-Magdalena P, Vieira E, Amaral ME, Cederroth CR, Nef S, et al. Short-term treatment with bisphenol-A leads to metabolic abnormalities in adult male mice. *PLoS ONE.* (2012) 7:e33814. doi: 10.1371/journal.pone.0033814
103. Moon MK, Jeong IK, Jung Oh T, Ahn HY, Kim HH, Park YJ, et al. Long-term oral exposure to bisphenol A induces glucose intolerance and insulin resistance. *J Endocrinol.* (2015) 226:35–42. doi: 10.1530/JOE-14-0714
104. Foulds CE, Trevino LS, York B, Walker CL. Endocrine-disrupting chemicals and fatty liver disease. *Nat Rev Endocrinol.* (2017) 13:445–457. doi: 10.1038/nrendo.2017.42
105. Trevino LS, Katz TA. Endocrine disruptors and developmental origins of nonalcoholic fatty liver disease. *Endocrinology.* (2018) 159:20–31. doi: 10.1210/en.2017-00887
106. Mellor CL, Steinmetz FP, Cronin MT. The identification of nuclear receptors associated with hepatic steatosis to develop and extend adverse outcome pathways. *Crit Rev Toxicol.* (2016) 46:138–52. doi: 10.3109/10408444.2015.1089471
107. Al-Eryani L, Wahlang B, Falkner KC, Guardiola JJ, Clair HB, Prough RA, et al. Identification of environmental chemicals associated with the development of toxicant-associated fatty liver disease in rodents. *Toxicol Pathol.* (2015) 43:482–97. doi: 10.1177/0192623314549960
108. Wei J, Sun X, Chen Y, Li Y, Song L, Zhou Z, et al. Perinatal exposure to bisphenol A exacerbates nonalcoholic steatohepatitis-like phenotype in

male rat offspring fed on a high-fat diet. *J Endocrinol.* (2014) 222:313–25. doi: 10.1530/JOE-14-0356

109. Strakovsky RS, Wang H, Engeseth NJ, Flaws JA, Helferich WG, Pan YX, et al. Developmental bisphenol A (BPA) exposure leads to sex-specific modification of hepatic gene expression and epigenome at birth that may exacerbate high-fat diet-induced hepatic steatosis. *Toxicol Appl Pharmacol.* (2015) 284:101–12. doi: 10.1016/j.taap.2015.02.021
110. Claus SP, Guillou H, Ellero-Simatos S. The gut microbiota: a major player in the toxicity of environmental pollutants? *NPJ Biofilms Microbiomes.* (2016) 2:16003. doi: 10.1038/npjbiofilms.2016.3
111. Brestoff JR, Artis D. Immune regulation of metabolic homeostasis in health and disease. *Cell.* (2015) 161:146–60. doi: 10.1016/j.cell.2015.02.022
112. O'Brien E, Dolinoy DC, Mancuso P. Perinatal bisphenol A exposures increase production of pro-inflammatory mediators in bone marrow-derived mast cells of adult mice. *J Immunotoxicol.* (2014) 11:205–12. doi: 10.3109/1547691X.2013.822036
113. Miao S, Gao Z, Kou Z, Xu G, Su C, Liu N. Influence of bisphenol a on developing rat estrogen receptors and some cytokines in rats: a two-generational study. *J Toxicol Environ Health. Part A.* (2008) 71:1000–8. doi: 10.1080/15287390801907467
114. Bansal, Henao-Mejia J, Simmons RA. Immune system: an emerging player in mediating effects of endocrine disruptors on metabolic health. *Endocrinology.* (2018) 159:32–45. doi: 10.1210/en.2017-00882
115. Mauvais-Jarvis F. Sex differences in metabolic homeostasis, diabetes, and obesity. *Biol Sex Diff.* (2015) 6:14. doi: 10.1186/s13293-015-0033-y
116. Gonzalez-Garcia A, Contreras C, Estevez-Salguero A, Ruiz-Pino F, Colsh B, Pensado I, et al. Estradiol regulates energy balance by ameliorating hypothalamic ceramide-induced ER Stress. *Cell Rep.* (2018) 25:413–23 e5. doi: 10.1016/j.celrep.2018.09.038
117. Shi H, Strader AD, Sorrell JE, Chambers JB, Woods SC, Seeley RJ. Sexually different actions of leptin in proopiomelanocortin neurons to regulate glucose homeostasis. *Am J Physiol Endocrinol Metabol.* (2008) 294:E630–9. doi: 10.1152/ajpendo.00704.2007
118. Torre D, Lolli F, Ciana P, Maggi A. Sexual dimorphism and estrogen action in mouse liver. *Adv Exp Med Bio.* (2017) 1043:141–51. doi: 10.1007/978-3-319-70178-3_8
119. Palmer BF, Clegg DJ. The sexual dimorphism of obesity. *Mol Cell Endocrinol.* (2015) 402:113–9. doi: 10.1016/j.mce.2014.11.029
120. Rebuli ME, Patisaul HB. Assessment of sex specific endocrine disrupting effects in the prenatal and pre-pubertal rodent brain. *J Steroid Biochem Mol Biol.* (2016) 160:148–59. doi: 10.1016/j.jsbmb.2015.08.021
121. Rubin BS, Soto AM. Bisphenol A: perinatal exposure and body weight. *Mol Cel Endocrinol.* (2009) 304:55–62. doi: 10.1016/j.mce.2009.02.023
122. Newbold RR. Prenatal exposure to diethylstilbestrol (DES). *Fertil Steril.* (2008) 89:e55–6. doi: 10.1016/j.fertnstert.2008.01.062
123. Johnson SA, Painter MS, Javurek AB, Ellersieck MR, Wiedmeyer CE, Thyfault JP, et al. Sex-dependent effects of developmental exposure to bisphenol A and ethinyl estradiol on metabolic parameters and voluntary physical activity. *J Dev Orig Health Dis.* (2015) 6:539–52. doi: 10.1017/S2040174415001488
124. Heindel JJ, Newbold R, Schug TT. Endocrine disruptors and obesity. *Nat Rev Endocrinol.* (2015) 11:653–61. doi: 10.1038/nrendo.2015.163
125. Hazlehurst JM, Tomlinson JW. Non-alcoholic fatty liver disease in common endocrine disorders. *Eur J Endocrinol.* (2013) 169:R27–37. doi: 10.1530/EJE-13-0296
126. Bonde JP, Flachs EM, Rimborg S, Glazer CH, Giwercman A, Ramlau-Hansen CH, et al. The epidemiologic evidence linking prenatal and postnatal exposure to endocrine disrupting chemicals with male reproductive disorders: a systematic review and meta-analysis. *Hum Reproduct update.* (2016) 23:104–25. doi: 10.1093/humupd/dmw036
127. Goodman M, Naiman DQ, LaKind JS. Systematic review of the literature on triclosan and health outcomes in humans. *Crit Rev Toxicol.* (2018) 48:1–51. doi: 10.1080/10408444.2017.1350138
128. Goodman M, Lakind JS, Mattison DR. Do phthalates act as obesogens in humans? A systematic review of the epidemiological literature. *Crit Rev Toxicol.* (2014) 44:151–75. doi: 10.3109/10408444.2013.860076
129. Lakind JS, Goodman M, Mattison DR. Bisphenol A and indicators of obesity, glucose metabolism/type 2 diabetes and cardiovascular disease: a systematic review of epidemiologic research. *Crit Rev Toxicol.* (2014) 44:121–50. doi: 10.3109/10408444.2013.860075
130. Leonardi A, Cofini M, Rigante D, Lucchetti L, Cipolla C, Penta L, et al. The effect of Bisphenol A on puberty: a critical review of the medical literature. *Int J Environ Res Pub Health.* (2017) 14:E1044 doi: 10.3390/ijerph14091044
131. Lee DH, Jacobs DR Jr. Methodological issues in human studies of endocrine disrupting chemicals. *Rev Endocr Metabol Disord.* (2015) 16:289–97. doi: 10.1007/s11154-016-9340-9
132. Lee DH. Evidence of the possible harm of endocrine-disrupting chemicals in humans: ongoing debates and key issues. *Endocrinol Metabol.* (2018) 33:44–52. doi: 10.3803/EnM.2018.33.1.44
133. Ruzzin J, Petersen R, Meugnier E, Madsen L, Lock EJ, Lillefosse H, et al. Persistent organic pollutant exposure leads to insulin resistance syndrome. *Environ Health Perspect.* (2010) 118:465–71. doi: 10.1289/ehp.0901321
134. Lagarde F, Beausoleil C, Belcher SM, Belzunces LP, Emond C, Guerbet M, et al. Non-monotonic dose-response relationships and endocrine disruptors: a qualitative method of assessment. *Environ Health.* (2015) 14:13. doi: 10.1186/1476-069X-14-13

20

The Case for BPA as an Obesogen: Contributors to the Controversy

Beverly S. Rubin*, Cheryl M. Schaeberle and Ana M. Soto*

Department of Immunology, Tufts University School of Medicine, Boston, MA, United States

***Correspondence:**
Beverly S. Rubin
beverly.rubin@tufts.edu
Ana M. Soto
ana.soto@tufts.edu

Since the inception of the term endocrine disruptor, the idea that the environment is an important determinant of phenotype has motivated researchers to explore the effect of low dose exposure to BPA during organogenesis. The syndrome observed was complex, affecting various endpoints such as reproduction and reproductive tissues, behavior, mammary gland development and carcinogenesis, glucose homeostasis, and obesity. This constellation of impacted endpoints suggests the possibility of complex interactions among the multiple effects of early BPA exposure. One key finding of our rodent studies was alterations of energy and amino-acid metabolism that were detected soon after birth and continued to be present at all time points examined through 6 months of age. The classical manifestations of obesity and associated elements of metabolic disease took a longer time to become apparent. Here we examine the validity of the often-mentioned lack of reproducibility of obesogenic effects of BPA, starting from the known environmental causes of variation, which are diverse and range from the theoretical like the individuation process and the non-monotonicity of the dose-response curve, to the very pragmatic like housing, feed, and time and route of exposure. We then explore environmental conditions that may hinder reproducibility and discuss the effect of confounding factors such as BPA-induced hyperactivity. In spite of all the potential sources of variation, we find that some obesogenic or metabolic effects of BPA are reproducibly observed when study conditions are analogous. We recommend that study authors describe details of their study conditions including the environment, husbandry, and feed. Finally, we show that when experimental conditions are strictly maintained, reproducibility, and stability of the obese phenotype is consistently observed.

Keywords: Bisphenol A, non-monotonic dose response, metabolome, adiposity, exposure windows, exposure route, perinatal

INTRODUCTION

The incidence of obesity and associated elements of metabolic disease has increased rapidly during the last 30–40 years (1–3) reaching epidemic proportions in the industrialized world. This phenomenon has stimulated scientists to ponder about novel environmental factors that could contribute to this sudden change (4). These include chemicals referred to as "obesogens" (5), that inappropriately foster lipid accumulation and adipogenesis and lead to obesity. Bisphenol A (BPA) is just one compound on a growing list of possible obesogens; however, due to the ubiquitous nature of BPA exposure, it may represent an important compound among the putative contributors to the obesity epidemic. In fact, BPA was detected in the urine of over 92% of a representative sample of the US population (6), and positive associations have been found between urinary BPA levels and several adverse outcomes, including obesity and associated elements of metabolic disease (7–9). In addition to a putative obesogen, based on the data available, BPA may also be considered a metabolic disruptor (10) and a diabesogenic compound (11).

There has been some level of controversy regarding the effects of BPA exposure on obesity and metabolic disease. The purpose of this review is to delineate potential factors underlying seemingly discrepant outcomes in animal studies. We posit that these factors encompass differences like the species and strain, developmental stage at the time of BPA exposure, the ages at which animals were examined, as well as the doses tested, the routes of exposure, and the environment surrounding the animals. Of particular importance is the shape of the dose-response curve, which for endocrinology is often non-monotonic regardless of whether the hormonally active agent is a natural hormone or an endocrine disruptor. In addition, there are theoretical reasons that can account for different responses.

A Brief Theoretical Primer

In contrast to inert objects, living objects are not generic (interchangeable); they are individuals. Hence, what we measure as variation is the composite of an intrinsic and irreducible variation, since each animal is a unique individual, and a measurement error. Biologists address this problem by trying to make biological objects as "generic" as possible by using clonal cell lines and inbred strains, removing runts, culling litters, providing food of standardized composition, controlling the number of animals/cage, etc (12, 13). These procedures force a type of "invariance" or conservation into the system, allowing researchers to apply the mathematical tool of statistics. However, there is no mathematical theory of individuals, and thus biologists use statistics knowing that it has no way to contend with intrinsic variation. In addition, differences that are not statistically significant could be of utmost biological relevance. For example, Dolly the sheep was one clone that materialized from an enormous number of attempts. This also applies to the goat studied by Slijper that was born with paralysis of its front legs and soon learned to move by hopping on its hind legs. This behavioral accommodation resulted in dramatic morphological changes in bones of the hind legs and pelvis and changes in the morphology of the pelvic muscles (14) that were reminiscent of those present in bipeds. The mere fact that these singular results happen is sufficient to establish their relevance.

In this manuscript we analyze the effect of perinatal BPA exposure on adiposity and associated elements of metabolic disease and will show that when experimental conditions are kept constant to reduce variation (**Table 1**), the effect of BPA is reproducible. We also demonstrate that consideration of intrinsic individual variation allowed separation of two distinct phenotypes among females exposed perinatally to BPA (15).

BPA AS AN OBESOGEN: OUR LABORATORY

We initially chose BPA as the model endocrine disruptor for study in our lab because of its estrogenic activity and its structural resemblance to diethylstilbestrol (DES). Therefore, we expected to find alterations of the reproductive system and reproductive physiology in offspring exposed to BPA *in utero* and during lactation, as had been described in the DES-induced syndrome (16). We found reproductive alterations, but the earliest difference we noted between BPA-exposed and control offspring was on body weight (17), an effect that had been reported 2 years earlier in female mice by Howdeshell et al. (18) and was later reported in mice exposed neonatally to DES (19).

Body Weight and Adiposity

In the reproductive study mentioned above, we noticed differences in body weight in Sprague Dawley rats born to mothers that received BPA in their drinking water from gestational day 6 through weaning (17). Based on water consumption measurements, the exposure to the dams was estimated to be ~0.1 and 1.2 mg BPA/kg BW/day. The increase in body weight was modest, but significant. A similar study was performed by Somm et al. (20) using the same rat strain and only the lower BPA dose in drinking water. Both male and female BPA-exposed offspring were heavier at birth, and the females remained heavier through the termination of the study at 14 weeks.

TABLE 1 | Our experimental practices for consistent conditions.

Mice	Cages	#Animals/cage	Water	Diet	Exposure	Environment at the animal facility
CD-1	Polysulfone	Culling at PND2: 4 ♀ and 4 ♂	Glass water bottles	Harlan Teklad, 2018; non-irradiated	Subcutaneous osmotic minipumps (Alzet)	Light cycle: 14–10
Charles River	Static racks to allow pheromone exchange	Weaning at PND21, separation of ♀ and ♂	Stainless steel sipper; rubber stopper	Each lot tested for estrogenicity levels prior to purchase	GD8 to PND16	Lights on at 4 a.m. EST
Supplier Facility: Raleigh until site closed, then Kingston	Corn cob bedding	4/cage at weaning; 2–4 depending on weight thereafter	Filtered water		0.025, 0.25, 2.5, 25, 250 µg BPA/kg BW/day	Temperature: 20–24°C
	Cotton enrichment		Water tested for estrogenic activity		Internal dose: <0.3 ng/ml BPA in serum	

Increased perigonadal white adipose tissue weight and increased expression of adipogenic and lipogenic genes were observed in the females demonstrating that BPA exposure during gestation and lactation increased adipose storage and adipogenesis in a sex specific manner. Both BPA-exposed male and female offspring had increased body weights relative to controls when fed a high fat diet (HFD).

Subsequent studies in our lab using outbred CD-1 mice also examined the effects of perinatal BPA exposure on female reproduction and reproductive tissues (21–25). As in our previous rat study, we could not help but notice the increase in body weight in our BPA exposed mice. Also, when performing ovariectomies, we noted increased adiposity and ovarian fat pad size in the females born to mothers exposed to low levels of BPA. The BPA exposure for these studies was provided via osmotic minipumps that were implanted subcutaneously into pregnant females on GD-8 and released BPA through postnatal day 16; they provided continuous delivery of low levels of BPA (ranging from 0.025 μg/kg to 250 μg/kg BW/day) with great precision. Levels of unconjugated BPA in blood samples were below the detectability of the BPA assay (0.3 ng/ml) at all doses tested (15), and thus they are below or within human levels of exposure as measured in serum or plasma by analytical chemistry [adults: a range of 0–1 ng/ml [reviewed in Vandenberg et al. (26)]; umbilical cord blood: median = 1.03 ng/ml (27).

In later studies undertaken to examine the effects of perinatal BPA exposure on body weight and adiposity, we continued to observe increased body weight and fat pad weights, adipocyte hypertrophy, and an increased number of white adipocytes in the intrascapular brown fat depot. Most recently we reported increased body weight and fat mass measured by echoMRI in male and female mice exposed perinatally to BPA. This outcome was exacerbated in females exposed to BPA both perinatally and peripubertally, particularly when exposures were 2.5 and 25 μg BPA/kg BW/day (15). The additional peripubertal exposure increased insulin resistance, fat mass, BW, and inflammation in females in a dose dependent manner. Although the males showed significant increases in body weight and fat mass with perinatal BPA exposure, they did not show increased detrimental effects with the additional peripubertal exposure. This suggests that the specific extended period of BPA treatment was more damaging in females, or that females were more sensitive to harmful metabolic effects of BPA during the peripubertal window of exposure. Evidence of inflammation of fat pads was observed in BPA exposed male and female mice. Also observed was lipid accumulation in liver (15, 28) and increased serum leptin levels (15).

Metabolome Data

Metabolomics is the measurement of the set of small molecules (metabolites) that result from metabolism (29). The integration of metabolomics and physiopathological studies provides valuable information for understanding endocrine disruption and is expected to produce useful data for risk assessment of endocrine disruptors such as BPA. Metabolic fingerprints based on nuclear magnetic resonance (NMR) spectroscopy, can detect slight changes in the metabolome of cells, tissues, or organisms exposed to endocrine disruptors (EDs) opening the way to examine whether exposure to an ED results in global alterations of metabolism, whether these changes persist after cessation of exposure, and whether further changes arise in aging. Additionally, and in contrast with other omics, the interpretation of metabolomics is straightforward as most metabolic pathways are known, and metabolic network analysis can be used to understand how a given set of metabolites in a metabolomic profile are linked (30).

Metabolomics was used in our studies to examine global metabolites in our BPA exposed mice and rats (31, 32). In all cases, at all ages studied, metabolomic profiles differed in BPA exposed and control animals. Our first metabolome study involved male mice exposed to 0.025, 0.25, or 25 μg BPA/kg body weight/day from GD8 to PND16 (32). Aqueous extracts of PND2 animals and of livers, brains, and serum samples from PND21 animals were examined by 1H nuclear magnetic resonance spectroscopy. Endogenous metabolic fingerprints revealed changes in the global metabolism in PND2 extracts. Consistent with the findings of Alonso-Magdalena et al. (33) demonstrating that BPA exposure during fetal development in mice leads to disruption of glucose homeostasis that manifested at 6-months of age, the metabolomic profile in our study revealed that glucose was already affected by perinatal exposure to BPA at PND2. Additional alterations at PND2 included variations in pyruvate, amino acids, and neurotransmitters. Regarding PND21, statistical analysis successfully discriminated among treatment groups in liver, serum, and brain samples. Variations in glucose, pyruvate, amino acids, and neurotransmitters (γ-aminobutyric acid and glutamate) were identified. The fact that these alterations occurred well before the manifestation of the classical pathophysiological signs of metabolic disease suggests that metabolic pathways are an early target of BPA, rather than a consequence of obesity. Studies in female rats, also revealed alterations of energy, and amino-acid metabolism in the BPA exposed animals at all ages examined (31).

FACTORS THAT CAN INFLUENCE EFFECTS OF BPA EXPOSURE ON BODY WEIGHT AND ADIPOSITY

Although our studies in CD-1 mice have consistently suggested that BPA is an obesogen, there is considerable controversy in the literature that has caused many to question whether there is adequate evidence of the obesogenic properties of BPA. Several animal studies have noted increased BW and/or adiposity in their early BPA exposure models (15, 17, 18, 20, 34–43) while other studies have reported a decrease in BW and/or adiposity (40, 44–47) or no change (48, 49). Reviews of the data from human studies have also generated some controversy regarding the association between BPA exposure and obesity and metabolic disease (50–52). It is clear from the mouse studies in our lab that the effects of perinatal exposure to BPA on body weight, and fat mass, and associated parameters of metabolic disease are sex-dependent, dose dependent, and influenced by the precise window of exposure as well as the time of examination.

Route of exposure, diet, and housing conditions as well as other environmental factors undoubtedly play a role in the manifestation of increased adiposity and could potentially mask effects of BPA exposure. For example, accidental BPA exposure from damaged polycarbonate cages (53) led to meiotic disturbances including aneuploidy in oocytes in the mouse colony maintained by Pat Hunt. This finding demonstrates how external conditions could interfere with the ability to detect the effects of early BPA exposure on BW and adiposity or any other measurements. In order to facilitate comparisons of data from different laboratories, the factors mentioned above should be included in materials and methods (**Table 2**). Our practices for keeping the living conditions of our animals as constant as possible are summarized in **Table 1**.

Gender

There are several reports of increased adipogenesis in BPA exposed females relative to males particularly at young ages (20, 43). We initially noticed increased body weight and fat mass in our CD-1 mice with females showing more of an increase than males; however, that finding was influenced by changes in the environment and in housing conditions. For example, when males were singly housed to facilitate measurements of food intake and metabolism, the male data showed less variability allowing a clearer pattern to emerge. Whether the decrease in variability was influenced by the absence of a dominance hierarchy typically observed in group housed males, remains to be determined. In contrast to the males, when females were individually housed at 8 weeks of age, many of the BPA exposed females showed a tendency to lose weight. Overall compilation of recent data revealed that increased body weight and fat mass were more consistently apparent in perinatally exposed male than female CD-1 mice. This finding may be attributed, in part, to the hyperactivity observed in a subset of our BPA exposed females that represents a strong confounding factor when studying body weight and body composition and will be discussed below (15).

A recent study by Desai et al. (42), reported significant increases in BW and fat mass at 3 and 24 weeks of age in male but not female Sprague Dawley rats born to mothers exposed to BPA in their drinking water from 2 weeks prior to mating through pregnancy and lactation (5 mg BPA/liter which provided 500–900 μg/kg BW/day during pregnancy and ~1500 μg/kg BW/day during lactation). Further study of the BPA exposed males at 3 weeks of age revealed an increase in adipocyte size, lipogenic factors (SrebP1 and C/EBP alpha), and inflammation in the retroperitoneal fat pad. Sex also has a large impact on the effects of early BPA exposure on elements of metabolic disease. This is particularly apparent regarding the regulation of glucose/insulin homeostasis which has been extensively documented by Nadal and colleagues (54–56). They have clearly shown effects of gestational exposure to BPA on glucose regulation in male offspring that is not apparent in their female siblings at the times examined (33). Wistar rat offspring born to mothers exposed to 50 μg BPA/kg BW/day from GD0–PND 21 (by oral gavage) showed increased body weight on a chow diet. When fed a high fat diet (HFD), the body weight of males was increased before females (9 weeks vs. 15 weeks). This pattern was also seen in serum insulin levels that were increased at 15 weeks in males and 26 weeks in females (34).

TABLE 2 | Conditions that should be made explicit in Materials and Methods sections of research papers.

Strain and supplier	Specify the supplier's facility where animals were raised wherever possible
Feed and supplier	Specify which type of diet (casein-based, soy-based, other?) catalog number and supplier
	Specify if feed was tested for estrogenicity** and by which method
	Was the chemical of interest tested for its presence in feed?
	If the nutrient composition cannot be easily accessed, provide a short description (Calories from fat, % fat,% protein)
Water and water bottle	Filtered or tap?
	Glass or plastic bottle?
	If plastic what type of plastic?
	Stopper, sipper materials
	Was water tested for estrogenicity**?
Caging materials	What type of plastic? Was it tested for estrogenicity**?
	Static or ventilated racks?
	Enrichment? What materials?
	Bedding type (wood shavings, corn cob, etc)
	Number of animals/cage
Overall facility	Temperature range
	Humidity range
	Light/dark cycle
Animals	How many per litter
	Sex ratio
	Culled? To what number on what day
	Weaning day For Mice: exposure to pheromones by presence of males and females in alternate cages
Exposure	Route
	Period
	Dose
	Vehicle
	Internal circulating dose if possible
Timepoints	When were samples collected or measurements taken?

***Estrogenicity testing is a good measure even when the ED tested is not estrogenic, because of the ubiquity of contaminants with estrogenic activity that could be preset in food, plastics and water. Estrogenic activity could affect metabolism and interfere with the development of obesity.*

Hyperactivity

As mentioned above, increased activity has been reported in rodents exposed perinatally to BPA (15, 40, 44). Hyperactivity represents a serious confound to the assessment of increased body weight and adiposity and metabolic parameters in BPA exposed offspring. Although others have reported hyperactivity in both BPA- exposed males and females (57–60), in our studies, hyperactivity was more extreme and far more prevalent in BPA exposed females. A subset of females showed flipping or running behavior; both are repetitive behaviors that served no obvious function but were persistent in the affected animals (15). They remained lean despite a significant increase in food intake. If their data were included with the other females, no differences were noted in mean BW and mean estimates of adiposity as there was too much variability to allow statistically significant findings. If the data from the flippers were eliminated as outliers, the remaining data showed a pattern of increased body weight and adiposity in the non-affected females (15). It will be important to identify the factors involved in causing hyperactivity in a subset of the BPA exposed female offspring and to determine how widespread this phenomenon may be in other laboratories. Of interest, in their studies of C57Bl6 mice, van Esterik et al. reported increased body weights in their BPA exposed males and not their females although they did mention increased activity in their females (40). Similarly, Anderson et al. (44), reported decreased body weight and adiposity in their BPA exposed A^{vy} mice that was most pronounced in females, and when their movements were tracked, the females showed clear evidence of hyperactivity (44). In a study by Ryan et al. (49), when examined at 9–14 weeks of age, perinatally BPA exposed female CD-1 mice (but not their male siblings) consumed more calories and had less body fat than control females. These data would be consistent with increased activity levels or increased energy expenditure in the BPA exposed females. Hyperactivity was not measured in this study, and it can easily be overlooked as the hours of observation typically fall during the light cycle when the animals are sleeping.

Early BPA exposure has been found to alter cortical organization (61) and change dopaminergic projections in the neocortex which may play a role in activity changes. In our studies it is not clear why a subset of the females with identical BPA treatments show pronounced hyperactivity while others including their female siblings do not. This is an important observation to pursue and understand, particularly when one is attempting to study obesity and associated metabolic disease as it will have profound effects on the interpretation of the compiled data. Consistent with the results in rodents discussed above, it should be noted that there is a growing body of evidence suggesting an association between urinary BPA levels and increased activity in children (57, 62, 63).

Diet

We have routinely used a soy protein-based diet for our studies (Harlan-Teklad 2018). The estrogenicity of all food batches are tested in our laboratory prior to purchase using the ESCREEN assay (64). Only those found to have minimal estrogenic activity (<20 pmol of estrogen equivalents per gram) were purchased. Based on evaluation of available studies in the literature, casein based diets appear to be less likely to show the effects of BPA on several parameters (65) including body weight and adiposity (44, 48, 49, 66). Increased body weight and fat mass in BPA exposed rodents tended to be observed in animals eating a soy-based diet and not necessarily in a casein diet (44, 48, 49, 66). Ruhlen et al. have reported that a casein based diet elevated body weights of control animals and could therefore mask the effects of BPA on BW and adiposity in mice (65). In contrast, Cao et al. have reported that in their study in rats, it was soy and not BPA that caused increased body weight (48). However, in our studies with soy-based chow, we saw consistent effects of BPA. Unfortunately, many studies in the literature fail to provide information on diet; these omissions make it difficult to compare data between studies to formulate accurate conclusions.

Exposure Level: Low Doses, Monotonic and Non-monotonic Dose Response Curves (NMDRCs)

Exposure level is very important when studying the effects of early BPA exposure. BPA does not show a monotonic dose response curve for many endpoints including effects on BW and adiposity. The importance of the BPA dose on body weight and adiposity is clearly illustrated in a study by Wei et al. in rats (34). In that study, the lowest BPA dose administered by oral gavage through gestation and lactation (50 μg/kg BW/day, the current EPA reference dose) was obesogenic and predisposed the animals to elements of metabolic disease. The two higher doses (250 and 1250 μg/kg BW/day) did not produce these effects. Therefore, if only the higher doses had been examined, the report would conclude that BPA had no effect on BW, adiposity, and associated elements of metabolic syndrome. In another study in male CD-1 mice, animals were provided with 1 of 5 doses of BPA during the period of preadipocyte differentiation (GD9-GD 18) ranging from 5 μg to 5,000 μg/kg BW/day (35). The lower doses were more likely to increase BW and adiposity including adipocyte number and adipocyte size. In fact, no significant effects on these parameters were noted at the highest dose. Of interest, the studies of Tyl in mice (46) and in rats (47) revealed a very significant decrease in body weights in males and females exposed to the highest levels of BPA (500 mg or 600 mg/kg BW/day) during development. These levels were extremely high relative to the current EPA reference dose (67) and would not be considered environmentally relevant exposure levels. The toxicological model that presumes that the highest doses will provide the greatest effects is not typically applicable to endocrine disruptors or natural hormones.

A dose-response curve plots the intensity of a given effect over a range of doses examined. A monotonic response is characterized by a slope that does not change sign. In contrast, a non-monotonic dose response curve is characterized by a slope that changes sign within the dose-range tested. Some curves are U-shaped, others have an inverted U-shape and in others, the sign of the curve may change in multiple points along the range of doses examined. Non-monotonic dose-response curves are frequently seen in endocrinology. They range from proliferative effects observed in cell culture studies to whole organ, organismal effects and are even observed in epidemiological studies (68, 69).

Some processes leading to non-monotonicity have been identified in cell culture. Natural hormones like estrogens (70) and androgens (71–73) affect proliferation in a biphasic dose-response. At low doses, for example, sex steroids induce cell proliferation by neutralizing a plasma-borne inhibitor. At high doses, sex steroids block cell proliferation by inducing intracellular inhibitors (74) or by inducing cell death (75).

Natural hormones and endocrine disruptors also display non-monotonic dose-response curves when assessed *in vivo*. The vom

Saal group observed non monotonic effects of estradiol and DES on prostate weight (76). Our group demonstrated that estradiol produces a monophasic dose response curve when the endpoint measured is gene induction or the expression of a protein. In contrast, at higher levels of organization the uterus displays a monotonic dose–response whereas the mammary gland exhibits a non-monotonic response to increasing levels of estradiol (77). From a theoretical point of view, monotonic phenomena can be easily modeled due to their simplicity, by assuming that each step in a linear pathway behaves according to the law of mass action (78); thus, high doses will give predictable high effects. On the contrary, modeling a non-monotonic effect is not possible without first obtaining results from experiments using a complex experimental design to separate the components of such NMDRCs.

Exposure Window

Exposure windows must be considered when reviewing data on early exposure to BPA. Liu et al. published a study in C57Bl6 mice (38) in which the BPA exposure windows were dissected to include the following time intervals: GD 1-6; GD6-PND0; PND0-PND21; and GD6-PND21. Gestational exposure from GD6 to birth resulted in decreased body weights in males and females, and the postnatal exposure from birth to weaning resulted in a significant increase in body weight in the males. In contrast, for glucose tolerance and for insulin tolerance, the most consistent and persistent problem was seen in animals exposed from GD6 to PND0. This study delineates distinct differences in the exposure windows that affect BW and glucose homeostasis. These windows are reminiscent of the work of Cederroth and Nef (79) who observed that the beneficial effects of dietary soy and phytoestrogens on adiposity were noted only in postnatally treated CD-1 mice whereas improvements in glucose tolerance were restricted to animals that had fetal exposure.

When considering obesity and metabolic disease, it is important to realize that the metabolic circuits for food intake and metabolism in the hypothalamus are established primarily after birth. Therefore, neonatal BPA exposure could influence the development of these important circuits. The exquisitely timed postnatal leptin surge is essential for the proper development of neural circuits for food intake and metabolism (80), and MacKay et al. have provided evidence that peak leptin secretion is delayed in mice exposed perinatally to BPA (81). Disruption to the timing of the leptin surge impaired development of the melanocortin system resulting in alterations in the hypothalamic feeding circuitry that could contribute to metabolic disturbances in adulthood.

Route of Exposure

The route of exposure to BPA may have a significant effect on the outcomes observed. Although diet is considered the main source of BPA exposure in humans and ingestion the main route of intake, it is not the only source of exposure (82, 83). BPA exposure can occur through food and water, dermal absorption as occurs with BPA-laden register receipts (84–87), and via inhalation of air and dust. Moreover, BPA levels remain measurable in fasting individuals (88) suggesting the potential for non-oral sources of exposure, longer half- life, or storage in the body that differs from the idea of a relatively rapid clearance rate for this compound following ingestion. Of interest, urinary BPA excretion was elevated 84% in volunteers who handled thermal receipts and the delayed return to normal pre-exposure levels suggested a potential difference in bioavailability of BPA following dermal absorption relative to oral exposure (89). Some suggest that the non-oral exposures, although they are considered to occur at significantly lower levels, may be more potent as they avoid the first pass metabolism of BPA by conjugation and therefore dermal sources may have far higher toxicological relevance than expected (83). In a controlled experiment, handling of cash register receipt paper plus still wet hand sanitizer elevated unconjugated BPA serum levels (84) to those found after oral exposure to 50 μg/kg BW (90). Dermal contact may be the main contributor when both unconjugated and conjugated BPA are considered (82).

Exposure routes for BPA differ widely in the numerous studies reported. Whether animals receive their BPA once a day as a bolus or throughout the day could conceivably alter the impact of the same daily dose. Studies that use a single daily dose have provided BPA in a single subcutaneous injection, or by oral gavage, or less intrusively, in a drop of oil on the tongue or dispensed on a cookie. Although most studies aim to provide BPA levels in the range of human exposures, humans are not exposed to a single daily dose of BPA. In contrast, other studies provide BPA throughout the day by incorporating it into the food or the drinking water or via silastic capsules or osmotic minipumps. Although they may afford the same daily dose as that provided by bolus delivery, these more continuous or intermittent exposure paradigms could have a different effect on the animal (91, 92). In most of our studies, animals were exposed to continuous low levels of BPA via osmotic minipumps. This method allowed us to provide very low BPA doses (beginning at 0.025 μg BPA/kg BW/day) with a precision that would not be technically possible in other non-bolus dosing regimens.

In one study that compared subcutaneous and oral exposure of BPA, neonatal male rats (3-day old) received 10 μg BPA/kg BW in oil. The same preparation was administered as a subcutaneous injection or as an oral bolus. As expected, the maximal serum concentration of free and total BPA was higher with subcutaneous administration (91). A second study compared an oral bolus of BPA with administration via diet in mice. The authors reported different patterns of BPA concentration. Bolus administration was found to peak faster (1 h) than administration through food (6 h); however, bioavailability in the form of unconjugated BPA was higher when administered in food (92). Therefore, the route of administration may have significant effects on study outcomes.

Age of Outcome Measurement

Many effects of early BPA exposure do not manifest until later in life while others are apparent early in life. For example in the study by Somm (20), both male and female pups exposed to BPA *in utero* were heavier at birth than controls; however, at PND 21, only the females remained significantly heavier. Both males and females were heavier than controls when fed a high fat diet. Ryan et al. (49) found that males and females were heavier at weaning, but the increase in BW did not persist through week 14 when the study was terminated Several studies end at weaning or soon after and report no differences in BW or adiposity (45), but it is possible that such findings might have been observed in adulthood if they were examined. Malaise et al. reported (93) that relative to controls, mice exposed perinatally to BPA (50 μg/kg BW/day) were significantly leaner at PND 25, and they had decreased gonadal fat at PND 45. However, additional measurements from PND 70 to the end of the study at PND 170 revealed a significant increase in body weight and adiposity in BPA exposed mice relative to controls. Similarly in the study by Wei et al. (34), rats exposed perinatally to BPA (50 μg/kg BW/day) showed significant increases in body weight on a standard chow diet beginning at 17–19 weeks of age.

IN SUMMARY

The purpose of this article was to examine the controversy surrounding BPA as an obesogen. To address this issue, we focused on obesity and adiposity and only peripherally touched on its metabolic effects on glucose homeostasis and lipid metabolism, as these subjects are addressed by other articles in this issue. To assess the controversy, we focused on perinatal exposures in rodents since our own data from this window of exposure could be used to illustrate consistent results over 10 years of attempting to maintain a constant environment. Moreover, we found that departing from these stringent conditions resulted in measurable changes.

If one examines the existing publications on exposure to a relatively "low dose" of BPA during a window that includes gestational and lactational exposure in rodents, most references show some indication of increased BW and/or increased adiposity and/or elements of obesity-associated metabolic disease. This is true even though the endpoints collected, and the windows of observation may be diverse. Some papers not showing such an outcome reported potential confounds that could preclude increased body weight and adiposity such as hyperactivity, a feature that may go undetected unless animals are observed close to the start of the dark cycle. We also found that the trajectory of increased body weight and adiposity was more clearly defined when males were singly housed rather than group housed. Diet appears to be another contributor to phenotype. A review of the literature suggests that animals exposed to a soy-based diet were more likely to reveal the obesogenic properties of BPA than those fed a casein-based diet. Moreover, in some studies, obesogenic properties of BPA were enhanced or brought out by feeding a HFD. From our overall analysis, we posit that these interactions may explain the lack of concordance among apparently similar experiments, pointing to the need for investigators to publish detailed descriptions of housing, diet, caging materials, culling practices, and other crucial methodological details that are often omitted from the materials and methods (**Table 2**).

One striking result from our metabolomic studies is that as early as 2 days after birth there are clear changes in amino-acid and energy metabolism, including glucose in the BPA exposed animals. These alterations precede the clinical manifestations of obesity and associated elements of metabolic disease including altered glucose homeostasis. Differences in the metabolic fingerprints between control and BPA exposed offspring persist through life. The precocity of altered metabolomic profiles suggest that they may play a causal role in the manifestation of elements of metabolic disease in adulthood.

The shape of the dose response curve may sometimes explain divergence between two studies, because non-monotonicity is a frequent feature of BPA effects. If the effect studied has a non-monotonic dose response curve, and only one or two BPA doses are tested, it is likely that one or more of the multiple effects of BPA could be missed. It is expected that because BPA targets distinct receptors and various organs the resulting syndrome would be complex (94). However, it is important to keep in mind that animals are individuals, and therefore, not all animals will be affected identically. If one considers all the sources of variation described above, the fact that obesity and/or alterations of metabolism are observed in the majority of studies with some equivalency of exposure times and levels argues for the robustness of the effect.

Although we reviewed studies of early (fetal and neonatal) BPA exposure here, studies of BPA exposure in adult rodents have revealed effects on adiposity and elements of metabolic disease (95–97). One particularly interesting finding was observed in females exposed to BPA (10 or 100 μg/kg BW/day) during days 9–16 of pregnancy (33, 95). When examined on days 16–18 of pregnancy, females exposed to BPA revealed glucose intolerance and elevated levels of plasma insulin, triglycerides, and leptin relative to controls (33). By 4 months postpartum, BPA exposed mothers had increased body weights and at 6.5 months they had increased body weights, and increased perigonadal fat pad weights (95). Alterations in glucose and insulin tolerance were observed by 4 months postpartum, worsened at 5 months, and became even more pronounced at 6 months. In contrast, non-pregnant females exposed to the same level and length of exposure to BPA showed no changes in glucose or insulin tolerance when examined at 4, 5, or 6 months after treatment. These data reveal harmful long- term implications for BPA exposure during pregnancy.

Epidemiological studies have found a positive association between urinary BPA levels and obesity and diabetes in adults, (7–9, 98–100) children, and adolescents (101–108); others have questioned the strength of the association (50, 51). Of particular interest, a recent and rare planned exposure study in humans provided oral administration of the reference BPA dose to volunteers and measured the insulin/C-peptide response to administered glucose. Although this study had a small sample size, BPA exposure was found to alter this response (90).

What are the important messages that one can glean from these studies? The most urgent one concerns public health. The studies addressed here bolster the notion that BPA is an obesogen and metabolic disruptor. The incidence of obesity and obesity-associated metabolic disease including diabetes is increasing to alarming proportions, and human data shows a positive association between BPA level and health effects (109).

Given the fact that BPA exposure is ubiquitous, we need to conclude that BPA is a public health concern and take action to limit our exposure. European countries are reducing exposure by banning BPA in food packing materials, and a new law in France will ban the use of plastic in direct contact with food in school cafeterias (110).

A second issue in need of exploration is how BPA triggers these effects. The biological explanation of the syndrome produced by early BPA exposure is undoubtedly complex. It is worth remembering that the path from receptor binding to phenotype is not an obvious straight line. This complexity suggests it will take a long time to determine precisely how the BPA phenotype is determined. Organogenesis involves more than molecular interactions. As organs form, we observe supracellular phenomena such as cell to cell interactions, electrical gradients, mechanical forces, cell migration, and more (111). Additionally, the external environment co-constructs the phenotype (112) and the factors discussed above can modulate and affect the response to BPA. Therefore, we need to explore multiple pathways and processes that include all relevant levels of biological organization and we need to carefully control and report the conditions of our animals in the process. Unraveling the complexity of the BPA syndrome will provide us with a global understanding of how a very simple molecule derails development creating phenotypes prone to the development of multiple pathologies.

AUTHOR CONTRIBUTIONS

All authors listed have made a substantial, direct and intellectual contribution to the work, and approved it for publication.

FUNDING

Support was provided by Grant R01ES08314, 5RC2ES18781 and R21ES026283 from NIEHS. The findings and conclusions in this report are those of the authors and do not necessarily represent the views of the U. S. National Institute of Environmental Health Sciences or NIH.

ACKNOWLEDGMENTS

Thank you to Nafis Hasan for his critical reading of the manuscript.

REFERENCES

1. Flegal KM, Carroll MD, Kit BK, Ogden CL. Prevalence of obesity and trends in the distribution of body mass index among US adults, 1999-2010. *JAMA* (2012) 307:491–7. doi: 10.1001/jama.2012.39
2. Hales CM, Caroll MD, Fryar CD, Ogden CL. Prevalence of obesity among adults and youth: United States 2015-2016. *NCHS Data Brief* (2017) 1–8. Available online at: https://www.cdc.gov/nchs/data/databriefs/db288.pdf
3. Baillie-Hamilton PF. Chemical toxins: a hypothesis to explain the global obesity epidemic. *J Alter Complement Med.* (2002) 8:185–92. doi: 10.1089/107555302317371479
4. Heindel JJ, Blumberg B. Environmental obesogens: mechanisms and controversies. *Annu Rev Pharmacol Toxicol.* (2018) 59:89–106. doi: 10.1146/annurev-pharmtox-010818-021304
5. Grun F, Blumberg B. Endocrine disrupters as obesogens. *Mol Cell Endocrinol.* (2009) 304:19–29. doi: 10.1016/j.mce.2009.02.018
6. Calafat AM, Ye X, Wong LY, Reidy JA, Needham LL. Exposure of the U.S. population to bisphenol A and 4-tertiary-Octylphenol: 2003-2004. *Environ Health Perspect.* (2008) 116:39–44. doi: 10.1289/ehp.10753
7. Carwile JL, Michels KB. Urinary bisphenol A and obesity: NHANES 2003-2006. *Environ Res.* (2011) 111:825–30. doi: 10.1016/j.envres.2011.05.014
8. Lang IA, Galloway TS, Scarlett A, Henley WE, Depledge M, Wallace RB, Melzer D. Association of urinary bisphenol A concentration with medical disorders and laboratory abnormalities in adults. *J Am Med Assoc.* (2008) 300:1303–10. doi: 10.1001/jama.300.11.1303
9. Wang T, Li M, Chen B, Xu M, Xu Y, Huang Y, et al. Urinary bisphenol A (BPA) concentration associates with obesity and insulin resistance. *J Clin Endocrinol Metab.* (2012) 97:E223–7. doi: 10.1210/jc.2011-1989
10. Heindel JJ, Blumberg B, Cave M, Machtinger R, Mantovani A, Mendez MA, et al. Metabolism disrupting chemicals and metabolic disorders. *Reprod Toxicol.* (2017) 68:3–33. doi: 10.1016/j.reprotox.2016.10.001
11. Alonso-Magdalena P, Quesada I, Nadal A. Prenatal exposure to BPA and offspring outcomes: the diabesogenic behavior of BPA. *Dose Response* (2015) 13 15:59325815590395. doi: 10.1177/1559325815590395
12. Longo G, Soto AM. Why do we need theories? *Prog Biophys Mol Biol.* (2016) 122:4–10. doi: 10.1016/j.pbiomolbio.2016.06.005
13. Montévil M. *Biological Time and Extended Critical Transitions:Towards an Objectivization of the Living State of Matter.* École Doctorale 474 — Frontières du Vivant, Université de Paris V — René Descartes (2011). Paris.
14. West-Eberhard MJ. Phenotypic accommodation: adaptive innovation due to developmental plasticity. *J Exp Zool B Mol Dev Evol.* (2005) 304:610–8. doi: 10.1002/jez.b.21071
15. Rubin BS, Paranjpe M, DaFonte T, Schaeberle C, Soto AM, Obin M, et al. Perinatal BPA exposure alters body weight and composition in a dose specific and sex specific manner: the addition of peripubertal exposure exacerbates adverse effects in female mice. *Reprod Toxicol.* (2017) 68:130–44. doi: 10.1016/j.reprotox.2016.07.020
16. Newbold RR, Jefferson WN, Padilla-Banks E, Haseman J. Developmental exposure to diethylstilbestrol (DES) alters uterine response to estrogens in prepubescent mice: low versus high dose effects. *Reprod Toxicol.* (2004) 18:399–406. doi: 10.1016/j.reprotox.2004.01.007
17. Rubin BS, Murray MK, Damassa DA, King JC, Soto AM. Perinatal exposure to low doses of bisphenol-A affects body weight, patterns of estrous cyclicity and plasma LH levels. *Environ Health Perspect.* (2001) 109:675–80. doi: 10.1289/ehp.01109675
18. Howdeshell KL, Hotchkiss AK, Thayer KA, Vandenbergh JG, vom Saal FS. Exposure to bisphenol A advances puberty. *Nature* (1999) 401:763–4. doi: 10.1038/44517
19. Newbold RR, Padilla-Banks E, Snyder RJ, Jefferson WN. Developmental exposure to estrogenic compounds and obesity. *Birth Defects Res A Clin Mol Teratol.* (2005) 73:478–80. doi: 10.1002/bdra.20147
20. Somm E, Schwitzgebel VM, Toulotte A, Cederroth CR, Combescure C, Nef S, et al. Perinatal exposure to bisphenol a alters early adipogenesis in the rat. *Environ Health Perspect.* (2009) 117:1549–55. doi: 10.1289/ehp.11342
21. Markey CM, Wadia PR, Rubin BS, Sonnenschein C, Soto AM. Long-term effects of fetal exposure to low doses of the xenoestrogen bisphenol-A in the female mouse genital tract. *Biol Reprod.* (2005) 72:1344–51. doi: 10.1095/biolreprod.104.036301
22. Cabaton NJ, Wadia PR, Rubin BS, Zalko D, Schaeberle CM, Askenase MH, et al. Perinatal exposure to environmentally relevant levels of Bisphenol-A decreases fertility and fecundity in CD-1 mice. *Environ Health Perspect.* (2011) 119:547–52. doi: 10.1289/ehp.1002559
23. Markey CM, Coombs MA, Sonnenschein C, Soto AM. Mammalian development in a changing environment: exposure to endocrine disruptors

reveals the developmental plasticity of steroid-hormone target organs. *Evolu Dev.* (2003) 5: 67–75. doi: 10.1046/j.1525-142X.2003.03011.x

24. Acevedo N, Rubin BS, Schaeberle CM, Soto AM. Perinatal BPA exposure and reproductive axis function in CD-1 mice. *Reprod Toxicol.* (2018) 79:39–46. doi: 10.1016/j.reprotox.2018.05.002
25. Soto AM, Brisken C, Schaeberle CM, Sonnenschein C. Does cancer start in the womb? altered mammary gland development and predisposition to breast cancer due to *in utero* exposure to endocrine disruptors. *J Mammary Gland Biol Neoplasia* (2013) 18:199–208. doi: 10.1007/s10911-013-9293-5
26. Vandenberg LN, Chauhoud I, Heindel JJ, Padmanabhan V, Paumgartten FJ, Schoenfelder G. Urinary, circulating and tissue biomonitoring studies indicate widespread exposure to Bisphenol A. *Environ Health Perspect.* (2010) 118:1055–70. doi: 10.1289/ehp.0901716
27. Gerona RR, Woodruff TJ, Dickenson CA, Pan J, Schwartz JM, Sen S, et al. Bisphenol-A (BPA), BPA glucuronide, and BPA sulfate in midgestation umbilical cord serum in a northern and central California population. *Environ Sci Technol.* (2013) 47:12477–85. doi: 10.1021/es402764d
28. Shimpi PC, More VR, Paranjpe M, Donepudi AC, Goodrich JM, Dolinoy DC, et al. Hepatic lipid accumulation and Nrf2 expression following perinatal and peripubertal exposure to bisphenol A in a mouse model of nonalcoholic liver disease. *Environ Health Perspect.* (2017) 125:087005. doi: 10.1289/EHP664
29. Ramsden JJ. *Bioinformatics.* London:Springer-Verlag (2009).
30. Cottret L, Frainay C, Chazalviel M, Cabanettes F, Gloaguen Y, Camenen E, et al. MetExplore: collaborative edition and exploration of metabolic networks. *Nucleic Acids Res.* (2018) 46:W495–502. doi: 10.1007/s00204-015-1488-7
31. Tremblay-Franco M, Cabaton NJ, Canlet C, Gautier R, Schaeberle CM, Fabien J, et al. Dynamic metabolic disruption in rats perinatally exposed to low doses of bisphenol-A. *PLoS ONE* (2015) 10:e0141698. doi: 10.1371/journal.pone.0141698
32. Cabaton NJ, Canlet C, Wadia PR, Tremblay-Franco M, Gautier R, Molina J, et al. Effects of low doses of bisphenol A on the metabolome of perinatally exposed CD-1 mice. *Environ Health Perspect.* (2013) 121:586–93. doi: 10.1289/ehp.1205588
33. Alonso-Magdalena P, Vieira E, Soriano S, Menes L, Burks D, Quesada I, et al. Bisphenol A exposure during pregnancy disrupts glucose homeostasis in mothers and adult male offspring. *Environ Health Perspect.* (2010) 118:1243–50. doi: 10.1289/ehp.1001993
34. Wei J, Lin Y, Li Y, Ying C, Chen J, Song L, et al. Perinatal exposure to bisphenol A at reference dose predisposes offspring to metabolic syndrome in adult rats on a high-fat diet. *Endocrinology* (2011) 152:3049–61. doi: 10.1210/en.2011-0045
35. Angle BM, Do RP, Ponzi D, Stahlhut RW, Drury BE, Nagle SC, et al. Metabolic disruption in male mice due to fetal exposure to low but not high doses of bisphenol A (BPA): evidence for effects on body weight, food intake, adipocytes, leptin, adiponectin, insulin and glucose regulation. *Reprod Toxicol.* (2013) 42:256–68. doi: 10.1016/j.reprotox.2013.07.017
36. Nikaido Y, Yoshizawa K, Danbara N, Tsujita-Kyutoku M, Yuri T, Uehara N, et al. Effects of maternal xenoestrogen exposure on development of the reproductive tract and mammary gland in female CD-1 mouse offspring. *Reprod Toxicol.* (2004) 18:803–11. doi: 10.1016/j.reprotox.2004.05.002
37. Garc¡a-Arevalo M, Alonso-Magdalena P, Rebelo Dos Santos J, Quesada I, Carneiro EM, Nadal A. Exposure to bisphenol-A during pregnancy partially mimics the effects of a high-fat diet altering glucose homeostasis and gene expression in adult male mice. *PLoS ONE* (2014) 9:e100214. doi: 10.1371/journal.pone.0100214
38. Liu J, Yu P, Qian W, Li Y, Zhao J, Huan F, et al. Perinatal bisphenol A exposure and adult glucose homeostasis: identifying critical windows of exposure. *PLoS ONE* (2013) 10:e64143. doi: 10.1371/journal.pone.0064143
39. Patisaul HB, Bateman HL. Neonatal exposure to endocrine active compounds or an ERbeta agonist increases adult anxiety and aggression in gonadally intact male rats. *Horm Behav.* (2008) 53:580–8. doi: 10.1016/j.yhbeh.2008.01.008
40. van Esterik JC, Dollé ME, Lamoree MH, van Leeuwen SP, Hamers T, Legler J, et al. Programming of metabolic effects in C57BL/6JxFVB mice by exposure to bisphenol A during gestation and lactation. *Toxicology* (2014) 321:40–52. doi: 10.1016/j.tox.2014.04.001
41. Taylor JA, Shioda K, Mitsunaga S, Yawata S, Angle BM, Nagel SC, et al. Prenatal exposure to bisphenol A disrupts naturally occurring bimodal DNA methylation at proximal promoter of fggy, an obesity-relevant gene encoding a carbohydrate kinase, in gonadal white adipose tissues of CD-1 mice. *Endocrinology* (2018) 159:779–94. doi: 10.1210/en.2017-00711
42. Desai M, Ferrini MG, Jellyman JK, Han G, Ross MG. *In vivo* and *in vitro* bisphenol A exposure effects on adiposity. *J Dev Orig Health Dis.* (2018). doi: 10.1017/S2040174418000600. [Epub ahead of print].
43. Miyawaki J, Sakayama K, Kato H, Yamamoto H, Masuno H. Perinatal and postnatal exposure to bisphenol a increases adipose tissue mass and serum cholesterol level in mice. *J Atheroscl Thromb.* (2007) 14:245–52. doi: 10.5551/jat.E486
44. Anderson OS, Peterson KE, Sanchez BN, Zhang Z, Mancuso P, Dolinoy DC. Perinatal bisphenol A exposure promotes hyperactivity, lean body composition, and hormonal responses across the murine life course. *FASEB J.* (2013) 27:1784–92. doi: 10.1096/fj.12-223545
45. Ferguson SA, Law CD Jr, Abshire JS. Developmental treatment with bisphenol A or ethinyl estradiol causes few alterations on early preweaning measures. *Toxicol Sci.* (2011) 124:149–60. doi: 10.1093/toxsci/kfr201
46. Tyl RW, Myers CB, Marr MC, Sloan CS, Castillo NP, Veselica MM, et al. Two-generation reproductive toxicity study of dietary bisphenol A in CD-1 (Swiss) mice. *Toxicol Sci.* (2008) 104:362–84. doi: 10.1093/toxsci/kfn084
47. Tyl RW, Myers CB, Marr MC, Thomas BF, Keimowitz AR, Brine DR, et al. Three-generation reproductive toxicity study of dietary bisphenol A in CD Sprague-Dawley rats. *Toxicol Sci.* (2002) 68:121–46. doi: 10.1093/toxsci/68.1.121
48. Cao J, Echelberger R, Liu M, Sluzas E, McCaffery K, Buckley B, et al. Soy but not bisphenol A (BPA) or the phytoestrogen genistin alters developmental weight gain and food intake in pregnant rats and their offspring. *Reprod Toxicol.* (2015) 58:282–94. doi: 10.1016/j.reprotox.2015.07.077
49. Ryan KK, Haller AM, Sorrell JE, Woods SC, Jandacek RJ, Seeley RJ. Perinatal exposure to bisphenol-a and the development of metabolic syndrome in CD-1 mice. *Endocrinology* (2010) 151:2603–12. doi: 10.1210/en.2009-1218
50. Lakind JS, Goodman M, Mattison DR. Bisphenol A and indicators of obesity, glucose metabolism/type 2 diabetes and cardiovascular disease: a systematic review of epidemiologic research. *Crit Rev Toxicol.* (2014) 44:121–50. doi: 10.3109/10408444.2013.860075
51. Mirmira P, Evans-Molina C. Bisphenol A, obesity, and type 2 diabetes mellitus: genuine concern or unnecessary preoccupation? *Transl Res.* (2014) 164:13–21. doi: 10.1016/j.trsl.2014.03.003
52. Oppeneer SJ, Robien K. Bisphenol A exposure and associations with obesity among adults: a critical review. *Public Health Nutr.* (2015) 18:1847–63. doi: 10.1017/S1368980014002213
53. Hunt PA, Koehler KE, Susiarjo M, Hodges CA, Ilagan A, Voigt RC, et al. Bisphenol A exposure causes meiotic aneuploidy in the female mouse. *Curr Biol.* (2003) 13:546–53. doi: 10.1016/S0960-9822(03)00189-1
54. Ropero AB, Alonso-Magdalena P, Garcia-Garcia E, Ripoll C, Fuentes E, Nadal A. Bisphenol-A disruption of the endocrine pancreas and blood glucose homeostasis. *Int J Androl.* (2008) 31:194–200. doi: 10.1111/j.1365-2605.2007.00832.x
55. Nadal A, Obesity: fat from plastics? Linking bisphenol A exposure and obesity. *Nat Rev Endocrinol.* (2013) 9:9–10. doi: 10.1038/nrendo.2012.205
56. Nadal A, Quesada I, Tudur E, Nogueiras R, Alonso-Magdalena P. Endocrine-disrupting chemicals and the regulation of energy balance. *Nat Rev Endocrinol.* (2017) 13:536–46. doi: 10.1038/nrendo.2017.51
57. Rochester JR, Bolden AL, Kwiatkowski CF. Prenatal exposure to bisphenol A and hyperactivity in children: a systematic review and meta-analysis. *Environ Int.* (2018) 114:343–56. doi: 10.1016/j.envint.2017.12.028
58. Nojima K, Takata T, Masuno H. Prolonged exposure to a low-dose of bisphenol A increases spontaneous motor activity in adult male rats. *J Physiol Sci.* (2013) 63:311–5. doi: 10.1007/s12576-013-0265-8
59. Ishido M, Masuo Y, Kunimoto M, Oka S, Morita M. Bisphenol A causes hyperactivity in the rat concomitantly with impairment of tyrosine hydroxylase immunoreactivity. *J Neurosci Res.* (2004) 76:423–33. doi: 10.1002/jnr.20050

60. Ishido M, Masuo Y, Terasaki M, Morita M. Rat hyperactivity by bisphenol A, but not by its derivatives, 3-hydroxybisphenol A or bisphenol A 3,4-quinone. *Toxicol Lett.* (2011) 206:300–5. doi: 10.1016/j.toxlet.2011.08.011
61. Komada M, Itoh S, Kawachi K, Kagawa N, Ikeda Y, Nagao T. Newborn mice exposed prenatally to bisphenol A show hyperactivity and defective neocortical development. *Toxicology* (2014) 323:51–60. doi: 10.1016/j.tox.2014.06.009
62. Harley KG, Gunier RB, Kogut K, Johnson C, Bradman A, Calafat AM, et al. Prenatal and early childhood bisphenol A concentrations and behavior in school-aged children. *Environ Res.* (2013) 126:43–50. doi: 10.1016/j.envres.2013.06.004
63. Braun JM, Kalkbrenner AE, Calafat AM, Yolton K, Ye X, Dietrich KN, et al. Impact of early-life bisphenol A exposure on behavior and executive function in children. *Pediatrics* (2011) 128:873–82. doi: 10.1542/peds.2011-1335
64. Soto AM, Sonnenschein C, Chung KL, Fernandez MF, Olea N, Olea-Serrano MF. The E-SCREEN assay as a tool to identify estrogens: an update on estrogenic environmental pollutants. *Environ Health Perspect.* (1995) 103:113–22.
65. Ruhlen RL, Howdeshell KL, Mao J, Taylor JA, Bronson FH, Newbold RR, et al. Low phytoestrogen levels in feed increase fetal serum estradiol resulting in the "fetal estrogenization syndrome" and obesity in CD-1 mice. *Environ Health Perspect.* (2008) 116:322–8. doi: 10.1289/ehp.10448
66. Mackay H, Patterson ZR, Khazall R, Patel S, Tsirlin D, Abidzaid A. Organizational effects of perinatal exposure to bisphenol-A and diethylstilbestrol on arcuate nucleus circuitry controlling food intake and energy expenditure in male and female CD-1 mice. *Endocrinology* (2013) 154:1465–75. doi: 10.1210/en.2012-2044
67. Krishnan K, Gagne M, Nong A, Aylward LL, Hays SM. Biomonitoring equivalents for bisphenol A (BPA). *Regul Toxicol Pharmacol.* (2010) 58:18–24. doi: 10.1016/j.yrtph.2010.06.005
68. Vandenberg LN, Colborn T, Hayes TB, Heindel JJ, Jacobs DR Jr, Lee DH, et al. Hormones and endocrine disrupting chemicals: low dose effects and non-monotonic dose responses. *Endocr Rev.* (2012) 33:378–455. doi: 10.1210/er.2011-1050
69. Vandenberg LN. Non-monotonic dose responses in studies of endocrine disrupting chemicals: bisphenol a as a case study. *Dose Response* (2014) 12:259–76. doi: 10.2203/dose-response.13-020.
70. Amara JF, Dannies PS. 17 á-Estradiol has a biphasic effect on GH cell growth. *Endocrinology* (1983) 112:1141 3. doi: 10.1210/endo-112-3-1141
71. Sonnenschein C, Olea N, Pasanen ME, Soto AM. Negative controls of cell proliferation: human prostate cancer cells and androgens. *Cancer Res.* (1989) 49:3474–81.
72. Geck P, Szelei J, Jimenez J, Lin TM, Sonnenschein C, Soto AM. Expression of novel genes linked to the androgen-induced, proliferative shutoff in prostate cancer cells. *J Steroid Biochem Mol Biol.* (1997) 63:211–8. doi: 10.1016/S0960-0760(97)00122-2
73. Soto AM, Lin TM, Sakabe K, Olea N, Damassa DA, Sonnenschein C. Variants of the human prostate LNCaP cell line as a tool to study discrete components of the androgen-mediated proliferative response. *Oncol Res.* (1995) 7:545–58.
74. Geck P, Maffini MV, Szelei J, Sonnenschein C, Soto AM. Androgen-induced proliferative quiescence in prostate cancer: the role of AS3 as its mediator. *Proc Natl Acad Sci USA.* (2000) 97:10185–90. doi: 10.1073/pnas.97.18.10185
75. Soto AM, Sonnenschein C. The two faces of Janus: sex steroids as mediators of both cell proliferation and cell death. *J Ntl Cancer Institute* (2001) 93:1673–5. doi: 10.1093/jnci/93.22.1673
76. vom Saal FS, Timms BG, Montano MM, Palanza P, Thayer KA, Nagel SC, et al. Prostate enlargement in mice due to fetal exposure to low doses of estradiol or diethylstilbestrol and opposite effects at high doses. *Proc Natl Acad Sci USA.* (1997) 94:2056–61. doi: 10.1073/pnas.94.5.2056
77. Vandenberg LN, Wadia PR, Schaeberle CM, Rubin BS, Sonnenschein C, Soto AM. The mammary gland response to estradiol: monotonic at the cellular level, non-monotonic at the tissue-level of organization? *J Steroid Biochem Mol Biol.* (2006) 101:263–74. doi: 10.1016/j.jsbmb.2006.06.028
78. Kohn MC, Melnick RL. Biochemical origins of the non-monotonic receptor-mediated dose-response. *J Mol Endocrinol.* (2002) 29:113–23. doi: 10.1677/jme.0.0290113
79. Cederroth CR, Nef S. Fetal programming of adult glucose homeostasis in mice. *PLoS ONE* (2009) 4:e7281. doi: 10.1371/journal.pone.0007281
80. Bouret SG, Draper SJ, Simerly RB. Trophic action of leptin on hypothalamic neurons that regulate feeding. *Science* (2004) 304:108–10. doi: 10.1126/science.1095004
81. Mackay H, Patterson ZR, Abizaid A. Perinatal exposure to low-dose bisphenol-A disrupts the structural and functional development of the hypothalamic feeding circuitry. *Endocrinology* (2017) 158:768–77. doi: 10.1210/en.2016-1718
82. Lu S, Yu Y, Ren L, Zhang X, Liu G, Yu Y. Estimation of intake and uptake of bisphenols and triclosan from personal care products by dermal contact. *Sci Total Environ.* (2018) 621:1398–6. doi: 10.1016/j.scitotenv.2017.10.088
83. von Goetz N, Pirow R, Hart A, Bradley E, Poças F, Arcella D, et al. Including non-dietary sources into an exposure assessment of the European Food Safety Authority: The challenge of multi-sector chemicals such as Bisphenol A. *Regul Toxicol Pharmacol.* (2017) 85:70–8. doi: 10.1016/j.yrtph.2017.02.004
84. Hormann AM, vom Saal FS, Nagel SC, Stahlhut RW, Moyer CL, Ellersieck MR, et al. Holding thermal receipt paper and eating food after using hand sanitizer results in high serum bioactive and urine total levels of bisphenol A (BPA). *PLoS ONE* (2014) 9:e110509. doi: 10.1371/journal.pone.0110509
85. Ehrlich S, Calafat AM, Humblet O, Smith T, Hauser R. Handling of thermal receipts as a source of exposure to bisphenol A. *J Am Med Assoc.* (2014) 311:859–60. doi: 10.1001/jama.2013.283735
86. Biedermann S, Tschudin P, Grob K. Transfer of Bisphenol A from thermal printer paper to the skin. *Anal Bioanal Chem.* (2010) 398:571–6. doi: 10.1007/s00216-010-3936-9
87. Zalko D, Jacques C, Duplan H, Bruel S, Perdu E. Viable skin efficiently absorbs and metabolizes bisphenol A. *Chemosphere* (2011) 82:424–30. doi: 10.1016/j.chemosphere.2010.09.058
88. Stahlhut RW, Welshons WV, Swan SH. Bisphenol A data in NHANES suggest longer than expected half-life, substantial nonfood exposure, or both. *Environ Health Perspect.* (2009) 117:784–9. doi: 10.1289/ehp.0800376
89. Lv Y, Lu S, Dai Y, Rui C, Wang Y, Zhou Y, et al. Higher dermal exposure of cashiers to BPA and its association with DNA oxidative damage. *Environ Int.* (2017) 98:69–74. doi: 10.1016/j.envint.2016.10.001
90. Stahlhut RW, Myers JP, Taylor JA, Nadal A, Dyer JA, vom Saal FS. Experimental BPA exposure and glucose-stimulated insulin response in adult men and women. *J Endo Soc.* (2018) 2: 1173–87. doi: 10.1210/js.2018-00151
91. Prins GS, Ye SH, Birch L, Ho SM, Kannan K. Serum bisphenol A pharmacokinetics and prostate neoplastic responses following oral and subcutaneous exposures in neonatal Sprague-Dawley rats. *Reprod Toxicol.* (2011) 31:1–9. doi: 10.1016/j.reprotox.2010.09.009
92. Sieli PT, Jasarevic E, Warzak DA, Mao J, Ellersieck MR, Liao C, et al. Comparison of serum bisphenol A concentrations in mice exposed to bisphenol A through the diet versus oral bolus exposure. *Environ Health Perspect.* (2011) 119:1260–5. doi: 10.1289/ehp.1003385
93. Malais Y, Menard S, Cartier C, Gaultier E, Lasserre F, Lencina C, et al. Gut dysbiosis and impairment of immune system homeostasis in perinatally-exposed mice to Bisphenol A precede obese phenotype development. *Sci Rep.* (2017) 7:14472. doi: 10.1038/s41598-017-15196-w
94. Sonnenschein C, Wadia PR, Rubin BS, Soto AM. Cancer as development gone awry: the case for bisphenol-A as a carcinogen. *J Dev Orig Health Dis.* (2011) 2:9–16. doi: 10.1017/S2040174411000043
95. Alonso-Magdalena P, Garcįa-Arevalo M, Quesada I, Nadal A. Bisphenol-A treatment during pregnancy in mice: a new window of susceptibility for the development of diabetes in mothers later in life. *Endocrinology* (2015) 156:1659–70. doi: 10.1210/en.2014-1952
96. Yang M, Chen M, Wang J, Xu M, Sun J, Ding L, et al. Bisphenol A promotes adiposity and inflammation in a nonmonotonic dose-response way in five-week old male and female C57BL/6J mice fed a low-calorie diet. *Endocrinology* (2016) 157:2333–45. doi: 10.1210/en.2015-1926
97. Batista TM, Alonso-Magdalena P, Vieira E, Amaral ME, Cederroth CR, Nef S, et al. Short-term treatment with bisphenol-A leads to metabolic abnormalities in adult male mice. *PLoS ONE.* (2012) 7:e33814. doi: 10.1371/journal.pone.0033814
98. Klimentidis YC, Beasley TM, Lin HY, Murati G, Glass GE, Guyton M, et al. Canaries in the coal mine: a cross-species analysis of the plurality of obesity epidemics. *Proc Biol Sci.* (2011) 278:1626–32. doi: 10.1098/rspb.2010.1890

99. Shankar A, Teppala S, Sabanayagam C. Urinary bisphenol a levels and measures of obesity: results from the national health and nutrition examination survey 2003-2008. *ISRN Endocrinol.* (2012) 2012:965243. doi: 10.5402/2012/965243
100. Rancière F, Lyons JG, Loh HY, Botton J, Galloway T, Wang T, et al. Bisphenol A and the risk of cardiometabolic disorders: a systematic review with meta-analysis of the epidemiological evidence. *Environ Health* (2015) 14:46. doi: 10.1186/s12940-015-0036-5
101. Valvi D, Casas M, Mendez MA, Ballesteros-Gmez A, Luque N, Rubio S, et al. Prenatal bisphenol a urine concentrations and early rapid growth and overweight risk in the offspring. *Epidemiology* (2013) 24:791–9. doi: 10.1097/EDE.0b013e3182a67822
102. Vafeiadi M, Roumeliotaki T, Myridakis A, Chalkiadaki G, Fthenou E, Dermitzaki E, et al. Association of early life exposure to bisphenol A with obesity and cardiometabolic traits in childhood. *Environ Res.* (2016) 146:379–87. doi: 10.1016/j.envres.2016.01.017
103. Hoepner LA, Whyatt RM, Widen EM, Hassoun A, Oberfield SE, Mueller NT, et al. BPA and adiposity in inner city birth cohort. *Environ Health Perspect.* (2016) 124:1644–50. doi: 10.1289/EHP205
104. Trasande L, Attina TM, Blustein J. Association between urinary bisphenol A concentration and obesity prevalence in children and adolescents. *J Am Med Assoc.* (2012) 308:1113–21. doi: 10.1001/2012.jama.11461
105. Amin MM, Ebrahim K, Hashemi M, Shoshtari-Yeganeh B, Rafiei N, Mansourian M, et al. Association of exposure to Bisphenol A with obesity and cardiometabolic risk factors in children and adolescents. *Int J Environ Health Res.* (2018) 29:94–106. doi: 10.1080/09603123.2018.155896
106. Li DK, Miao M, Zhou Z, Wu C, Shi H, Liu X, et al. Urine bisphenol-A level in relation to obesity and overweight in school-age children. *PLoS ONE* (2013) 8:e65399. doi: 10.1371/journal.pone.0065399
107. Bhandari R, Xiao J, Shankar A. Urinary bisphenol A and obesity in U.S. children. *Am J Epidemiol.* (2013) 177:1263–70. doi: 10.1093/aje/kws391
108. Eng DS, Lee JM, Gebrmariam A, Meeker JD, Peterson K, Padmanabhan V. Bisphenol A and chronic disease risk factors in US childrens. *Pediatrics* (2013) 132:e637–45. doi: 10.1542/peds.2013-0106
109. Legeay S, Faure S. Is bisphenol A an environmental obesogen? *Fundam Clin Pharmacol.* (2017) 31:594–609. doi: 10.1111/fcp.12300
110. French Law. *French Law # 2018-938.* 28. Available online at: https://www.legifrance.gouv.fr/eli/loi/2018/10/30/AGRX1736303L/jo/texte
111. Soto AM, Longo G, Miquel PA, Montévil M, Mossio M, Perret N, et al. Toward a theory of organisms: three founding principles in search of a useful integration. *Prog Biophys Mol Biol.* (2016) 122:77–82. doi: 10.1016/j.pbiomolbio.2016.07.006
112. Gilbert SF. Ecological developmental biology: environmental signals for normal animal development. *Evolu Dev.* (2012) 14:20–8. doi: 10.1111/j.1525-142X.2011.00519.x

Permissions

All chapters in this book were first published by Frontiers; hereby published with permission under the Creative Commons Attribution License or equivalent. Every chapter published in this book has been scrutinized by our experts. Their significance has been extensively debated. The topics covered herein carry significant findings which will fuel the growth of the discipline. They may even be implemented as practical applications or may be referred to as a beginning point for another development.

The contributors of this book come from diverse backgrounds, making this book a truly international effort. This book will bring forth new frontiers with its revolutionizing research information and detailed analysis of the nascent developments around the world.

We would like to thank all the contributing authors for lending their expertise to make the book truly unique. They have played a crucial role in the development of this book. Without their invaluable contributions this book wouldn't have been possible. They have made vital efforts to compile up to date information on the varied aspects of this subject to make this book a valuable addition to the collection of many professionals and students.

This book was conceptualized with the vision of imparting up-to-date information and advanced data in this field. To ensure the same, a matchless editorial board was set up. Every individual on the board went through rigorous rounds of assessment to prove their worth. After which they invested a large part of their time researching and compiling the most relevant data for our readers.

The editorial board has been involved in producing this book since its inception. They have spent rigorous hours researching and exploring the diverse topics which have resulted in the successful publishing of this book. They have passed on their knowledge of decades through this book. To expedite this challenging task, the publisher supported the team at every step. A small team of assistant editors was also appointed to further simplify the editing procedure and attain best results for the readers.

Apart from the editorial board, the designing team has also invested a significant amount of their time in understanding the subject and creating the most relevant covers. They scrutinized every image to scout for the most suitable representation of the subject and create an appropriate cover for the book.

The publishing team has been an ardent support to the editorial, designing and production team. Their endless efforts to recruit the best for this project, has resulted in the accomplishment of this book. They are a veteran in the field of academics and their pool of knowledge is as vast as their experience in printing. Their expertise and guidance has proved useful at every step. Their uncompromising quality standards have made this book an exceptional effort. Their encouragement from time to time has been an inspiration for everyone.

The publisher and the editorial board hope that this book will prove to be a valuable piece of knowledge for researchers, students, practitioners and scholars across the globe.

List of Contributors

Nicolas J. Cabaton, Nathalie Poupin, Marc Audebert, Jean-Pierre Cravedi, Anne Riu, Fabien Jourdan and Daniel Zalko
Toxalim (Research Centre in Food Toxicology), Université de Toulouse, INRA, ENVT, INP-Purpan, UPS, Toulouse, France

Cécile Canlet and Marie Tremblay-Franco
Toxalim (Research Centre in Food Toxicology), Université de Toulouse, INRA, ENVT, INP-Purpan, UPS, Toulouse, France
Axiom Platform, MetaToul-MetaboHub, National Infrastructure for Metabolomics and Fluxomics, Toulouse, France

Eva Tudurí, Laura Marroqui, Reinaldo S. Dos Santos, Iván Quesada, Esther Fuentes and Paloma Alonso-Magdalena
Centro de Investigación Biomédica en Red de Diabetes y Enfermedades Metabólicas Asociadas and Instituto de Biología Molecular y Celular, Universidad Miguel Hernández de Elche, Alicante, Spain

Sarah G. Howard
Diabetes and Environment Program, Commonweal, Bolinas, CA, United States

Victoria D. Balise and Susan C. Nagel
Department of Obstetrics, Gynecology and Women's Health, University of Missouri, Columbia, MO, United States
Department of Biological Sciences, University of Missouri, Columbia, MO, United States

Jennifer N. Cornelius-Green, Brittany Parmenter and Sierra Baxter
Department of Obstetrics, Gynecology and Women's Health, University of Missouri, Columbia, MO, United States

R. Scott Rector
Department of Nutrition and Health Exercise Physiology, University of Missouri, Columbia, MO, United States
Division of Gastroenterology and Hepatology, School of Medicine, University of Missouri, Columbia, MO, United States
Research Service, Harry S. Truman Memorial Veterans Medical Center, Columbia, MO, United States

Raquel Chamorro-Garcia
Department of Developmental and Cell Biology, University of California, Irvine, Irvine, CA, United States

John P. Thyfault
Department of Molecular and Integrative Physiology, University of Kansas Medical Center, Kansas City, KS, United States
Kansas City VA Medical Center, Research Service, Kansas City, MO, United States

Silvia Paterlini and Paola Palanza
Unit of Neuroscience, Department of Medicine and Surgery, University of Parma, Parma, Italy

Daniel Ruiz and Robert Sargis
Department of Medicine, University of Illinois at Chicago, Chicago, IL, United States

Bruce Blumberg
Department of Developmental and Cell Biology, University of California, Irvine, Irvine, CA, United States
Department of Pharmaceutical Sciences, University of California, Irvine, Irvine, CA, United States
Department of Biomedical Engineering, University of California, Irvine, Irvine, CA, United States

Robert B. Hamanaka and Gökhan M. Mutlu
Section of Pulmonary and Critical Care Medicine, Department of Medicine, The University of Chicago, Chicago, IL, United States

Christopher M. Carmean
Division of Molecular and Metabolic Medicine, Department of Physiology and Cell Biology, Kobe University Graduate School of Medicine, Kobe, Japan
Division of Endocrinology, Diabetes, and Metabolism, Department of Medicine, University of Illinois at Chicago, Chicago, IL, United States

Susumu Seino
Division of Molecular and Metabolic Medicine, Department of Physiology and Cell Biology, Kobe University Graduate School of Medicine, Kobe, Japan
Division of Endocrinology, Diabetes, and Metabolism, Department of Medicine, University of Illinois at Chicago, Chicago, IL, United States

Ahmed Khalil
Department of Environmental Health Sciences, University of Massachusetts Amherst, Amherst, MA, United States
Medical Biotechnology Department, Genetic Engineering & Biotechnology Research Institute, City of Scientific Research & Technological Applications, Alexandria, Egypt

Sebnem E. Cevik, Stephanie Hung, Sridurgadevi Kolla, Monika A. Roy and Alexander Suvorov
Department of Environmental Health Sciences, University of Massachusetts Amherst, Amherst, MA, United States
Medical Biotechnology Department, Genetic Engineering & Biotechnology Research Institute, City of Scientific Research & Technological Applications, Alexandria, Egypt

Ayushi Priyam, Pushplata Prasad Singh and Shweta Gehlout
TERI Deakin Nanobiotechnology Centre, The Energy and Resources Institute, New Delhi, India

Brigitte Le Magueresse-Battistoni, Hubert Vidal and Danielle Naville
Univ Lyon, CarMeN Laboratory, INSERM U1060, INRA U1397, INSA Lyon, Université Claude Bernard Lyon1, Oullins, France

Yu-Mi Lee
Department of Preventive Medicine, School of Medicine, Kyungpook National University, Daegu, South Korea

David R. Jacobs Jr.
Division of Epidemiology and Community Health, School of Public Health, University of Minnesota, Minneapolis, MN, United States

Duk-Hee Lee
Department of Preventive Medicine, School of Medicine, Kyungpook National University, Daegu, South Korea
BK21 Plus KNU Biomedical Convergence Program, Department of Biomedical Science, Kyungpook National University, Daegu, South Korea

Liana Bastos Sales, Marja H. Lamoree and Timo Hamers
Department of Environment and Health, Vrije Universiteit Amsterdam, Amsterdam, Netherlands

Joantine C. J. van Esterik
Department of Pathobiology, Faculty of Veterinary Medicine, Utrecht University, Utrecht, Netherlands

Hennie M. Hodemaekers and Leo T. M. van der Ven
Center for Health Protection, National Institute for Public Health and the Environment (RIVM), Bilthoven, Netherlands

Juliette Legler
Institute for Risk Assessment Sciences (IRAS), Utrecht University, Utrecht, Netherlands
Utrecht Institute for Pharmaceutical Sciences, Utrecht University, Utrecht, Netherlands

Jerrold J. Heindel
Program on Endocrine Disruption Strategies, Commonweal, Bolinas, CA, United States

Abby F. Fleisch
Pediatric Endocrinology and Diabetes, Maine Medical Center, Portland, ME, United States
Center for Outcomes Research and Evaluation, Maine Medical Center Research Institute, Portland, ME, United States

Izzuddin M. Aris
Division of Chronic Disease Research Across the Lifecourse, Department of Population Medicine, Harvard Medical School and Harvard Pilgrim Health Care Institute, Boston, MA, United States
Department of Obstetrics and Gynecology, Yong Loo Lin School of Medicine, National University of Singapore, Singapore, Singapore

Sheryl L. Rifas-Shiman
Division of Chronic Disease Research Across the Lifecourse, Department of Population Medicine, Harvard Medical School and Harvard Pilgrim Health Care Institute, Boston, MA, United States

Brent A. Coull
Department of Biostatistics, Harvard School of Public Health, Boston, MA, United States

Heike Luttmann-Gibson, Petros Koutrakis and Joel D. Schwartz
Department of Environmental Health, Harvard School of Public Health, Boston, MA, United States

Itai Kloog
Department of Environmental Health, Harvard School of Public Health, Boston, MA, United States
Department of Geography and Environmental Development, Ben-Gurion University of the Negev, Beersheba, Israel

Diane R. Gold
Department of Environmental Health, Harvard School of Public Health, Boston, MA, United States
Channing Laboratory, Brigham and Women's Hospital, Boston, MA, United States

Emily Oken
Division of Chronic Disease Research Across the Lifecourse, Department of Population Medicine, Harvard Medical School and Harvard Pilgrim Health Care Institute, Boston, MA, United States
Department of Nutrition, Harvard School of Public Health, Boston, MA, United States

Marilena Marraudino, Brigitta Bonaldo, Alice Farinetti, GianCarlo Panzica and Stefano Gotti
Neuroscience Institute Cavalieri Ottolenghi, Turin, Italy
Department of Neuroscience "Rita Levi-Montalcini", University of Turin, Turin, Italy

Giovanna Ponti
Neuroscience Institute Cavalieri Ottolenghi, Turin, Italy
Department of Veterinary Sciences, University of Turin, Turin, Italy

Christopher D. Kassotis and Heather M. Stapleton
Nicholas School of the Environment, Duke University, Durham, NC, United States

Robert M. Sargis
Department of Medicine, University of Illinois at Chicago, Chicago, IL, United States

Vasantha Padmanabhan
Department of Pediatrics, University of Michigan, Ann Arbor, MI, United States

Olga Papalou, Eleni A. Kandaraki and Evanthia Diamanti-Kandarakis
Department of Endocrinology & Diabetes, Hygeia Hospital, Athens, Greece

George Papadakis
STEPS Stoffwechselzentrum, Biel/Bienne, Switzerland

Beverly S. Rubin, Cheryl M. Schaeberle and Ana M. Soto
Department of Immunology, Tufts University School of Medicine, Boston, MA, United States

Index

www.ingramcontent.com/pod-product-compliance
Lightning Source LLC
LaVergne TN
LVHW082126200926
848484LV00008B/2011